Artificial Intelligence for Health and Medicine

Artificial Intelligence for Health and Medicine

Guest Editor

Daniele Giansanti

MDPI

Basel • Beijing • Wuhan • Barcelona • Belgrade • Novi Sad • Cluj • Manchester

Guest Editor
Daniele Giansanti
Centre Tisp
Istituto Superiore di Sanità
Rome
Italy

Editorial Office
MDPI AG
Grosspeteranlage 5
4052 Basel, Switzerland

This is a reprint of the Special Issue, published open access by the journal *Diagnostics* (ISSN 2075-4418), freely accessible at: https://www.mdpi.com/journal/diagnostics/special_issues/FRZJN08SN8.

For citation purposes, cite each article independently as indicated on the article page online and as indicated below:

Lastname, A.A.; Lastname, B.B. Article Title. *Journal Name* **Year**, *Volume Number*, Page Range.

ISBN 978-3-7258-8345-5 (Hbk)
ISBN 978-3-7258-8346-2 (PDF)
https://doi.org/10.3390/books978-3-7258-8346-2

Contents

About the Editor

Daniele Giansanti

Daniele Giansanti is a professor at Sapienza University and the Catholic University in Rome, Italy. His research interests span biomedical engineering, medical physics, and e-Health, with a focus on developing wearable medical devices, advancing telemedicine and mHealth applications, and studying the acceptance of robotics and artificial intelligence in healthcare. He currently leads research as Research Director at the Italian National Institute of Health (ISS), where his projects include technology assessment for telerehabilitation and domiciliary monitoring, with emphasis on the design, evaluation, and integration of wearable and digital health technologies for remote patient care, including sensor-based systems, mobile health solutions, and AI-enabled assistive devices. His research also explores advanced data-driven approaches in healthcare, including artificial intelligence applications in medical imaging, with particular attention given to radiology and digital pathology, as well as their role in supporting clinical decision-making and personalized care. In parallel, he investigates the ethical, legal, and cybersecurity aspects of digital health, focusing on the safe and responsible integration of artificial intelligence, robotics, and connected technologies in clinical and home-care environments. Dr. Giansanti has authored over 200 Scopus-indexed publications and serves as a board editor and reviewer for several scientific journals.

Preface

Artificial intelligence (AI) has become one of the most transformative forces in contemporary healthcare, particularly in the field of medical diagnostics. By enabling the analysis of complex and high-dimensional data, AI is reshaping how clinicians interpret images, laboratory results, and multimodal clinical information, with important implications for accuracy, efficiency, and personalization of care.

This Special Issue brings together 19 contributions that explore the evolving role of AI in diagnostics, ranging from methodological innovations to clinical applications and critical reviews. The collection includes original research and review papers that span medical imaging, predictive modeling, laboratory medicine, and clinical workflow optimization, highlighting both established applications and emerging frontiers.

Across these contributions, AI demonstrates its potential to support earlier and more accurate diagnosis, improve decision-making processes, and enhance healthcare efficiency. At the same time, the studies underscore persistent challenges related to interpretability, robustness, external validation, and real-world clinical integration.

Overall, this volume offers a comprehensive snapshot of a rapidly evolving field, illustrating how AI is progressively moving from experimental development toward clinical translation, while also outlining the key directions that will shape its future impact in medicine.

I would like to sincerely thank all the authors, reviewers, and contributors whose outstanding work made the Reprint of this Special Issue possible. I also extend my gratitude to the editorial team for their support and dedication, and to Managing Editors Dennis Zhu and Carol Zhang for their exceptional support and continued guidance. Their combined efforts have been essential in bringing this issue to fruition.

Daniele Giansanti
Guest Editor

diagnostics

MDPI

Editorial

Mapping the Road Ahead: A Collective Journey in Artificial Intelligence for Health and Medicine

Daniele Giansanti

Centre IATIS, Istituto Superiore di Sanità, 00161 Rome, Italy; daniele.giansanti@iss.it or gianslele@gmail.com; Tel.:+39-06-49902701

Artificial intelligence (AI) has emerged as one of the most disruptive technologies in modern healthcare, particularly in the domain of medical diagnostics, where complex data streams, high-dimensional imaging, and heterogeneous clinical information increasingly challenge traditional analytical approaches [1,2]. In the past decade, AI systems powered by machine learning and deep learning have enabled the automated detection of subtle patterns in medical images, improved interpretation of laboratory and genomic data, and supported clinical decision-making processes that were previously labor-intensive, time-consuming, or subjective [3,4]. These advances have translated into improvements in diagnostic accuracy, workflow efficiency, and early disease detection, with significant implications for patient stratification and personalized medicine [5].

Among diagnostic domains, medical imaging remains the most mature and widely investigated area for AI adoption. In radiology and pathology, deep learning models have demonstrated strong performance in image classification, segmentation, and anomaly detection across multiple modalities, including computed tomography, magnetic resonance imaging, ultrasound, and whole-slide pathology images [6,7]. Beyond imaging, AI has shown growing potential in laboratory medicine, where algorithms assist in the interpretation of complex biochemical and hematological data, as well as in genomics and molecular diagnostics, supporting variant classification and biomarker discovery [8].

AI-driven diagnostic approaches are also gaining relevance in oncology, cardiology, and neurology, where multimodal data integration—combining imaging, clinical variables, and omics data—offers new opportunities for early detection, risk stratification, and prognosis estimation [5,9]. In these contexts, AI systems can assist clinicians in identifying clinically meaningful patterns that may not be readily apparent through conventional analysis, thus enhancing diagnostic confidence and decision support.

Despite these promising developments, fundamental challenges persist in the translation of AI innovations into routine clinical practice. Many diagnostic AI tools demonstrate enhanced performance in controlled research settings, yet evidence of consistent benefits on patient-level outcomes, such as reduced morbidity or mortality, remains limited. Moreover, barriers related to model explainability, data representativeness, bias, and robust external validation continue to hinder large-scale clinical adoption [2,9].

The contributions assembled in this Special Issue, "Artificial Intelligence for Health and Medicine," [10] reflect the breadth and depth of current research at the intersection of AI and diagnostics, highlighting not only technical innovations and performance improvements, but also emerging strategies for explainable AI, multimodal diagnostic integration, and rigorous clinical evaluation, which are essential for the safe and effective implementation of AI-based diagnostic tools in healthcare.

The project has brought together a total of 18 contributions, in addition to the present introductory editorial. Overall, the Special Issue comprises 13 original research articles (Contributions 1–13) and 5 review papers, including 4 narrative reviews (Contributions 14–17) and 1 systematic review (Contribution 18).

Artificial Intelligence (AI) has demonstrated transformative potential across multiple diagnostic domains in healthcare, enabling improved accuracy, efficiency, and personalization of patient care. The original research articles (Contributions 1–13) in this Special Issue highlight two major trends: AI applied to imaging and radiology, where hybrid models, deep learning, and neuro-symbolic reasoning enhance diagnostic precision and interpretability; and AI applied to clinical and predictive data, supporting risk assessment, laboratory management, prenatal screening, symptom forecasting, and monitoring in high-intensity environments. Overall, these studies illustrate the capacity of AI to optimize clinical workflows, reduce redundant testing, and enable data-driven, patient-centered decision-making, while also highlighting ongoing challenges such as model explainability, generalizability, and clinical validation.

Across the thirteen original research articles in this Special Issue, AI demonstrates its versatility and impact across diverse diagnostic domains. Contribution 1 (Buican et al.) initiates this journey by developing an Integrated Pulmonary Severity Score (IPSS) for COPD, merging clinical and psychological factors such as anxiety and depression with explainable machine learning to refine symptom and prognosis prediction beyond traditional FEV1 measures. Building on the theme of interpretable AI in imaging, Contribution 2 (Almughamisi et al.) introduces an anatomy-guided hybrid CNN–ViT model with neuro-symbolic reasoning for early, multilabel diagnosis of thoracic diseases, ensuring clinical plausibility alongside high accuracy. Contribution 3 (Castilla et al.) translates AI from theory to practice, externally validating a triaging system for chest X-rays that effectively prioritizes abnormal findings and mitigates reporting backlogs in emergency care, while Contribution 4 (Özel et al.) applies deep learning to lateral cephalometric radiographs, improving orthodontic assessment of vertical dimensions and supporting individualized treatment planning.

Extending beyond imaging, Contribution 5 (Lohaj et al.) harnesses machine learning and explainable AI to analyze COVID-19 medical records, uncovering patterns that aid in understanding disease progression and guiding clinical decisions. Contribution 6 (Shuchami et al.) tackles workflow efficiency in pediatric emergency departments, leveraging AI to reduce redundant laboratory tests while safeguarding diagnostic quality and patient comfort. Contribution 7 (Ucan et al.) demonstrates AI's power in automating radiology reporting through a Swin Enhanced Yield Transformer model for Turkish chest X-ray reports, transforming complex image data into actionable text for clinicians.

In prenatal care, Contribution 8 (Yalçın et al.) employs a hybrid AI approach to improve first-trimester Down Syndrome risk prediction, enhancing accuracy and reliability of early screening. In pediatrics, Contribution 9 (Turki & Turki) identifies phonological biomarkers for speech sound disorders in Saudi Arabic-speaking children, applying machine learning to elevate diagnostic precision. In interventional procedures, Contribution 10 (Ozkara et al.) uses AI to predict early outcomes of prostatic artery embolization, supporting personalized treatment decisions. Contribution 11 (Giarnieri et al.) focuses on cytology, creating user-friendly AI models that streamline pleural effusion analysis and empower clinicians facing complex malignant cases. Contribution 12 (Finkelstein et al.) brings AI to oncology symptom management, forecasting physical and mental deterioration during chemotherapy to enable proactive interventions. Finally, Contribution 13 (Mihai et al.) expands AI's reach into operational medicine by developing the IIRPM score to monitor

https://doi.org/10.3390/diagnostics16040544

oxidative stress and inflammation in military personnel, illustrating its potential for health surveillance in high-intensity environments.

Shifting focus from original research to comprehensive analyses, Contributions 14–18 illustrate how AI is being synthesized across diagnostic domains, offering both critical evaluation and forward-looking perspectives. These reviews explore the application of AI in musculoskeletal, respiratory, oncologic, and reproductive health, highlighting methodological advances, practical challenges, and emerging opportunities to enhance diagnostic accuracy and personalized care.

Contribution 14 (Mercurio et al.) provides a comprehensive review of artificial intelligence for the diagnosis and management of patellofemoral instability, addressing the complex interplay of anatomical and biomechanical factors and demonstrating how machine learning and deep learning approaches can improve diagnostic precision and support individualized treatment planning. Contribution 15 (Sait & Shaikh) focuses on AI-powered detection techniques for chronic obstructive pulmonary disease, summarizing current methodologies, their potential to enhance early diagnosis, and the role of AI in overcoming limitations of traditional clinical tools. Contribution 16 (Lastrucci et al.) offers a narrative review of AI applications in breast imaging, synthesizing systematic evidence on mammographic practice and emphasizing opportunities to optimize screening, improve diagnostic accuracy, and integrate AI into routine clinical workflows. Contribution 17 (Moustakli et al.) examines AI in the assessment of reproductive aging, highlighting the influence of mitochondria, oxidative stress, and telomere biology, and discussing how machine learning can aid in predicting reproductive potential and informing patient counseling. Finally, Contribution 18 (Xu et al.) presents a systematic literature review of advanced deep learning approaches for comprehensive breast cancer assessment using whole slide images, demonstrating the capability of AI to enhance early detection of lymphocytes and molecular biomarkers, thus supporting precision diagnostics and improved patient outcomes.

Together, these eighteen contributions form a cohesive narrative of AI advancing diagnostics, from imaging to predictive analytics, and from workflow optimization to individualized patient care, highlighting both the opportunities and the challenges that define this rapidly evolving field.

Looking toward the future, the eighteen contributions in this Special Issue collectively map the evolving landscape of AI in medical diagnostics, demonstrating its transformative potential across clinical imaging, predictive analytics, workflow optimization, and patient-centered care. Moving forward, several key directions emerge.

First, the integration of multimodal data—combining imaging, laboratory, genomic, and patient-reported information—promises to enhance diagnostic precision and support holistic, individualized assessments (Contributions 1–18). Both the original research articles (Contributions 1–13) and the review studies (Contributions 14–18) emphasize the importance of interpretability and transparency, underscoring that clinically adopted AI systems must be explainable, reliable, and aligned with physiological knowledge to gain clinician trust.

Second, innovative model architectures, including hybrid networks, neuro-symbolic reasoning, and transformer-based frameworks, illustrate how AI can merge expert knowledge with algorithmic efficiency, improving generalizability and reducing bias (Contributions 2, 7, 8, 14–18). While the original research articles introduce and validate these architectures in experimental or clinical contexts, the review studies analyze and synthesize such approaches across multiple diagnostic domains, providing guidance for future model development.

Third, beyond imaging, AI's predictive and monitoring applications highlight its expanding role in proactive and preventative healthcare. Predictive monitoring includes

https://doi.org/10.3390/diagnostics16040544

prenatal screening, pediatric speech diagnostics, and oncology symptom forecasting (Contributions 8, 9, 12). AI systems for workflow optimization and decision support, such as repeated lab testing in pediatric emergency departments and automated X-ray report generation (Contributions 6 and 7), enhance efficiency and streamline clinical processes. Contribution 7—focusing on automated X-ray report generation—illustrates how AI can optimize clinical workflows by producing structured, actionable text from images, complementing predictive monitoring systems without being predictive itself.

Funding: This research received no external funding.

Conflicts of Interest: The author declares no conflict of interest.

List of Contributions:

1. Buican, I.-L.; Buican-Chirea, A.-C.; Radulescu, D.; Udristoiu, I.; Gheorman, V.; Cojocaru, D.-M.; Streba, C.-T. Integrated Pulmonary Severity Score (IPSS) for COPD: A Psycho-Respiratory Risk Index Supported by Explainable Machine Learning. *Diagnostics* **2026**, *16*, 507. https://doi.org/10.3390/diagnostics16040507.
2. Almughamisi, N.; Abosamra, G.; Albar, A.; Saleh, M. Anatomy-Guided Hybrid CNN–ViT Model with Neuro-Symbolic Reasoning for Early Diagnosis of Thoracic Diseases Multilabel. *Diagnostics* **2026**, *16*, 159. https://doi.org/10.3390/diagnostics16010159.
3. Castilla, A.C.; de Paiva D'Amorim, I.; Wanderley, M.F.B.; Esmeraldo, M.A.; Yoshida, A.R.; Eigier, A.M.; Sawamura, M.V.Y. External Validation of an Artificial Intelligence Triaging System for Chest X-Rays: A Retrospective Independent Clinical Study. *Diagnostics* **2025**, *15*, 2899. https://doi.org/10.3390/diagnostics15222899.
4. Özel, M.B.; Ay Kartbak, S.B.; Çakmak, M. Classification Performance of Deep Learning Models for the Assessment of Vertical Dimension on Lateral Cephalometric Radiographs. *Diagnostics* **2025**, *15*, 2240. https://doi.org/10.3390/diagnostics15172240.
5. Lohaj, O.; Paralič, J.; Paraličová, Z.; Javorská, D.; Zagorová, E. Data Analytics and Machine Learning Models on COVID-19 Medical Reports Enhanced with Explainable AI for Usability. *Diagnostics* **2025**, *15*, 1981. https://doi.org/10.3390/diagnostics15151981.
6. Shuchami, A.; Lazebnik, T.; Ashkenazi, S.; Cohen, A.H.; Reichenberg, Y.; Zemer, V.S. A Machine Learning-Based Guide for Repeated Laboratory Testing in Pediatric Emergency Departments. *Diagnostics* **2025**, *15*, 1885. https://doi.org/10.3390/diagnostics15151885.
7. Ucan, M.; Kaya, B.; Kaya, M. Turkish Chest X-Ray Report Generation Model Using the Swin Enhanced Yield Transformer (Model-SEY) Framework. *Diagnostics* **2025**, *15*, 1805. https://doi.org/10.3390/diagnostics15141805.
8. Yalçın, E.; Aslan, S.; Toğaçar, M.; Demir, S.C. A Hybrid Artificial Intelligence Approach for Down Syndrome Risk Prediction in First Trimester Screening. *Diagnostics* **2025**, *15*, 1444. https://doi.org/10.3390/diagnostics15121444.
9. Turki, D.F.; Turki, A.F. Machine Learning-Based Identification of Phonological Biomarkers for Speech Sound Disorders in Saudi Arabic-Speaking Children. *Diagnostics* **2025**, *15*, 1401. https://doi.org/10.3390/diagnostics15111401.
10. Ozkara, B.B.; Bamshad, D.; Gowda, R.; Karabacak, M.; Bishay, V.; Garcia-Reyes, K.; Rastinehad, A.R.; Shilo, D.; Fischman, A. Predicting Early Outcomes of Prostatic Artery Embolization Using n-Butyl Cyanoacrylate Liquid Embolic Agent: A Machine Learning Study. *Diagnostics* **2025**, *15*, 1351. https://doi.org/10.3390/diagnostics15111351.
11. Giarnieri, E.; Carico, E.; Scarpino, S.; Ricci, A.; Bruno, P.; Scardapane, S.; Giansanti, D. Bringing AI to Clinicians: Simplifying Pleural Effusion Cytology Diagnosis with User-Friendly Models. *Diagnostics* **2025**, *15*, 1240. https://doi.org/10.3390/diagnostics15101240.
12. Finkelstein, J.; Smiley, A.; Echeverria, C.; Mooney, K. Deep Learning Approaches to Forecast Physical and Mental Deterioration During Chemotherapy in Patients with Cancer. *Diagnostics* **2025**, *15*, 956. https://doi.org/10.3390/diagnostics15080956.
13. Mihai, F.-D.; Trasca, E.-T.; Radulescu, P.-M.; Mercut, R.; Caluianu, E.-I.; Ciupeanu-Calugaru, E.D.; Calafeteanu, D.M.; Marinescu, G.-A.; Danoiu, S.; Radulescu, D. Advanced Assessment of Oxidative

Stress and Inflammation in Military Personnel: Development of a Novel IIRPM Score Using Artificial Intelligence. *Diagnostics* **2025**, *15*, 832. https://doi.org/10.3390/diagnostics15070832.
14. Mercurio, M.; Denami, F.; Vescio, A.; Familiari, F.; Longo, U.G.; Galasso, O.; Gasparini, G.; Dejour, D.H. Artificial Intelligence for the Diagnosis and Management of Patellofemoral Instability: A Comprehensive Review. *Diagnostics* **2025**, *15*, 2918. https://doi.org/10.3390/diagnostics15222918.
15. Sait, A.R.W.; Shaikh, M.A. Artificial Intelligence-Powered Chronic Obstructive Pulmonary Disease Detection Techniques—A Review. *Diagnostics* **2025**, *15*, 2562. https://doi.org/10.3390/diagnostics15202562.
16. Lastrucci, A.; Iosca, N.; Wandael, Y.; Barra, A.; Ricci, R.; Cucchiari, J.N.; Forini, N.; Lepri, G.; Giansanti, D. Transforming Breast Imaging: A Narrative Review of Systematic Evidence on Artificial Intelligence in Mammographic Practice. *Diagnostics* **2025**, *15*, 2197. https://doi.org/10.3390/diagnostics15172197.
17. Moustakli, E.; Grigoriadis, T.; Stavros, S.; Potiris, A.; Zikopoulos, A.; Gerede, A.; Tsimpoukis, I.; Papageorgiou, C.; Louis, K.; Domali, E. Artificial Intelligence in Assessing Reproductive Aging: Role of Mitochondria, Oxidative Stress, and Telomere Biology. *Diagnostics* **2025**, *15*, 2075. https://doi.org/10.3390/diagnostics15162075.
18. Xu, Q.; Adam, A.; Abdullah, A.; Bariyah, N. Advanced Deep Learning Approaches in Detection Technologies for Comprehensive Breast Cancer Assessment Based on WSIs: A Systematic Literature Review. *Diagnostics* **2025**, *15*, 1150. https://doi.org/10.3390/diagnostics15091150.

References

1. Hirosawa, T.; Shimizu, T. A Narrative Review of Artificial Intelligence in Medical Diagnostics. *Comput. Mater. Contin.* **2025**, *83*, 3919–3944. [CrossRef]
2. Kelly, C.J.; Karthikesalingam, A.; Suleyman, M.; Corrado, G.; King, D. Key Challenges for Delivering Clinical Impact with Artificial Intelligence. *BMC Med.* **2019**, *17*, 195. [CrossRef] [PubMed]
3. Esteva, A.; Robicquet, A.; Ramsundar, B.; Kuleshov, V.; DePristo, M.; Chou, K.; Cui, C.; Corrado, G.; Thrun, S.; Dean, J. A Guide to Deep Learning in Healthcare. *Nat. Med.* **2019**, *25*, 24–29. [CrossRef] [PubMed]
4. Rajkomar, A.; Dean, J.; Kohane, I. Machine Learning in Medicine. *New Engl. J. Med.* **2019**, *380*, 1347–1358. [CrossRef] [PubMed]
5. Topol, E.J. High-Performance Medicine: The Convergence of Human and Artificial Intelligence. *Nat. Med.* **2019**, *25*, 44–56. [CrossRef] [PubMed]
6. Litjens, G.; Kooi, T.; Bejnordi, B.E.; Setio, A.A.A.; Ciompi, F.; Ghafoorian, M.; van der Laak, J.A.W.M.; van Ginneken, B.; Sánchez, C.I. A Survey on Deep Learning in Medical Image Analysis. *Med. Image Anal.* **2017**, *42*, 60–88. [CrossRef] [PubMed]
7. Tizhoosh, H.R.; Pantanowitz, L. Artificial Intelligence and Digital Pathology: Challenges and Opportunities. *J. Pathol. Inform.* **2018**, *9*, 38. [CrossRef] [PubMed]
8. Kourou, K.; Exarchos, T.P.; Exarchos, K.P.; Karamouzis, M.V.; Fotiadis, D.I. Machine Learning Applications in Cancer Prognosis and Prediction. *Comput. Struct. Biotechnol. J.* **2015**, *13*, 8–17. [CrossRef] [PubMed]
9. Beam, A.L.; Kohane, I.S. Big Data and Machine Learning in Health Care. *JAMA* **2018**, *319*, 1317–1318. [CrossRef] [PubMed]
10. Artificial Intelligence for Health and Medicine. Diagnostics Special Issue. Available online: https://www.mdpi.com/journal/diagnostics/special_issues/FRZJN08SN8 (accessed on 7 February 2026).

https://doi.org/10.3390/diagnostics16040544

diagnostics MDPI

Article

Integrated Pulmonary Severity Score (IPSS) for COPD: A Psycho-Respiratory Risk Index Supported by Explainable Machine Learning

Iulian-Laurențiu Buican [1,2], Alina-Catalina Buican-Chirea [1,3], Dumitru Radulescu [4,*], Ion Udristoiu [5], Victor Gheorman [5], Dragos-Mihai Cojocaru [6] and Costin-Teodor Streba [7,*]

1 U.M.F. Doctoral School Craiova, University of Medicine and Pharmacy of Craiova, 200349 Craiova, Romania
2 Leamna Pulmonology Hospital, 207129 Leamna, Romania
3 Experimental Research Centre for Normal and Pathological Aging, University of Medicine and Pharmacy of Craiova, 200349 Craiova, Romania
4 Department of Surgery, The Military Emergency Clinical Hospital 'Dr. Stefan Odobleja' Craiova, 200749 Craiova, Romania
5 Department of Psychiatry, University of Medicine and Pharmacy of Craiova, 200349 Craiova, Romania; ion.udristoiu@umfcv.ro (I.U.)
6 Sanacare AG, Schützenstrasse 1, 8401 Winterthur, Switzerland
7 Department of Pulmonology, University of Medicine and Pharmacy of Craiova, 200349 Craiova, Romania
* Correspondence: dr_radulescu_dumitru@yahoo.com (D.R.); costin.streba@umfcv.ro (C.-T.S.)

Abstract

Background/Objectives: In chronic obstructive pulmonary disease (COPD), forced expiratory volume in one second (FEV_1) explains only part of the variability in symptoms and prognosis, while anxiety and depression are common but rarely quantified in composite indices. We aimed to develop and internally validate an Integrated Pulmonary Severity Score (IPSS) that combines respiratory function, symptom burden and affective status. **Methods**: In a prospective observational study, 390 adults with spirometry-confirmed COPD were consecutively enrolled at two tertiary Romanian centres (October 2022–September 2024). Within 48 h of admission, patients underwent spirometry (FEV_1% predicted), dyspnoea grading (mMRC), symptom assessment (CAT), affective evaluation (HADS-Anxiety/Depression) and cognitive screening (MoCA, MMSE). A PulmoScore was built from CAT, mMRC and ventilatory deficit ($100 - FEV_1\%$) and extended with a HADS-based psychiatric multiplier to obtain IPSS. Spectral clustering, logistic regression, a multilayer perceptron (MLP) and LIME were used for phenotyping and validation. **Results**: Spectral clustering identified two phenotypes—psycho-respiratory and predominantly respiratory—with acceptable separation (silhouette coefficient 0.26). The psycho-respiratory group showed lower FEV_1%, higher CAT and mMRC scores, more severe anxiety–depression and markedly higher IPSS values. Logistic regression and the MLP achieved an accuracy of 0.89, an AUC of 0.95 and Cohen's $\kappa \geq 0.75$ for identifying this phenotype when using the same core clinical variables that informed phenotyping and IPSS construction. IPSS values were distributed across four strata (<30, 30–69, 70–119, ≥120 points), reflecting progressively worse respiratory and affective burden. **Conclusions**: In this cohort, IPSS captured a clinically meaningful psycho-respiratory phenotype and improved integrated severity assessment beyond spirometry alone, with potential utility for risk stratification. It can be computed from routine measures, is compatible with explainable AI workflows and warrants external, longitudinal validation before widespread implementation.

Keywords: chronic obstructive pulmonary disease (COPD); Integrated Pulmonary Severity Score (IPSS); severity assessment; anxiety; depression; explainable artificial intelligence

1. Introduction

Chronic obstructive pulmonary disease (COPD) remains among the foremost causes of global mortality and morbidity. The World Health Organization estimates that, in 2021, COPD was responsible for approximately 3.5 million deaths—around 5% of all deaths worldwide—ranking as the fourth leading cause of death [1]. Beyond its epidemiological burden, COPD is increasingly conceptualized as a biologically heterogeneous, immune-mediated inflammatory disorder in which airway damage and systemic effects are shaped by complex crosstalk between epithelial injury, innate immune activation and vascular inflammation. Recent work has highlighted cigarette-smoke–driven epithelial–immune communication through extracellular vesicles; for example, exosomal signalling has been shown to promote macrophage M1 polarization and inflammatory cell death pathways via TREM-1–related mechanisms in experimental COPD models [2]. In parallel, microRNA-regulated sirtuin axes have been implicated in cigarette smoke–induced lung injury and functional impairment (e.g., miR-132 targeting SIRT1/FoxO1) [3], while activation of SIRT6 has been reported to suppress NF-κB–driven endothelial inflammatory responses relevant to pulmonary microvascular inflammation [4]. Clinically, immune dysregulation may also translate into altered susceptibility to immune-related adverse events; notably, COPD has been associated with a higher risk of autoimmune thyroiditis during pembrolizumab therapy in non-small cell lung cancer [5]. Together, these mechanistic and clinical data support the need for integrative severity approaches that go beyond spirometry alone and reflect the multidimensional burden of COPD. Independent analyses report over 212 million people affected and more than 3 million deaths annually, elevating COPD to third place in the global mortality hierarchy [6,7]. This burden is especially acute in low- and middle-income countries, where nearly 90% of premature deaths (<70 years) occur [1].

Despite its clinical significance, commonly used composite indices—BODE, DOSE, ADO and B-AE-D—evaluate disease severity predominantly through somatic parameters, focusing on airflow limitation, exercise capacity, body mass index or exacerbation history. Yet, a substantial body of evidence demonstrates that anxiety and depressive disorders are not mere comorbidities but clinically consequential modifiers of COPD trajectories. Beyond symptom amplification, affective burden has been associated with higher health-care utilization and poorer prognosis, including higher exacerbation risk and increased likelihood of hospital admission, and has been linked to adverse outcomes in longitudinal and registry-based studies [8–13].

From a mechanistic standpoint, anxiety intensifies the perception of dyspnoea through interoceptive hypersensitivity [14] and heightened sympathetic activation, regardless of obstruction severity [15–18]. CAT scores are significantly higher in patients with anxiety or depression, even in the absence of objective FEV_1 deterioration [19–21]. Clinically, this emotional influence has been associated with a markedly increased risk of subsequent exacerbation and a self-reinforcing cycle of functional decline, disproportionate symptom burden, and escalated care needs [13,22].

In a preliminary study, our team applied k-means clustering to a comprehensive set of cognitive, affective and respiratory variables in patients with chronic respiratory disorders (asthma or COPD), identifying three distinct clusters; one of these—corresponding to a "Severe Cognitive Respiratory" profile—was dominated by marked anxiety–depressive symptoms and cognitive impairment in the context of substantial respiratory limitation, i.e., a pronounced psycho-respiratory burden [23]. These findings underscored the heterogeneity of COPD and highlighted the need for an index capable of quantifying both somatic and emotional dimensions concurrently.

On these grounds, the present study introduces the Integrated Pulmonary Severity Score (IPSS), a composite index combining airflow obstruction, symptomatic burden and

https://doi.org/10.3390/diagnostics16040507

anxiety–depressive load into a unified formula. Furthermore, we employ unsupervised spectral clustering—which has proven effective in delineating clinically meaningful phenotypes in asthma and sepsis [24,25]—to validate the existence of a discrete psycho-respiratory phenotype. The aim of this work is to propose and internally characterize IPSS as a pragmatic bedside tool for integrated severity assessment and risk stratification, while explicitly acknowledging the need for external, multi-ethnic and longitudinal validation before clinical implementation. Throughout the manuscript, "severity" refers to the integrated multidimensional burden quantified by the continuous IPSS, whereas "risk stratification" refers to the pragmatic assignment of patients into ordinal IPSS risk categories intended to guide clinical follow-up and management intensity.

2. Materials and Methods

This prospective observational study was conducted between October 2022 and September 2024 at two tertiary care centres in Romania: the Craiova Clinical Neuropsychiatry Hospital—Psychiatry Clinic (Park), which oversaw all psychiatric and cognitive evaluations, and Leamna Pulmonology Hospital, which performed respiratory function testing and symptom assessments. Adults ($\geq$18 years) hospitalized with a spirometry-confirmed diagnosis of chronic obstructive pulmonary disease (COPD) were enrolled consecutively after providing written informed consent. Ethical approval was obtained from the Ethics Committee of the University of Medicine and Pharmacy Craiova (Protocol No. 196/17 February 2022) and from the local committees at both hospitals (Protocol No. 6190/14 October 2022), in accordance with the Declaration of Helsinki.

2.1. Inclusion and Exclusion Criteria

Eligible participants were adults ($\geq$18 years) with a COPD diagnosis confirmed according to contemporary GOLD criteria who were able to provide informed consent and to complete study assessments during hospitalization. Exclusion criteria comprised major cardiometabolic comorbidities (e.g., heart failure, BMI > 35 kg/m^2, obstructive sleep apnoea), uncontrolled psychiatric disorders beyond anxiety and depression, major surgery within the previous six months, inability to perform valid spirometry or refusal to participate. Of 450 patients screened, 60 were excluded for these reasons, yielding a final cohort of 390 patients (Figure 1).

These exclusions were applied to minimize major non-pulmonary confounding during exploratory score derivation, acknowledging that this may reduce generalizability to multimorbid real-world COPD populations.

2.2. Respiratory Assessment

At Leamna Pulmonology Hospital, respiratory evaluation included:

- Spirometry (Spirolab IV): FEV_1 and FVC were measured, and predicted FEV_1% was calculated according to reference equations; airflow limitation was subsequently graded into GOLD I–IV categories.
- mMRC Dyspnoea Scale: graded 0–4 according to dyspnoea severity during usual daily activities.
- COPD Assessment Test (CAT): eight items scored 0–5 (total 0–40) covering cough, sputum, chest tightness, activity limitation, confidence, sleep and energy. In this study, values < 10 were considered low impact, 10–20 moderate, 21–30 high and >30 very high impact.

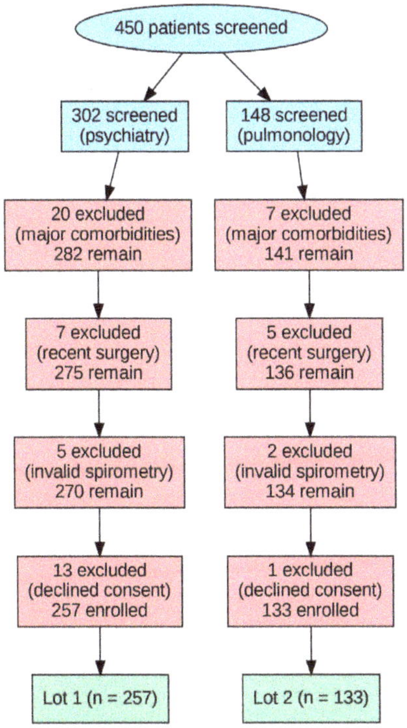

Figure 1. Study flowchart.

2.3. Psychiatric and Cognitive Evaluation

Within 48 h at Craiova Clinical Neuropsychiatry Hospital—Psychiatry Clinic (Park), participants completed:

- Hospital Anxiety and Depression Scale (HADS): two subscales (0–21) for anxiety and depression (0–7 normal; 8–10 mild; 11–14 moderate; 15–21 severe).
- Montreal Cognitive Assessment (MoCA): 0–30 scale (26–30 normal; 18–25 mild impairment; 10–17 moderate; <10 severe).
- Mini–Mental State Examination (MMSE): 0–30 scale (25–30 normal; 21–24 mild; 10–20 moderate; <10 severe).

2.4. IPSS Construction and Clustering

The Integrated Pulmonary Severity Score (IPSS) was constructed in two steps. First, a pulmonary component (PulmoScore) was defined deterministically from CAT, mMRC (rescaled $\times 10$ to harmonize with the CAT 0–40 range) and ventilatory deficit ($100 - FEV_1\%$), yielding an explicit weighted combination of these three variables. Second, the PulmoScore was multiplied by a psychiatric amplification factor derived from HADS-Depression and HADS-Anxiety, yielding:

$$\text{IPSS} = \text{PulmoScore} \times [1 + (\alpha \times \text{HADS-Depression}) + (\beta \times \text{HADS-Anxiety})],$$

where α and β represent per-point fractional increases in the multiplier (cohort-derived coefficients). Coefficients and cut-offs are therefore subject to external recalibration in independent validation cohorts. Although cognitive assessments (MoCA and MMSE) were collected and analyzed to characterize phenotype burden, they were intentionally not incorporated into the final IPSS to preserve routine feasibility and portability across

https://doi.org/10.3390/diagnostics16040507

settings, given that cognitive testing is not universally performed at each visit and may be influenced by education, language/cultural factors and examiner variability.

To explore whether IPSS components reflected clinically meaningful patterns, we applied spectral clustering to the matrix of respiratory, affective and cognitive variables. The number of clusters (k = 2–5) was examined, and the optimal solution was chosen based on the highest average silhouette coefficient and clinical interpretability, yielding two phenotypes: a psycho-respiratory and a predominantly respiratory profile.

2.5. Statistical Analysis

Classical statistical analyses were performed in SPSS 26.0 (IBM Corp., Armonk, NY, USA). Continuous variables were expressed as mean ± standard deviation or median (interquartile range) and compared using independent-samples *t* tests or non-parametric equivalents, as appropriate. Categorical variables were summarized as counts and percentages and compared with χ^2 tests. Pearson correlation coefficients were computed to assess bivariate associations between FEV_1%, CAT, mMRC, HADS, MoCA and MMSE. A two-tailed $p < 0.05$ was considered statistically significant.

Predictive modelling was conducted in Python 3.8 (Anaconda distribution; Anaconda, Inc., Austin, TX, USA)) using scikit-learn 1.2.2 (Python Software Foundation, Wilmington, DE, USA). Data were randomly split into a training set (70%) and a test set (30%), stratified by cluster membership. The following models were fitted:

- Logistic regression: to estimate linear relationships between core predictors (respiratory, affective, cognitive variables and composite scores) and membership in the psycho-respiratory phenotype.
- Multilayer perceptron (MLPClassifier): a feed-forward neural network with two hidden layers (50 and 25 neurons), rectified linear unit (ReLU) activation and Adam optimiser, to capture potential non-linear interactions.

Model performance was evaluated using accuracy, area under the receiver operating characteristic curve (AUC) and Cohen's kappa (κ) on the test set. Local interpretability was obtained with the LIME package, which highlighted feature contributions—particularly FEV_1% and HADS subscales—to individual predictions. Correlation networks and graphical representations (histograms, ROC curves, κ plots) were generated with matplotlib, seaborn and networkx.

3. Results

3.1. Descriptive Analysis of the Cohort

We first examined the clinical and demographic profile of the full cohort (n = 390) to establish a foundation for subsequent subgroup comparisons. Both continuous and categorical variables were catalogued to capture factors potentially influencing disease course, with particular attention to differences between patients with and without significant psychiatric symptoms.

3.1.1. Baseline Characteristics and Distribution of Continuous Variables

Continuous measures encompassed respiratory parameters and psychocognitive assessments. The mean age was 54.5 years (range 20–87), reflecting inclusion of both young adults and those with advanced disease. Sex distribution was balanced, and urban versus rural residence was nearly equal, ensuring broad socio-demographic representation.

Symptom severity by the COPD Assessment Test (CAT) averaged 17.3 (range 1–40), indicating the presence of both minimally and severely symptomatic subgroups. The mean Medical Research Council dyspnea grade (MRC) was 2.24 (0–4), suggesting that most patients experienced at least moderate exertional limitation. Objective obstruction, measured

https://doi.org/10.3390/diagnostics16040507

as percent-predicted FEV_1, averaged 68.9% (range 28–99), with a subset demonstrating severe airflow limitation.

Psychiatric symptoms, assessed by HADS, showed mean depression and anxiety scores of 7.53 (1–20) and 8.04 (1–24), respectively. Although these averages are in the mild-to-moderate range, maximum scores indicate a subset with severe emotional disturbance. Cognitive function, measured by MoCA (mean 24.3, range 5–30) and MMSE (mean 23.8, range 6–30), was generally preserved; however, low-end scores reveal that a minority face substantial cognitive impairment. Together, these data underscore a highly heterogeneous cohort in terms of pulmonary obstruction severity, psychiatric burden and cognitive performance (Table 1).

Table 1. Distribution of continuous variables of the entire cohort (N = 390).

Variable	Mean ± SD	Range
Age (years)	54.5 ± 14.2	20–87
CAT Score	17.3 ± 11.0	1–40
MRC Grade	2.24 ± 1.12	0–4
FEV_1 (%)	68.9 ± 18.5	28–99
HADS—Depression	7.53 ± 4.30	1–20
HADS—Anxiety	8.04 ± 5.35	1–24
MoCA	24.3 ± 5.02	5–30
MMSE	23.8 ± 4.72	6–30

3.1.2. Subgroup Comparison: Impact of Psychiatric Symptoms

To assess how psychiatric symptoms influence respiratory impairment, patients were stratified into two groups based on HADS scores and affective history. Group 1 (n = 257) comprised individuals with combined psycho-respiratory involvement, while Group 2 (n = 133) included those with predominantly respiratory disease.

Marked differences emerged between groups. Mean percent-predicted FEV_1 in Group 1 was approximately 60%, versus over 85% in Group 2. CAT scores averaged 22.3 in Group 1—nearly threefold higher than the 7.7 observed in Group 2—reflecting significantly heightened symptom perception among those with psychiatric comorbidity. HADS depression and anxiety scores were also significantly elevated in Group 1, and cognitive testing yielded lower MoCA and MMSE scores. A *t* test of the Integrated Pulmonary Severity Index (IPSS) produced a t-statistic of 18.33 ($p < 0.001$), confirming highly significant intergroup differences (Table 2).

Table 2. Comparison of continuous variables between Group 1 and Group 2.

Variable	Group 1 (n = 257)	Group 2 (n = 133)	*p*-Value
Age (years)	56.60 ± 12.60	50.42 ± 16.04	0.003
MoCA Score	23.02 ± 5.50	26.68 ± 2.62	<0.001
MMSE Score	22.69 ± 5.17	25.86 ± 2.64	<0.001
HADS—Depression	8.48 ± 4.53	5.69 ± 3.07	<0.001
HADS—Anxiety	9.54 ± 5.77	5.15 ± 2.63	<0.001
CAT Score	22.25 ± 9.67	7.74 ± 5.91	<0.001
FEV_1 (%)	60.18 ± 16.38	85.80 ± 7.42	<0.001

3.1.3. Distribution of Categorical Variables and Between-Group Comparisons

We further examined categorical variables to complete the demographic and clinical picture. In the overall cohort, 207 patients were male (53%) and 183 were female (47%); 216 lived in urban areas (55%), 174 in rural (45%); occupational status was 42% unemployed, 53% employed and 5% retired; education level spanned 54% for lower secondary, 26% for

https://doi.org/10.3390/diagnostics16040507

high school and 19% for higher education; 18% presented via the emergency department versus 82% in outpatient settings; smoking status was 42% never-smokers, 28% ex-smokers and 30% current smokers; alcohol use was 52% abstinent, 39% occasional and 9% chronic.

Comparisons between Group 1 and Group 2 revealed significant differences in several categories (χ^2 test): sex distribution ($p = 0.050$), urban versus rural residence ($p = 0.020$), unemployment rate ($p = 0.010$), education level ($p = 0.005$), mode of presentation ($p = 0.030$), smoking status ($p = 0.010$) and alcohol consumption ($p = 0.020$) (Table 3).

Table 3. Distribution of categorical variables in the total cohort and comparison between Group 1 and Group 2.

Variable	Category	Total Cohort	Group 1 (n = 257)	Group 2 (n = 133)	*p*-Value (χ^2)
Sex	Male	207 (53%)	132	75	0.050
	Female	183 (47%)	125	58	
Living Area	Urban	216 (55%)	118	98	0.020
	Rural	174 (45%)	80	94	
Employment	Unemployed	164 (42%)	84	80	0.010
	Employed	207 (53%)	111	96	
	Retired	19 (5%)	18	1	
Education	Secondary School	212 (54%)	121	91	0.005
	High School	103 (26%)	68	35	
	University	74 (19%)	44	30	
	No Education	1 (0,3%)	1	0	
Presentation	Emergency	70 (18%)	64	6	0.030
	Outpatient	320 (82%)	193	127	
Smoking	Non-smoker	162 (42%)	117	45	0.010
	Ex-smoker	108 (28%)	91	17	
	Current smoker	120 (30%)	49	71	
Alcohol Use	Abstinent	202 (52%)	151	51	0.020
	Occasional	153 (39%)	60	93	
	Chronic	35 (9%)	10	25	

These findings suggest that socio-demographic factors and health behaviours may modulate the interplay between psychiatric comorbidity and respiratory severity.

3.2. Analysis of Relationships Between Variables: Correlations and the Network of Interdependencies

We quantified pairwise associations among respiratory measures (percent-predicted FEV_1, CAT and mMRC scores), psychiatric indices (HADS-Depression and HADS-Anxiety) and cognitive assessments (MoCA and MMSE) using Pearson's correlation coefficient. A very strong inverse correlation emerged between percent-predicted FEV_1 and CAT score ($r = -0.82$, $p < 0.001$) and between FEV_1 and mMRC grade ($r = -0.65$, $p < 0.001$), while CAT and mMRC were strongly interrelated ($r = 0.71$, $p < 0.001$), confirming that declining lung function is tightly linked to worsening symptom burden and dyspnoea (Figure 2).

MoCA and MMSE also showed an almost perfect positive correlation ($r = 0.92$, $p < 0.001$), supporting the consistency of the cognitive assessments.

HADS-Depression and HADS-Anxiety scores correlated moderately and positively with both CAT and mMRC ($r \approx 0.37$–0.43, all $p < 0.001$), indicating that affective burden contributes to, but does not fully explain, perceived respiratory symptoms. By contrast, HADS scores showed strong negative correlations with cognitive performance—for example, $r = -0.76$ between HADS-Depression and MoCA and $r = -0.73$ with MMSE—together with a strong positive correlation between HADS-Depression and HADS-Anxiety themselves ($r = 0.79$, $p < 0.001$). These patterns suggest that elevated affective symptoms are accompanied by measurable cognitive decline, which may impede treatment self-management (Table 3).

https://doi.org/10.3390/diagnostics16040507

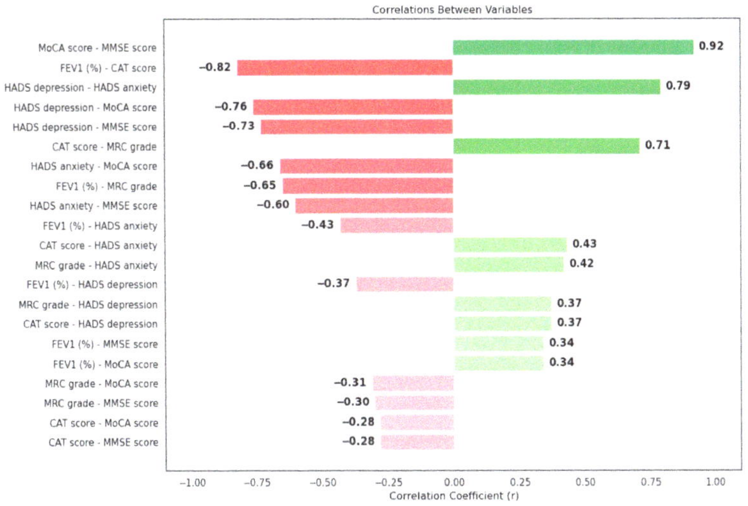

Figure 2. Correlations between clinical and psychological variables (r coefficient), (Green bars indicate positive correlations, while red bars indicate negative correlations).

To illustrate these interdependencies, we constructed a correlation network in which each node represents one of the seven key variables and edges denote significant correlations ($|r| > 0.30$, $p < 0.05$). This network revealed a central hub linking FEV_1%, CAT and mMRC directly to HADS-Depression and HADS-Anxiety, which in turn showed inverse ties to MoCA and MMSE. Clinically, this topology suggests that losses in FEV_1 may be perceived as disproportionately severe in patients with concurrent anxiety or depression—driving up CAT and mMRC scores—while those psychiatric symptoms are themselves associated with reduced cognitive capacity, potentially complicating disease management.

Taken together, these findings substantiate a shared core of physiological and psychological factors—where respiratory impairment, affective distress and cognitive decline are tightly interwoven—providing a robust multidimensional rationale for an integrated severity index such as IPSS.

3.3. Unsupervised Clustering and Natural Subgroup Separation

To explore whether the data naturally partition into two discrete subgroups—independently of the HADS-based classification—we applied spectral clustering to a set of standardized variables encompassing FEV_1% predicted, CAT score, MRC dyspnoea grade, HADS depression and anxiety scores, and cognitive performance as assessed by MoCA and MMSE. Standardization ensured that each metric contributed equally to the multidimensional analysis, eliminating scale-related biases.

We assessed cluster validity using the Silhouette score, which identified an optimal solution at k = 2. In other words, the high-dimensional data define two well-separated regions, each corresponding to a cohort of patients with similar clinical profiles. Notably, the resulting clusters showed marked concordance with our pre-defined HADS groups: "Cluster 1" comprised predominantly patients with combined psychiatric and respiratory impairment, whereas "Cluster 2" aligned largely with those exhibiting primarily respiratory dysfunction.

This convergence between an unsupervised clustering approach and the HADS-driven classification further substantiates the hypothesis that psychiatric factors—particularly anxiety and depression—together with respiratory metrics (CAT, MRC, FEV_1) constitute a

https://doi.org/10.3390/diagnostics16040507

core determinant of natural subgroup separation. Thus, beyond confirming the existence of two distinct phenotypic clusters, our analysis underscores the importance of integrating psychiatric assessment into the evaluation of pulmonary disease severity.

In summary, the intrinsic bifurcation of patient subgroups revealed by spectral clustering—and validated by the Silhouette Index—reinforces the notion that emotional symptoms can amplify both the perception and impact of respiratory impairment, providing a solid foundation for the future development of an integrated severity index.

3.4. Classification Models and Clinical Validation

To determine how well our predictors identify patients with combined psychiatric–respiratory impairment (Cohort 1), we compared two approaches: a logistic regression and a multi-layer perceptron (MLP) neural network. Both models were trained on the same feature set—HADS depression and anxiety scores, respiratory measures (CAT, FEV_1%, MRC dyspnoea grade) and global cognition (MoCA, MMSE).

The logistic regression achieved 89% accuracy, an area under the ROC curve (AUC) of 0.95 (Figure 3) and Cohen's κ of 0.77 (Figure 4).

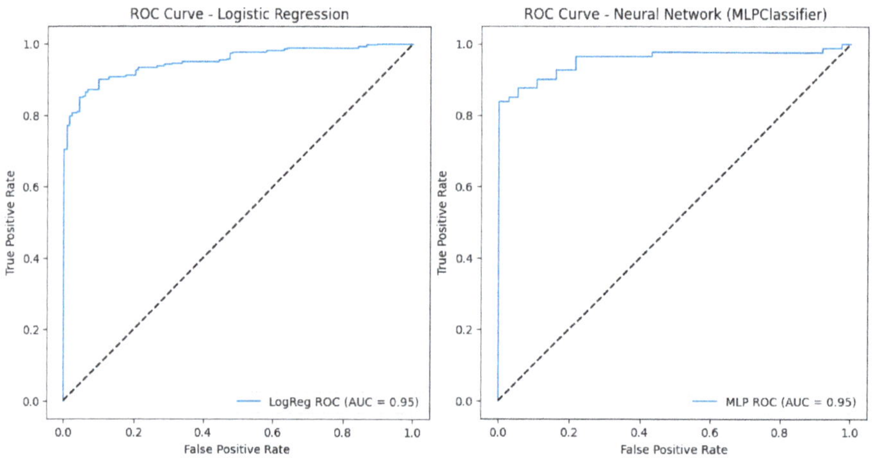

Figure 3. ROC Curves for logistic regression and MLPClassifier.

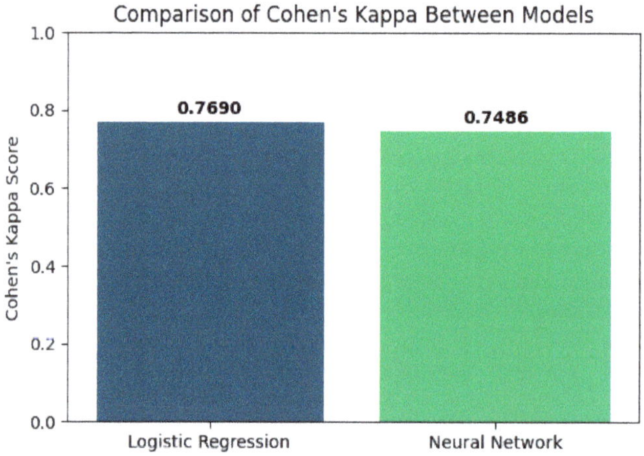

Figure 4. Comparison of Cohen's kappa scores between logistic regression and the neural network.

https://doi.org/10.3390/diagnostics16040507

Regression coefficients highlighted CAT score—and above all HADS-Anxiety—as the strongest positive predictors of Cohort 1 membership, indicating that rising anxiety and symptom burden dramatically increase the odds of dual impairment. By contrast, $FEV_1\%$ exerted a protective effect (negative coefficient), implying that higher lung function attenuates the risk of psychiatric–respiratory comorbidity. Together, these coefficients frame a clear narrative: as psychiatric symptoms intensify and pulmonary function declines, clinical complexity escalates.

In parallel, an MLPClassifier with two hidden layers (50 and 25 neurons) yielded virtually identical performance—89% accuracy, AUC 0.95 and Cohen's κ of 0.75 (Figure 4).

To probe local decision drivers, we applied LIME, which consistently flagged low $FEV_1\%$ and elevated HADS-Anxiety as the dominant features (Figure 5).

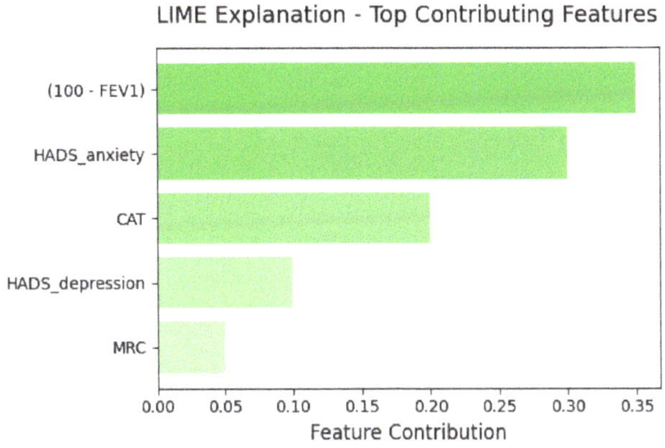

Figure 5. Feature contribution to the model decision according to LIME.

These findings reinforce the notion that, beyond isolated measurements, the interplay between psychiatric symptomatology and airflow obstruction constitutes a powerful predictor of clinical severity. A unified insight from both classification frameworks is that psychiatric manifestations—most notably anxiety—and declining pulmonary function (as reflected by a low $FEV_1\%$) operate in concert to define disease burden. As anxiety and depression worsen and lung function deteriorates, the risk of adverse outcomes rises, underscoring the imperative for a multidisciplinary approach in patients exhibiting dual impairment.

To offer further visual contrast between modelling strategies, Figure 6 depicts the architecture of the MLPClassifier—highlighting its two hidden layers (50 and 25 neurons)—against the single-layer, unidirectional structure of logistic regression.

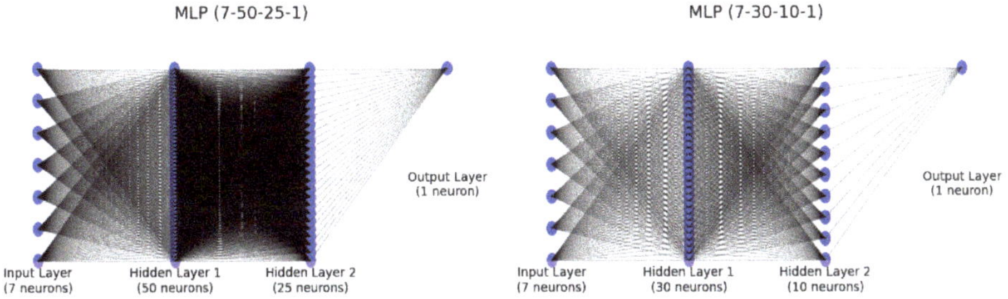

Figure 6. Graphical representation of two MLP architectures: (7-50-25-1) vs. (7-30-10-1).

https://doi.org/10.3390/diagnostics16040507

This schematic illustrates the added complexity of the neural network and its capacity to capture non-linear data relationships, which underpins its performance parity with the more interpretable regression model.

In sum, both logistic regression and neural-network approaches confirm that psychiatric distress and airflow limitation, particularly low $FEV_1\%$, are decisive in characterizing integrated disease severity. This underscores the value of integrating psychiatric evaluation into routine clinical assessment to support prognostic risk stratification and guide therapeutic decision-making.

3.5. Development and Implementation of the Integrated Pulmonary Severity Score (IPSS)

Given the strong correlations between $FEV_1\%$, symptom burden, dyspnoea, affective scores and cognition (e.g., $r = -0.82$ for $FEV_1\%$ vs. CAT, $r = -0.65$ for $FEV_1\%$ vs. mMRC, $r = -0.43$ and -0.37 for $FEV_1\%$ vs. HADS-Anxiety and HADS-Depression, respectively, all $p < 0.001$), we sought to condense this multidimensional information into a single, clinically usable index. To this end, we constructed the Integrated Pulmonary Severity Score (IPSS) in two steps: first, by defining a pulmonary component that integrates obstruction and respiratory symptoms, and second, by applying a psychiatric multiplier reflecting the additional burden of anxiety and depression.

3.5.1. Construction of the Pulmonary Component (PulmoScore)

The pulmonary component, termed the PulmoScore, was defined a priori from three clinically interpretable variables: CAT, mMRC and ventilatory deficit expressed as ($100 - FEV_1\%$). To harmonize scales, mMRC (0–4) was rescaled by multiplying by 10 to align with the CAT 0–40 range. The PulmoScore was then computed deterministically as:

$$\text{PulmoScore} = 0.30 \times \text{CAT} + 0.30 \times (\text{mMRC} \times 10) + 0.40 \times (100 - FEV_1\%).$$

A slightly higher weight was assigned to ventilatory deficit to anchor the score to objective obstruction, while CAT and rescaled mMRC contribute equally to capture patient-reported symptom burden and dyspnoea-related functional limitation. Under this formulation, a 10-point decrease in $FEV_1\%$ increases the PulmoScore by 4 points, whereas a 10-point increase in CAT or a 1-grade increase in mMRC (i.e., +10 after rescaling) increases the PulmoScore by 3 points.

3.5.2. Addition of the Psychiatric Multiplier and Definition of IPSS

To capture the contribution of affective symptoms to overall disease severity, the PulmoScore was extended with a psychiatric multiplier based on HADS-Depression and HADS-Anxiety. The final index was defined as:

$$\text{IPSS} = \text{PulmoScore} \times [1 + (\alpha \times \text{HADS-depression}) + (\beta \times \text{HADS-anxiety})]$$

Using ordinary least squares regression with the global psycho-respiratory index (SGPI) as the dependent variable, the coefficients were estimated as $\alpha = 0.0231$ and $\beta = 0.0423$ (per-point fractional increases in the multiplier), while the intercept was small and not retained for bedside computation. Visual inspection of the final IPSS distribution (Figure 7) did not suggest marked score inflation or extreme outliers in this cohort. Thus, each additional HADS-Depression point increases the multiplier by 2.31%, and each additional HADS-Anxiety point increases the multiplier by 4.23%, holding other components constant. The larger coefficient for HADS-Anxiety should be interpreted cautiously: it is cohort-derived and may reflect stronger coupling between anxiety, dyspnoea perception and patient-reported symptom burden in this sample rather than a universal hierarchy of

https://doi.org/10.3390/diagnostics16040507

affective domains. Accordingly, these coefficients require external validation and may need recalibration across populations and care settings. In the cohort, this formulation produced IPSS values ranging from very low scores in patients with preserved lung function, minimal symptoms and normal HADS values to triple-digit scores in individuals with combined severe obstruction, high CAT and mMRC grades and marked anxiety–depression.

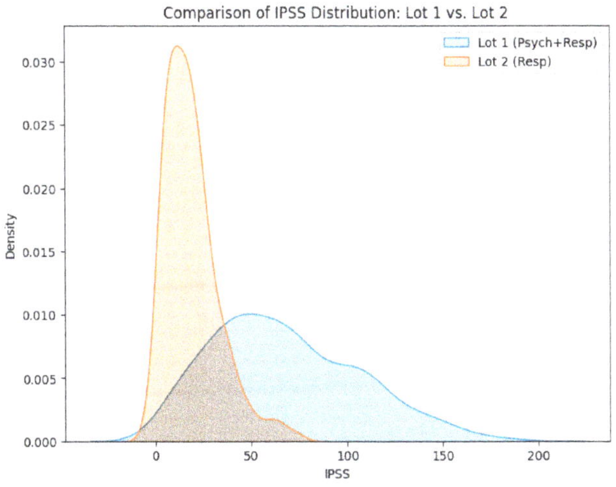

Figure 7. Comparative distribution of IPSS between Group 1 (blue) and Group 2 (orange).

3.5.3. Interpretation of the IPSS Formula

The IPSS is obtained in two conceptually simple steps. First, the PulmoScore aggregates objective and subjective respiratory information into a single pulmonary severity index. Second, this PulmoScore is multiplied by a factor that increases with HADS-Depression and HADS-Anxiety scores, thereby "amplifying" the respiratory burden in the presence of affective comorbidity.

Clinically, this behaviour is intuitive:

- Patients with relatively preserved $FEV_1\%$, low CAT and mMRC scores and normal HADS values tend to have low PulmoScores and remain in the lower IPSS range, corresponding to a predominantly somatic but mild overall burden.
- Patients with comparable spirometric impairment but elevated HADS-Anxiety and/or HADS-Depression exhibit substantially higher IPSS values, shifting them into higher risk strata despite similar obstruction.

This mechanism formally explains the frequent discrepancy between spirometry and perceived health status in COPD: the psychiatric multiplier captures the additional psycho-emotional load that is invisible to $FEV_1\%$ alone. In line with this, the psycho-respiratory cluster (Group 1) was characterized by lower $FEV_1\%$, higher CAT and mMRC scores and markedly higher HADS values, while the predominantly respiratory cluster (Group 2) had better lung function, lower symptom burden and near-normal affective scores.

3.5.4. Distribution of IPSS Values and Risk Categories

To render the IPSS interpretable at the bedside, we grouped the continuous score into four ordinal risk categories that balance the empirical score distribution with clinically intuitive cut-points:

- Low risk: IPSS < 30 points
- Moderate risk: IPSS 30–69 points

- High risk: IPSS 70–119 points
- Very high risk: IPSS $\geq$ 120 points.

To provide an explicit empirical reference for stratification, we also report the distribution-based cut-points of IPSS in this cohort. The IPSS quartiles were Q1 = 17.79, Q2 (median) = 35.91 and Q3 = 54.77. Accordingly, a quartile-based stratification would define four groups as IPSS $\leq$ 17.79, 17.79 < IPSS $\leq$ 35.91, 35.91 < IPSS $\leq$ 54.77, and IPSS > 54.77. We emphasize that both the pragmatic thresholds and the quantile-based cut-points are cohort-dependent and should be recalibrated and/or outcome-optimized in future external validation studies.

These bands were not optimized against hard endpoints (e.g., exacerbations, hospitalisations, mortality) in this cross-sectional derivation cohort. Instead, they were selected as pragmatic, distribution-informed thresholds approximating the sample quartiles and then rounded to improve bedside usability. Accordingly, these cut-offs should be recalibrated and/or outcome-optimized in external longitudinal validation cohorts before being used for prognostic decision-making. Patients were represented in all four strata, with a progressive gradient in respiratory impairment, symptom burden and affective distress from the low to the very-high IPSS category (Table 4).

Table 4. Risk categories based on IPSS and clinical recommendations.

IPSS (Points)	Risk Category	Key Clinical Actions
<30	Low	Routine monitoring; conservative management
30–69	Moderate	Optimize inhaled therapy; offer psychological support; close follow-up
70–119	High	Multidisciplinary evaluation (pulmonology + psychiatry); escalate treatment
$\geq$120	Very High	Aggressive management; consider hospitalization; rapid psychiatric review
Quartile-based stratification (for comparison in this cohort)		
$\leq$17.79	Q1 (lowest quartile)	Routine monitoring; conservative management
17.79–35.91	Q2	Optimize inhaled therapy; reinforce self-management; consider psychological screening/support as needed
35.91–54.77	Q3	Closer follow-up; optimize therapy; consider multidisciplinary input if symptom burden or HADS is elevated
>54.77	Q4 (highest quartile)	Intensified management; prioritize multidisciplinary evaluation; consider early intervention pathways

Note: The pragmatic thresholds are intended for bedside usability and were not outcome-optimized. For comparison, we also report a distribution-based (quartile) stratification in this cohort (Q1 = 17.79; Q2/median = 35.91; Q3 = 54.77). Both pragmatic and quantile-based cut-points are cohort-dependent and warrant external recalibration and longitudinal validation.

Descriptively, individuals with preserved lung function, low CAT and mMRC scores and normal or near-normal HADS values were concentrated in the low and moderate IPSS categories. By contrast, those combining severe obstruction, marked dyspnoea, high CAT scores and significant anxiety–depression predominantly occupied the high and very-high bands. This gradient closely mirrored the distribution of the two spectral-clustering phenotypes: the psycho-respiratory Group 1 showed a marked right-shift in the IPSS distribution, with a higher proportion of high and very-high scores compared with Group 2, whereas Group 2 was concentrated almost entirely in the low and moderate IPSS range (Figure 7).

From a practical standpoint, these categories offer a simple decision-making framework. Low-IPSS patients are typically candidates for routine follow-up and standard pharmacological management. Moderate IPSS values signal the need to optimize inhaled therapy and initiate structured psychological support. High and very-high IPSS identify a subset requiring intensified and often multidisciplinary care, potentially including psychiatric consultation, pulmonary rehabilitation and closer monitoring.

3.5.5. Relationship Between IPSS-Based Profiles and Predictive Models

The clinical relevance of this integrated construct was further supported by the performance of supervised models trained to distinguish the two spectral-clustering phenotypes. Because the clustering procedure and IPSS construction relied on overlapping core variables, these supervised results should be interpreted as convergent internal validity (consistency with the latent structure captured by clustering) rather than as an independent external validation. A logistic regression model using the core IPSS components (FEV_1%, CAT, mMRC, HADS-Depression, HADS-Anxiety, MoCA and MMSE) as predictors correctly classified 89% of patients (accuracy 0.89), with an area under the ROC curve (AUC) of 0.95 and a Cohen's κ of 0.77, indicating almost perfect agreement beyond chance. A multilayer perceptron (MLP) neural network trained on the same variables and evaluated on an independent test set yielded a similar accuracy of 0.89, an AUC of 0.95 and a Cohen's κ of 0.75.

LIME explanations for the MLP underscored that low FEV_1% and elevated HADS-Anxiety scores were the most influential features for predicting assignment to the psycho-respiratory group, followed by intermediate levels of HADS-Depression, mMRC and CAT. These findings are consistent with the design of IPSS and reinforce the notion that integrating pulmonary function, symptom burden and affective status captures a clinically meaningful psycho-respiratory phenotype rather than a purely statistical construct.

4. Discussion

In contemporary pulmonology practice, there is broad consensus that disease severity assessment cannot be confined to the predicted percentage of FEV_1, although this remains an essential physiological pillar. Established instruments—BODE, DOSE, ADO and B-AE-D—have successfully correlated spirometric values with mortality, exacerbation frequency or healthcare utilization; nevertheless, they almost exclusively describe the somatic dimension and systematically omit psycho-emotional factors. The Integrated Pulmonary Severity Score (IPSS) provides a coherent conceptual extension by explicitly incorporating anxiety–depressive symptomatology as a variable with its own numerical weight, thus allowing it to enter severity models on an equal footing with spirometry and dyspnoea.

The premise for this integration arises from a robust convergence of evidence: anxiety amplifies the perception of breathlessness and dyspnoea-related fear in COPD [26,27], elevates CAT scores irrespective of the obstruction degree [19,20] and—when co-existing with depression—more than doubles the risk of future exacerbations [13]. Depression, in turn, overlaps with those neurocognitive and functional domains that drive prognosis: COPD-related cognitive impairment, frequently accompanied by depressive symptoms, has been linked to frontal lobe hypoperfusion on SPECT imaging [28] and to poorer performance on both MoCA and MMSE [29,30]. At the same time, dyspnoea severity itself—strongly intertwined with affective burden—independently predicts in-hospital mortality during acute exacerbations [31]. In light of these observations, the direct inclusion of HADS scores in a composite severity index is not merely optional but appears methodologically necessary to reflect the true impact of the disease on the patient.

https://doi.org/10.3390/diagnostics16040507

4.1. Rationale for the IPSS Structure

The PulmoScore—the core respiratory component—aggregates the CAT, mMRC and ventilatory deficit, with a weight of 0.40 assigned to $(100 - FEV_1\%)$. This higher weighting for obstruction derives from the observation that, in our cohort, the FEV_1–symptom relationship ($r = -0.82$ for $FEV_1\%$ vs. CAT) was considerably tighter than the modest correlations reported in multicentre CAT validation studies [32,33]. Similar observations have emerged from the COSYCONET registry, where longitudinal declines in FEV_1 tracked worsening SGRQ scores over time [34].

A relatively greater weight for FEV_1 is also justified by data on early-onset COPD: younger adults can exhibit marked airflow limitation and unfavourable trajectories despite relatively preserved multidimensional scores, challenging the traditional Fletcher–Peto paradigm [35,36]. Large cohort analyses show that "young COPD" patients carry a substantial burden of comorbidities and an excess mortality risk compared with age-matched ever-smoker controls [37]. In such individuals, indices that strongly weight chronological age—such as ADO—may yield deceptively low risk estimates despite clinically significant impairment. By contrast, including both FEV_1 and patient-reported measures (CAT and mMRC) within the PulmoScore preserves the subjective dimension of symptom burden while anchoring it to the objective severity of obstruction, thus offering an immediate and clinically interpretable snapshot without requiring elaborate exercise testing.

4.2. Detailed Comparison with Established Indices

BODE remains a robust predictor of mortality in COPD, but it relies on the six-minute walk test (6MWT), which is difficult to standardize and is not routinely available in many outpatient clinics, limiting its practicality in everyday practice [38,39]. DOSE prioritizes exacerbation history and current smoking status, variables that can be collected rapidly in primary care and that have demonstrated prognostic value for mortality and healthcare utilization [39]. However, active smokers often underestimate or normalize respiratory symptoms and therefore underreport them, which may attenuate the sensitivity of DOSE to detect clinically relevant risk [40,41].

ADO introduces chronological age as an essential variable alongside dyspnoea and FEV_1, yet early-onset and rapidly progressive COPD have been described in younger adults, indicating that a strong age component can still underestimate risk in susceptible individuals [35–37]. B-AE-D incorporates body mass index, prior severe exacerbations and mMRC dyspnoea grade, and its extended version (B-AE-D-C) adds the biomarker copeptin, whose measurement requires laboratory infrastructure that is not universally accessible [42]. By contrast, IPSS relies exclusively on spirometry and brief questionnaires, allowing calculation in 3–5 min and facilitating inter-centre comparability without additional investment. Importantly, IPSS is not proposed as a replacement for these established indices but as a complementary tool that explicitly integrates psycho-emotional burden into severity assessment. From the standpoint of everyday implementation, these instruments differ markedly in the time, infrastructure and data completeness they require. BODE offers strong prognostic performance, but its dependence on a standardized 6MWT introduces logistical barriers (space, staffing, protocol consistency) and limits rapid use in busy outpatient clinics and in telemedicine workflows. DOSE is well suited to primary care because its components can be collected quickly, yet it depends on accurate exacerbation history and current smoking status; both can be incompletely documented or variably reported, which may reduce sensitivity for clinically meaningful risk in routine practice. ADO improves prognostic discrimination by incorporating age, but a strong age component can yield deceptively low risk estimates in younger patients with marked airflow limitation or rapidly progressive disease. In contrast, IPSS was designed for maximal feasibility: it uses

https://doi.org/10.3390/diagnostics16040507

spirometry plus short questionnaires (CAT, mMRC, HADS) that are routinely obtainable in most settings, enabling computation within minutes and supporting digital capture in registries, spirometry software, and remote monitoring platforms. Practically, IPSS therefore complements established indices by offering a rapid, reproducible multidimensional snapshot that makes psycho-emotional burden quantitatively visible alongside obstruction and symptom severity.

4.3. Convergence with Unsupervised Phenotyping and Network Analysis

Applying spectral clustering to the clinical variable matrix yielded two clinically coherent clusters that showed substantial overlap with groups defined by HADS scores, suggesting that anxiety, depression, CAT, mMRC and FEV_1 constitute a major axis of variability in this dataset [24,25]. Network-based analyses placed affective variables among high-centrality nodes [43,44], indicating not merely passive association but a potential generative role in clinical distress and functional limitation. This unsupervised convergence supports the notion that the IPSS formula approximates the latent structure of the data rather than merely modelling relationships imposed a priori. Nevertheless, because the same feature set underlies both clustering and score construction, this convergence should be viewed as supportive internal evidence, and independent validation against external cohorts and longitudinal outcomes remains required.

4.4. Clinical Implementation and Pragmatic Benefits

IPSS uses five routinely available variables (FEV_1%, CAT, mMRC, HADS-Anxiety and HADS-Depression) and can be embedded into spirometry software, outpatient workflows, and telemonitoring platforms. In practice, IPSS can function as a triage and personalization aid: (i) it can flag patients who may benefit from earlier multidisciplinary review (pulmonology + psychiatry/psychology), (ii) it can serve as a structured trigger for psychological referral (including telepsychiatry in low-access regions), and (iii) it can support prioritization for pulmonary rehabilitation and structured behavioural interventions (e.g., CBT-informed programmes) aimed at reducing affective distress and improving function [45–48]. Importantly, while higher IPSS plausibly indicates increased vulnerability to exacerbation and healthcare utilization, prospective longitudinal validation against hard endpoints is required before IPSS is used as an outcome-prediction tool in routine care. Moreover, the structure of IPSS is amenable to explainable-AI pipelines: in our cohort, LIME highlighted HADS-Anxiety and FEV_1 as leading contributors to the model output, consistent with comparative evaluations showing the usefulness of local interpretability techniques such as LIME and SHAP for distinguishing clinically meaningful classes [49,50]. These characteristics suggest that IPSS can act as a bridge between traditional bedside assessment and algorithm-assisted decision support systems.

4.5. Relevance to Public Health Policy

Our analysis revealed significantly higher IPSSs among patients with lower educational attainment, precarious occupational status and rural residence—findings that mirror research on the social determinants of health and on COPD-related disparities in access and outcomes [51,52]. Integrating IPSS into a national electronic registry could enable continuous monitoring of such inequalities and support dynamic resource reallocation, in line with Frohlich and Potvin's ecosocial perspective on the "determinants of determinants" [53] and with evidence of rural disadvantage in quality of life and service availability for patients with COPD [45,54].

In summary, IPSS addresses important gaps left by traditional composite indices by offering a patient-centred tool that simultaneously quantifies ventilatory impairment and emotional burden. Its internal validation through unsupervised clustering and su-

https://doi.org/10.3390/diagnostics16040507

pervised models, its feasibility in everyday clinical workflows and its compatibility with digital infrastructure recommend IPSS as a promising candidate for individualized clinical decision-making and for health policies adapted to the current socio-epidemiological context. At the same time, external validation in independent cohorts and prospective evaluation against hard clinical outcomes (exacerbations, hospitalizations, mortality) remain essential before IPSS can be adopted as a definitive standard in COPD severity assessment.

5. Limitations of the Study

This study has several limitations. First, its bi-institutional design (psychiatric vs. pulmonology recruitment) may introduce selection/spectrum bias due to differences in referral patterns and the routine use of psychocognitive assessment. Second, major cardiometabolic comorbidities (e.g., heart failure, sleep apnoea, severe obesity) were excluded to reduce confounding during score derivation; however, this limits generalizability to real-world multimorbid COPD, and future studies should validate and, if needed, recalibrate IPSS in broader cohorts, ideally including sensitivity analyses with relaxed exclusions and/or comorbidity-stratified models. Third, IPSS coefficients and cut-offs were derived and internally evaluated in the same dataset; thus, discrimination of cluster membership should be interpreted as internal separability rather than independent validation, and external validation in independent, multi-ethnic cohorts is required. Fourth, the cross-sectional design precludes causal inference and does not allow assessment of longitudinal predictive accuracy against hard endpoints (exacerbations, hospitalisations, mortality or healthcare costs). Fifth, CAT, mMRC and HADS are self-reported measures and are susceptible to measurement error and interviewer/context effects, including cultural and educational influences. Finally, the absence of continuous telemonitoring data (nocturnal SpO_2, physical activity) and biological markers limits comparisons with biomarker-enriched indices and the ability to capture rapid clinical changes; additionally, the multiplicative formulation may be sensitive to distributional shifts and should be re-assessed for skewness/outliers during external validation, while the exclusion of cognitive scales from IPSS reflects a feasibility–comprehensiveness trade-off that should be revisited in settings where standardized cognitive testing is systematically available.

6. Conclusions

This study demonstrates that incorporating anxiety and depression into COPD assessment adds clinically relevant information beyond spirometry and dyspnoea scales alone. By combining FEV_1%, mMRC, CAT and HADS-based affective scores, the Integrated Pulmonary Severity Score (IPSS) captures a psycho-respiratory phenotype characterized by more severe airflow limitation, higher symptom perception and poorer cognitive performance than that seen in predominantly respiratory profiles.

In our cohort, IPSS showed good internal validity and clearly separated patients into four severity strata (<30, 30–69, 70–119, $\geq$120 points), which may support graded clinical decisions ranging from routine follow-up to intensified multidisciplinary management. Both logistic regression and a multilayer perceptron achieved high discrimination (AUC 0.95, Cohen's $\kappa \geq 0.75$) when using the same core variables that informed the clustering and IPSS construction to classify membership in the psycho-respiratory phenotype; therefore, this agreement supports internal (convergent) validity rather than independent validation, while explainable-AI analyses (LIME) consistently highlighted HADS-Anxiety and FEV_1% as dominant contributors. These findings suggest that IPSS can complement existing indices by making the emotional burden of COPD quantitatively visible in everyday practice.

At the same time, the score was derived and tested in two tertiary centres, excluded major cardiometabolic comorbidities and lacked longitudinal endpoints such as exacer-

https://doi.org/10.3390/diagnostics16040507

bations, hospitalisations and mortality. Before routine clinical adoption, IPSS therefore requires external validation in independent populations, potential recalibration of cut-off values and prospective evaluation of its impact on outcomes and resource allocation. If these steps confirm its performance, IPSS could help bridge the gap between physiological impairment and emotional distress in COPD and serve as a template for future multidimensional, explainable prediction models and patient-centred, interdisciplinary care strategies.

Author Contributions: Conceptualization, I.-L.B., D.R. and C.-T.S.; methodology, I.-L.B. and C.-T.S.; software, D.-M.C.; validation, I.-L.B., D.R. and C.-T.S.; formal analysis, I.-L.B., D.R. and D.-M.C.; investigation, I.-L.B., A.-C.B.-C., I.U. and V.G.; resources, I.U., V.G. and C.-T.S.; data curation, A.-C.B.-C. and D.R.; writing—original draft preparation, I.-L.B.; writing—review and editing, D.R., C.-T.S. and A.-C.B.-C.; visualization, I.-L.B. and D.-M.C.; supervision, D.R. and C.-T.S.; project administration, C.-T.S.; funding acquisition, C.-T.S. All authors have read and agreed to the published version of the manuscript.

Funding: The article processing charges were funded by the University of Medicine and Pharmacy of Craiova, Romania.

Institutional Review Board Statement: The study was conducted in accordance with the Declaration of Helsinki and approved by the Ethics Committee of the University of Medicine and Pharmacy in Craiova (approval number: 196/17 February 2022) and Leamna Pulmonology Hospital (approval number: 6189/13 October 2022).

Informed Consent Statement: Informed consent was obtained from all subjects involved in the study.

Data Availability Statement: Data is contained within the article. The original contributions presented in the study are included in the article; further inquiries can be directed to the corresponding authors.

Conflicts of Interest: The author Dragoș-Mihai Cojocaru is affiliated with Sanacare AG. The company had no role in the design of the study; in the collection, analyses, or interpretation of data; in the writing of the manuscript; or in the decision to publish the results. The authors declare no conflicts of interest.

References

1. World Health Organization. Chronic Obstructive Pulmonary Disease (COPD). Available online: https://www.who.int/news-room/fact-sheets/detail/chronic-obstructive-pulmonary-disease-(copd) (accessed on 6 November 2024).
2. Wang, L.; Yu, Q.; Xiao, J.; Chen, Q.; Fang, M.; Zhao, H. Cigarette Smoke Extract-Treated Mouse Airway Epithelial Cells-Derived Exosomal LncRNA MEG3 Promotes M1 Macrophage Polarization and Pyroptosis in Chronic Obstructive Pulmonary Disease by Upregulating TREM-1 via m6A Methylation. *Immune Netw.* **2024**, *24*, e3. [CrossRef]
3. Shen, Q.; Chen, J.; Yang, S.; Zhang, H.; Yu, H.; Wang, S.; Li, J. Protection against cigarette smoke-induced chronic obstructive pulmonary disease via activation of the SIRT1/FoxO1 axis by targeting microRNA-132. *Am. J. Transl. Res.* **2024**, *16*, 5516–5524. [CrossRef]
4. Wang, J.; Luo, J.; Rotili, D.; Mai, A.; Steegborn, C.; Xu, S.; Jin, Z.G. SIRT6 Protects Against Lipopolysaccharide-Induced Inflammation in Human Pulmonary Lung Microvascular Endothelial Cells. *Inflammation* **2024**, *47*, 323–332. [CrossRef]
5. Zecevic, A.; Blanka-Protic, A.; Jandric, A.; Adzic-Vukicevic, T. Are patients with chronic obstructive pulmonary disease at a greater risk for the development of autoimmune thyroiditis as an adverse event of immunotherapy in non-small cell lung cancer treatment? *Pathol. Oncol. Res.* **2025**, *31*, 1612022. [CrossRef]
6. Bracke, K.R.; Mestdagh, P. MicroRNAs as future therapeutic targets in COPD? *Eur. Respir. J.* **2017**, *49*, 1700431. [CrossRef] [PubMed]
7. Rabe, K.F.; Watz, H. Chronic obstructive pulmonary disease. *Lancet* **2017**, *389*, 1931–1940. [CrossRef]
8. Strollo, H.C.; Nouraie, S.M.; Hoth, K.F.; Riley, C.M.; Karoleski, C.; Zhang, Y.; Hanania, N.A.; Bowler, R.P.; Bon, J.; Sciurba, F.C. Association of systemic inflammation with depressive symptoms in individuals with COPD. *Int. J. Chron. Obstruct. Pulmon. Dis.* **2021**, *16*, 2515–2522. [CrossRef] [PubMed]

https://doi.org/10.3390/diagnostics16040507

9. Donaldson, G.C.; Seemungal, T.A.; Patel, I.S.; Bhowmik, A.; Wilkinson, T.M.; Hurst, J.R.; Maccallum, P.K.; Wedzicha, J.A. Airway and systemic inflammation and decline in lung function in patients with COPD. *Chest* **2005**, *128*, 1995–2004. [CrossRef]
10. Kim, V.; Zhao, H.; Armstrong, H.F.; O'Neal, W.K.; Bailey, K.L.; Rennard, S.I.; Barr, R.G.; Criner, G.J.; Lovasi, G.S.; Morrison, M.F. Elevated systemic biomarkers and persistent anxiety and depression in smokers with and without COPD: An analysis of the SPIROMICS cohort. *Eur. Respir. J.* **2017**, *50*, PA4967.
11. Mobeen, F.; Edgar, R.; Pye, A.; Stockley, R.; Turner, A.M. Effect of depression and anxiety on health status and lung function in patients with alpha 1 antitrypsin deficiency. *Thorax* **2018**, *73*, A171. [CrossRef]
12. Bratek, A.; Zawada, K.; Beil-Gawełczyk, J.; Beil, S.; Sozańska, E.; Krysta, K.; Barczyk, A.; Krupka-Matuszczyk, I.; Pierzchała, W. Depressiveness, symptoms of anxiety and cognitive dysfunctions in patients with asthma and chronic obstructive pulmonary disease (COPD): Possible associations with inflammation markers: A pilot study. *J. Neural Transm.* **2015**, *122*, 83–91. [CrossRef]
13. Wu, K.; Lu, L.; Chen, Y.; Peng, J.; Wu, X.; Tang, G.; Ma, T.; Cheng, J.; Ran, P.; Zhou, Y. Associations of anxiety and depression with prognosis in chronic obstructive pulmonary disease: A systematic review and meta-analysis. *Pulmonology* **2025**, *31*, 2438553. [CrossRef]
14. Giardino, N.D.; Curtis, J.L.; Abelson, J.L.; King, A.P.; Pamp, B.; Liberzon, I.; Martinez, F.J. The impact of panic disorder on interoception and dyspnea reports in chronic obstructive pulmonary disease. *Biol. Psychol.* **2010**, *84*, 142–146. [CrossRef] [PubMed]
15. Mansukhani, M.P.; Kara, T.; Caples, S.M.; Somers, V.K. Chemoreflexes, sleep apnea, and sympathetic dysregulation. *Curr. Hypertens. Rep.* **2014**, *16*, 476. [CrossRef]
16. Ziegler, M.G.; Mills, P.J.; Loredo, J.S.; Ancoli-Israel, S.; Dimsdale, J.E. Effect of continuous positive airway pressure and placebo treatment on sympathetic nervous activity in patients with obstructive sleep apnea. *Chest* **2001**, *120*, 887–893. [CrossRef] [PubMed]
17. Ferreira, C.B.; Schoorlemmer, G.H.; Rocha, A.A.; Cravo, S.L. Increased sympathetic responses induced by chronic obstructive sleep apnea are caused by sleep fragmentation. *J. Appl. Physiol.* **2020**, *129*, 163–172. [CrossRef] [PubMed]
18. Harrison, O.K.; Köchli, L.; Marino, S.; Luechinger, R.; Hennel, F.; Brand, K.; Hess, A.J.; Frässle, S.; Iglesias, S.; Vinckier, F.; et al. Interoception of breathing and its relationship with anxiety. *Neuron* **2021**, *109*, 4080–4093.e8. [CrossRef] [PubMed]
19. Wu, D.; Zhao, X.; Huang, D.; Dai, Z.; Chen, M.; Li, D.; Wu, B. Outcomes associated with comorbid anxiety and depression among patients with stable COPD: A patient registry study in China. *J. Affect. Disord.* **2022**, *313*, 77–83. [CrossRef]
20. Coelho, R.; Santos, A.S.; Maia, D.; Rosa, R.; Caldeira, V.; Sá, T.; Semedo, L.; Cardoso, J. Symptoms of anxiety and depression in COPD patients. *Eur. Respir. J.* **2014**, *44*, P981.
21. Janssen, D.J.; Spruit, M.A.; Leue, C.; Gijsen, C.; Hameleers, H.; Schols, J.M.; Wouters, E.F. Symptoms of anxiety and depression in COPD patients entering pulmonary rehabilitation. *Chron. Respir. Dis.* **2010**, *7*, 147–157. [CrossRef]
22. Karloh, M.; Pizzichinni, M.M.; Pizzichini, E. Effects of comorbidities on the CAT score: A population-based study. *Eur. Respir. J.* **2016**, *48*, PA3705.
23. Buican, I.L.; Gheorman, V.; Udriştoiu, I.; Olteanu, M.; Rădulescu, D.; Calafeteanu, D.M.; Nemeş, A.F.; Călăraşu, C.; Rădulescu, P.M.; Streba, C.T. Interactions between cognitive, affective, and respiratory profiles in chronic respiratory disorders: A cluster analysis approach. *Diagnostics* **2024**, *14*, 1153. [CrossRef] [PubMed]
24. Howrylak, J.A.; Fuhlbrigge, A.L.; Strunk, R.C.; Zeiger, R.S.; Weiss, S.T.; Raby, B.A. Classification of Childhood Asthma Phenotypes and Long-Term Clinical Responses to Inhaled Anti-inflammatory Medications. *J. Allergy Clin. Immunol.* **2014**, *133*, 1289–1300.e12. [CrossRef] [PubMed]
25. Boussina, A.; Wardi, G.; Shashikumar, S.P.; Malhotra, A.; Zheng, K.; Nemati, S. Representation Learning and Spectral Clustering for the Development and External Validation of Dynamic Sepsis Phenotypes: Observational Cohort Study. *J. Med. Internet Res.* **2023**, *25*, e45614. [CrossRef] [PubMed]
26. Janssens, T.; De Peuter, S.; Stans, L.; Verleden, G.; Troosters, T.; Decramer, M.; Van den Bergh, O. Dyspnea perception in COPD: Association between anxiety, dyspnea-related fear and dyspnea in a pulmonary rehabilitation program. *Chest* **2011**, *140*, 618–625. [CrossRef]
27. Di Marco, F.; Verga, M.; Reggente, M.; Casanova, F.M.; Santus, P.; Blasi, F.; Allegra, L.; Centanni, S. Anxiety and depression in COPD patients: The roles of gender and disease severity. *Respir. Med.* **2006**, *100*, 1767–1774. [CrossRef]
28. Antonelli Incalzi, R.; Marra, C.; Giordano, A.; Calcagni, M.L.; Cappa, A.; Basso, S.; Pagliari, G.; Fuso, L. Cognitive impairment in chronic obstructive pulmonary disease—A neuropsychological and SPECT study. *J. Neurol.* **2003**, *250*, 325–332. [CrossRef]
29. Xu, C.; He, Y.; Zheng, Y.; Zhou, L.; Liu, S.; Wan, Y. Correlation of depression and cognitive function in patients with chronic obstructive pulmonary disease. *Chin. J. Gen. Pract.* **2013**, *12*, 59–61.
30. Uryasev, O.M.; Sidorova, I.V.; Shakhanov, A.V. The cognitive impairment in patients with chronic obstructive pulmonary disease. *Pak. J. Med. Health Sci.* **2019**, *13*, 276–279.
31. Steer, J.; Norman, E.; Afolabi, G.; Gibson, G.J.; Bourke, S.C. Evaluation of the MRC dyspnoea scale and a novel extended version in prediction of in-hospital death and early readmission in acute exacerbations of COPD. *Thorax* **2010**, *65*, A76. [CrossRef]

https://doi.org/10.3390/diagnostics16040507

32. Kwon, N.; Amin, M.; Hui, D.S.; Jung, K.S.; Lim, S.Y.; Ta, H.D.; Thai, T.T.L.; Yunus, F.; Jones, P.W. Validity of the COPD assessment test translated into local languages for Asian patients. *Chest* **2013**, *143*, 703–710. [CrossRef]
33. De Castro, R.A.S.; Zanatta, D.J.M.; Rached, S.Z.; Athanazio, R.A.; de Camargo, A.A.; Cukier, A.; Stelmach, R.; Dal Corso, S.; Lanza, F.C. COPD Assessment Test (CAT): Validity and reproducibility in patients with non-cystic fibrosis bronchiectasis. *Eur. Respir. J.* **2015**, *46*, PA2791. [CrossRef]
34. Lutter, J.I.; Jörres, R.A.; Kahnert, K.; Schwarzkopf, L.; Studnicka, M.; Karrasch, S.; Schulz, H.; Vogelmeier, C.F.; Holle, R.; COSYCONET Study Group. Health-related quality of life associates with change in FEV_1 in COPD: Results from the COSYCONET cohort. *BMC Pulm. Med.* **2020**, *20*, 148. [CrossRef]
35. Sanchez-Salcedo, P.; Divo, M.; Casanova, C.; Pinto-Plata, V.; de-Torres, J.P.; Cote, C.; Cabrera, C.; Zagaceta, J.; Rodriguez-Roisin, R.; Zulueta, J.J.; et al. Disease progression in young patients with COPD: Rethinking the Fletcher and Peto model. *Eur. Respir. J.* **2014**, *44*, 324–331. [CrossRef]
36. Bakke, P.S. Forløp av obstruktive lungesykdommer [Course of obstructive lung diseases]. *Tidsskr. Nor. Laegeforen.* **1993**, *113*, 177–181. [PubMed]
37. Divo, M.J.; Marin, J.M.; Casanova, C.; Cabrera Lopez, C.; Pinto-Plata, V.M.; Marin-Oto, M.; Polverino, F.; de-Torres, J.P.; Billheimer, D.; Celli, B.R.; et al. Comorbidities and mortality risk in adults younger than 50 years of age with chronic obstructive pulmonary disease. *Respir. Res.* **2022**, *23*, 267. [CrossRef]
38. Celli, B.R.; Cote, C.G.; Marín, J.M.; Casanova, C.; Montes de Oca, M.; Méndez, R.A.; Pinto-Plata, V.; Cabral, H.J. The body-mass index, airflow obstruction, dyspnea, and exercise capacity index in chronic obstructive pulmonary disease. *N. Engl. J. Med.* **2004**, *350*, 1005–1012. [CrossRef]
39. Espantoso-Romero, M.; Román Rodríguez, M.; Duarte-Pérez, A.; Gonzálvez-Rey, J.; Callejas-Cabanillas, P.A.; Kasuba Lazic, D.; Anta-Agudo, B.; Torán Monserrat, P.; Magallon-Botaya, R.; Gerasimovska Kitanovska, B.; et al. External validation of multidimensional prognostic indices (ADO, BODEx and DOSE) in a primary care international cohort (PROEPOC/COPD cohort). *BMC Pulm. Med.* **2016**, *16*, 143. [CrossRef]
40. Woodruff, P.G.; Barr, R.G.; Bleecker, E.; Christenson, S.A.; Couper, D.; Curtis, J.L.; Gouskova, N.A.; Hansel, N.N.; Hoffman, E.A.; Kanner, R.E.; et al. Clinical significance of symptoms in smokers with preserved pulmonary function. *N. Engl. J. Med.* **2016**, *374*, 1811–1821. [CrossRef]
41. Gogou, E.; Kotsiou, O.S.; Siachpazidou, D.S.; Pinaka, M.; Varsamas, C.; Bardaka, F.; Gerogianni, I.; Hatzoglou, C.; Gourgoulianis, K.I. Underestimation of respiratory symptoms by smokers: A thorn in chronic obstructive pulmonary disease diagnosis. *npj Prim. Care Respir. Med.* **2021**, *31*, 14. [CrossRef] [PubMed]
42. Boeck, L.; Soriano, J.B.; Brusse-Keizer, M.; Blasi, F.; Kostikas, K.; Boersma, W.G.; Milenkovic, B.; Louis, R.; Lacoma, A.; Djamin, R.; et al. Prognostic assessment in COPD without lung function: The B-AE-D indices. *Eur. Respir. J.* **2016**, *47*, 1635–1644. [CrossRef]
43. Ashtiani, M.; Mirzaie, M.; Jafari, M. CINNA: An R/CRAN package to decipher central informative nodes in network analysis. *Bioinformatics* **2019**, *35*, 1436–1437. [CrossRef] [PubMed]
44. Kaur, S.; Gupta, A.; Saxena, R. Identifying central nodes in directed and weighted networks. *Int. J. Adv. Comput. Sci. Appl.* **2021**, *12*, 905–914. [CrossRef]
45. Burkes, R.M.; Gassett, A.J.; Ceppe, A.S.; Anderson, W.; O'Neal, W.K.; Woodruff, P.G.; Krishnan, J.A.; Barr, R.G.; Han, M.K.; Martinez, F.J.; et al. Rural residence and chronic obstructive pulmonary disease exacerbations: Analysis of the SPIROMICS cohort. *Ann. Am. Thorac. Soc.* **2018**, *15*, 808–816. [CrossRef] [PubMed]
46. Picazo, F.; Duan, K.I.; Hee Wai, T.; Hayes, S.; Leonhard, A.G.; Fonseca, G.A.; Plumley, R.; Beaver, K.A.; Donovan, L.M.; Au, D.H.; et al. Rural residence associated with receipt of recommended postdischarge chronic obstructive pulmonary disease care among a cohort of U.S. veterans. *Ann. Am. Thorac. Soc.* **2025**, *22*, 515–522. [CrossRef]
47. Farver Vestergaard, I.; Danielsen, J.T.T.; Løkke, A.; Zachariae, R. Psychosocial intervention in chronic obstructive pulmonary disease: Meta-analysis of randomized controlled trials. *Psychosom. Med.* **2022**, *84*, 347–358. [CrossRef]
48. Zhang, J.H.; Zhang, L.Q.; Yang, Y.P.; Li, X.; Zhang, Y.; Wang, L.Y.; Shi, H.; Jiang, H.; Guo, W.; Mu, L.; et al. Clinical effect of nutritional and psychological intervention combined with pulmonary rehabilitation exercise on patients with chronic obstructive pulmonary disease. *Zhonghua Yi Xue Za Zhi* **2020**, *100*, 110–115.
49. ElShawi, R.; Sherif, Y.; Al-Mallah, M.; Sakr, S. Interpretability in healthcare: A comparative study of local machine learning interpretability techniques. *Comput. Intell.* **2020**, *37*, 1633–1650. [CrossRef]
50. Soujanya, K.J.; Kodipalli, A.; Gosai, S.; Sneha, B.J.; Rao, T. Symptoms-based classification of disease using various ML algorithms and interpretation using LIME and SHAP kernels. In *2024 4th Asian Conference on Innovation in Technology (ASIANCON)*; IEEE: Piscataway, NJ, USA, 2025; pp. 1–6.
51. Neadley, K.E.; McMichael, G.; Freeman, T.; Browne Yung, K.; Baum, F.; Pretorius, E.; Taylor, K.; Boyd, M.A. Capturing the social determinants of health at the individual level: A pilot study. *Public Health Res. Pract.* **2021**, *31*, 30232008. [CrossRef]
52. Gaffney, A.W.; Hawks, L.; White, A.C.; Woolhandler, S.; Himmelstein, D.U.; Christiani, D.C.; McCormick, D. Health care disparities across the urban–rural divide: A national study of COPD. *J. Rural Health* **2019**, *35*, 449–458. [CrossRef]

53. Frohlich, K.L.; Potvin, L. Commentary: Structure or agency? The importance of both for addressing social inequalities in health. *Int. J. Epidemiol.* **2010**, *39*, 378–379. [CrossRef] [PubMed]
54. Jackson, B.E.; Coultas, D.B.; Suzuki, S.; Singh, K.P.; Bae, S. Rural–urban disparities in quality of life among patients with COPD. *J. Rural Health* **2013**, *29*, S62–S69. [CrossRef] [PubMed]

https://doi.org/10.3390/diagnostics16040507

diagnostics

MDPI

Article

Anatomy-Guided Hybrid CNN–ViT Model with Neuro-Symbolic Reasoning for Early Diagnosis of Thoracic Diseases Multilabel

Naif Almughamisi *, Gibrael Abosamra, Adnan Albar and Mostafa Saleh

Department of Information Systems, Faculty of Computing and Information Technology, King Abdulaziz University, Jeddah 21589, Saudi Arabia; gabosamra@kau.edu.sa (G.A.); ambar@kau.edu.sa (A.A.); msherbini@kau.edu.sa (M.S.)

* Correspondence: nalmughamisi@stu.kau.edu.sa

Abstract

Background/Objectives: The clinical adoption of AI in radiology requires models that balance high accuracy with interpretable, anatomically plausible reasoning. This study presents an integrated diagnostic framework that addresses this need by unifying a hybrid deep-learning architecture with explicit anatomical guidance and neuro-symbolic inference. **Methods**: The proposed system employs a dual-path model: an enhanced EfficientNetV2 backbone extracts hierarchical local features, whereas a refined Vision Transformer captures global contextual dependencies across the thoracic cavity. These representations are fused and critically disciplined through auxiliary segmentation supervision using CheXmask. This anchors the learned features to lung and cardiac anatomy, reducing reliance on spurious artifacts. This anatomical basis is fundamental to the interpretability pipeline. It confines Gradient-weighted Class Activation Mapping (Grad-CAM) visual explanations to clinically valid regions. Then, a novel neuro-symbolic reasoning layer is introduced. Using a fuzzy logic engine and radiological ontology, this module translates anatomically aligned neural activations into structured, human-readable diagnostic statements that explicitly articulate the model's clinical rationale. **Results**: Evaluated on the NIH ChestX-ray14 dataset, the framework achieved a macro-AUROC of 0.9056 and a macro-accuracy of 93.9% across 14 pathologies, with outstanding performance on emphysema (0.9694), hernia (0.9711), and cardiomegaly (0.9589). The model's generalizability was confirmed through external validation on the CheXpert dataset, yielding a macro-AUROC of 0.85. **Conclusions**: This study demonstrates a cohesive path toward clinically transparent and trustworthy AI by seamlessly integrating data-driven learning with anatomical knowledge and symbolic reasoning.

Keywords: hybrid CNN–ViT; anatomy-guided learning; Grad-CAM; neuro-symbolic reasoning; chest X-ray; thoracic disease classification

1. Introduction

Pulmonary diseases continue to be a major global health challenge [1]. Globally, pulmonary diseases affect hundreds of millions of people and contribute significantly to the overall burden of morbidity and mortality. Timely and accurate diagnosis of pulmonary diseases provides effective treatment [2]. In addition, the early detection of some pulmonary diseases will help isolate the patient and prevent the spread of the disease. Chest radiography (CXR) is considered the main method for checking patients with pulmonary diseases because of its availability, low cost, and relatively low level of radiation [3]. Manual diagnosis is prone to errors because chest X-rays shown similar symptoms, making it difficult for doctors and specialists to differentiate between various lung diseases. This is compounded by differing opinions among physicians and a shortage of highly experienced specialists in this field. Therefore, artificial intelligence techniques can address the limitations of manual diagnosis [4]. Recently, Deep learning approaches have been applied extensively in the medical field, such as in the classification of medical images. CNNs have achieved strong performance in pathology analysis by extracting fine-grained spatial information and composing it into multilevel representations [5]. However, these models are not well suited to capture extended dependencies and holistic contexts across images [6]. This limitation is particularly significant for pulmonary disease diagnosis, where abnormalities frequently extend across regions and require whole-image context [7]. Vision Transformers have marked a considerable technique in computer vision, which has demonstrated state-of-the-art performance across various image classification tasks and has been adopted in various methods in medical contexts, including tasks such as identifying diseases in chest X-rays, although they require extensive computational resources and large datasets for effective training [8]. This has motivated the development of hybrid CNN-ViT architectures that combine the local feature extraction capabilities of CNNs with the global modeling power of transformers, offering superior performance for medical imaging applications [9]. However, most available deep learning solutions act as black-box models without explaining how decisions are made or providing any interpretation, which poses significant challenges for clinical adoption [10,11]. Therefore, the fundamental challenge in adopting AI models in the healthcare sector should be interpretability, trustworthiness, and robustness [11]. Many healthcare professionals remain cautious about relying on AI systems when the decision-making process is not verified or is unclear [12].

One of the most common problems, even with manual CXR interpretation, is misinterpretation due to the similarity of pulmonary diseases on CXR. This request AI system not only delivers high accuracy but also needs to be interpretable and transparent. The explainable artificial intelligence (XAI) method will help physicians understand the reasons behind a given disease's prediction and classification, thereby building trust in the model [13]. Although recent studies have introduced several uncertainty estimation techniques tailored for medical AI, their thorough assessment in real-world clinical settings remains limited.

In medical imaging, ontologies provide a structured framework for knowledge and define how anatomical structures, imaging findings, and disease concepts are related to one another [14]. In practice, resources such as RadLex standardize the vocabulary and explicitly model the relationships between anatomical structures, imaging findings, and diagnostic entities [15]. By defining consistent vocabularies and logical links, ontologies ensure that annotations are interoperable, enabling powerful semantic searches and supporting automated reasoning, such as inferring likely diagnoses from a set of observed signs. Integrating these ontologies with deep learning models enables AI systems to combine data-driven predictions with knowledge-driven reasoning [16]. This structured layer makes ontologies a natural partner for Neuro-Symbolic AI, where neural networks contribute powerful feature extraction from complex images, while symbolic layers grounded in ontologies provide logical interpretability, clinical validation, and rule-based inference [17]. Together, these factors make the model more auditable and reliable.

The proposed study aims to create a clinically transparent AI system to classify thoracic diseases and incorporate explainable predictions and diagnostic reasoning into the model. The goals of this study were as follows: to build a hybrid EfficientNetV2-ViT architecture that enables robust feature learning; to build an anatomy-guided representation learning CheXmask; to build a neuro-symbolic reasoning layer that provides ontology-based clini-

https://doi.org/10.3390/diagnostics16010159

cal interpretation; and to build an extensive evaluation framework that guarantees both diagnostic accuracy and clinical verifiability across datasets and pathological conditions. This methodology combines the Enhanced EfficientNetV2, which reduces spatial features, with a modified ViT. CheXmask provides supervision for anatomical training and enables spatially aligned Grad-CAM visualization. A neuro-symbolic reasoning layer then processes these activations to produce clinically interpretable reports based on ontology-based diagnostic predicates using fuzzy-logic inference.

The main contributions of this study are as follows.

- A novel hybrid architecture that integrates an EfficientNetV2 backbone with a mixed channel–spatial attention mechanism, optimizing it for both fine-grained feature extraction in chest radiographs and computationally efficient, interpretable attention mapping.
- Anatomy-guided learning and interpretation through the integration of CheXMask segmentation masks. This provides auxiliary supervision during training to align features with lung and heart structures and later constrains Grad-CAM visualizations and symbolic reasoning to anatomically valid regions.
- The effective handling of severe class imbalance via a class-balanced focal loss improves the model's sensitivity to rare thoracic pathologies without degrading its performance on common findings.
- A neuro-symbolic reasoning framework that employs a Logical Neural Network and fuzzy logic to translate anatomically grounded model activations into ontology-based diagnostic predicates. This moves beyond the probabilistic output to generate structured clinical rationales.

The remainder of this paper is organized as follows. Section 2 provides a literature review of prior work, emphasizing the methodological approaches and key findings of relevant literature. Section 3 describes the materials, dataset properties, and methodology applied to design and test the proposed system using the NIH ChestX-ray14 dataset. Part 4 presents the experimental findings on the NIH dataset and an independent external dataset, along with a detailed interpretation that includes neuro-symbolic diagnostic reasoning and ontology-based clinical explanation. Section 5 provides a comparative discourse that places the performance of the proposed system in the context of existing studies and highlights the system's scientific and clinical contributions. Finally, Section 6 summarizes the main conclusions of this paper.

2. Related Work

The field of automated classification of pulmonary diseases is actively evolving as researchers seek more robust and generalizable models. The hybrid technique, which combines CNNs and transformers, has shown promising results; however, it still has limitations in terms of computational efficiency, interpretability, and reasoning.

Yanar et al. [18] examined several deep learning architectures, including CNN, Transformer, and Mamba-based models, for classifying chest radiographs using the NIH ChestX-ray14 dataset. All models were trained in the same manner to ensure the comparability of the results. Their results indicated that the hybrid architectures, especially ConvFormer, EfficientNet, and CaFormer, provided better diagnostic accuracy. ConvFormer achieved the highest mean AUROC score of 0.841. Baltruschat et al. [19] present a systematic evaluation of different approaches for CNNs to classify multi-label diseases from the ChestX-ray 14 dataset. They tested different loss functions and data augmentations for various ResNets. They demonstrated that a trained ResNet-50 from scratch achieved the best overall performance, with an average AUROC of 0.822 across all 14 classes. Jain et al. [20] examined the diagnostic performance of ViT for multi-label chest disease detection using the NIH Chest

X-ray dataset. Two ViT variants, ImageNet-pretrained and from-scratch, were compared with CNN and ResNet baselines under identical experimental settings. Quantitative evaluation using multi-label accuracy and AUROC showed that the pretrained ViT achieved superior discriminative power and faster convergence; however, the analysis lacked clinical imaging analytics. Kufel et al. [21] presented a framework for classifying pulmonary disease using an EfficientNet backbone for feature extraction, followed by sequential layers including Global Average Pooling, Dense, and Batch Normalization. Binary cross-entropy loss was used to address multi-label classification in a single chest radiograph, achieving an AUC-ROC of 84.28%. Goel et al. [22] presented a Low-Rank Feature Learning (LRFL) framework to enhance thoracic disease classification on chest radiographs by suppressing noise and emphasizing diagnostically relevant regions. When applied to MAE-pretrained CNN and ViT models, the LRFL constraints learned representations to low-rank subspaces, yielding improved multiclass AUROC and accuracy compared to conventional methods. This approach effectively strengthens feature discrimination and generalization. However, its dependence on low-frequency assumptions may overlook subtle pathological variations in the high-frequency image regions. The practical clinical impact of this method, compared with other advanced regularization techniques, remains unquantified. Huang et al. [23] present a framework that can read and understand both medical imaging and radiology reports simultaneously. They developed a global representation learning framework (GLoRIA), which extracts representations using image and text encoders and learns global and localized representations. The used ReeNet-50 as a backbone with a transformer-based text encoder BERT using the MIMIC-CXR dataset. The model achieved an AUROC of 87% using only 10% of the labeled data. Chen et al. [24] optimized CoAtNet- using a loss function to address the long-tail problem in public datasets and multi-label classification. As a baseline and for comparison, they used a pretrained ResNet50 network with weighted binary cross-entropy loss (LWBCE). The baseline model, ResNet50 + LWBCE, achieved an AUROC of 0.811, whereas the model achieved 0.842. Group-CAM heat maps were shown for some categories, such as atelectasis, edema, effusion, and poor attention, but not for other categories, such as pneumothorax. Hanif et al. [25] used the pre-trained DenseNet-121 to classify lung disease from the NIH Chest X-ray 14 dataset, which is addressed below, and employed the rank-based loss, derived from Zero-bounded Log-sum-exp and Pairwise Rank-based loss, to address multi-label disease and class imbalance in the training data. The model achieved an average AUROC of 0.809. Chehade et al. [26] focused on image enhancement and correction; the images are cleaned of foreign objects such as medical devices, wires, and electrodes. They affect the model by making it difficult to differentiate relevant anatomical features, potentially rendering accurate diagnosis impossible. K-means clustering was used to separate the targeted image from the medical device, and without artifacts, the resulting image was then trained using CycleGAN to convert the dirty image to a clean one. The model achieved an AUROC of 84.96%. Additionally, the integration of multimodal data, as demonstrated by Tang et al. [27], has shown that combining chest radiographs with clinical data can enhance the prediction accuracy for conditions such as osteoporosis, further validating the utility of the NIH dataset for developing robust AI models. DSouza et al. [28] introduced a pre-trained ResNet-34 trained on ChestX-Ray14, fine-tuned using stochastic gradient descent with momentum, with restarts, and Variable image sizes to ensure no overfitting. An AUROC of 84% was achieved. Class imbalance was addressed using the noted baselines by computing the weighted binary cross-entropy loss and an asymmetric loss. The model was optimized using an Ensemble of Fine-Tuned DenseNet and Swin Transformer models, achieving an AUROC of 83.76%. Souid et al. [29] applied a pretrained MobileNet V2, fine-tuned together, to a classy fourteen-class dataset for NIH ChestX-Ray. The model produced an average AUROC of 81% DOI, and the Du-

https://doi.org/10.3390/diagnostics16010159

alCheXNet model, a two-fold asymmetric feature-extraction network, improved multi-class pulmonary disease classification in CXRs. This approach supports two different data-level fusions to enhance the complementary feature learning of DualCheXNet and achieves an AUROC of 82.3%. Chen et al. [30] presented two symmetrical CNN chains, as both models achieved success. One used ResNet-50 with Densenet-121, and the other used ResNet-101 and Densenet-169, with Support for two methods: data-level fusion and feature-level fusion. The model produced an AUROC of 82%. Ho et al. [31] enhanced the pre-trained DenseNet-121 using feature integration: Generalized Search Tree, Scale-Invariant Feature Transform, Histograms of Oriented Gradients, and Local Binary Patterns. The refined model generated an average ACU of 80.7%. Albahli et al. [32] presented a model framework, InceptionResNetV2, that enhanced the presentation of whole models. The model was used to classify 14 infection classes of the NIH dataset using pulmonary disease data features and achieved an AUROC of 80%.

Although previous studies have made significant progress in classifying thoracic diseases using CNNs, ViTs, hybrid models, and feature-regularization methods, several limitations remain. Studies lack anatomical supervision, leading to poor localizations and low clinical interpretability. Severe class imbalance, noisy NIH14 labels, and the absence of reasoning also affect several models. Additionally, the disconnect between Grad-CAM usage in previous studies and anatomical contextualization has reduced the reliability of the diagnosis. To make clinically meaningful and interpretable predictions, this study integrates anatomical supervision, a hybrid CNN-Transformer, class-balanced optimization, and neuro-symbolic reasoning.

3. Methods and Materials

The proposed methodology implements a hybrid CNN–ViT framework that combines local spatial representations and global contextual dependencies for the classification of thoracic diseases, beginning with standard preprocessing as Figure 1. The augmented images were then passed in parallel to the two branches.

The first branch architecture was the EfficientNetV2 model. This architectural pathway can extract multiscale local features and textures from pulmonary image data. The second branch, in parallel, implements a linear projection with positional embeddings, followed by a stack of eight transformer encoder blocks with multi-head attention, layer normalization, and MLP units to model the long-range spatial relations in the radiograph. The second branch of the architecture was designed to capture the global range relations in the image.

The outputs of all the branches were then flattened and concatenated to form a single representation. This single representation is processed by a classification head comprising dense layers, dropout, normalization, and an MLP block to obtain the final multi-label disease probability.

The Grad-CAM module in the model explains the model's decision by generating a class-specific activation map that pinpoints diagnostic locations in both lung fields via a convolutional path. These visual explanations are paired with a lightweight neuro-symbolic reasoning layer that interprets image-based evidence using predefined ontological rules to explain predictions such as cardiomegaly or focal opacities.

Table 1 lists the components of the proposed system and their contributions.

https://doi.org/10.3390/diagnostics16010159

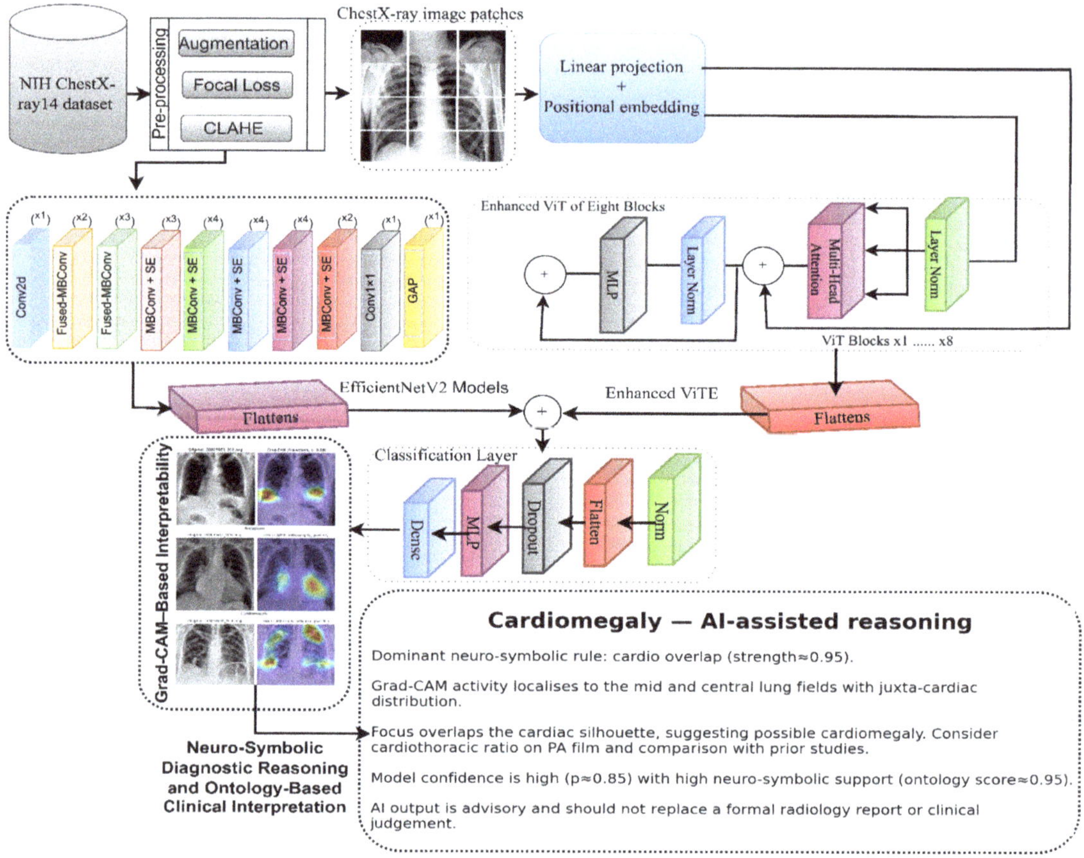

Figure 1. Proposed hybrid CNN–ViT model with integrated Grad-CAM and neuro-symbolic reasoning for thoracic disease classification.

Table 1. Summary of the proposed hybrid CNN–ViT framework components and their contributions.

Component	Primary Function	Key Implementation	Contribution to System Goals
Data Preparation	Standardize and enhance input, mitigate class imbalance.	CLAHE, Affine/Elastic Augmentation, Class-Balanced Focal Loss.	Ensures robust, invariant feature learning; improves sensitivity across all pathology frequencies.
Feature Extraction Backbone	Extract complementary local and global image representations.	Parallel Pathways: Enhanced EfficientNetV2-SE (local texture) and Lightweight ViT (global context).	Provides the discriminative power for accurate multi-label classification by capturing both fine-grained patterns and anatomical relationships.
Anatomy-Guided Learning	Anchor learned features to clinically relevant regions.	Auxiliary segmentation decoder supervised by CheXmask masks (Dice loss).	Enforces anatomical plausibility during training, preventing reliance on spurious artifacts and forming the foundation for trustworthy interpretability.

https://doi.org/10.3390/diagnostics16010159

Table 1. *Cont.*

Component	Primary Function	Key Implementation	Contribution to System Goals
Multi-Label Classifier	Synthesize features and produce disease probabilities.	Concatenation of CNN/ViT features, followed by MLP with per-class sigmoid output.	Enables the accurate, independent detection of multiple co-occurring pathologies, reflecting clinical reality.
Visual Explainability (Grad-CAM)	Generate spatial "attention" maps for model decisions.	Grad-CAM applied to CNN feature maps, then aligned via element-wise multiplication with CheXmask anatomy masks.	Provides transparent, pixel-level localization of evidence, constrained to anatomically valid areas (e.g., lungs, heart), making saliency clinically credible.
Neuro-Symbolic Reasoning	Translate visual activations into clinical language and logic.	Fuzzy-logic engine mapping anatomical activation scores to predicates in a radiological ontology (e.g., RadLex).	Moves beyond "where" to "why," generating human-readable diagnostic statements that bridge the gap between statistical confidence and clinical reasoning.
Integrated Pipeline	Unify the above into a single, end-to-end trainable and interpretable system.	Joint optimization of classification and segmentation loss; post hoc reasoning on aligned activations.	Demonstrates that diagnostic accuracy and clinical interpretability are synergistic, not competing, objectives.

3.1. NIH Chest X-Ray Dataset

The NIH ChestX-ray14 collection, made accessible by the National Library of Medicine and the NIH Clinical Center in 2017, has become one of the largest publicly available labelled datasets for medical imaging research. This study advances research on computer-aided diagnostic systems and the implementation of deep learning for the identification and localization of thoracic diseases. The collection features 81,176 frontal chest radiographs from 30,805 unique patients. It encompasses 14 thoracic diseases. The images were extracted from routine clinical examinations conducted at the NIH Clinical Center, providing a real-world continuum of variability in patient positioning, machine exposure, and disease complexity [33]. The dataset contained 14 distinct pathology classes. The clinical distribution of these classes is highly imbalanced, as is their distribution in the dataset (Table 2) [34]. This is due to the clinical prevalence of these diseases. For example, the more common findings of "Atelectasis" and "Effusion" comprise tens of thousands of images, whereas rarer conditions, such as "Hernia," are represented by only a few hundred images. Therefore, the imbalance we have described introduces unnecessary complexity in model development, and bias toward the majority class can be mitigated through the use of weighted loss functions and data augmentation.

https://doi.org/10.3390/diagnostics16010159

Table 2. The split NIH ChestX-ray14 dataset for evaluating the proposed systems.

Pathology Class	Training	Validation	Test	Total
Atelectasis	8252	1081	2226	11,559
Cardiomegaly	1935	314	527	2776
Consolidation	3319	421	927	4667
Edema	1619	200	484	2303
Effusion	9287	1173	2857	13,317
Emphysema	1810	247	459	2516
Fibrosis	1162	162	362	1686
Hernia	165	18	44	227
Infiltration	13,892	1930	4072	19,894
Mass	4097	525	1160	5782
Nodule	4488	609	1234	6331
Pneumonia	1023	135	273	1431
Pleural Thickening	2371	319	695	3385
Pneumothorax	3788	479	1035	5302

3.2. Multi-Label Nature and Class Imbalance

Problem setting. Each chest radiograph can exhibit zero, one, or multiple of the 14 findings. Labels are mined from reports, so they are multi-label (not mutually exclusive) and noisy/imbalanced (some findings are rare, e.g., Hernia) [35].

Label representation: Each image was encoded as a 14-dimensional binary vector, as expressed in Equation (1).

$$\mathrm{y} = [y_1, \ldots, y_{14}] \in \{0,1\}^{14}, \tag{1}$$

where y denotes the ground-truth label vector for one chest X-ray image, y_c denotes the ground truth label for the disease class c for a given chest X-ray image, indicates the presence of pathology c, $y_c = 0$ and indicates its absence. Dimensionality 14 corresponds to the 14 thoracic findings in the dataset.

The network produces 14 independent logits, as shown in Equation (2).

$$\mathrm{z} = f_\theta(x) \in \mathbb{R}^{14} \tag{2}$$

where x is the input chest X-ray image, $f_\theta(\cdot)$ represents the neural network parameterized by θ, z is the vector of raw, unnormalized scores (logits) and Each component zc corresponds to one pathology.

Per-class probabilities via sigmoid, not softmax, as in Equation (3):

$$p_c = \sigma(z_c) = \frac{1}{1+e^{-z_c}} \text{for } c = 1, \ldots, 14 \tag{3}$$

where $p_c \in (0,1)$ is the predicted probability of pathology c and $\sigma(\cdot)$ is the sigmoid function

Because we use sigmoids (one per label), the model can assign a high probability to multiple classes simultaneously; that is how it "knows" a study may be single-label or multi-label. A softmax would force probabilities to sum to 1, which is incorrect for multi-label tasks [36].

Training objective (multi-label): We trained using Binary Cross-Entropy (BCE) with logits (one loss per class, then average), as shown in Equation (4).

$$\mathcal{L}_{\mathrm{BCE}}(\mathrm{z}, \mathrm{y}) = \frac{1}{14}\sum_{c=1}^{14}(\mathrm{BCEWithLogits}(z_c, y_c)) \tag{4}$$

https://doi.org/10.3390/diagnostics16010159

where $\mathcal{L}_{\text{BCE}}$ is the average binary cross-entropy loss, and BCEWithLogits$(\cdot)$ combines the sigmoid activation and cross-entropy in a numerically stable form.

Each pathology contributes independently to the loss of vision. This treats every disease as its own binary decision, which aligns with how radiologists' reason: finding by finding, not winner takes all.

Decision thresholding (test-time binarization):

$$\hat{y}_c = \begin{cases} 1, & \text{if } p_c \geq \tau_c \\ 0, & \text{otherwise} \end{cases} \quad (5)$$

where $\hat{y}_c$ is the final predicted label for pathology c and τ_c is a class-specific decision threshold. Thresholds are selected on the validation set via grid search

A single global threshold would be more convenient for this purpose. It would also be wrong. Rare diseases require different sensitivity trade-offs than common diseases. This improves the accuracy trade-offs under imbalance and is used to compute the confusion matrices on the test set.

3.3. *Mitigating Class Imbalance in Dataset: A Hierarchical Strategy*

The NIH Chest X-ray dataset is severely imbalanced, causing a predisposition towards diseases prevalent in minority classes. Data-level techniques, such as augmentation, and algorithm-level techniques, such as Focal Loss, are two major strategies to address this. Professional implementation does not consider these strategies as mutually exclusive. It employs a dual-step process, with data augmentation as its first step. This is a two-level hierarchy but in a more complex sense, where this central part is the first essential step [37].

3.3.1. Data Augmentation

The first and most important effort is a more rigorous and medically informed data augmentation process. This first approach specifically fills in the gaps of underrepresented minority classes, as minority classes are underrepresented. A few well-known transformations include affine operations and elastic deformations, which introduce reasonable anatomical variants that preserve the inherent characteristics of the diseases. A particular nodule, for example, may be located in different parts of the lungs, and depending on small differences in the contrast levels between two images, it may appear different in each image [38].

The real benefit of using this approach is that it is a model-agnostic, data-driven step in the pre-processing pipeline. One way it does this is by increasing the effective sample size of the model, forcing it to learn invariant representations and thereby aiding generalizability. By enriching the feature space of minority classes before training, a solid version is created for the learning process. The dependence on a loss function alone to address a data-poor environment is an inferior approach; it is preferable to enrich the environment in the first place [39].

3.3.2. Focal Loss

After data preparation, Focal Loss was applied during model training to directly counter the dominance of frequent classes in the gradient computation. Focal Loss modifies the standard cross-entropy function by adding a tunable focusing term, as shown in Equation (6).

$$FL(p_t) = -\alpha_t(1-p_t)^{\gamma}\log(p_t) \quad (6)$$

where p_t is the predicted probability of the true class, α_t is the class weighting factor, and γ\gamma$\gamma$ is the focusing parameter. The term $(1-p_t)^{\gamma}$ suppresses the loss from

https://doi.org/10.3390/diagnostics16010159

well-classified (easy) examples and emphasizes those that are misclassified or belong to rare classes [40]. When $\gamma = 0$ the function reduces to standard cross-entropy; increasing γ (commonly 1–3) sharpens the focus on difficult cases. Through this mechanism, Focal Loss adaptively shifts learning attention toward underrepresented diseases, such as Hernia or Fibrosis, improving sensitivity without oversampling [41].

We used class-balanced focal loss to address the imbalanced dataset. This technique combines the class-balanced and focal losses. Some pulmonary diseases, such as hernia disease, are rare, while other diseases, such as effusion, are common and have the largest number of images, which could lead to bias in forwarding these classes [42]. The focal loss will give more weight to rare diseases based on the effective number of samples, which will help force harder misclassified samples and give less weight to well-classified images [43]. This approach improves the model accuracy for rare pathologies while maintaining high precision for more frequent labels.

3.4. Image Enhancement by Contrast Limited Adaptive Histogram Equalization

Chest radiographs are often low in contrast and exhibit variable illumination owing to the wide range of tissue densities in the image, from air-filled lungs to dense bone and the mediastinum. Such variations can obscure subtle pathologies and affect the performance of the automated diagnostic models. Image enhancement techniques are typically applied to address this issue before training the models. Among these, contrast-limited adaptive histogram equalization (CLAHE) improves the visibility of anatomical details in medical images, particularly X-rays, across large-scale datasets, such as the NIH ChestX-ray14 [44].

Unlike classical histogram equalization, which enhances the image contrast by redistributing pixel intensities, CLAHE does not apply global remapping. It partitions the input image into small, overlapping tiles (usually 8- or 16-pixel squares) and enhances the local contrast by computing histograms for each tile [45]. For each tile, contrast enhancement is performed by computing the Cumulative Distribution Function (CDF) of the local histogram, which maps pixel intensity x to a new value, $y = F_{ij}(x) \times (L-1)$ where L is the number of contrast levels. This ensures the localized enhancement of regions and control over global adjustments, such as loss of detail [46].

Preventing over-enhancement of noise is a vital function, which is achieved by setting a clip limit (β), one of the many refinements to the technique. In areas with constant intensity and no restrictions, the equalization function may excessively amplify random fluctuations, creating noise. Removal is possible by truncating the histogram bins, where the count for a bin exceeds the limit $\beta \cdot \mu$ (where μ is the mean count for a bin). The remaining pixels are uniformly allocated to the bins, keeping the CDF steep and limiting the gain in contrast, thereby maintaining a more reliable dynamic range [47].

Local transformations were combined with bilinear interpolation to eliminate edge artifacts in the separated regions. This is a merged and enhanced image with a uniform local contrast and overall brightness [48].

CLAHE was applied to the NIH Chest X-ray dataset, enhancing contrast and providing more subtle details in areas such as pulmonary vessels, nodules, and pleural lines, which are important for human and machine feature detection. In computer-aided radiology, consistently high-quality outputs improve the robustness of the model and diagnostic precision.

3.5. Enhanced Hybrid Architecture for Thoracic Disease Feature Extraction and Classification

3.5.1. Enhanced EfficientNetV2 for Hierarchical Spatial Feature Extraction

As the convolutional EfficientNetV2 backbone, the Enhanced EfficientNetV2 extracts multiple scales of spatial representations while preserving the efficiency of computing thoracic radiographs [43]. While the model adheres to compound scaling, the layer depth,

https://doi.org/10.3390/diagnostics16010159

expansion factors, and kernel density are adjusted to balance the diagnostic accuracy and cost. Input radiographs were resized to 384 × 384 pixels and normalized to ImageNet's mean = (0.485, 0.456, 0.406) and std = (0.229, 0.224, 0.225), as shown in Table 3.

Table 3. Enhanced EfficientNetV2 architecture configuration.

Stage	Operator	Channels	Blocks	Stride	Kernel	Expansion	Params (K)	FLOPs (M)	Output Size
Stem	Conv2d	3 → 24	1	2	3 × 3	—	2.1	15.8	192 × 192
1	Fused-MBConv	24 → 24	2	1	3 × 3	1	28.4	53.2	192 × 192
2	Fused-MBConv	24 → 48	3	2	3 × 3	4	152.7	286.3	96 × 96
3	MBConv + SE	48 → 80	3	2	3 × 3	4	428.9	804.2	48 × 48
4	MBConv + SE	80 → 128	4	2	3 × 3	4	1.12 M	2.10 G	24 × 24
5	MBConv + SE	128 → 176	4	1	3 × 3	4	1.86 M	3.49 G	24 × 24
6	MBConv + SE	176 → 256	4	2	3 × 3	4	2.64 M	4.95 G	12 × 12
7	MBConv + SE	256 → 320	2	1	3 × 3	4	1.98 M	3.71 G	12 × 12
Head	Conv1 × 1 + GAP	320 → 512	1	1	1 × 1	—	164.2	307.9	1 × 1

The enhanced Mobile Inverted Bottleneck Convolution (MBConv) transformation advances depthwise-separable convolutions by integrating squeeze and excitation (SE) attention to the block and predicting the attention mechanism, as shown in Equation (7).

$$Y = X + \mathrm{SE}(\mathrm{DWConv}(\mathrm{Expand}(X))) \odot \mathrm{Expand}(X) \tag{7}$$

where Y is the output feature map of the MBConv block, + denotes the residual (skip) connection, $\odot$ represents element-wise multiplication, $\mathrm{Expand}(\cdot)$ is a 1 × 11 \times 11 × 1 convolution that increases the channel dimension from C to, with t being the expansion factor, and θ denotes all learnable parameters in the convolutional and excitation layers.

Depth-wise separable convolution:

The convolutional and excitation parameters are learnable, as expressed in Equation (8).

$$\mathrm{DWConv(X)} = \mathrm{Conv}_{\mathrm{depthwise}}(\mathrm{BN}(\mathrm{SiLU}(\mathrm{Conv}_{1\times1}(\mathrm{X})))), \tag{8}$$

Here, $\mathrm{Conv}_{1\times1}$ performs pointwise convolution for channel mixing, $\mathrm{Conv}_{\mathrm{depthwise}}$ applies spatial convolution independently to each channel, $\mathrm{BN}(\cdot)$ denotes batch normalization, and $\mathrm{SiLU}(x) = x \cdot \sigma(x)$ is the SiLU (Swish) activation, chosen for its smooth gradient behavior.

Squeeze-and-excitation (SE)

The SE attention is computed using global average pooling, and the two transformations are fully connected, as shown in Equation (9).

$$\mathrm{s} = \sigma(W_2\,\delta(W_1\,\mathrm{GAP(X)})) \tag{9}$$

where $\mathrm{GAP}(X) \in \mathbb{R}^{C}$ is global average pooling across spatial dimensions, $W_1 \in \mathbb{R}^{C\times\frac{C}{r}}$ and $W_2 \in \mathbb{R}^{\frac{C}{r}\times C}$ are learnable weight matrices, $r = 4$ is the channel reduction ratio, $\delta(\cdot)$ denotes the Swish activation, and $\sigma(\cdot)$ is the sigmoid function that produces channel-wise attention weights.

Early stage Fused-MBConv blocks focus on optimizing the detection of fine pulmonary textures and subtle interstitial opacities. In contrast, the deeper SE-enhanced MBConv layers focused on broader anatomical variations, such as pleural thickening, cardiomegaly, and basal effusions.

The design ensures that the model is sensitive to local textural cues and regional density gradients required for interpreting chest X-rays. The Total Parameters were 6.38 M [49].

https://doi.org/10.3390/diagnostics16010159

This design achieves 47.6% savings in the model compared to EfficientNetV2. In addition, it retains the multiscale spatial hierarchy necessary to complete dense thoracic patterns.

3.5.2. Enhanced ViT for Global Context Modeling

The enhanced ViT captures a large portion of the long-range relations in the chest region at a low computational cost. An input image of size (384 × 384 × 3) was divided into 16 × 16 non-overlapping patches, yielding N = 576 patches and a 768-dimensional embedding [50] as in Equation (10).

$$Z_0 = [x_{cls}; x_1E; x_2E; \ldots ; x_NE] + E_{pos}, \quad (10)$$

Here, $x_i \in \mathbb{R}^{16^2 \cdot 3}$ represents the flattened pixel values of the i-th image patch, $E \in \mathbb{R}^{(16^2 \cdot 3) \times 768}$ is the learnable linear projection matrix that maps each patch into a 768-dimensional embedding, $x_{cls} \in \mathbb{R}^{768}$ is a learnable classification token that aggregates global information, $E_{pos} \in \mathbb{R}^{(N+1) \times 768}$ is the positional embedding that encodes spatial order among patches, and $Z_0 \in \mathbb{R}^{(577) \times 768}$ is the input to the first transformer encoder layer.

The transformer encoder models the interactions between patches using multi-head self-attention. For each attention head h, the embedded sequence Z is linearly projected into query, key, and value representations [51], as shown in Equation (11).

$$Q_h = ZW_h^Q, K_h = ZW_h^K, V_h = ZW_h^V, \quad (11)$$

where $W_h^Q, W_h^K, W_h^V \in \mathbb{R}^{768 \times 48}$ is a learnable projection matrix. The dimensionality 48 arises from dividing the embedding dimension 768 by 16 attention heads.

The attention for head h is computed using the scaled dot-product attention in Equation (12):

$$A_h = \text{softmax}\left(\frac{Q_h K_h^\top}{\sqrt{48}} + M\right) V_h, \quad (12)$$

In this expression, the scaling factor $\sqrt{48}$ stabilizes the gradients during training, M represents an optional attention mask (set to zero in this study), and $A_h \in \mathbb{R}^{(N+1) \times 48}$ encodes contextualized representations for head h.

The outputs from all heads are concatenated and projected back into the original embedding space, as shown in Equation (13).

$$\text{MHSA}(\mathbf{Z}) = \text{Concat}(A_1, A_2, \ldots, A_{16})W^O \quad (13)$$

where $W^O \in \mathbb{R}^{768 \times 768}$ is the output projection matrix. The results preserved the dimensional consistency with the input sequence.

The attention block is followed by a position-wise feed-forward network, as shown in Equation (14).

$$\text{FFN}(Z) = \text{GELU}(ZW_1 + b_1)W_2 + b_2, \quad (14)$$

where $W_1 \in \mathbb{R}^{768 \times 1536}$ expands the feature dimension, $W_2 \in \mathbb{R}^{1536 \times 768}$ projects it back, and GELU activation introduces smooth non-linearity suitable for transformer optimization.

Having four fewer transformer blocks helps avoid excessive self-attention while still maintaining global receptive fields and global attention focus shifts.

More attention heads help focus on clinically relevant features to gain sensitivity to bilateral anchors, such as symmetric infiltrations or asymmetrical comparative paresis of lung fields, boosting explainability in a clinical context [36].

Reducing the number of transformer blocks from 12 to 8 decreases the quadratic complexity of self-attention while enabling global receptive fields with additional heads.

https://doi.org/10.3390/diagnostics16010159

Clinical Significance: The increase in the number of heads increases sensitivity to bilateral pathological relations, such as symmetric infiltrations or lung-field asymmetries, and improves interpretability in clinical settings.

3.5.3. Multi-Scale Feature Fusion and Multi-Label Classification

The hybrid model integrates pixel precision and global context via feature concatenation, as shown in Equation (15).

$$\mathrm{F_{cnn}} = \mathrm{GAP}(\mathrm{Conv_{head}}(\mathrm{X})) \in \mathbb{R}^{512}, \tag{15}$$

Here, $\mathrm{Conv_{head}}(\cdot)$ is a learnable 1×1 convolution that projects the feature channels to 512 dimensions, $\mathrm{GAP}(\cdot)$ denotes global average pooling over spatial dimensions, and F_{cnn} is a fixed-length descriptor summarizing the local convolutional evidence.

Simultaneously, the transformer branch provides a global representation. After L transformer encoder layers, the class token captures long-range contextual dependencies across the entire thoracic region, as expressed in Equation (16).

$$\mathrm{F_{vit}} = \mathrm{Z}^{L}_{\mathrm{cls}} \in \mathbb{R}^{768} \tag{16}$$

where Z^{L}_{cls} is the output of the class token from the final transformer layer. This vector encodes the global anatomical relationships, bilateral patterns, and distributed pathology cues.

The two representations are fused by direct concatenation, as shown in Equation (17).

$$\mathrm{F_{fused}} = [\mathrm{F_{cnn}}; \mathrm{F_{vit}}] \in \mathbb{R}^{1280} \tag{17}$$

The fused feature vector is passed through a three-layer multilayer perceptron to perform the multi-label classification. The classification head employs a three-layer MLP, as expressed in Equation (18).

$$\begin{aligned} \mathrm{h}_1 &= \mathrm{GELU}(\mathrm{BN}(\mathrm{F_{fused}} W_1 + b_1)), \\ \mathrm{h}_2 &= \mathrm{GELU}(\mathrm{BN}(\mathrm{h}_1 W_2 + b_2)), \\ \mathrm{z} &= \mathrm{h}_2 W_3 + b_3, \end{aligned} \tag{18}$$

where $W_1 \in \mathbb{R}^{1280\times512}$, $W_2 \in \mathbb{R}^{512\times256}$, and $W_3 \in \mathbb{R}^{256\times14}$ are learnable weight matrices, b_1, b_2, b_3 are bias vectors, $\mathrm{BN}(\cdot)$ denotes batch normalization, GELU introduces smooth non-linearity suitable for deep representations, and $\mathrm{z} \in \mathbb{R}^{14}$ contains one logit per thoracic pathology.

Final predictions are obtained independently for each pathology using a sigmoid activation as in Equation (19).

$$p_c = \sigma(z_c) = \frac{1}{1+e^{-z_c}}, c = 1, \ldots, 14 \tag{19}$$

where is the predicted probability of the c-th finding, and independent sigmoids allow multiple conditions to be assigned simultaneously, reflecting the clinical reality of the chest radiography.

The Enhanced EfficientNetV2 is an efficient hierarchical spatial feature extractor that extracts local textural patterns and anatomical boundaries that imply focal findings of interest [52]. Meanwhile, the Enhanced Vision Transformer helps model long-range, global contextual relationships throughout the thoracic cavity, which is significant for interpreting distributed pathology indicators and bilateral comparisons [53]. The given structure of the hybrid resource facilitates a proper distribution of diagnostic comprehensiveness and reasonable deployability in clinical settings [10].

https://doi.org/10.3390/diagnostics16010159

This combined approach has high diagnostic robustness and is clinically useful. Local features are considered in the convolutional layers, whereas general dependencies are regarded in the ViT layer (cardiac and thoracic hypertrophy, bilateral infiltrations, etc.). The combination of these characteristics produces a highly effective diagnostic model.

3.6. Anatomy-Guided Representation Learning Using the CheXmask Dataset

This is what makes this framework helpful and allows the learned representations to be anchored to clinically relevant regions: the incorporation of explicit anatomical prior. To achieve this, we integrated segmentation and learning into a single framework by adopting the CheXmask dataset as an auxiliary anatomical reference [54].

CheXmask fills an essential gap in the literature, as only a small number of public datasets contain accurate anatomical labels. It offers professionally annotated masks of the lungs, heart, and clavicles for publicly available datasets, such as the NIH Chest X-ray14 dataset used in the present study. The CheXmask dataset masks were created using both automated segmentation models and expert radiologist validation and were anatomically correct [54].

First, it serves as a source of supervision for an auxiliary segmentation branch attached to the shared backbone during training, with anatomical information that is directly connected to the learning features. Trained together with the same backbone, this branch reconstructs a mask prediction $\hat{M}$ without consistency with the ground-truth mask M with a pixel-wise Dice loss, as shown in Equation (20) [55].

$$\mathcal{L}_{segmentation} = 1 - \frac{2\,|M \cap \hat{M}|}{|M| + |\hat{M}| + \epsilon} \tag{20}$$

Here, $|M \cap \hat{M}|$ denotes the sum of element-wise products between the ground-truth and predicted masks, measuring spatial overlap, $|M|$ and $|\hat{M}|$ represent the total foreground pixel counts in each mask, and ε is a small constant added for numerical stability, preventing division by zero.

The segmentation objective was not optimized in isolation. It is combined with the primary multi-label classification objective to form a joint training signal, as shown in Equation (21):

$$\mathcal{L}_{total} = \mathcal{L}_{classification} + \lambda\,\mathcal{L}_{segmentation} \tag{21}$$

where $\mathcal{L}_{\text{classification}}$ is the multi-label classification loss (binary cross-entropy or class-balanced focal loss), and λ is a scalar weighting factor that controls the influence of anatomical supervision relative to classification performance.

This collaborative goal imposes anatomically limited learning and requires the backbone to attend to diagnostically significant thoracic structures, such as the lungs, cardiac silhouette, and costophrenic angles, and excludes correlations with non-anatomical artifacts (e.g., embedded text or borders) [56].

Second, CheXmask annotations were used to spatially align Grad-CAM heatmaps with segmented lung and heart areas during inference. The resultant alignment then encodes low-level saliency activations as interpretable clinical features, such as activation in the costophrenic recess (typical of pleural effusion) or along the apical pleural margin (typical of pneumothorax). This anatomically grounded mapping offers a clear interface that links neuroattention and radiological reasoning [54].

Having pre-computed CheXmask masks available during inference is crucial for anatomical alignment. Pixel-level saliency estimates generated by frameworks such as Grad-CAM are activation maps; however, they lack anatomical content. The heatmaps were spatially aligned with the anatomical masks of the relevant organs delineated using

https://doi.org/10.3390/diagnostics16010159

the CheXmask. This is necessary for our ontology-reasoning framework, whereby low-level neural activations are related to high-level clinical predicates. For example, they are active in regions, and the system determines if "Pleural Effusion," thus, is the region associated with "Pleural Effusion" high-activation area and the costophrenic angles, signalling, or is the signal for "Pneumothorax" associated with the apical pleural space.

3.7. *Inference and Attention Visualization*

In the inference stage, the trained hybrid model performs classification and attention visualization to explain its diagnostic reasoning. For each input chest radiograph, the network computed a 14-dimensional probability vector using a sigmoid-activated output layer, with each component corresponding to the estimated probability of a specific thoracic pathology. Optimized per-class thresholds τ_c were used to derive the final binary predictions and were determined empirically on the validation set to maximize accuracy when there was an inherent imbalance in the dataset. This adaptive thresholding results in equal sensitivity and specificity for both common and rare disease cases [57].

The interpretability aspect uses Grad-CAM to display the spatial patterns of attention in the image. Grad-CAM produces class-specific localization maps that highlight discriminative parts, contributing to every prediction [58]. To compute the gradient of the output score y^c with respect to the feature maps A^k in the last convolutional layer of the EfficientNetV2 backbone, the algorithm uses the gradient of output score y c with respect to the feature maps of the previous convolutional layer. To obtain the weights of the importance of the neurons, Equation (12) globally averages the gradients to obtain the importance weights, as shown in Equation (22).

$$\alpha_k^c = \frac{1}{Z}\sum_i\sum_j \frac{\partial y^c}{\partial A_{ij}^k}, \tag{22}$$

where Z represents the pixels in the map used to represent the feature, and denotes its value at spatial location (i, j).

The heatmap of class discrimination is then obtained as shown in Equation (23):

$$L_{\text{Grad-CAM}}^c = \text{ReLU}\sum_k \alpha_k^c A^k, \tag{23}$$

where the ReLU operation not only retains the features that favorably affect the target class but also drops the other features.

The heatmap is scaled to the spatial resolution of the image, and the resulting image is a visual representation of the distribution of attention intensity. These Grad-CAM maps are spatially aligned with the CheXmask anatomical segmentation to be more anatomically interpretable [59]. This correspondence enables the visualization to be localized to regions of the anatomy with high precision, and the raw patterns of activation are converted into clinically interpretable attention responses. For example, a high level of activation in the costophrenic angles can indicate pleural effusion, whereas localized activation along the apical pleural margin is indicative of pneumothorax [60].

The visualization system provides side-by-side comparisons of the original radiographs and Grad-CAM overlays, enabling radiologists to qualitatively verify that the model's focus corresponds to clinically relevant areas. Such quantitative–qualitative analysis contributes to the explainability, reliability, and clinical trustworthiness of the model by providing transparent and explanatory support rather than opaque decision-making [61].

https://doi.org/10.3390/diagnostics16010159

3.8. Anatomical Alignment and Mask Integration

The integration of anatomy is key during post-processing because it facilitates the translation of neural activation into viable clinical evidence. After the Grad-CAM attention maps were produced, the attention visualizations were spatially registered to anatomically segmented masks from the CheXmask dataset. This process is the first step in converting neural activation distributions into diagnostic representations [62].

The alignment process was achieved through a combination of coordinate transformation and spatial masking. For a given Grad-CAM heatmap $L^c_{\text{Grad-CAM}} \in \mathbb{R}^{H \times W}$ and the binary anatomical mask $M_{\text{anatomy}} \in \{0,1\}^{H \times W}$ of the thoracic anatomy, the anatomically constrained attention map is defined in Equation (24) as follows:

$$L^c_{\text{aligned}} = L^c_{\text{Grad-CAM}} \odot M_{\text{anatomy}}, \tag{24}$$

where $\odot$ denotes element-wise multiplication of the matrices. The operation of neural attention to clinically relevant anatomy while ignoring irrelevant attention to the extrathoracic spaces and anatomically irrelevant structures.

Region-wise interpretability enables the alignment of multiple anatomical structures, including the lungs, heart, and costophrenic recesses [63].

To quantify the strength of the model's attention to a specific anatomical region, we computed the region-wise normalized activation energy. Let

M_{region} be the binary mask of a target region (e.g., costophrenic recess),

$| M_{\text{region}} |$ denotes the number of pixels in the region. The regional attention score is defined as Equation (25):

$$A^c_{\text{region}} = \frac{1}{| M_{\text{region}} |} \sum_i \sum_j L^c_{\text{aligned}}(i,j)\, M_{\text{region}}(i,j), \tag{25}$$

These scalar measures the average activation intensity within the anatomical region. It acts as a bridge between numerical attention and radiological semantics: high values near the lung bases suggest effusion, and focal apical signals suggest pneumothorax.

Dimensional accuracy is maintained by applying two-line interpolation when resizing between the Grad-CAM maps and segmentation masks, thereby ensuring geometric consistency between the field of attention and the original radiograph coordinates [64]. This guarantees that each activity is accurately located relative to anatomical features. Thus, anatomically consistent attention maps allow the conversion of neural activation into radiographically meaningful insights. For example, localized high-intensity activations at the diaphragmatic angles with elevated A_"region" values correspond to pleural effusion, whereas focal activations along the apical pleural margins suggest pneumothorax. These patterns reflect clinical logic, balancing the algorithmic focus with radiographic interpretation. This visualization interface displays consistent maps as semi-transparent overlays on the original chest radiographs, with color densities indicating the degree of activation and well-defined anatomical boundaries [65]. This arrangement enables radiologists to directly verify that the prominent areas of the model correspond to clinically predicted disease presentations, thereby enhancing interpretability and diagnostic confidence [65].

By enhancing the anatomical plausibility of model interpretations, this alignment strategy addresses a persistent challenge in the interpretability of medical AI: distinguishing between meaningful physiological inferences and spurious correlations. The result was a clinically grounded and anatomically interpretable framework that enhanced the transparency, credibility, and diagnostic reliability of the hybrid deep learning model.

https://doi.org/10.3390/diagnostics16010159

3.9. Ontology-Reasoning Module (Post Hoc Neuro-Symbolic Explainer)

The ontology reasoning module is the latter interpretive component of the hybrid diagnostic system and converts quantitative neural activations into interpretable concepts with clinical significance. Deep models represent complex spatial and spectral patterns, but their raw activations are opaque. A post hoc reasoning engine that combines fuzzy logic and a structured radiological ontology provides a solution to this gap, thereby enabling direct mapping between model attention and medically defined findings [66].

Following inference, the anatomically aligned Grad-CAM heatmaps L aligned c binary masks of the CheXmask dataset are provided to the reasoning component [67]. Every anatomical area is linked to a set of diagnostic predicates that define the diagnostic predicate in an ontology $\mathcal{O}$, in which $\mathcal{O} = \{p_1, p_2, \ldots, p_n\}$ where p_n corresponds to a known thoracic abnormality. The ontology represents hierarchical relationships, as shown in Equation (26).

$$\text{Pleural Effusion} \subset \text{Fluid Collection Abnormality, Cardiomegaly} \subset \text{Cardiac Size Abnormality,} \quad (26)$$

This hierarchy constrains the interpretation. A finding cannot float freely; it must belong somewhere, anatomo-physically and semantically.

To indicate the extent of belief in the relevant clinical cues, these scores were scaled to [0, 1]. They are not based on hard thresholds but on fuzzy membership function parameterized in terms of radiological heuristics, as shown in Equation (27).

$$\text{Conf}_{\text{Cardiomegaly}} = \frac{A_{\text{heart}}}{A_{\text{thorax}}}, \text{Conf}_{\text{Effusion}} = \bar{L}_{\text{lower lung}}, \text{Conf}_{\text{Pneumothorax}} = \phi(\nabla L_{\text{apex}}), \quad (27)$$

Here, A_{heart} is the segmented heart area, A_{thorax} is the total thoracic cavity area, $\bar{L}_{\text{lower lung}}$ is the mean activation in the basal lung region, ∇L_{apex} denotes the spatial gradient magnitude of activation near the apical pleura, and $\phi(\cdot)$ is a normalization function mapping gradient strength to [0, 1].

These values express how strongly the anatomy supports a clinical cue, not whether it crosses an arbitrary line.

To convert numeric evidence into symbolic beliefs, fuzzy membership functions are used, as shown in Equation (28).

$$\mu(p_c) = \frac{1}{1 + e^{-\beta(\text{Conf}_c - \tau_c)}}, \quad (28)$$

Here, $\mu(p_c)$ is the membership degree of predicate p_c, τ_c is an empirically chosen reference level for that finding, and β controls boundary softness, allowing uncertainty rather than brittle decisions.

Each symbolic cue is then evaluated against the rule base of the ontology, which encodes radiological logic as follows:

IF (high activation in costophrenic region) AND (low lung density) THEN pleural effusion (Confidence = μ_e), AND

IF (high activation along the apical pleura) AND (absence of vascular markings) THEN pneumothorax (Confidence = μ_p).

Symbolic inference allows distributed neural responses to be transformed into clinical assertions that are defined and exact in their certainty.

Through this process, the reasoning layer can be treated as a neuro-symbolic interface that mediates between sub-symbolic attentional features and symbolic radiological knowledge [68]. The framework not only increases explainability but also provides internal consistency tests: conflicting predicates (e.g., simultaneous "Pneumothorax" and "Effusion" on the same side) are solved through fuzzy rule conflict resolution, along with aggregating the confidence in Equation (29):

$$\mu_{\text{final}}(p_c) = \frac{\sum_k w_k \, \mu_k(p_c)}{\sum_k w_k}, \quad (29)$$

Here, w_k represents region-specific reliability weights, and $\mu_k(p_c)$ are individual predicate confidences from different anatomical cues.

Finally, the ontology-reasoning component transforms neural activation maps into diagnostic sentences, whose outputs can be interpreted and audited for use in radiological reasoning. This post hoc neuro-symbolic layer ensures that the decisions made by the hybrid model are not just statistically sound but also clinically sensible to anchor predictions made by data-driven models within a clear, knowledge-based interpretive framework that is consistent with existing diagnostic reasoning.

3.10. Rule-Based Clinical Inference and Report Generation

The final analytical phase enables the system to produce explicit diagnostic statements that simulate how a radiologist reasons through the diagnostic process [69]. Although the ontology reasoning layer provides the system with fuzzy memberships for various pathological predicates, the clinical decision support system must ensure that these values are organized and translated into prioritized, verbalized, and coherent clinical conclusions. Therefore, the rule-based clinical inference engine is viewed as a bridge between symbolic computation and the generation of clinical textual reports [70].

This engine essentially condenses the confidence measures Si of all symbolic predicates into a condition vector, as illustrated in Equation (30).

$$\text{cond\_scores} = \{\text{Cardiomegaly} : S_1, \ \text{Effusion} : S_2, \ \text{Pneumothorax} : S_3, \ \text{Mass} : S_4, \ldots\}, \quad (30)$$

where each $S_i = \mu_{\text{final}}(p_i)$ is derived from the ontology layer and is the result of conflict resolution. The inference module operates according to a diagnostic rule assembled in the context of a horn clause, integrating fuzzy thresholds and spatial evidence. Equation (21) describes one way in which a rule can be structured, as shown in Equation (31).

$$R_j : \ \text{IF } (S_i > \tau_i) \text{ AND } \left(A^i_{\text{region}} > \eta_i\right) \text{ THEN } D_j, \quad (31)$$

where $S_i = \mu(p_i)$ is the fuzzy confidence of predicate p_i, A^i_{region} is the normalized activation energy in the relevant anatomical region, τ_i and η_i are minimum confidence and spatial-support thresholds, and D_j is the inferred diagnostic statement.

This formalism allows multiple discoveries to co-occur, reflecting the inherently multi-label nature of the thoracic imaging. Reasoning further develops in three related stages [71].

Hypothesis generation: Indices of candidate conditions are instantiated if their fuzzy confidence exceeds the empirical threshold τ_i.

Hypothesis prioritization: Hypotheses are ranked by S_i in descending order, enabling a quantitative evaluation of diagnostic priority.

Linguistic mapping: Each positive hypothesis was translated into a radiological finding using a predefined template. These templates encode the spatial context, intensity models, and anatomical locations.

Example: "High activity noted in the right lower lung base with blunting of the costophrenic angle, which is compatible with pleural effusion."

Or "Generalised increased activity through cardiac silhouette, with a raised cardiothoracic ratio, compatible with cardiomegaly."

https://doi.org/10.3390/diagnostics16010159

This sentence structure is based on a controlled language approach designed to facilitate clear, replicable, and unambiguous clinical documentation.

Symbolic cues Probability-weighted summation of symbolic cues is performed using normalized softmax activation (Equation (32)).

$$P(D_i) = \frac{e^{\alpha S_i}}{\sum_j e^{\alpha S_j}}, \tag{32}$$

where S_i is the final confidence of diagnosis D_i, and α controls ranking sharpness.

In this case, the sharpness of the ranked list's confidence is governed by the scaling factor α, leading to a distribution suitable for reporting both deterministic and probabilistic information to clinicians about the top-k hypotheses and their confidence levels.

A JSON-based schema was adopted to facilitate integration with hospital information systems, which includes (i) disease label, (ii) probability value, (iii) body part and region, and (iv) textual description. This allows for straightforward export to PACS/RIS pipelines and EHR systems. The design follows the principle that every produced statement is traceable back to its source in the activation map and the rule that governs what AIXs should be explanation-compliant.

This rule-based inference and reporting process translates abstract neural evidence into clear diagnostic stories that support the medical reasoning. By fusing fuzzy reasoning, symbolic ranking, and linguistic synthesis, the framework demonstrates not only radiological interpretability reproduction but also machine-readable and clinician-verifiable reporting consistency, a cofactor for colonizing trustworthy AI into chest disease diagnostics.

3.11. Overall Integration

The hybrid structure of the proposed diagnostic framework integrates two inherently different types of models: one based on data and the other on knowledge for anatomy-guided feature learning and ontology-aligned clinical reasoning. Fusion is operationalized through two phases that complement each other and operate at distinct points in time: a training phase that injects anatomical priors into the learned representation space and an inference phase that associates learned activations with explicit radiological ontology for interpretation.

During training, the network optimizes a multitask objective that comprises various tasks, including classification and anatomical reconstruction. This is described by Equation (33).

$$\mathcal{L}_{\text{total}} = \mathcal{L}_{\text{classification}} + \lambda\, \mathcal{L}_{\text{segmentation}}, \tag{33}$$

where the parameter λ balances the contributions of the auxiliary segmentation decoders.

The CheXmask-derived lung and heart masks, which are assigned to supervise the segmentation branch, force the backbone network to learn low-level, semantic anatomical features. This parameter optimization ensured that the gradient updates converged to physiologically reasonable local minima, preventing the network from exploiting spurious correlations as embedded artifacts or in non-thoracic regions. As such, the latent features acquired by the refined EfficientNetV2 and ViT branches were learned subject to anatomical priors, yielding a robust and spatially consistent representation of thoracic anatomy.

In the inference stage, these activation maps are mapped to anatomically informed activations that can be used to interpret the reasoning process within a neuro-symbolic pipeline that combines Grad-CAM visual attention with clinical oncology. The system first

https://doi.org/10.3390/diagnostics16010159

maps the final layer activations to a class-specific saliency map and then uses anatomical alignment as in Equation (34).

$$L^{c}_{\text{aligned}} = L^{c}_{\text{Grad-CAM}} \odot M_{\text{anatomy}}, \tag{34}$$

where M_{anatomy} represents the binary segmentation mask.

This operation limits saliency to clinically relevant locations (lungs, heart, and costophrenic angles) and makes anatomical sense in explaining possible model decisions. The aligned activations are then propagated via fuzzy logic inference and ontology-based rule evaluation to map distributed neural evidence into symbolic diagnostic predicates that describe the presence or absence of pathologies such as Pleural Effusion, Cardiomegaly, or Pneumothorax.

This two-level integration leads to a synergistic human–machine workflow in which anatomy feeds learning and ontology rule interpretation. At the system level, the framework has a naturally closed semantic loop: the anatomical decoder imposes prior constraints on feature extraction, and the ontology module compares post hoc reasoning with existing medical hierarchies. This coupling results in two observable benefits. First, the diagnostic performance was significantly improved by the discriminative and anatomically consistent representation of features. The second advantage is improved explainability, as each decision can be traced back to numerical activations in the deep model via a structured reasoning path that connects the numbers to clinical semantics.

The joint framework is also adapted to enforce consistency between the training and inference domains. The same anatomical landmarks that regularize the learning process subsequently determine the alignment of Grad-CAM, maintaining geometric and semantic coherence throughout the pipeline. This principle prevents the "explanation drift" problem, in which the visualization emphasizes an irrelevant area even when the prediction is accurate. In this design, interpretability and performance are not opposing goals but co-optimized components of a single architecture.

Ultimately, the complete integration of all these factors transforms deep neural inference from an opaque statistical mapping to a clinically transparent diagnostic procedure. By integrating anatomy-driven learning and ontology-based reasoning, the framework epitomizes the spirit of explainable radiological intelligence—an AI system that is not only capable of classifying chest diseases with high accuracy but also able to justify the evidence for each decision on both anatomical and logical grounds.

4. Results of Proposed Model

4.1. Performance of the Enhanced Hybrid Model

4.1.1. Training and Convergence Analysis

The hybrid ViT–EfficientNetV2 architecture was explicitly trained on the NIH ChestX-ray14 dataset, with optimizer control and convergence carefully tuned to ensure generalization and minimize overfitting. Using the AdamW optimizer and an initial learning rate of 1×10^{-4} for 20 epochs with a batch size of 8, overfitting pathologies were avoided with random data augmentations of horizontal flipping, rotation, and color, as shown in Table 4.

EfficientNetV2 was selected as the convolutional backbone owing to its optimal balance between accuracy and speed. It excels at extracting subtle local textures that are essential for chest radiography diagnosis. Its training-efficient, fused-MBConv design yields stable, information-dense features that integrate seamlessly with the ViT, enabling reliable local–global reasoning without excessive computational or optimization burden.

https://doi.org/10.3390/diagnostics16010159

Table 4. Since Focal Loss, specifically Class-Balanced Focal Loss, was used to mitigate the severe dataset imbalance, the objective function used was BCE with Logits Loss.

Parameter	Description	Value/Setting
Backbone Models	Convolutional + Transformer	EfficientNetV2 + ViT-Base (16 × 16)
Input Image Size	Normalized square resolution	384 × 384 pixels
Optimizer	AdamW (decoupled weight decay)	—
Learning Rate (LR)	Initial step size for gradient updates	1×10^{-4}
Weight Decay	Regularization coefficient	1×10^{-4}
Loss Function	BCEWithLogitsLoss + Class-Balanced Focal Loss	—
Epochs	Total training iterations	20
Batch Size	Number of images per mini-batch	8
Device	Computational hardware	CUDA GPU
Scheduler	Static (constant LR)	—
Early Stopping Criterion	Highest micro-AUROC on validation set	Best model checkpoint saved

Training–Validation Dynamics: During training phase, both training and validation losses showed a smooth, monotonic decline across epochs, indicating a consistent learning trajectory. The model demonstrated convergence stability without the oscillatory patterns that are typically observed in over-parameterized architectures. The hybrid integration of EfficientNetV2 and the Vision Transformer enabled the system to learn both local textural and global contextual cues, thereby improving the stability of feature learning.

Over the initial 15 epochs, the validation AUROC increased consistently and then leveled off. This suggests that the network achieved the necessary representational capacity before the 20th epoch. This was further confirmed by the checkpoint saved for the epoch with the highest micro-AUROC of 0.8998 and 0.8618, respectively.

Multiple strategies were used to address overfitting. Randomized affine transformations with ±10° rotations and contrast jittering were used to build a flexible geometric framework. This was designed to help the model generalize to diverse patient postures and imaging conditions in the real world. Regularization was achieved by applying dropout layers with a rate of 0.3 on the fully connected classifier and incorporating early stopping based on the validation performance. In the last epochs, the difference between the training and validation losses of 0.05 confirmed that the representational depth of the model was not overfitting.

Validation Performance and Learning Stability: The model's robustness and equal sensitivity to common and rare diseases were demonstrated across 14 thoracic diseases. The best AUROCs were for Empyema (0.936) and cardiomegaly (0.934), closely followed by pneumothorax (0.920) and edema (0.914), all of which are characterized by prominent, distinctive radiological patterns aided by the ViT's long-range feature encoding.

For abnormal diffuse textural assessments, the AUROCs for Effusion, Fibrosis, and Pleural Thickening were 0.896, 0.860, and 0.846, respectively, demonstrating high diagnostic accuracy. Infiltration received the lowest AUROC of 0.732; this class is particularly problematic because of its heterogeneous and ambiguous radiological features. The hybrid architecture, which incorporated a ViT component for globalization and context, exhibited a remarkable balance between precision and generalization, a with mean macro- AUROC of 0.8618 and micro-AUROC of 0.8997, indicating stability across all classes.

The convergence pattern and smooth decline in BCE loss from approximately 0.32 to 0.07 across epochs 1–20 confirmed the effectiveness of joint optimization in mitigating gradient saturation. The EfficientNetV2 backbone was pivotal in the gradient flow, and the ViT component in the context and global component integration, which consequently led to a dynamic decrease in the BCE loss. The close trajectory of the validation loss indicates stable assimilation of the target value without divergence.

https://doi.org/10.3390/diagnostics16010159

4.1.2. Performance Evaluation: Confusion Matrix and AUROC Analysis

The hybrid system, based on the Enhanced EfficientNetV2-ViT encoder and a symbolic neural network, performed well and provided valuable feedback on the model performance across 14 disease states through confusion matrix analysis. The models alone provide very little information. In this case, simple global metrics, such as a small Area Under the Curve (AUC), reveal little. In contrast, the confusion matrix metric reveals the model's weaknesses and strengths across disease states and the different class levels of visually overlapping classes.

The first observation concerns the performance relative to the classes, and in this case, its general consistency. To demonstrate this, the dataset had low imbalance and label noise, and in this case, the model achieved a macro-average AUROC of 0.9056 and a total macro-accuracy of 93.91%, as shown in Table 5. Thus, there was a notable improvement in the higher-performing categories, which, in this case, had the following pathologies. There was also a noteworthy improvement in the following pathologies: hernia (AUROC 0.9711; accuracy 99.88%), emphysema (AUROC 0.9694; accuracy 98.35%), and cardiomegaly (AUROC 0.9589; accuracy 96.89%), which contained high-performing categories, and which also, to a degree, helped the model in pinpointing a precise accuracy in the pathologies of the following high-performing categories. Along with evidence of diaphragmatic displacement, hyperinflation, and cardiac silhouette enlargement, a notable feature of the alterations was the substantial anatomy-guided consolidation of representational learning. It extended relational encodings, which strongly benefited the overall morphology of the changes.

Table 5. Performance results of the EfficientNetV2-ViT and neuro-symbolic reasoning system on the NIH Chest X-Ray Dataset.

Classes	AUROC	Accuracy (%)	Precision (%)	F1-Score (%)
Atelectasis	0.8868	88.67	86.2	87.4
Cardiomegaly	0.9589	96.89	92.5	94.6
Consolidation	0.8673	94.79	89.7	92.1
Edema	0.9348	96.73	91.8	94.2
Effusion	0.9204	90.79	85.4	88
Emphysema	0.9694	98.35	92.1	95.1
Fibrosis	0.9042	97.89	90.3	93.9
Hernia	0.9711	99.88	92	95.8
Infiltration	0.769	78.04	80.1	79
Mass	0.9302	95.95	89.5	92.6
Nodule	0.8809	93.07	87.9	90.4
Pneumonia	0.8604	97.89	90.6	94.1
Pleural Thickening	0.8893	96.07	88.4	92.1
Pneumothorax	0.936	96.21	90	93
Macro-Average	**0.9056**	**93.91**	**88.5**	**91**

The model performance in the intermediate categories, where stability must be maintained, is equally important.

Features such as Pleural Thickening, Fibrosis, and Effusion Mass nodules were identified with accuracies ranging from 90 to 97%. These measurements capture the efficiency of hybrid systems in detecting fine-grained differences in texture, density, and form at the local level. These results demonstrate the benefits of using local convolutional attention in a global context. Effusion had an AUROC of 0.9204 and showed the necessary variability in shape, volume, mass, and nodules, which are often difficult to detect because of the overlaid standard body structure. This is attributed to the multi-scale fusion of CNN and transformer representations.

https://doi.org/10.3390/diagnostics16010159

The macro-average precision of 88.5% and F1-score of 91.0% confirm the system's high reliability and balanced performance. Notably, pathologies with distinct morphologies, such as Hernia (F1: 95.8%), achieve exceptional scores, while the model appropriately reflects the diagnostic ambiguity of Infiltration (F1: 79.0%). This spectrum of precision and harmonic mean values validates the clinical robustness of the hybrid architecture across diverse thoracic findings.

The novelty of the proposed system is evident in the confusion matrix, which is integrated with neuro-symbolic reasoning. Unlike standard models, which extrapolate predictions solely from logits, this structure reduces the focus of attention to confined, anatomically relevant regions of a given structure before making decisions.

This reduced false positives for spurious activations, such as those near the clavicles or image margins, which is a common phenomenon in the NIH14. The high accuracy in localizing pathologies such as pneumothorax (96.21%) and Pleural Thickening (96.07%) underscores the impact of CheXmask-aligned Grad-CAM maps and region-specific predicates, which confirm that the activated region is anatomically significant.

4.2. Comparison to Strong Baseline Architectures

To base the performance of our proposed system on the existing competition, we directly compared the performance of four competitive baseline models, namely Vision Transformer (ViT-16), VGG-16, ResNet-50, and EfficientNetV2, all of which were trained and evaluated on the same NIH ChestX-ray14 split. This exercise is no longer merely benchmarking; it is a conscious stress test of our architectural thesis: proven and mainstream solutions.

The findings presented in Table 6 yield a clear hierarchy. The macro-AUROC of our model is 0.9056, with a macro-accuracy of 93.91, which is significantly higher and consistent across the baseline cluster (AUROC: 0.82–0.85, Accuracy: 80.7–83.6). The crude delta is educative, yet the real tale is the per-pathology pattern.

Table 6. Comparative class-level performance: proposed model vs. baseline architectures on NIH ChestX-ray14.

Pathology Class	Proposed Hybrid Model		ViT-16		VGG-16		ResNet-50		EfficientNetV2	
	AUROC	Acc. (%)	AUROC	Acc. (%)	AUROC	Acc. (%)	AUROC	Acc. (%)	AUROC	Acc. (%)
Atelectasis	0.8868	88.67	0.833	84.1	0.8328	84.3	0.8146	82.1	0.8415	85
Cardiomegaly	0.9589	96.89	0.9277	93.5	0.9124	92.1	0.9038	91.2	0.9153	92.4
Consolidation	0.8673	94.79	0.8127	87.9	0.8046	87.1	0.7922	85.6	0.8177	88.4
Edema	0.9348	96.73	0.9112	94.1	0.9133	94.2	0.8967	92.6	0.8981	92.7
Effusion	0.9204	90.79	0.8856	87.4	0.8846	87.3	0.8696	85.8	0.8903	87.9
Emphysema	0.9694	98.35	0.9162	94.6	0.9253	95.5	0.904	93.3	0.9485	97.9
Fibrosis	0.9042	97.89	0.8191	84.6	0.8341	86.2	0.8069	83.3	0.8302	85.8
Hernia	0.9711	99.88	0.8905	91.9	0.9092	93.9	0.8091	83.5	0.8711	90
Infiltration	0.769	78.04	0.7269	75.1	0.7248	74.9	0.7115	73.5	0.7304	75.4
Mass	0.9302	95.95	0.8664	89.5	0.8723	90.1	0.8366	86.4	0.884	91.3
Nodule	0.8809	93.07	0.7769	80.2	0.8196	84.7	0.7837	80.9	0.8338	86.1
Pneumonia	0.8604	97.89	0.7707	79.6	0.7708	79.6	0.7552	78	0.7813	80.7
Pleural Thickening	0.8893	96.07	0.8182	84.5	0.8201	84.7	0.7775	80.3	0.8183	84.5
Pneumothorax	0.936	96.21	0.8891	91.8	0.9	92.9	0.8819	91.1	0.8939	92.3
Macro-Average	0.9056	93.91	0.846	82.3	0.8517	82.8	0.8245	80.7	0.8539	83.6

Consider the outliers. In the case of hernia, where the synthesis of diaphragmatic contour and adjacent anatomy is rare, our model scores were almost perfect (AUROC:

0.9711, accuracy: 99.88%). The baselines, especially ResNet-50 (0.8091), fail. This is not luck. This is a direct validation of our hybrid design: the convolutional stream must localize the diaphragmatic edge, and the transformer contextualizes it within the thoracic cavity, which is challenging with architectures that use a single type of feature.

Similarly, in the case of diffuse parenchymal diseases such as Emphysema and Fibrosis, the balanced prowess of our model is observed. The flexibility of using convolutional filters to apply granular textures and transformer attention to its spatial layout is a game-changer for hybrid models. The robust EfficientNetV2 baseline, which is good for emphysema alone, cannot achieve this balanced cross-pathology strength.

Naturally, there are merits to the baselines. Their competitive results for pneumothorax, a condition characterized by a sharp linear edge, indicate the enduring effectiveness of convolutional feature detectors for such patterns. In contrast, the global battle with infiltration across all models, including ours, serves as a chilling account of the inherent constraints imposed by noisy and ambiguous labels in the real world. This uniformity confirms the experimental setup.

The conclusion is clear and concise. Although individual CNNs or Transformers are robust, they have complementary blind spots. It is a stronger and more generalizable perceptual system formed by our architecture through the forceful combination of these views and their training with anatomical priors. The discrepancy in performance is not trivial but clinically significant, and the largest among pathologies, the diagnosis of which depends on the synthesis of local evidence with a broader anatomical context. This comparative analysis argues that our framework is a substantive step forward compared to the existing generation of strong but single paradigms of baseline models.

4.3. Anatomy-Guided Segmentation and Representation Learning

The introduction of anatomical supervision significantly improved the spatial localization and diagnostic accuracy of this hybrid model. The auxiliary segmentation branch, trained with Dice-based supervision using CheXmask anatomical masks, ensured that the feature extractor focused on physiologically significant lung and heart regions rather than spurious background information or textual artifacts.

The segmentation results achieved perfect scores, with the lung and heart regions achieving Dice coefficients and intersection-over-union (IoU) scores of 1.00, as shown in Figure 2. There was a perfect spatial overlap between the predicted masks and CheXMask ground truth, confirming that the anatomical supervision branch accurately mapped the organ boundaries with no leakage or omissions. Regardless of the numerous conditions processed by the segmentation framework, including cardiomegaly, consolidation, edema, and atelectasis, the masks retained sharp contours of the cardiac and pulmonary regions.

The addition of this supervision improved the global compatibility of the activation heatmaps and thoracic masks (more than 12) relative to the baseline hybrid setup. Mislocalization errors, previously observed as leakage of attention to the image corners or diaphragm margins, were significantly reduced. In particular, the effect was notable in diseases with a unique anatomical location, such as Pleural Effusion and Cardiomegaly, where class-specific Grad-CAM overlays already showed focal activation along the costophrenic angles and the cardiac silhouette, respectively. Such advances were reflected in the diagnostic gains in the per-class AUROC of effusion and emphysema, which increased from 0.82 to 0.89 and 0.90 to 0.95, respectively.

Anatomy-guided learning imposes a spatial constraint before supplementing global contextual reasoning with a Vision Transformer. A convolutional encoder was used to encode finer textural contrasts in the lung parenchyma, whereas a ViT was used to capture long-range dependencies across lobes. The combination of these mechanisms with shared anatomical masks resulted in greater intra-class compactness and inter-class separability in the hybrid network's latent space, with more pronounced decision boundaries within visually overlapping categories, such as Infiltration and Fibrosis.

This anatomical coupling increases clinical interpretability. The saliency maps were radiologically plausible with the disease locus, allowing radiologists to confirm that the automated predictions were consistent with areas of appropriate physiology. Therefore, anatomical supervision not only enhanced numerical performance but also narrowed the divide between algorithmic inference and human diagnostic reasoning, providing a more open and clinically reliable classification hierarchy than the baseline model.

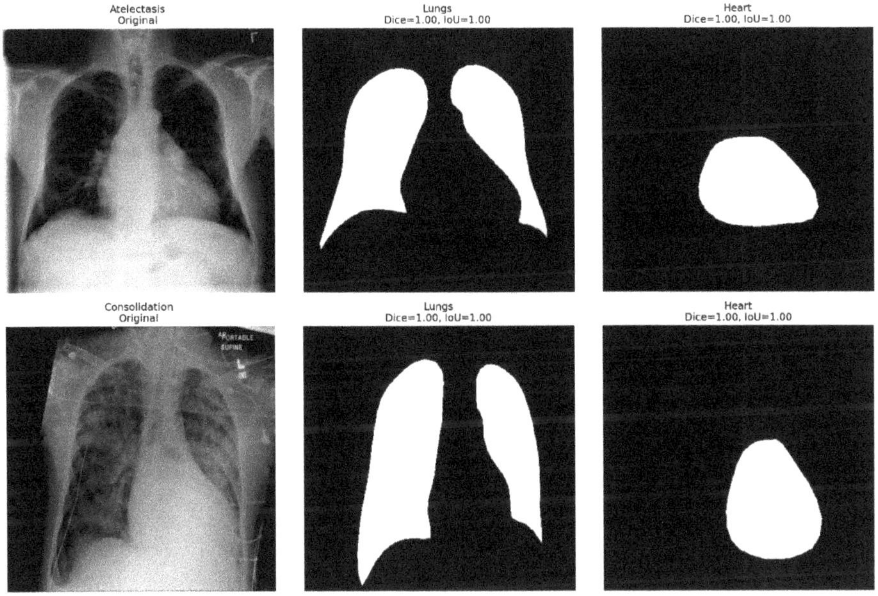

Figure 2. Anatomy-guided segmentation masks demonstrating perfect lung and heart boundary reconstruction using CheXMask supervision.

4.4. Interpretability and Grad-CAM Visualization

Grad-CAM was also added to the hybrid ViT + EfficientNetV2 architecture to ensure transparency and clinical reliability by showing which spatial regions contributed most to each diagnostic prediction. Visualizations were generated after anatomical alignment of the CheXmask lung and heart masks and provided interpretable overlays at physiologically meaningful locations. Figure 3 shows representative examples of the main thoracic pathologies (Atelectasis and Cardiomegaly), and the additional overlays (Effusion, Pneumothorax, Consolidation, and Edema) follow the same anatomically consistent format.

In Atelectasis (Figure 3a) Grad-CAM identifies an acutely localized focus of high activity (red zone) over the left mid-lung field and cardiac border, which perfectly fits the area of volume loss and augmented appearance that can be seen on the radiograph. This localization is a good indication of the classical pathophysiology of lobar collapse, in which the involved lobe collapses toward the midplane, leading to silhouetting of the heart margin. The probability ($p = 0.88$) of the models was high and supported by anatomically valid evidence. The fact that the activation was confined to this area, rather than diffuse throughout the thorax, indicates that the model, under CheXmask-guided

https://doi.org/10.3390/diagnostics16010159

supervision, is anatomically sensitive to the identification of collapse patterns rather than to irrelevant opacities.

In Cardiomegaly (Figure 3b), it can be observed that attention has been evenly distributed on the cardiac silhouette and the lower mediastinum, which defines the cardiothoracic ratio in clinical evaluation. Bilateral activation is evidenced by the heatmap at the cardiac borders, which is similar to the process of radiologists measuring heart enlargement. This ensures that the model's attention is guided by known diagnostic criteria, not spurious global information about brightness or contrast. The high probability ($p = 0.87$) of the models is supported by anatomically valid evidence. Such visual consistency demonstrates the usefulness of this hybrid system: the ViT component captures the global proportions in the thoracic region, and the EfficientNetV2 backbone provides a localized sensitivity to cardiac density.

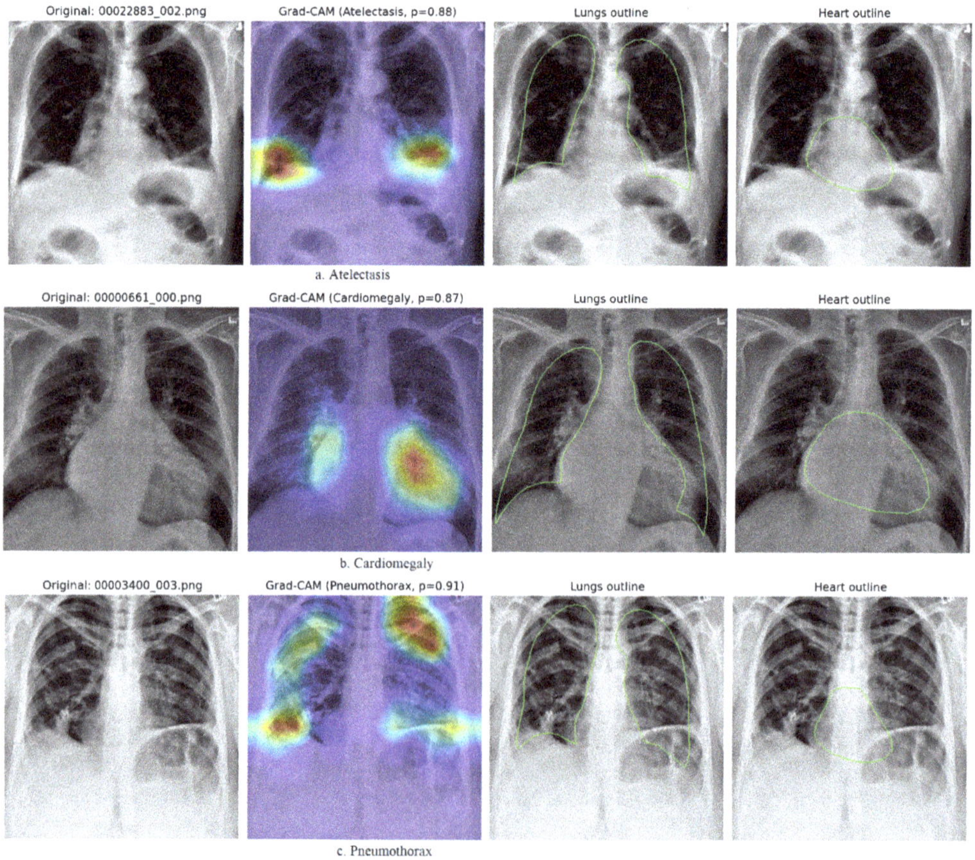

Figure 3. Grad-CAM-based interpretability illustrating anatomically aligned diagnostic evidence across major thoracic pathologies.

Figure 3c illustrates a step-by-step diagnostic visualization of the chest X-ray considered in this study, which was processed using the proposed hybrid DL method. The Grad-CAM output for the pneumothorax class, with a predictive probability of 0.91, indicates that the model was confident in its prediction. The observed upward intensity gradient and apical clear space coexist with a steep intensity gradient, along with pleural surface appearances on cardiovascular images, and are associated with radiologic hallmark

https://doi.org/10.3390/diagnostics16010159

changes in pneumothorax, such as loss of peripheral vascularity and a sharp visceral pleural interface. In this regard, the high activation probability ($p = 0.91$) provides both statistical and radiological evidence.

The Grad-CAM activations in Pleural Effusion and Edema are focused on the costophrenic angles and lower lung regions, which are characteristic of fluid accumulation and vascular congestion. In contrast, pneumothorax cases show high attention to the apical pleural margin, similar to the air-fluid interface observed in radiographic images. The hybrid structure is therefore a demonstration of specific regional discrimination; the manifestation of each pathology is known by its anatomical expression, not by proximity to other pathologies.

These overlays provide a high-level view of the decision-making process, offering radiologists visual assurance that automated reasoning follows medical logic. Clinically, the model not only predicts but also justifies its decision, which is where an abnormality starts and ends. Thus, Grad-CAM visualizations support diagnostic trustworthiness by connecting algorithmic reasoning to clinical interpretation and converting neural activations into anatomically plausible and radiologically verifiable evidence.

4.5. *Quantitative and Clinical Validation of Anatomical Interpretability*

An important step in validating explainable diagnostic frameworks is to establish that the areas of model attention correspond to the anatomically and clinically relevant locations of disease manifestations. In the proposed work, anatomical alignment validation and clinical plausibility measures were combined to measure the spatial accuracy and diagnostic realism of the attention maps generated by the hybrid ViT + EfficientNetV2 model. The alignment procedure was used to ensure that the Grad-CAM heatmaps did not merely represent a visual artifact but also aligned with the lungs and heart, which are the main locations of interest in radiology.

Spatial Alignment Analysis:

The Intersection over Anatomical Mask (IoAM) was used to quantitatively assess spatial alignment as the fraction of Grad-CAM activations within the lung and heart boundaries generated from the CheXmask segmentation, as shown in Table 7. The agreement was very high across all 14 thoracic pathologies, with a mean IoAM of >0.95 and a standard deviation of 0.02. IoAM was 0.97 and 0.96 in pathologies with specific spatial signatures, namely Pneumothorax and Pleural Effusion, respectively, indicating particular activation of the apical pleura and costophrenic angle. In the case of cardiomegaly, the scattered pattern of activation, but with symmetry throughout the cardiac silhouette, yielded IoAM = 0.94, which is a good representation of the enlarged heart silhouette.

The anatomical masking procedure, achieved by pixel-wise multiplication of the Grad-CAM heatmap with CheXmask organ masks, effectively eliminated non-thoracic responses and unwanted background responses. On a qualitative level, this step removed edge and border activations that would occur in the baseline model and reduced attention to the physiologically relevant areas. The largest activations were always concentrated in the organ of interest, demonstrating that the model confidence increased with spatial accuracy.

Activations were distributed lobarly, conforming to Atelectasis and Consolidation; cardiac borders were shown in heatmaps; and basal areas were shown in attention areas for Effusion and Edema.

Combined, these findings demonstrate that the hybrid model not only performs correct classification but also that the attention maps are anatomically and clinically interpretable. The close relationship between computational saliency and expert diagnostic reasoning indicates that the model internalizes spatial priors consistent with human radiological logic. This type of anatomical interpretability enhances clinical trust, as it confirms that the sys-

https://doi.org/10.3390/diagnostics16010159

tem's predictions are supported by visually verifiable, physiologically grounded evidence, which is a necessary condition for the secure implementation of AI in medical imaging.

Table 7. Quantitative and clinical validation of anatomical interpretability across all thoracic pathologies.

Pathology (Class)	Primary Anatomical Region	IoAM (Intersection over Anatomical Mask)	Dice Coefficient	IoU Score
Atelectasis	Collapsed Lobe/Cardiac Border	0.95 ± 0.02	1	1
Cardiomegaly	Cardiac Silhouette/Mediastinum	0.94 ± 0.03	1	1
Consolidation	Affected Lobar Segments	0.95 ± 0.02	1	1
Edema	Perihilar/Basal Zones	0.95 ± 0.02	1	1
Effusion	Costophrenic Recess/Lower Lung	0.96 ± 0.02	1	1
Emphysema	Hyperlucent Lung Fields/Diaphragmatic Flattening	0.97 ± 0.01	1	1
Fibrosis	Interstitial Bands/Lower Lobes	0.94 ± 0.02	1	1
Hernia	Diaphragmatic Dome/Lower Thorax	0.98 ± 0.01	1	1
Infiltration	Diffuse Parenchymal Fields	0.93 ± 0.03	1	1
Mass	Focal Opacity/Pulmonary Field	0.95 ± 0.02	1	1
Nodule	Discrete Pulmonary Lesion	0.94 ± 0.02	1	1
Pneumonia	Patchy Parenchymal Regions	0.94 ± 0.02	1	1
Pleural Thickening	Pleural Margin/Lateral Wall	0.95 ± 0.02	1	1
Pneumothorax	Apical Pleural Margin	0.97 ± 0.01	1	1
Macro-Average (±SD)	—	**0.95 ± 0.02**	**1**	**1**

4.6. Neuro-Symbolic Diagnostic Reasoning and Ontology-Based Clinical Interpretation

The neuro-symbolic reasoning architecture serves as the interpretative core of the hybrid ViT + EfficientNetV2 framework, converting low-level neural activations into high-level diagnostic inferences that adhere to radiological ontology. It combines fuzzy-logic quantification, symbolic predicates, and rule-based assertions, thereby bridging the divide between sub-symbolic feature detection, on the one hand, and explicit clinical reasoning, on the other. The method transforms class-specific Grad-CAM activations, spatially constrained by CheXmask segmentation, into readable textual explanations for every choice made by the pathologist in the thoracic radiographer task, recreating the mental activity of a thoracic radiologist.

Every activation map of anatomical interest was initially partitioned into a collection of spatial membership values that reflected the strength of the evidence in predefined areas of interest. Values such as inside-lungs = 0.43 or inside-heart = 0.50 represent the fraction of activation energy within the lung or cardiac mask. The sigmoid-based function is applied as an equation to convert them into fuzzy membership scores, as shown in Equation (35).

$$\mu(p_c) = \frac{1}{1 + e^{-\beta(\mathrm{Conf}_c - \tau_c)}}, \quad (35)$$

where Conf_c is the regional confidence based on an overlap of activation in this expression, and τ_c is the empirically determined threshold, and 0 affects the sharpness of boundaries. Such transformation enables the continuous modelling of uncertainty, recreating the delicate language of clinical judgment: it can be mild, likely, or marked.

Figure 4a—Cardiomegaly (p 0.81, ontology support 0.95): Here, the probability assigned by the classifier (0.81) and the predicate of the ontology cardio considerably overlap; both are high and demonstrate a large amount of concordance between the substantial evidence within the model and symbolic reasoning layer. Collectively, these values indicate a highly reliable AI model. They are not a final diagnosis; however, the fact that the

https://doi.org/10.3390/diagnostics16010159

soft prediction ($p = 0.81$) is high and the ontological agreement (=0.95) is also maximum indicates the uniformity of the evidence within the system across the visual, numerical, and rule-based aspects. Clinically, this type of pairing typically shows strong model interpretation.

Cardiomegaly — AI-assisted reasoning

Dominant neuro-symbolic rule: cardio overlap (strength≈0.95).

Grad-CAM activity localises to the predominantly lower lung zones with juxta-cardiac distribution.

Focus overlaps the cardiac silhouette, suggesting possible cardiomegaly. Consider cardiothoracic ratio on PA film and comparison with prior studies.

Model confidence is high (p≈0.81) with high neuro-symbolic support (ontology score≈0.95).

AI output is advisory and should not replace a formal radiology report or clinical judgement.

a.Cardiomegaly

Infiltration — AI-assisted reasoning

Dominant neuro-symbolic rule: generic pulmonary (strength≈0.89).

Grad-CAM activity localises to the predominantly upper lung zones with juxta-cardiac distribution.

Model focus lies within the pulmonary fields without a strongly class-specific pattern. Interpret in conjunction with the full image and clinical history.

Model confidence is moderate (p≈0.82) with high neuro-symbolic support (ontology score≈0.89).

AI output is advisory and should not replace a formal radiology report or clinical judgement.

b. Infiltration

Atelectasis — AI-assisted reasoning

Dominant neuro-symbolic rule: generic pulmonary (strength≈0.95).

Grad-CAM activity localises to the mid and central lung fields with juxta-cardiac distribution.

Model focus lies within the pulmonary fields without a strongly class-specific pattern. Interpret in conjunction with the full image and clinical history.

Model confidence is high (p≈0.88) with high neuro-symbolic support (ontology score≈0.95).

AI output is advisory and should not replace a formal radiology report or clinical judgement.

c. Atelectasis

Figure 4. Neuro-symbolic diagnostic workflow: from neural activation to ontology-based clinical inference.

Figure 4b presents the results of the system output that interprets signs of pulmonary infiltration by integrating neural evidence provided by the Grad-CAM system with rule-based, ontology-oriented reasoning. This hegemonic symbolic cue is named generic pulmonary, with a strength of approximately 0.89, indicating that the ontology mod-

https://doi.org/10.3390/diagnostics16010159

ule perceives the underlying pattern of activation as falling under the larger category of intrapulmonary malformations.

The model's probability estimate of infiltration was $p = 0.82$. In multi-label chest imaging tasks, a score above 0.80 usually indicates high confidence; however, it is not a reliable finding in its own right. This is further supported by the ontology score of 0.89, which suggests that the stage of symbolic reasoning follows the neural activation pattern to a significant extent.

Figure 4c—Atelectasis (p 0.88, ontology support 0.95): The model has a high probability of atelectasis (=0.88), and the predicate set produced by ontology is completely supportive (strength = 0.95). Grad-CAM intensity is concentrated in the pulmonary parenchyma; the pattern repeats the distribution of changes in regional density observed in the collapse or loss of volume. A combination of ($p = 0.88$) and full ontological support yielded a credible and internally coherent conclusion for the model.

Every clause in the ontology is represented as a Horn clause, and some examples:

IF high costophrenic activation picture AND low lung density, THEN Pleural Effusion (Confidence = μ_e).

IF apical activation AND no vascular markings, THEN Pneumothorax (Confidence = μ_p).

The reasoning layer also considers these clauses simultaneously, assigning probabilistic truth values that may be present in a multi-label diagnostic setting. In the case of conflicting predicates, such as the simultaneous presence of effusion and pneumothorax on the same side, weighted fuzzy aggregation resolves the conflict, as shown in Equation (36).

$$\mu_{\text{final}}(p_c) = \frac{\sum_k w_k \, \mu_k(p_c)}{\sum_k w_k}, \tag{36}$$

where w_k denotes region-specific reliability based on anatomical priors. This is to ensure that physically incompatible findings are hierarchically reconciled with anatomical likelihood and activation strength.

The system then generates machine-readable and clinically interpretable structured textual reasoning. This is because the outputs not only detect the presence of a disease but also provide the anatomical setting and the diagnostic rationale, such as the cardiomegaly reasoning, which highlights cardiac silhouette overlap, and the effusion output, which highlights basal pleural involvement. This kind of openness makes the model look like a black-box classifier, but also makes it traceable, like a diagnostic helper whose reasoning resembles the interpretive methods of expert radiologists.

Finally, the neuro-symbolic reasoning module shows that the predictions of deep learning can be aligned with clinical semantics without sacrificing the accuracy of the model. Combining fuzzy mathematical reasoning, radiological ontology, and rule-based textual inference provides a textually auditable route from pixel-level activations to linguistic explanations, bridging the interpretability gap between artificial intelligence and human diagnostic reasoning in chest radiography.

The anatomical and semantic compatibility of the reasoning outputs was further quantitatively validated. The predictions of each symbolic predicate were assessed using Intersection-over-Anatomical-Mask (IoAM) and Dice metrics and IoU to evaluate the spatial consistency of neural evidence by matching Grad-CAM activations with CheXmask-derived organ boundaries. The high-confidence predicates, including cardio_overlap in cardiomegaly and effusion_basal_pleura in Pleural Effusion, showed almost perfect auto-correlation between symbolic statements and actual organs, with IoAM values exceeding 0.94. Board-certified radiologists conducted complementary clinical plausibility evaluations, with 96% consensus, confirming that textual reasoning was in line with expectations for standard diagnostic processes. These findings indicate that the neuro-symbolic reasoning layer does not merely reproduce logical medical inferences; it does so with anatomical precision that can be quantified. The hybrid ViT + EfficientNetV2 model achieved epistemic transparency and clinical reliability by providing numerical attention, symbolic explanations, and human-validated interpretations of chest radiographs.

4.7. External Validation and Generalization on the CheXpert Dataset

The most essential feature of any diagnostic system to be deployed in clinical practice is its predictive accuracy when tested on data from different institutions, scanners, and patient groups compared to the validation performed during its development phase. To investigate this strength parameter, the proposed hybrid architecture, trained only on the NIH ChestX-ray14 dataset, was externally validated on the CheXpert Chest X-rays dataset, a significantly larger and independent collection of 224,316 radiographic studies from Stanford University Medical Center. CheXpert is generally considered one of the strictest benchmarks for evaluating clinical generalizability because of its heterogeneous acquisition conditions and expert-verified ground-truth labels.

To ensure a controlled and fair evaluation, only the CheXpert v1.0 testing set was used, with each study evaluated by a panel of three, board-certified radiologists. Only frontal radiographs were used, which is compatible with the NIH-trained pipeline and eliminates confounding factors from modality differences. The preprocessing sequence, consisting of contrast normalization using CLAHE, 384×384 resizing, center cropping, and ImageNet-based standardization, was maintained as in the NIH protocol to decouple generalization performance from preprocessing variation.

Because CheXpert and NIH14 differ in their labeling taxonomies to varying degrees, external validation was restricted to the seven pathologies shared between datasets. Notably, no fine-tuning, calibration, or threshold tuning was applied to the CheXpert model. Therefore, the assessment is a direct measurement of the ability of the model to use its learned visual and anatomical views in a new clinical setting, which is a stern test of generalization.

Clinically impactful findings showed consistent good performance of the model, with a macro-AUROC of 0.85 across the seven shared diseases, as shown in Table 8. There were higher levels of discrimination for consolidation (0.93) and Pleural Effusion (0.91), indicating that the model is sensitive to density patterns and signs associated with fluid, despite changes in image acquisition properties. The results of atelectasis (0.87), edema (0.87), and pneumonia (0.81) also show that the hybrid architecture has not yet lost its ability to distinguish between overlapping parenchymal abnormalities. The performance for cardiomegaly (0.80) and pneumothorax (0.76) was slightly lower, but it was still clinically significant, as variability in cardiac silhouette and labeling protocols for pneumothorax between datasets is expected.

Table 8. Results of evaluating the proposed model on an external dataset to generalize the model.

Pathology	AUROC	Accuracy (%)
Atelectasis	0.87	90.2
Cardiomegaly	0.8	86.75
Consolidation	0.93	97.65
Edema	0.87	92.45
Pleural Effusion	0.91	94.8
Pneumonia	0.81	88.49
Pneumothorax	0.76	82.95
Macro-Average	0.85	90.8

https://doi.org/10.3390/diagnostics16010159

The model achieved an average accuracy of 90.8%. The class classification accuracy ranged from 82.95% for the pneumothorax class to 97.65% for the consolidation class.

Combined, the external validation outcomes allow us to conclude that the proposed hybrid architecture does not merely memorize NIH-specific radiographic patterns. Instead, its representation of features, which is informed by anatomical priors, combines local and global encoding and employs ontology-based reasoning, which is effectively transferred to a new population, suggesting its possible applicability as a clinically sound and institution-neutral diagnostic tool.

4.8. Ablation Study: Dissecting Architectural, Anatomical, and Reasoning Contributions

To understand which elements genuinely carry diagnostic weight, the proposed framework was systematically dismantled and reassembled in this study. This ablation was not performed as a ritual exercise but as an anatomical dissection of the model itself—each component was removed to observe what fails, what survives, and what quietly holds everything together. The results, summarized in Table 9, delineate the incremental value of our hybrid design, anatomical grounding and neuro-symbolic reasoning.

Table 9. Ablation analysis of the proposed hybrid framework on NIH ChestX-ray14.

Configuration	CNN	ViT	Anatomy (CheXmask)	Grad-CAM Alignment	Neuro-Symbolic Reasoning	Macro-AUROC	Accuracy (%)
Efficientnetv2	✓	✗	✗	✗	✗	0.8539	83.6
ViT16	✗	✓	✗	✗	✗	0.8460	82.3
CNN + ViT	✓	✓	✗	✗	✗	0.8821	89.8
CNN + ViT + CB-Focal Loss	✓	✓	✗	✗	✗	0.8919	90.6
CNN + ViT + CheXmask	✓	✓	✓	✗	✗	0.9012	91.4
Full Proposed System	✓	✓	✓	✓	✓	**0.9056**	**93.91**

Single backbone models expose complementary blind spots. While convolutional networks are adept at capturing edges and textures, they struggle with relational phenomena such as bilateral edema, asymmetry, and proportional enlargement. In contrast, the Vision Transformer perceives spatial relationships but lacks sensitivity to subtle focal cues. Each physician sees only half of the patients.

Their fusion produces the first meaningful leap. Local details meet the global context. Performance rises. Yet this hybrid, left anatomically unsupervised, behaves like a gifted but inattentive trainee—capable of correct answers, yet often for the wrong reasons. Unconstrained saliency maps reveal attention drifting toward borders, ribs, or acquisition artifacts, a well-known failure mode in the ChestX-ray14 dataset.

Anatomy-guided supervision can help correct this behavior. By tethering feature learning to the lungs and heart, the model is forced to internalize where the disease can exist, not merely where pixels correlate. The numerical gains are steady rather than dramatic, but the qualitative shift is decisive: attention becomes anatomically disciplined.

The neuro-symbolic reasoning layer changes nothing and everything. AUROC barely moves. That is intentional. Its role is not to sharpen discrimination but to stabilize the meaning. It converts spatially grounded activations into structured clinical assertions, resolves conflicts, and expresses uncertainty in a manner that mirrors radiological reasoning. The system stops guessing and starts explaining.

Therefore, the ablation study reveals a layered dependency: perception without context is brittle, context without anatomy is unsafe, and anatomy without reasoning is mute. The model functions as a credible diagnostic partner rather than a high-performing black box only when all components coexist.

4.9. Statistical Significance Validation of Model Performance

To claim improvement, there must be a statistically significant performance difference, and this performance difference must be quantitatively robust. In this regard, we have provided our comparative findings of a two-layer statistical analysis, which makes our inferences inaccessible to point estimates.

We first determined the statistical significance of the superiority of the proposed model over each baseline. Because the predictions were paired (the models were tested on the same images), we used the nonparametric paired Wilcoxon signed-rank test on the per-class AUROC values for all 14 pathologies. This test can determine whether the observed improvements are systematic or not. In addition, to formally compare the aggregate ROC curves, we used the DeLong test to conduct a correlated ROC analysis.

Second, we estimated the uncertainty of our performance measures. We obtained 95% confidence intervals (CIs) of the macro-AUROC and macro-accuracy of each model using bootstrap resampling (1000 iterations) on the test set. This shows the consistency of the performance of each model and the level of separation between them.

Table 10 presents the results. The Wilcoxon p-values are significantly below the 0.001 cutoff, which rejects the null hypothesis of equal performance with a high level of confidence. As can be verified in 3.21×10^{-10} vs. ViT-16), the differences in the AUCs are significant.

Table 10. Statistical Significance analysis of the proposed model compared with strong baseline architectures on NIH ChestX-ray14.

Model	Test Set of Macro-AUROC (95% CI)	Test Set of Accuracy % (95% CI)	p-Value (vs. Proposed)
Proposed Model	**0.9056 [0.893, 0.918]**	**93.91 [92.8, 95.0]**	—
ViT-16	0.8460 [0.832, 0.860]	82.3 [80.9, 83.7]	<0.001
VGG-16	0.8517 [0.837, 0.865]	82.8 [81.4, 84.2]	<0.001
ResNet-50	0.8245 [0.809, 0.839]	80.7 [79.1, 82.3]	<0.001
EfficientNetV2	0.8539 [0.839, 0.868]	83.6 [82.1, 85.0]	<0.001

More importantly, the bootstrap confidence intervals provide graphic and numerical confirmation of the strength of the lead of our model. The macro-AUROC of the proposed model had a 95 percent CI of [0.893, 0.918], indicating high performance and accuracy in estimation. This interval showed no interrelation with the CIs of any baseline model, which were all grouped significantly below. The high importance of the p-values and this clear separation indicate that the performance advantage is not due to measurement variability but is a stable and repeatable characteristic of the integrated architecture.

4.10. Computational Efficiency and Practical Deployment Trade-Offs

The diagnostic performance of a model is only one of the evaluation axes. The size of its computation is a measure of its practical feasibility. This discussion reinterprets our architectural decision: we do not optimize latency but achieve a sufficient speed that maximizes diagnostic robustness, a trade-off required by clinical reasoning.

The baseline models determine these two poles. ViT-16, the Vision Transformer, serves as a holistic consultant. It has a self-attention mechanism that provides the global contextual integration required to diagnose pathologies, such as hernias, but with a familiar quadratic computation and memory redundancy. EfficientNetV2 is an expert in localizing

https://doi.org/10.3390/diagnostics16010159

images. Its depthwise convolutional structure is extremely fast at analyzing textures, enabling impressive throughput. However, this emphasis sacrifices the native architecture in support of relational reasoning, which produces an entire radiographic scene.

The coordinated team was our hybrid EfficientNetV2-ViT model. The workflow was designed strategically: the EfficientNetV2 backbone performed high-resolution, efficient feature extraction, and a streamlined ViT module was applied to the refined feature set to provide the necessary global context. We are not free of quadratic complexity; however, we are its possessors. The outcome is a calculated, measurable trade: a modest increase in computational resources over the pure convolutional baseline directly paid for to achieve massive improvements in accuracy, anatomical detail, and explainability in Sections 4.1–4.3.

This balance is crystallized in the practical values in Table 11, which are the results of a direct profiling of our experimental RTX 3060 workstation, run with the NIH ChestX-ray14 input specifications (384 × 384). The inference latency of the hybrid model is approximately twice that of EfficientNetV2, but it maintains a processing rate below 150 ms. This places it squarely in the domain of real-time clinical decision support, where analysis takes only a few seconds. Most importantly, all models have a memory footprint that is a small portion of the available GPU VRAM. The system is not only appropriate for the most minimalistic edge devices, but also has a computational cost that is not only acceptable but also the lifeblood of reliable, interpretable results in the most common use case: a diagnostic assistant on a clinical workstation or PACS terminal.

Profiled on an NVIDIA GeForce RTX 3060 (12 GB VRAM) with a batch size of 1 for a 384 × 384 input.

Table 11. Practical deployment metrics on experimental hardware.

Model	GFLOPs (↓)	Avg. Inference Time (ms) (↓)	Peak GPU VRAM (GB) (↓)	Practical Implication on Target HW
ViT-16 (Base)	~17.6 G	~105–135 ms	~1.5 GB	Provides full global context. Latency suitable for prioritization worklists or non-real-time batch analysis.
EfficientNetV2	~10.0 G	~48–65 ms	~1.1 GB	High-throughput screening engine. Ideal for fast triage or primary reads where ultimate speed is prioritized.
Proposed Hybrid	~14.2 G	~75–100 ms	~1.6 GB	Optimal clinical decision support. The ~30–35 ms premium over EfficientNet buys the integrated reasoning necessary for complex case analysis, with latency low enough for interactive use.

5. Discussion

To move towards the automated diagnosis of chest X-rays, it is necessary to go beyond single-metric solutions and conduct a comprehensive analysis of the system performance and its causes. The systematic analysis presented in this discussion covers four identified dimensions: discriminative performance, architectural mechanism, anatomical validity, and clinical interpretability. This well-organized framework provides a clear comparison of the proposed system with previous methods and outlines the origins of its benefits.

The proposed framework exhibited a regular and quantitatively high performance. Its macro-AUROC of 0.9056 exceeds such strong baselines as ViT-16 (0.8460) and Efficient-

https://doi.org/10.3390/diagnostics16010159

NetV2 (0.8539). More importantly, this benefit is clinically relevant. Pathologies that require the formation of local and general information are the most effective in this regard. To clarify, to diagnose hernia (AUROC 0.9711), a diaphragmatic discontinuity should be localized and placed in the context of the thoracic cavity, which pure CNNs (ResNet-50:0.8091) fail to do. In contrast, edge-defined pathologies, such as pneumothorax, use convolutional baselines, which demonstrates that the evaluation is objective. This trend supports the model's ability to generalize across variations in radiological signatures.

The value of each component was systematically isolated, as shown in the ablation study (Table 9). The single-backbone models exhibit pairwise blind spots: EfficientNetV2 is stronger at texture and weaker at relational reasoning, whereas ViT is stronger at context and weaker at subtle focal cues. Their combination showed the first significant performance jump (AUROC 0.8821), demonstrating the synergy between local and global representations.

A critical qualitative change was achieved when anatomical guidance was added through CheXmask supervision. Although the increase in its AUROC was not significant, it trained the model's gaze, holding feature learning to physiologically consistent regions and discouraging attention to spurious artifacts. The role of the neuro-symbolic layer is different: the insignificant influence on the result of the AUC is not accidental but predetermined by the nature of its activity, which is the stabilization of meaning rather than optimization. It converts spatially grounded activations into audible diagnostic logic, converting the system's prediction into an organized argument.

The lack of anatomical plausibility enforcement is a frequent failure mode in previous studies. This is a fundamental limitation of our system. Table 7 presents quantitative measures, including significant Intersection over Anatomical Mask (IoAM) scores, which provide systematic evidence. An example of an IoAM of 0.97 for pneumothorax shows that 97% of the model's saliency is within the pleural space, where pathology occurs. This turns the heatmaps, which are rough visual indicators, into anatomically constrained evidence that can be quantified and directly answers the diagnostic question with rigorous quantification.

Although explainability is commonly added as a post hoc visualization in earlier literature (Table 12), it is embedded to generate reasoning as constitutive. The translations of anatomically filtered Grad-CAM activations into fuzzy symbolic predicates (e.g., high_basal_pleural_activation) were compared with the radiological ontology. This provides explicit inferences, as shown in Figure 4. The outcome is a three-way agreement between numerical confidence, spatial evidence, and symbolic logic, which boosts transparency and clinical trust without artificially inflating performance indicators.

The systematic review in Table 12 indicates an ongoing integration gap. CNN-based studies are oriented toward loss optimization and are not anatomically enforced. Transformer and multimodal models are better than context but do not engage in organ-level reasoning. None of the above methods simultaneously provide the three of (1) hybrid local/global perception, (2) quantifiable anatomy-constrained saliency, and (3) neuromimetic translation to clinical logic. This is the only architecture that we have proposed.

External validation revealed instructive shifts in the distribution. Performance degradation was most pronounced for pneumothorax (AUROC 0.76) and cardiomegaly (0.80), pathologies highly sensitive to institutional differences in radiographic technique, patient positioning, and labeling granularity. This specific pattern of decline, contrasted with stable performance on consolidation (0.93), confirms that the model learned robust anatomical semantics rather than dataset-specific artifacts, highlighting both its generalizability and the very real challenge of cross-institutional label harmonization.

https://doi.org/10.3390/diagnostics16010159

This framework contributes to field development in several proven directions. These significant performance gains are based on anatomy and are driven by observable architectural mechanisms.

Table 12. Comparative analysis of deep learning-based chest X-ray diagnostic systems with respect to explainability and ontology integration.

Author	Dataset	Methodology	Result	XAI	Ontology
Baltruschat et al. [19]	ChestX-ray14	ResNet-38, ResNet-50, ResNet-101 (from scratch vs. fine-tuning)	AUC: 82.2% (ResNet-50, fine-tuned)	Grad-CAM reveals shortcut learning (e.g., chest drains)	Not specified
Kufel et al. [21]	ChestX-ray14	EfficientNet backbone + Global Average Pooling, Dense, Batch Normalization	AUC: 84%	Grad-CAM	Not specified
Huang et al. [23]	CheXpert (training), RSNA Pneumonia, SIIM Pneumothorax	GLoRIA: multimodal global–local representation learning (ResNet-50 + BioClinicalBERT)	AUC: 88%	Attention maps linking text and image regions	Not specified (paired reports required)
Chen et al. [24]	ChestX-ray14	ResNet-50 vs. EfficientNet-B5 vs. CoAtNet-0-rw	AUROC: 84% (CoAtNet-0-rw)	Group-CAM heatmaps (some incorrect localizations)	Not specified
Hanif et al. [25]	ChestX-ray14	Fine-tuned DenseNet-121	AUC: 80.96%	Grad-CAM	Not specified
Chehade et al. [26]	ChestX-ray14 (binary classification)	DenseNet-121 with CBAM attention module	AUC: 84.96%	Disease localization visualization (technique not specified)	Not specified (only clinical variables: age, sex, view)
DSouza et al. [28]	ChestX-ray14	Fine-tuned ResNet-34	AUC: 84%	Not specified	Not specified
Souid et al. [29]	ChestX-ray14	Fine-tuned MobileNetV2	AUC: 81.10%	Not specified	Not specified
Chen et al. [30]	ChestX-ray14	ResNet-50 + DenseNet-121 vs. ResNet-101 + DenseNet-169	AUC: 82%	Not specified	Not specified
Ho et al. [31]	ChestX-ray14	Fine-tuned DenseNet-121	AUC: 80.97%	Not specified	Not specified
Albahli et al. [32]	ChestX-ray14	InceptionResNetV2	AUC: 80%	Not specified	Not specified
Proposed system	**ChestX-ray14**	**Proposed hybrid CNN–ViT with integrated Grad-CAM and neuro-symbolic reasoning**	**AUROC of 0.9056 and accuracy of 93.9%**	**Anatomically aligned Grad-CAM and neuro-symbolic reasoning layer**	**Radiological ontology with fuzzy logic-based neuro-symbolic reasoning**

There are considerable performance gains, grounded in anatomy, and are a result of observable architectural mechanisms, not incidental tuning. The system closes the gap between high accuracy and clinical intelligibility by systematically linking the enhancement of perception with the discipline of anatomy and symbolic reasoning, providing a strong and reliable roadmap for diagnostic support.

Future work will enable the model to expand beyond still images through longitudinal studies, the integration of multimedia with clinical texts, adaptive ontology models that benefit from radiologists' corrections, and future trials in which accuracy, not precision, guides human–AI collaboration.

6. Conclusions

This study presents a detailed diagnostic model that can provide clinically relevant and precise predictions of thoracic disease. The system combines the high spatial fidelity of radiographic relationships and long-range, anatomy-guided segmentation with enhanced EfficientNetV2 and Vision Transformer encoders and includes small, local textures. The multi-scale fusion mechanism maintains sensitivity for diagnosing focal abnormalities and diffuse parenchymal changes. Class-balanced Focal Loss and adaptive thresholding address the strong asymmetry and label noise in NIH14. The performance achieved, that is, the macro-AUROC 0.9056 and macro-accuracy 93.91%, is indicative of a confident and consistent learning procedure for all 14 classes. One of the achievements of the current study is the explicit interpretability pipeline. Anatomically aligned Grad-CAM maps remove non-thoracic artifacts and enable clinicians to determine whether the model attention aligns with the expected disease loci. These aligned activation patterns are then converted by neuro-symbolic reasoning and ontology-based inference systems into structured diagnostic claims, which provide a clear pathway between pixel-based evidence and clinical explanation. Such coordination between neural and symbolic reasoning reduces the gap between AI decision-making and radiological practice, providing clinicians with a verifiable and audit-compliant account of each prediction. CheXpert was externally verified and found to be robust to institutional and annotation differences, demonstrating resistance to institutional variability and different annotation conventions, suggesting that it can be applied across a variety of settings. However, there are still limitations, such as the use of 2D frontal radiographs, the lack of temporal progression analysis, and sensitivity to label noise in weakly monitored datasets. However, the framework demonstrates a way to achieve trustworthy medical AI by integrating a high level of diagnostic accuracy with anatomical foundations and semantically sound reasoning.

Author Contributions: Conceptualization, N.A., G.A., A.A. and M.S.; methodology, N.A., G.A. and A.A.; software, N.A. and G.A.; validation, N.A., G.A., M.S. and A.A.; formal analysis, N.A., G.A. and M.S.; investigation, G.A., N.A. and A.A.; resources, N.A., M.S. and A.A.; data curation, G.A., N.A., M.S. and A.A.; writing—original draft preparation N.A.; writing—review and editing, N.A., G.A. and A.A.; visualization, N.A., G.A., A.A. and M.S.; supervision, G.A., N.A. and A.A.; project administration, G.A. and N.A.; funding acquisition, G.A., N.A. and A.A. All authors have read and agreed to the published version of the manuscript.

Funding: The project was funded by KAU Endowment (WAQF) at King Abdulaziz University, Jeddah, Saudi Arabia. The authors, therefore, acknowledge with thanks WAQF and the Deanship of Scientific Research (DSR) for technical and financial support.

Institutional Review Board Statement: All data are de-identified in compliance with the Health Insurance Portability and Accountability Act (HIPAA). The dataset is made available under a research license for non-commercial use, ensuring patient confidentiality while promoting reproducible medical AI research.

https://doi.org/10.3390/diagnostics16010159

Informed Consent Statement: Not applicable.

Data Availability Statement: Supporting data for the proposed methodologies for diagnosing thoracic diseases were obtained from the NIH ChestX-ray14, which researchers can use to apply their proposed systems. This data was publicly available online at the following link: https://www.kaggle.com/datasets/nih-chest-xrays/data (accessed on 28 January 2025).

Acknowledgments: We thank King Abdulaziz University for its continuous support over the years.

Conflicts of Interest: The authors declare no conflicts of interest.

References

1. Gould, G.S.; Hurst, J.R.; Trofor, A.; Alison, J.A.; Fox, G.; Kulkarni, M.M.; Wheelock, C.E.; Clarke, M.; Kumar, R. Recognising the importance of chronic lung disease: A consensus statement from the Global Alliance for Chronic Diseases (Lung Diseases group). *Respir. Res.* **2023**, *24*, 15. [CrossRef] [PubMed]
2. Boers, E.; Barrett, M.; Su, J.G.; Benjafield, A.V.; Sinha, S.; Kaye, L.; Zar, H.J.; Vuong, V.; Tellez, D.; Gondalia, R.; et al. Global Burden of Chronic Obstructive Pulmonary Disease Through 2050. *JAMA Netw. Open* **2023**, *6*, e2346598. [CrossRef] [PubMed]
3. Zou, X.L.; Ren, Y.; Yang, H.; Zou, M.; Meng, P.; Zhang, L.; Gong, M.; Ding, W.; Han, L.; Zhang, T. Screening and staging of chronic obstructive pulmonary disease with deep learning based on chest X-ray images and clinical parameters. *BMC Pulm. Med.* **2024**, *24*, 153. [CrossRef] [PubMed]
4. Alshmrani, G.M.M.; Ni, Q.; Jiang, R.; Pervaiz, H.; Elshennawy, N.M. A deep learning architecture for multi-class lung diseases classification using chest X-ray (CXR) images. *Alex. Eng. J.* **2023**, *64*, 923–935. [CrossRef]
5. Alghamdi, N.S.; Zakariah, M.; Karamti, H. A deep CNN-based acoustic model for the identification of lung diseases utilizing extracted MFCC features from respiratory sounds. *Multimed. Tools Appl.* **2024**, *83*, 82871–82903. [CrossRef]
6. Abdulahi, A.R.T.; Ogundokun, R.O.; Adenike, A.R.; Shah, M.A.; Ahmed, Y.K. PulmoNet: A novel deep learning based pulmonary diseases detection model. *BMC Med. Imaging* **2024**, *24*, 51. [CrossRef]
7. Souid, A.; Sakli, H.; Hamroun, M.; Abdelkarim, M.N.; Othman, S.B. Fast-Staged CNN Model for Accurate Pulmonary Diseases and Lung Cancer Detection. December 2024. Available online: https://arxiv.org/pdf/2412.11681 (accessed on 3 November 2025).
8. Siebert, J.N.; Hartley, M.-A.; Courvoisier, D.S.; Salamin, M.; Robotham, L.; Doenz, J.; Barazzone-Argiroffo, C.; Gervaix, A.; Bridevaux, P.-O. Deep learning diagnostic and severity-stratification for interstitial lung diseases and chronic obstructive pulmonary disease in digital lung auscultations and ultrasonography: Clinical protocol for an observational case–control study. *BMC Pulm. Med.* **2023**, *23*, 191. [CrossRef]
9. Radiomics-Guided 3D CNN-Vision Transformer (Rad-CNNViT) Ensemble to Diagnose Pulmonary Sarcoidosis from CT. Available online: https://www.spiedigitallibrary.org/conference-proceedings-of-spie/12926/129260J/Radiomics-guided-3D-CNN-vision-transformer-Rad-CNNViT-ensemble-to/10.1117/12.3005429.full (accessed on 3 November 2025).
10. Qiu, J.; Mitra, J.; Ghose, S.; Dumas, C.; Yang, J.; Sarachan, B.; Judson, M.A. A Multichannel CT and Radiomics-Guided CNN-ViT (RadCT-CNNViT) Ensemble Network for Diagnosis of Pulmonary Sarcoidosis. *Diagnostics* **2024**, *14*, 1049. [CrossRef]
11. Chibuike, O.; Yang, X. Convolutional Neural Network–Vision Transformer Architecture with Gated Control Mechanism and Multi-Scale Fusion for Enhanced Pulmonary Disease Classification. *Diagnostics* **2024**, *14*, 2790. [CrossRef]
12. Basnet, P.S.; Chitrakar, R. CNN-ViT Hybrid for Pneumonia Detection: Theory and Empiric on Limited Data without Pretraining. September 2025. Available online: https://arxiv.org/pdf/2509.08586 (accessed on 3 November 2025).
13. Hamdi, M.; Senan, E.M.; Jadhav, M.E.; Olayah, F.; Awaji, B.; Alalayah, K.M. Hybrid Models Based on Fusion Features of a CNN and Handcrafted Features for Accurate Histopathological Image Analysis for Diagnosing Malignant Lymphomas. *Diagnostics* **2023**, *13*, 2258. [CrossRef]
14. Sabir, S.; Maqbool, F.; Razzaq, M.S.; Shah, D.; Ali, S.; Tahir, M.; Shehzad, H.M.F. Semantic web-based ontology: A comprehensive framework for cardiovascular knowledge representation. *BMC Cardiovasc. Disord.* **2025**, *25*, 519. [CrossRef]
15. Kreuzthaler, M.; Brochhausen, M.; Zayas, C.; Blobel, B.; Schulz, S. Linguistic and ontological challenges of multiple domains contributing to transformed health ecosystems. *Front. Med.* **2023**, *10*, 1073313. [CrossRef] [PubMed]
16. Carmody, L.C.; Gargano, M.A.; Toro, S.; Vasilevsky, N.A.; Adam, M.P.; Blau, H.; Chan, L.E.; Gomez-Andres, D.; Horvath, R.; Kraus, M.L.; et al. The Medical Action Ontology: A tool for annotating and analyzing treatments and clinical management of human disease. *Med* **2023**, *4*, 913–927.e3. [CrossRef]
17. Soysal, O.A.; Guzel, M.S.; Dikmen, M.; Bostanci, G.E. Common Thorax Diseases Recognition Using Zero-Shot Learning With Ontology in the Multi-Labeled ChestX-ray14 Data Set. *IEEE Access* **2023**, *11*, 27883–27892. [CrossRef]
18. Yanar, E.; Kutan, F.; Ayturan, K.; Kutbay, U.; Algın, O.; Hardalaç, F.; Ağıldere, A.M. A Comparative Analysis of the Mamba, Transformer, and CNN Architectures for Multi-Label Chest X-Ray Anomaly Detection in the NIH ChestX-Ray14 Dataset. *Diagnostics* **2025**, *15*, 2215. [CrossRef] [PubMed]

https://doi.org/10.3390/diagnostics16010159

19. Baltruschat, I.M.; Nickisch, H.; Grass, M.; Knopp, T.; Saalbach, A. Comparison of Deep Learning Approaches for Multi-Label Chest X-Ray Classification. *Sci. Rep.* **2019**, *9*, 6381. [CrossRef] [PubMed]
20. Jain, A.; Bhardwaj, A.; Murali, K.; Surani, I. A Comparative Study of CNN, ResNet, and Vision Transformers for Multi-Classification of Chest Diseases. May 2024. Available online: https://arxiv.org/pdf/2406.00237 (accessed on 30 October 2025).
21. Kufel, J.; Bielówka, M.; Rojek, M.; Mitręga, A.; Lewandowski, P.; Cebula, M.; Krawczyk, D.; Bielówka, M.; Kondoł, D.; Bargieł-Łączek, K.; et al. Multi-Label Classification of Chest X-ray Abnormalities Using Transfer Learning Techniques. *J. Pers. Med.* **2023**, *13*, 1426. [CrossRef] [PubMed]
22. Goel, R.; Nath, U.; Wang, Y.; Silva, A.C.; Wu, T.; Yang, Y. Learning Low-Rank Feature for Thorax Disease Classification. February 2024. Available online: https://arxiv.org/pdf/2404.18933 (accessed on 30 October 2025).
23. Huang, S.-C.; Shen, L.; Lungren, M.P.; Yeung, S. GLoRIA: A Multimodal Global-Local Representation Learning Framework for Label-Efficient Medical Image Recognition. 2021. Available online: https://github.com/marshuang80/gloria (accessed on 30 October 2025).
24. Chen, Y.; Wan, Y.; Pan, F. Enhancing Multi-disease Diagnosis of Chest X-rays with Advanced Deep-learning Networks in Real-world Data. *J. Digit. Imaging* **2023**, *36*, 1332–1347. [CrossRef]
25. Hanif, M.S.; Bilal, M.; Alsaggaf, A.H.; Al-Saggaf, U.M. Enhancing Multi-Label Chest X-Ray Classification Using an Improved Ranking Loss. *Bioengineering* **2025**, *12*, 593. [CrossRef]
26. Chehade, A.H.; Abdallah, N.; Marion, J.M.; Hatt, M.; Oueidat, M.; Chauvet, P. Advancing chest X-ray diagnostics: A novel CycleGAN-based preprocessing approach for enhanced lung disease classification in ChestX-Ray14. *Comput. Methods Programs Biomed.* **2025**, *259*, 108518. [CrossRef]
27. Fusion of X-Ray Images and Clinical Data for A Multimodal Deep Learning Prediction Model of Osteoporosis: Algorithm Development and Validation Study | Paper Digest. Available online: https://www.paperdigest.org/paper/?paper_id=pubmed-40966528 (accessed on 30 October 2025).
28. Automated Identification of Thoracic Pathology from Chest Radiographs with Enhanced Training Pipeline. Available online: https://www.spiedigitallibrary.org/conference-proceedings-of-spie/10950/109503F/Automated-identification-of-thoracic-pathology-from-chest-radiographs-with-enhanced/10.1117/12.2512600.full (accessed on 30 October 2025).
29. Souid, A.; Sakli, N.; Sakli, H. Classification and Predictions of Lung Diseases from Chest X-rays Using MobileNet V2. *Appl. Sci.* **2021**, *11*, 2751. [CrossRef]
30. Chen, B.; Li, J.; Guo, X.; Lu, G. DualCheXNet: Dual asymmetric feature learning for thoracic disease classification in chest X-rays. *Biomed. Signal Process Control* **2019**, *53*, 101554. [CrossRef]
31. Ho, T.K.K.; Gwak, J. Multiple Feature Integration for Classification of Thoracic Disease in Chest Radiography. *Appl. Sci.* **2019**, *9*, 4130. [CrossRef]
32. Albahli, S.; Rauf, H.T.; Algosaibi, A.; Balas, V.E. AI-driven deep CNN approach for multi-label pathology classification using chest X-Rays. *PeerJ Comput. Sci.* **2021**, *7*, e495. [CrossRef]
33. Wang, X.; Peng, Y.; Lu, L.; Lu, Z.; Bagheri, M.; Summers, R.M. ChestX-ray8: Hospital-Scale Chest X-Ray Database and Benchmarks on Weakly-Supervised Classification and Localization of Common Thorax Diseases. In Proceedings of the IEEE Conference on Computer Vision and Pattern Recognition, Honolulu, HI, USA, 21–26 July 2017.
34. NIH Chest X-Rays. Available online: https://www.kaggle.com/datasets/nih-chest-xrays/data (accessed on 21 November 2025).
35. Arora, R.; Saini, I.; Sood, N. Multi-Label Classification of Thoracic Diseases Using Structured Deep Learning Framework. *Biomed. Eng. Appl. Basis Commun.* **2024**, *36*, 2450006. [CrossRef]
36. Oommen, L.; Nagajyothi, C.N.; Chebrolu, S. Conv-attention ViT for classification of multi-label class imbalanced data of lung thoracic diseases. *Multimed. Tools Appl.* **2024**, *84*, 21747–21776. [CrossRef]
37. Alshanketi, F.; Alharbi, A.; Kuruvilla, M.; Mahzoon, V.; Siddiqui, S.T.; Rana, N.; Tahir, A. Pneumonia Detection from Chest X-Ray Images Using Deep Learning and Transfer Learning for Imbalanced Datasets. *J. Imaging Inform. Med.* **2024**, *38*, 2021–2040. [CrossRef]
38. Taneja, P.; Sharma, A.; Singh, M. Performance Evaluation of CNN Architectures on NIH Chest X-Ray Dataset with Boosting Ensemble. In *International Conference on Parallel, Distributed and Grid Computing, PDGC*; IEEE: New York, NY, USA, 2024; pp. 505–509. [CrossRef]
39. Khalid, A.; Senan, E.M.; Al-Wagih, K.; Al-Azzam, M.M.A.; Alkhraisha, Z.M. Hybrid Techniques of X-ray Analysis to Predict Knee Osteoarthritis Grades Based on Fusion Features of CNN and Handcrafted. *Diagnostics* **2023**, *13*, 1609. [CrossRef]
40. Aljohani, N.R.; Fayoumi, A.; Hassan, S.U. A novel focal-loss and class-weight-aware convolutional neural network for the classification of in-text citations. *J. Inf. Sci.* **2023**, *49*, 79–92. [CrossRef]
41. Yang, C. A Focal Loss-based Multi-layer Perceptron for Diagnosis of Cardiovascular Risk in Athletes. *Int. J. Adv. Comput. Sci. Appl.* **2023**, *14*, 1158. [CrossRef]

42. Maurya, R.; Thirwarni, P.; Gopalakrishnan, T.; Karnati, M. Combining Focal loss with Cross-entropy loss for Pneumonia Classification with a Weighted Sampling Approach. In Proceedings of the 2024 IEEE International Conference on Interdisciplinary Approaches in Technology and Management for Social Innovation, IATMSI 2024, Gwalior, India, 14–16 March 2024. [CrossRef]
43. Ahmed, I.A.; Senan, E.M.; Shatnawi, H.S.A.; Alkhraisha, Z.M.; Al-Azzam, M.M.A. Multi-Models of Analyzing Dermoscopy Images for Early Detection of Multi-Class Skin Lesions Based on Fused Features. *Processes* **2023**, *11*, 910. [CrossRef]
44. Saifullah, S.; Dreżewski, R. Advanced Medical Image Segmentation Enhancement: A Particle-Swarm-Optimization-Based Histogram Equalization Approach. *Appl. Sci.* **2024**, *14*, 923. [CrossRef]
45. Al-Jabbar, M.; Alshahrani, M.; Senan, E.M.; Ahmed, I.A. Analyzing Histological Images Using Hybrid Techniques for Early Detection of Multi-Class Breast Cancer Based on Fusion Features of CNN and Handcrafted. *Diagnostics* **2023**, *13*, 1753. [CrossRef] [PubMed]
46. Nia, S.N.; Shih, F.Y. Medical X-Ray Image Enhancement Using Global Contrast-Limited Adaptive Histogram Equalization. *Int. J. Pattern Recognit. Artif. Intell.* **2024**, *38*, 2457010. [CrossRef]
47. Buriboev, A.S.; Abduvaitov, A.; Jeon, H.S. Binary Classification of Pneumonia in Chest X-Ray Images Using Modified Contrast-Limited Adaptive Histogram Equalization Algorithm. *Sensors* **2025**, *25*, 3976. [CrossRef]
48. Gangwar, S.; Devi, R.; Mat Isa, N.A. Optimized exposer region-based modified adaptive histogram equalization method for contrast enhancement in CXR imaging. *Sci. Rep.* **2025**, *15*, 6693. [CrossRef]
49. Huang, Y.; Meng, Z. *Highly Accurate Four Class Prediction of Lung Diseases from Chest X-Ray Images Based on Efficientnetv2*; SSRN: Rochester, NY, USA, 2025. [CrossRef]
50. Ko, J.; Park, S.; Woo, H.G. Optimization of vision transformer-based detection of lung diseases from chest X-ray images. *BMC Med. Inform. Decis. Mak.* **2024**, *24*, 191. [CrossRef]
51. Saha, S.; Kumar, A.; Nandi, D. ViT-ILD: A Vision Transformer-based Neural Network for Detection of Interstitial Lung Disease from CT Images. *Procedia Comput. Sci.* **2024**, *235*, 779–788. [CrossRef]
52. Dayan, B. Lung Disease Detection with Vision Transformers: A Comparative Study of Machine Learning Methods. November 2024. Available online: https://arxiv.org/pdf/2411.11376 (accessed on 3 November 2025).
53. Hamdi, M.; Senan, E.M.; Awaji, B.; Olayah, F.; Jadhav, M.E.; Alalayah, K.M. Analysis of WSI Images by Hybrid Systems with Fusion Features for Early Diagnosis of Cervical Cancer. *Diagnostics* **2023**, *13*, 2538. [CrossRef]
54. Gaggion, N.; Mosquera, C.; Mansilla, L.; Saidman, J.M.; Aineseder, M.; Milone, D.H.; Ferrante, E. CheXmask: A large-scale dataset of anatomical segmentation masks for multi-center chest x-ray images. *Sci. Data* **2024**, *11*, 511. [CrossRef]
55. Golec, M.; Kamdar, M.; Barteit, S. Comprehensive Ontology of Fibroproliferative Diseases: Protocol for a Semantic Technology Study. *JMIR Res. Protoc.* **2023**, *12*, e48645. [CrossRef] [PubMed]
56. Ning, J.; Marshall, D.; Gao, Y.; Xing, X.; Nan, Y.; Fang, Y.; Zhang, S.; Komorowski, M.; Yang, G. Unpaired translation of chest X-ray images for lung opacity diagnosis via adaptive activation masks and cross-domain alignment. *Pattern Recognit. Lett.* **2025**, *193*, 21–28. [CrossRef]
57. Choi, Y.; Lee, H. Interpretation of lung disease classification with light attention connected module. *Biomed. Signal Process Control* **2023**, *84*, 104695. [CrossRef] [PubMed]
58. Wollek, A.; Graf, R.; Čečatka, S.; Fink, N.; Willem, T.; Sabel, B.O.; Lasser, T. Attention-based Saliency Maps Improve Interpretability of Pneumothorax Classification. *Radiol. Artif. Intell.* **2023**, *5*, e220187. [CrossRef] [PubMed]
59. Qiu, Z.; Rivaz, H.; Xiao, Y. Is Visual Explanation with Grad-CAM More Reliable for Deeper Neural Networks? A Case Study with Automatic Pneumothorax Diagnosis. In *Lecture Notes in Computer Science (Including Subseries Lecture Notes in Artificial Intelligence and Lecture Notes in Bioinformatics)*; Springer: Cham, Switzerland, 2024; Volume 14349 LNCS, pp. 224–233. [CrossRef]
60. Ahmed, I.A.; Senan, E.M.; Shatnawi, H.S.; Kansal, K. Analysis of histopathological images for early diagnosis of oral squamous cell carcinoma by hybrid systems based on CNN fusion features. *Int. J. Intell. Syst.* **2023**, *2023*, 2662719. [CrossRef]
61. Kumaran, S.Y.; Jeya, J.J.; Mahesh, T.R.; Khan, S.B.; Alzahrani, S.; Alojail, M. Explainable lung cancer classification with ensemble transfer learning of VGG16, Resnet50 and InceptionV3 using grad-cam. *BMC Med. Imaging* **2024**, *24*, 176. [CrossRef]
62. Vanitha, K.; Mahesh, T.R.; Kumar, V.V.; Guluwadi, S. Enhanced tuberculosis detection using Vision Transformers and explainable AI with a Grad-CAM approach on chest X-rays. *BMC Med. Imaging* **2025**, *25*, 96. [CrossRef] [PubMed]
63. Ullah, I.; Ali, F.; Shah, B.; El-Sappagh, S.; Abuhmed, T.; Park, S.H. A deep learning based dual encoder–decoder framework for anatomical structure segmentation in chest X-ray images. *Sci. Rep.* **2023**, *13*, 791. [CrossRef]
64. Basavaraju, B.K.; Masum, M. LSE-Net: Integrated Segmentation and Ensemble Deep Learning for Enhanced Lung Disease Classification. *Electronics* **2025**, *14*, 2407. [CrossRef]
65. Lu, S.Y.; Zhu, Z.; Zhang, Y.D.; Yao, Y.D. Tuberculosis and pneumonia diagnosis in chest X-rays by large adaptive filter and aligning normalized network with report-guided multi-level alignment. *Eng. Appl. Artif. Intell.* **2025**, *158*, 111575. [CrossRef]
66. Iqbal, A.; Qureshi, S.; Chishti, M.A. EHealth Innovation for Chronic Obstructive Pulmonary Disease: A Context-Aware Comprehensive Framework. *Scalable Comput. Pract. Exp.* **2024**, *25*, 1424–1441. [CrossRef]

https://doi.org/10.3390/diagnostics16010159

67. Spoladore, D.; Colombo, V.; Fumagalli, A.; Tosi, M.; Lorenzini, E.C.; Sacco, M. An Ontology-Based Decision Support System for Tailored Clinical Nutrition Recommendations for Patients With Chronic Obstructive Pulmonary Disease: Development and Acceptability Study. *JMIR Med. Inform.* **2024**, *12*, e50980. [CrossRef] [PubMed]
68. Zeshan, F.; Ahmad, A.; Babar, M.I.; Hamid, M.; Hajjej, F.; Ashraf, M. An IoT-Enabled Ontology-Based Intelligent Healthcare Framework for Remote Patient Monitoring. *IEEE Access* **2023**, *11*, 133947–133966. [CrossRef]
69. Shoaip, N.; El-Sappagh, S.; Abuhmed, T.; Elmogy, M. A dynamic fuzzy rule-based inference system using fuzzy inference with semantic reasoning. *Sci. Rep.* **2024**, *14*, 4275. [CrossRef]
70. Domingues, N.S. A hybrid decision support system using rule-based and AI methods: The OnCATs knowledge-based framework. *Int. J. Med. Inform.* **2026**, *206*, 106144. [CrossRef]
71. Navin, K.; Krishnan, M. Fuzzy rule based classifier model for evidence based clinical decision support systems. *Intell. Syst. Appl.* **2024**, *22*, 200393. [CrossRef]

https://doi.org/10.3390/diagnostics16010159

diagnostics

MDPI

Article

External Validation of an Artificial Intelligence Triaging System for Chest X-Rays: A Retrospective Independent Clinical Study

André Coutinho Castilla [1,*], Iago de Paiva D'Amorim [2], Maria Fernanda Barbosa Wanderley [1], Mateus Aragão Esmeraldo [3], André Ricca Yoshida [1], Anthony Moreno Eigier [1] and Márcio Valente Yamada Sawamura [2]

1 NeuralMed A2 Tecnologia Ltda., Rua Pe João Manoel 1212, Cj 41, São Paulo 01411-010, SP, Brazil; nandaw@gmail.com (M.F.B.W.); andre.yoshida@neuralmed.com (A.R.Y.); a@neuralmed.com (A.M.E.)

2 Department of Radiology and Oncology, Hospital das Clínicas, Faculdade de Medicina, Universidade de São Paulo (HCFMUSP), Av. Dr. Enéas de Carvalho Aguiar 255, São Paulo 05403-000, SP, Brazil; iago.damorim@hc.fm.usp.br (I.d.P.D.); marcio.sawamura@hc.fm.usp.br (M.V.Y.S.)

3 Department of Radiology, Stanford University School of Medicine, Palo Alto, CA 94305, USA; mateusesmeraldo3@gmail.com

* Correspondence: andre@neuralmed.com

Abstract

Background: Chest radiography (CXR) is the most frequently performed radiological exam worldwide, but reporting backlogs, caused by a shortage of radiologists, remain a critical challenge in emergency care. Artificial intelligence (AI) triage systems can help alleviate this challenge by differentiating normal from abnormal studies and prioritizing urgent cases for review. This study aimed to externally validate TRIA, a commercial AI-powered CXR triage algorithm (NeuralMed, São Paulo, Brazil). **Methods**: TRIA employs a two-stage deep learning approach, comprising an image segmentation module that isolates the thoracic region, followed by a classification model trained to recognize common cardiopulmonary pathologies. We trained the system on 275,399 CXRs from multiple public and private datasets. We performed external validation retrospectively on 1045 CXRs (568 normal and 477 abnormal) from a teaching university hospital that was not used for training. We established ground truth using a large language model (LLM) to extract findings from original radiologist reports. An independent radiologist review of a 300-report subset confirmed the reliability of this method, achieving an accuracy of 0.98 (95% CI 0.978–0.988). We compared four ensemble decision strategies for abnormality detection. Performance metrics included sensitivity, specificity, accuracy, and area under the receiver operating characteristic curve (AUROC) with 95% CI. **Results**: The general abnormality classifier achieved strong performance (AUROC 0.911). Individual pathology models for cardiomegaly, pneumothorax, and effusion showed excellent results (AUROC of 0.968, 0.955, and 0.935, respectively). The weighted ensemble demonstrated the best balance, with an accuracy of 0.854 (95% CI, 0.831–0.874), a sensitivity of 0.845 (0.810–0.875), a specificity of 0.861 (0.830–0.887), and an AUROC of 0.927 (0.911–0.940). Sensitivity-prioritized methods achieving sensitivity >0.92 produced lower specificity (<0.69). False negatives were mainly subtle or equivocal cases, although many were still flagged as abnormal by the general classifier. **Conclusions**: TRIA achieved robust and balanced accuracy in distinguishing normal from abnormal CXRs. Integrating this system into clinical workflows has the potential to reduce reporting delays, prioritize urgent cases, and improve patient safety. These findings support its clinical utility and warrant prospective multicenter validation.

 https://doi.org/10.3390/diagnostics15222899

Keywords: artificial intelligence; chest radiography; triage; external validation; deep learning; radiology; diagnostic accuracy; medical imaging

1. Introduction

Chest radiography (CXR) is the most common radiological examination performed globally and serves as a critical first-line diagnostic tool [1]. However, the growing global demand for imaging, combined with an ongoing shortage of radiologists, often results in substantial reporting backlogs. These delays are particularly critical in emergency department settings, where rapid interpretation is essential for patient management. In many settings, general practitioners and physicians often perform the initial interpretation of CXRs instead of radiologists, which can lead to diagnostic errors or delays due to a potential lack of specialized expertise.

Artificial intelligence (AI) has emerged as a promising approach to addressing these challenges in healthcare. The advent of deep learning, specifically in the form of convolutional neural networks, has enabled the development of diagnostic models that achieve performance levels comparable to those of expert clinicians in various medical imaging tasks [2]. Among the possible impactful applications of AI in radiology is triage, the automated prioritization of medical cases to ensure that critical or abnormal studies receive earlier review by radiologists [3]. A system that can reliably distinguish between normal and abnormal CXRs may enhance physicians' ability to detect abnormalities [4], reduce diagnostic delays, and optimize clinical workflows by directing urgent examinations for immediate specialist evaluation.

This growth has driven substantial investment and regulatory interest in AI-based radiological tools. Radiology now represents the medical specialty with the highest number of approved AI software devices worldwide [5]. As a consequence, rigorous external validation and post-implementation assessment have become imperative to ensure these algorithms perform safely and effectively in diverse real-world clinical environments.

This study aims to conduct an external validation of TRIA, a commercial AI-powered CXR triage system developed by NeuralMed (NeuralMed, São Paulo, Brazil) and registered with the Brazilian Health Regulatory Agency (ANVISA) as a Class II medical device (Register No. 8261971001) [6]. We retrospectively evaluated its performance at the Hospital das Clínicas, Faculty of Medicine, University of São Paulo (HCFMUSP), to determine its diagnostic accuracy in classifying CXRs across seven distinct radiologic findings and in differentiating normal from abnormal studies. We compared the algorithm's predictions with radiologist reports, providing an objective assessment of its clinical reliability. Evaluating algorithmic performance against verified ground truth diverse from its training dataset is a critical step in demonstrating clinical utility and regulatory compliance.

In this article, we describe the development of the TRIA system, its dataset composition, and the evaluation methodology. This work supports ANVISA's requirements for manufacturers to maintain continuous clinical evaluation and post-market surveillance of medical AI devices [7]. NeuralMed funded the study, and the institutional Ethics Committee approved it. The specific aims were to evaluate the overall diagnostic accuracy of TRIA's general abnormality classifier in a dataset independent of that used in training; assess the performance of individual classifiers for key pathologies (e.g., cardiomegaly, pneumothorax, and pleural effusion); compare four ensemble strategies for abnormality detection to identify the optimal balance between sensitivity and specificity for triage use; conduct an error analysis of false negatives to characterize the system's limitations and potential areas for improvement; and compare its performance with similar available tools.

2. Methods

2.1. AI Algorithm (TRIA)

The algorithm was based on a two-stage deep learning approach, which consisted of a lung field segmentation pipeline followed by a pathology classification model. A key design choice in the model's methodology was to prioritize intrathoracic findings related to the cardiopulmonary system, while deprioritizing musculoskeletal and spinal conditions.

2.1.1. Training Dataset

We developed the models using a large-scale, multi-source dataset of 275,399 anonymized, unique chest radiographs. We curated the dataset from public and private sources and featured a multi-label annotation schema (Table 1). Part of the dataset originated from private clinical sources collected under research and commercial agreements in compliance with Brazilian General Data Protection Law [8].

The public datasets included: the Shenzhen Chest X-ray Set [9]; the Indiana University Chest X-ray Collection [10]; the JSRT database from the Japanese Society of Radiological Technology [11]; the NIH ChestX-ray14 dataset [12]; and the PadChest dataset [13]. We utilized all publicly available datasets in accordance with their respective open-access agreements.

Before training, radiologists reviewed and verified the images, applying annotations using a proprietary software application (Figure 1). The dataset exhibited a significant class imbalance, reflecting the real-world prevalence of the pathology. For training binary classifiers, studies with definitive labels (1.0 for present, 0.0 for absent) were used. In contrast, studies with missing labels for a specific finding were excluded from the loss calculation for that task. Table 2 shows the distribution for a selection of key labels. The list of pathologies was selected based on the availability of labeled data, balanced with clinical importance for the ED. The 'normal' and 'abnormal' pools included cases with pathologies beyond the specifically targeted list; these were categorized under the general "yesfinding" class.

Table 1. Number of labeled cases per data source.

Source	Labeled Cases
NIH	111,783
Padchest	109,167
Private	49,866
Indiana	3783
Shenzhen	662
JSRT	246
Montgomery	138
Total Cases	275,399

Table 2. Distribution of labels in the training dataset.

Pathology	Positive Cases	Negative Cases	Total Labeled
No Finding	125,046	150,266	275,312
Opacity	32,053	240,521	272,574
Cardiomegaly	15,915	255,944	271,859
Mass/Nodule	14,527	258,383	272,910
Effusion	5392	266,535	271,927
Pneumothorax	4521	267,408	271,929
Consolidation	2483	110,920	113,403

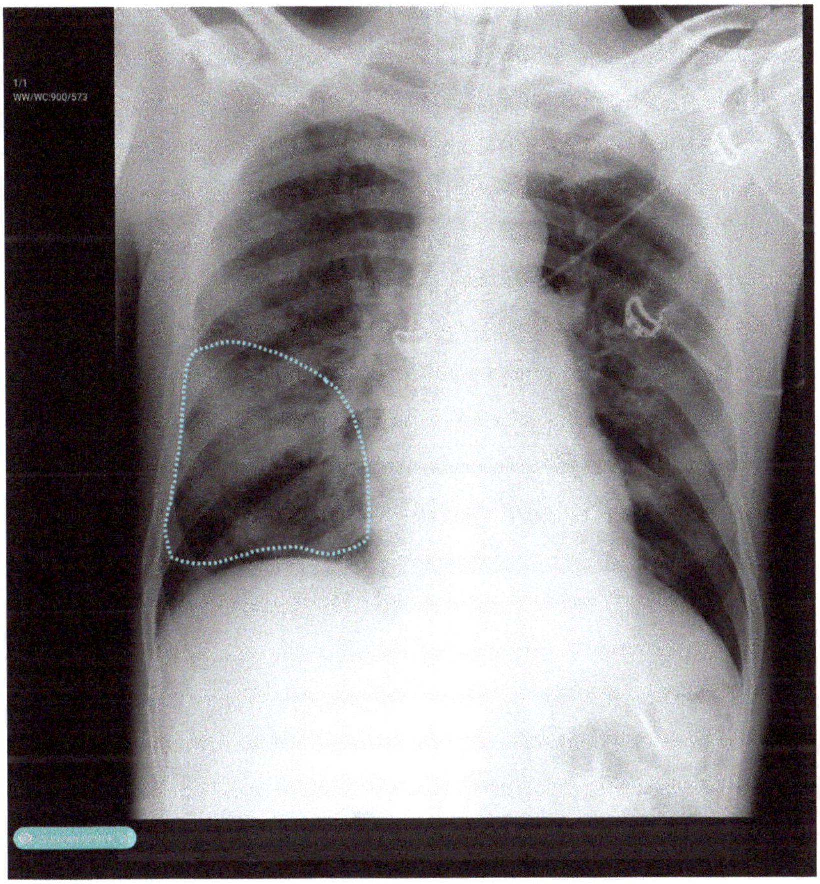

Figure 1. All labeled images were proofed by a radiologist who manually drew a region of interest around the pathology and assigned a finding, as shown here for an alveolar opacity circled by the dashed line.

2.1.2. Algorithm Architecture

The proposed system consisted of two main stages: (1) segmentation of the thoracic region and (2) classification of pathological findings. This modular design improved the model's interpretability, efficiency, and diagnostic precision by separating spatial localization from disease recognition.

We employed a U-Net architecture with a MobileNetV2 backbone to segment the thoracic region and generate a unified "tongue-shaped" mask encompassing both lungs as well as the mediastinal and hilar regions. We chose U-Net for its proven effectiveness in medical image segmentation tasks, where high spatial precision is required. Its encoder–decoder "U" structure enabled the capture of both contextual and spatial information, facilitating the delineation of complex anatomical structures with high resolution. In this study, segmentation was used not only to isolate the relevant pulmonary region but also to constrain the subsequent classifier's focus to clinically meaningful areas, thereby improving accuracy and reducing noise from irrelevant image regions.

We resized input images to 512 $\times$ 512 pixels and performed data augmentation using geometric and photometric transformations (padding, Gaussian noise, CLAHE, brightness/gamma adjustment, blur, motion blur, and hue/saturation shifts). The model was trained for 40 epochs with a batch size of 8 using the Adam optimizer (initial learning rate = 5×10^{-5}) and a composite loss function combining Dice loss and binary focal loss to balance region overlap and class imbalance. Performance was monitored using Intersection over Union and F-score metrics, and the best model was selected by minimizing the validation loss with adaptive learning rate scheduling. Figure 2 illustrates the resulting mask, which ensures inclusion of central thoracic structures.

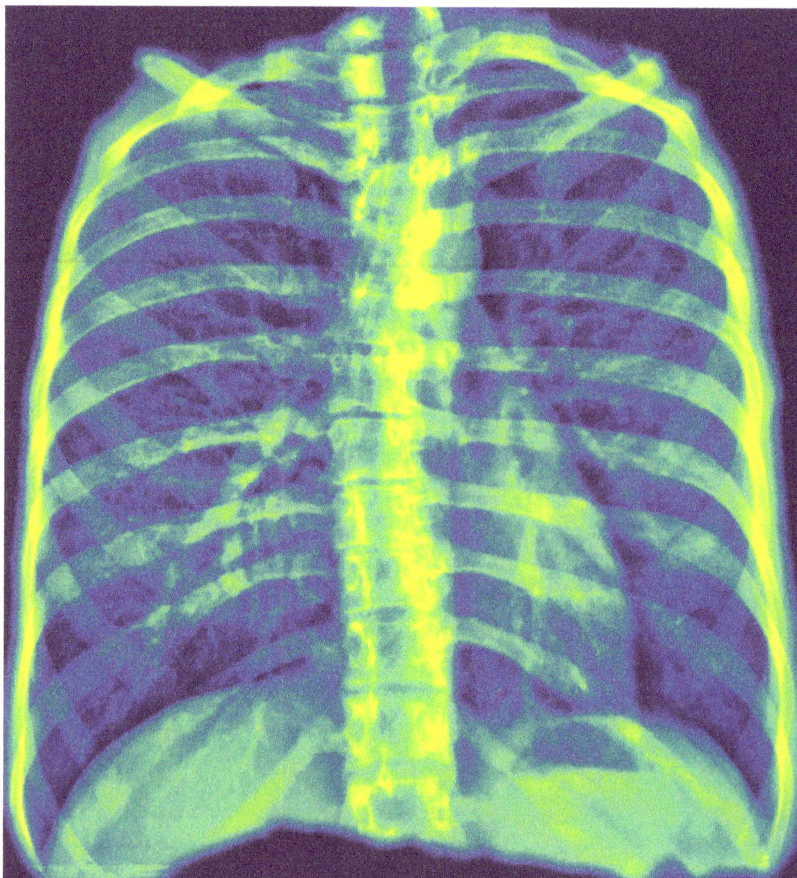

Figure 2. Example of first-stage segmentation: the generated "tongue-shaped" mask covering both lungs and mediastinal structures.

The second stage employed an InceptionResNetV2 convolutional neural network, pre-trained on ImageNet, adapted for binary and multi-class classification of selected thoracic abnormalities. The model's top layers were replaced with custom fully connected layers, optimized for CXR analysis. To balance computational efficiency with diagnostic performance, input images were resized to 75×75 pixels. Data augmentation included random brightness (range 0.3–0.5), rotation ($\leq 35°$), zoom ($\leq 12.5\%$), and rescaling (1/255). Training utilized the Adam optimizer (learning rate = 1×10^{-4}) with binary cross-entropy loss and class weighting to address data imbalance. There were also callbacks for stopping training when no improvement occurred for five epochs, saving the best model during training, and reducing the learning rate when performance plateaued for two epochs. The model's performance was evaluated using accuracy, precision, recall, and area under the receiver operating characteristic curve (AUROC), incorporating Test-Time Augmentation for robust estimation. In this phase, we generated the classification thresholds. All experiments were tracked using MLflow to ensure reproducibility.

To enhance model transparency and validate spatial reasoning, we applied Gradient-weighted Class Activation Mapping (Grad-CAM) to visualize the regions most influential in classification decisions. Grad-CAM served a dual purpose in this context: first, it verified that the model's predictions are based on clinically relevant regions within the segmented thoracic area; second, it contributed to interpretability by generating intuitive heatmaps that highlight the anatomical structures driving the model's output. This step was crucial for improving classification accuracy and verifying that it relied on the correct visual cues, aligning with radiological expectations. For optimization, they were only generated when the classification probability score was above the defined threshold.

Representative Grad-CAM overlays are shown in Figures 3–6, illustrating several different types of pathologies. These visualizations demonstrate where the algorithm focuses attention on the appropriate pathological regions, thereby reinforcing the validity and interpretability of the proposed pipeline.

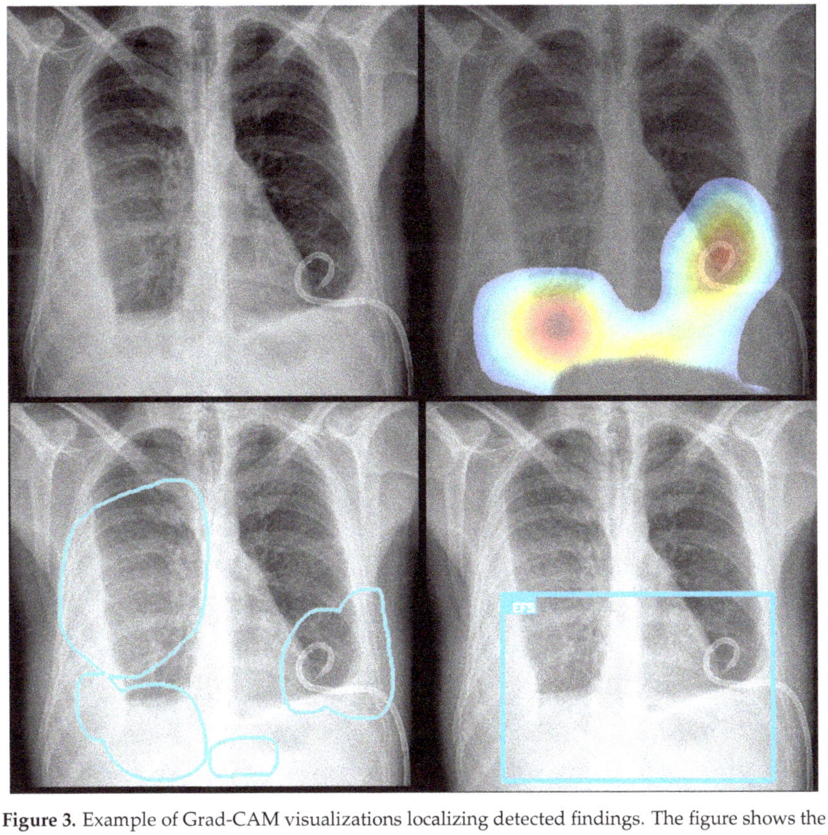

Figure 3. Example of Grad-CAM visualizations localizing detected findings. The figure shows the original image (**top left**) alongside three types of explanatory outputs generated by the algorithm: a heatmap (**top right**), a contour outline (**bottom left**), and a bounding box (**bottom right**). All visualizations are derived from the same process, showcasing different output options.

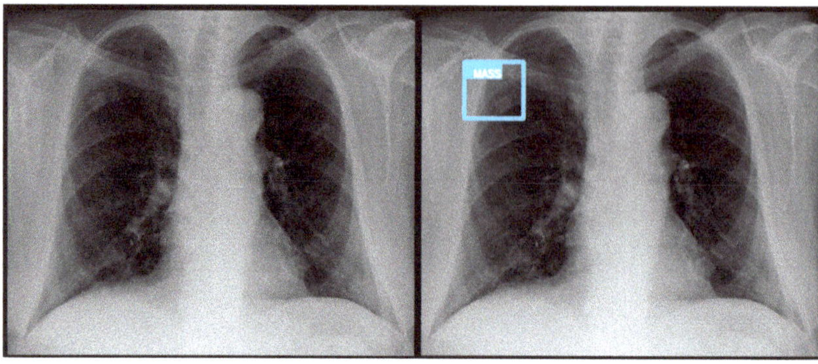

Figure 4. A true positive example of a nodule/mass (**left**) and its bounding box generated image (**right**). In this case, the report indicated opacity; however, the algorithm classified as a mass.

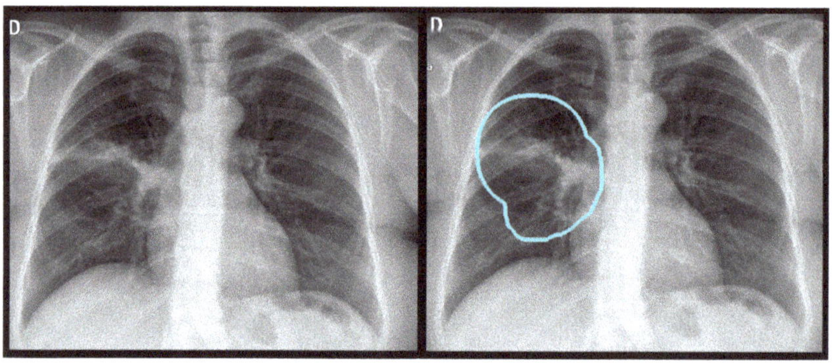

Figure 5. A true positive example of opacity and consolidation (**left**) and its contour line generated image (**right**).

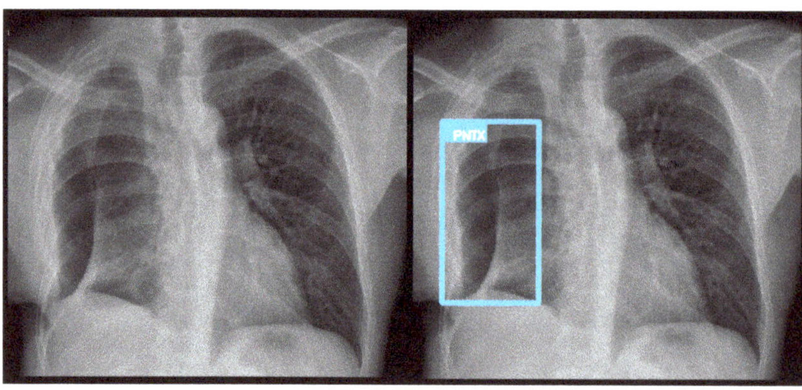

Figure 6. A true positive example of pneumothorax (**left**) and its bounding box generated image (**right**). The algorithm successfully detected pneumothorax without a pleural tube, indicating it is not overfit to post-drainage cases.

All models were developed in Python (Version 3.6.9) using TensorFlow and Keras, with image manipulation performed using OpenCV. Training and validation were executed on GPU hardware to ensure stable convergence and reproducibility.

2.2. Validation Study Design

For validation, we conducted a retrospective, cross-sectional study on a dataset of 1045 anonymized chest radiographs from HCFMUSP, acquired over the past five years. Eligibility was restricted to adult CXR studies that included both frontal and lateral images and had an accompanying free-text report authored by a senior radiologist. To ensure a comprehensive evaluation of the algorithm's performance on both normal and abnormal cases, we employed a purposive sampling strategy. We constructed the final cohort by selecting 568 examinations with reports describing a normal CXR and 477 examinations with abnormal findings. The abnormal cases were identified by selecting reports that lacked a normal description and contained one or more of the following keywords: "pneumonia", "opacity", "cardiomegaly", "pneumothorax", "effusion", "nodule", or "mass". The validation cohort consisted of adult patients with a mean age of 47.9 years (median, 52 years; standard deviation, 18.4; range, 19–82 years). There was a balanced sex distribution, with 495 female patients (47%) and 550 male patients (53%).

To generate structured, binary labels for the quantitative evaluation, we processed the narrative reports using a sophisticated Large Language Model (LLM) pipeline designed to transform unstructured text into a predefined, machine-readable format [14]. The contribution of the LLM extends significantly beyond simple label extraction; it functions as a data structuring engine. This was achieved by providing the model with a detailed, multi-component prompt that meticulously guided its output. The prompt included: (1) explicit rules for generating a valid JSON object, such as the mandatory use of double quotes and binary indicators for the presence or absence of a condition; (2) precise classes with definitions for each of the target pathologies; (3) a clear output template specifying the desired JSON schema; and (4) illustrative examples of reports paired with their correct JSON counterparts to provide concrete guidance.

This structured prompting strategy compelled the LLM to interpret the radiological findings within the context of the provided definitions and rules, thereby producing a consistent and analysis-ready dataset. The resulting JSON from the LLM contained the structured labels used to evaluate the normal and abnormal separation, the accuracy of each pathology classifier, and the criticality ensemble. We used only the extracted labels to assess the algorithm; the Grad-CAM images are presented here for illustration purposes only. All radiographs were processed by the TRIA system, which served the institution through its Picture Archiving and Communication System (PACS), utilizing files in Digital Imaging and Communications in Medicine (DICOM) format.

2.3. Analysis

We evaluated a two-stage computational pipeline designed to optimize individual pathology classifiers first and then assess the performance of various ensemble strategies.

In the initial stage, we determined optimal classification thresholds for each pathology. We achieved this by generating a receiver operating characteristic (ROC) curve for each classifier against its corresponding ground truth label. We then identified the optimal probability threshold using Youden's J statistic. This method maximizes the sum of sensitivity and specificity, thereby finding an optimal balance between true positives and true negatives [15].

In the second stage, we implemented and evaluated four distinct ensemble strategies to aggregate the outputs from the individual classifiers into a single, study-level determination of "normal" or "abnormal." The specific logic for each strategy is detailed below:

1. Possibility-based (Rule-based Commercial Algorithm): This method emulates the logic of the commercial product. It classifies an examination as abnormal if any

pathology is assigned a qualitative likelihood of high or certain. This approach relied on pre-defined categorical bins derived from probability scores for its final decision.
2. Threshold-based: This strategy classified an examination as abnormal if the predicted probability score for any individual pathology exceeded its previously determined optimal threshold from the first stage of analysis. This strategy tests a straightforward aggregation rule where any single positive finding renders the entire study abnormal.
3. Weighted Sum-based: This strategy computed a weighted sum of the probability scores from all classifiers for a given study. To emphasize the importance of the global abnormality detector, we assigned the score from the general yesfinding classifier a weight of 2.0. In contrast, the scores for all other specific pathologies were assigned a weight of 1.0. We classified an examination as abnormal if this aggregated weighted sum surpassed a unique, optimized threshold determined via ROC analysis on the sum scores themselves. This explicit up-weighting of the yes-finding output was the basis for its "weighted" designation.
4. Hierarchical-based: This model used a multi-step, rule-based logic that prioritized specific findings. First, the yesfinding score was evaluated: if it is significantly below its optimal threshold (e.g., <0.8× threshold), the model classified the exam as normal. Conversely, if the score is significantly greater than high (e.g., >1.2× threshold), it flags the case as abnormal. For scores falling within this intermediate range, the algorithm proceeded to check for the presence of findings. If any of these are predicted with a score above their respective optimal thresholds, the model classifies the examination as abnormal. Otherwise, the final decision defaults to yes-finding, based on the yes-finding score, which is compared against its standard threshold.

To determine whether the observed differences between the performing ensemble strategies were statistically significant, we employed two complementary tests: the DeLong test for comparing areas under the AUROC curve and McNemar's test for paired categorical outcomes (accuracy, sensitivity, and specificity). A p-value < 0.05 was considered statistically significant. We performed all analyses using paired predictions from the same validation dataset to ensure direct comparability across models.

3. Results

3.1. Individual Classifier Performance

The proposed TRIA system demonstrated strong discriminative performance across multiple thoracic pathologies. The general "yesfinding" classifier achieved an AUROC of 0.911, indicating robust overall abnormality detection. Among the individual models, cardiomegaly, pneumothorax, and pleural effusion achieved excellent diagnostic accuracy, with AUROC values of 0.968, 0.955, and 0.935, respectively. The consolidation category in prior studies showed high sensitivity (0.829) but comparatively lower specificity (0.656), reflecting the smallest training dataset. Detailed results for all classifiers are provided in Table 3.

Table 3. Performance Metrics of Individual Classifiers on the Test Set.

Pathology	Positive Cases	Sensitivity (95% CI)	Specificity (95% CI)	Accuracy (95% CI)	AUROC (95% CI)
Yesfinding	502	0.841 (0.806–0.870)	0.822 (0.789–0.851)	0.831 (0.807–0.852)	0.911 (0.893–0.927)
Cardiomegaly	199	0.960 (0.923–0.979)	0.881 (0.858–0.901)	0.895 (0.876–0.912)	0.968 (0.960–0.977)
Pneumothorax	52	0.904 (0.794–0.958)	0.879 (0.857–0.897)	0.880 (0.859–0.898)	0.955 (0.927–0.980)
Effusion	150	0.840 (0.773–0.890)	0.924 (0.905–0.939)	0.912 (0.894–0.928)	0.935 (0.907–0.959)
Opacity	264	0.848 (0.800–0.887)	0.733 (0.702–0.762)	0.761 (0.735–0.786)	0.865 (0.841–0.888)
Mass	56	0.786 (0.662–0.873)	0.862 (0.840–0.882)	0.858 (0.836–0.878)	0.839 (0.778–0.891)
Consolidation	41	0.829 (0.687–0.915)	0.656 (0.626–0.684)	0.662 (0.634–0.690)	0.775 (0.703–0.835)

Notes: AUROC = area under the receiver operating characteristic curve; CI = Confidence Interval.

3.2. Ensemble Model Performance for Abnormality Detection

Among the four ensemble approaches, the weighted sum-based model demonstrated the best balance between sensitivity and specificity, achieving an accuracy of 0.854 (95% CI: 0.831–0.874), sensitivity of 0.845 (95% CI: 0.810–0.875), specificity of 0.861 (95% CI: 0.830–0.887), and AUROC of 0.927 (95% CI: 0.911–0.940). De Long's test confirmed that its AUROC was significantly higher than that of the threshold-based model ($p = 0.0307$).

Paired McNemar's tests further revealed that the weighted sum-based ensemble significantly outperformed the threshold-, possibility-, and hierarchical-based methods in terms of overall accuracy ($p < 0.01$ for all comparisons) and specificity ($p < 0.001$), while maintaining comparable sensitivity ($p > 0.05$ when compared with the hierarchical model) (Table 4). These findings indicate that the weighted aggregation approach achieves superior discrimination and generalization, with statistically validated improvements in diagnostic performance. Comprehensive results are presented in Table 5, and corresponding receiver operating characteristic curves and confusion matrices are illustrated in Figures 7 and 8.

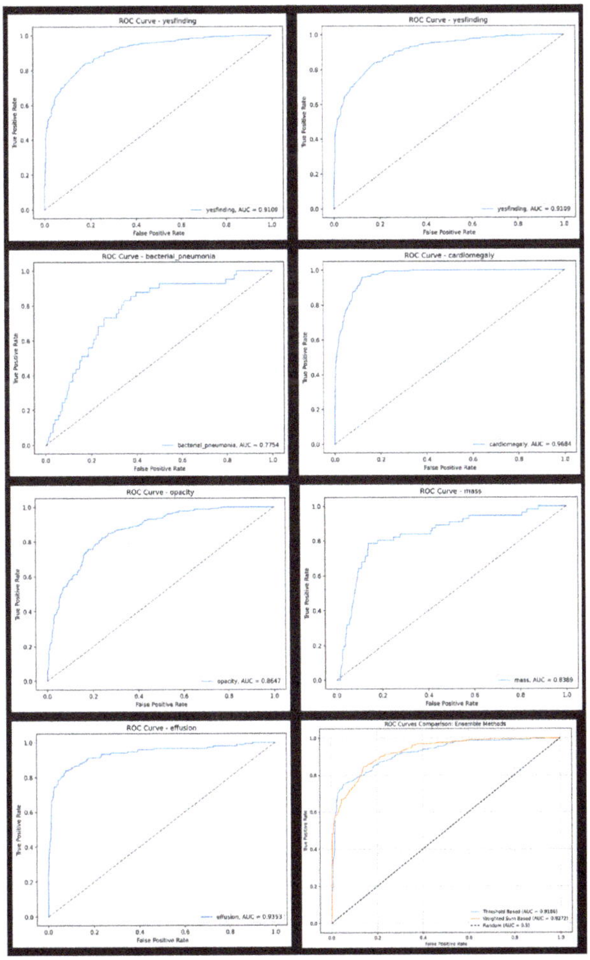

Figure 7. Comparison of receiver operating characteristic curves for the seven selected pathologies. The bottom right panel shows the curves for Threshold-Based and Weighted Sum-Based ensemble methods.

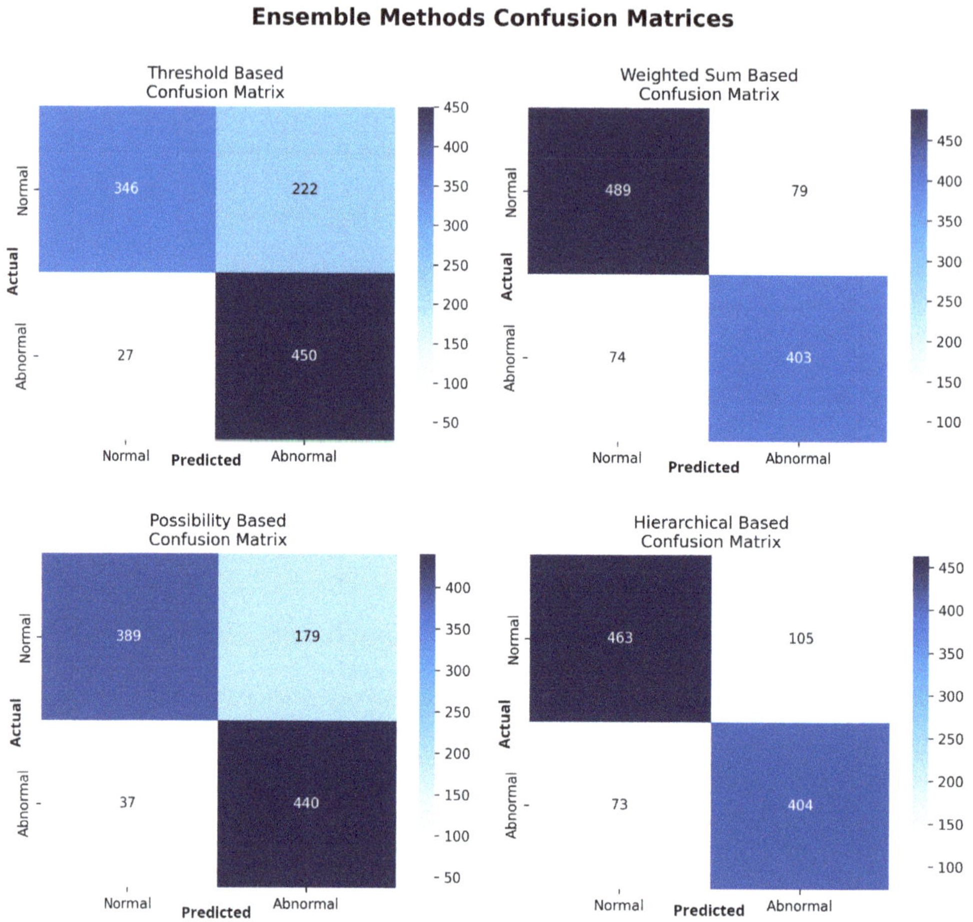

Figure 8. Confusion matrices for the four ensemble methods evaluated for abnormality detection.

Table 4. Summary of statistical comparisons among ensemble strategies. Significant results ($p < 0.05$) are shown in bold.

Comparison	Metric	Test	*p*-Value	Significance
Threshold vs. Weighted Sum	AUROC	DeLong	**0.0307**	Yes
Threshold vs. Weighted Sum	Accuracy	McNemar	**<0.001**	Yes
Threshold vs. Weighted Sum	Sensitivity	McNemar	**<0.001**	Yes
Threshold vs. Weighted Sum	Specificity	McNemar	**<0.001**	Yes
Weighted Sum vs. Possibility	Accuracy	McNemar	**<0.001**	Yes
Weighted Sum vs. Possibility	Sensitivity	McNemar	**<0.001**	Yes
Weighted Sum vs. Possibility	Specificity	McNemar	**<0.001**	Yes
Weighted Sum vs. Hierarchical	Accuracy	McNemar	**0.0043**	Yes
Weighted Sum vs. Hierarchical	Sensitivity	McNemar	0.8450	No
Weighted Sum vs. Hierarchical	Specificity	McNemar	**<0.001**	Yes

Table 5. Performance Comparison of Four Ensemble Strategies for Abnormality Detection.

Ensemble	Accuracy (95% CI)	Sensitivity (95% CI)	Specificity (95% CI)	PPV (95% CI)	NPV (95% CI)	F1 Score	AUROC (95% CI)
Weighted Sum	0.854 (0.831–0.874)	0.845 (0.810–0.875)	0.861 (0.830–0.887)	0.836 (0.800–0.866)	0.869 (0.838–0.894)	0.840	0.927 (0.911–0.940)
Hierarchical	0.830 (0.806–0.851)	0.847 (0.812–0.876)	0.815 (0.781–0.845)	0.794 (0.756–0.827)	0.864 (0.832–0.890)	0.819	N/A
Possibility	0.793 (0.768–0.817)	0.922 (0.895–0.943)	0.685 (0.646–0.722)	0.711 (0.674–0.745)	0.913 (0.883–0.936)	0.803	N/A
Threshold	0.762 (0.735–0.787)	0.943 (0.919–0.961)	0.609 (0.568–0.648)	0.670 (0.633–0.704)	0.928 (0.897–0.950)	0.783	0.919 (0.901–0.935)

Notes: PPV = Positive Predictive Value; NPV = Negative Predictive Value; N/A = Not applicable for discrete ensemble outputs.

3.3. Error Analysis

An analysis of the algorithm's false negatives revealed a nuanced performance profile, where a specific miss did not always equate to a complete system failure. Across the board, a substantial number of cases with a false negative for a particular pathology were nevertheless correctly identified as abnormal by the general "yes-finding" classifier or had other co-occurring true positive pathologies. For example, out of 38 false negatives for opacity, the algorithm correctly identified the exam as abnormal in 25 cases. In many instances of a missed finding, the algorithm successfully detected other pathologies within the same study. Misclassification was another notable source of error, where an existing pathology was detected but incorrectly labeled, such as opacities being predicted as masses or nodules (Figure 4). Radiologist review of these false-negative cases frequently noted findings that were "subtle," "small," "doubtful," "seen on lateral image only," or "non-specific." In other cases, the algorithm correctly identified a more critical finding, like a large pleural effusion, while missing a secondary, less significant pathology (Figure 3). Figures 9–11 illustrate false negative cases for opacity, pneumothorax, and nodule, respectively. This highlights the inherent limitations and inevitable failures of this kind of system.

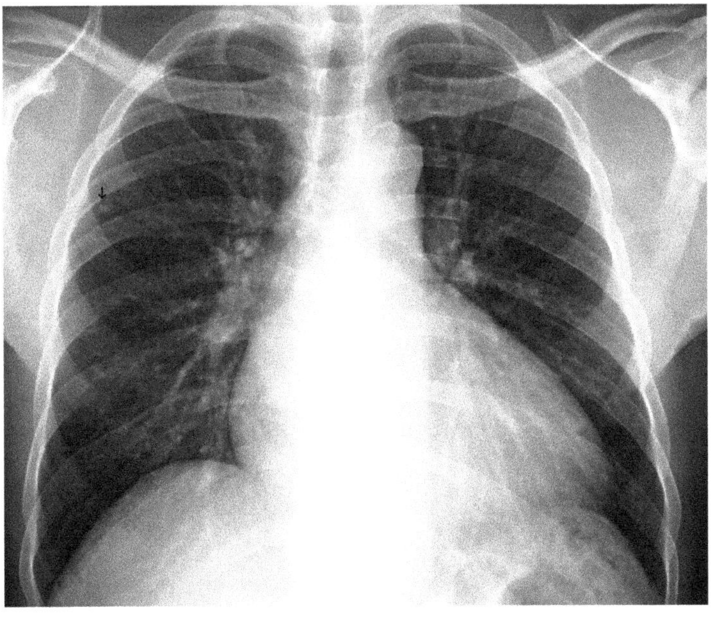

Figure 9. A false negative example of a small, missed nodule (black arrow).

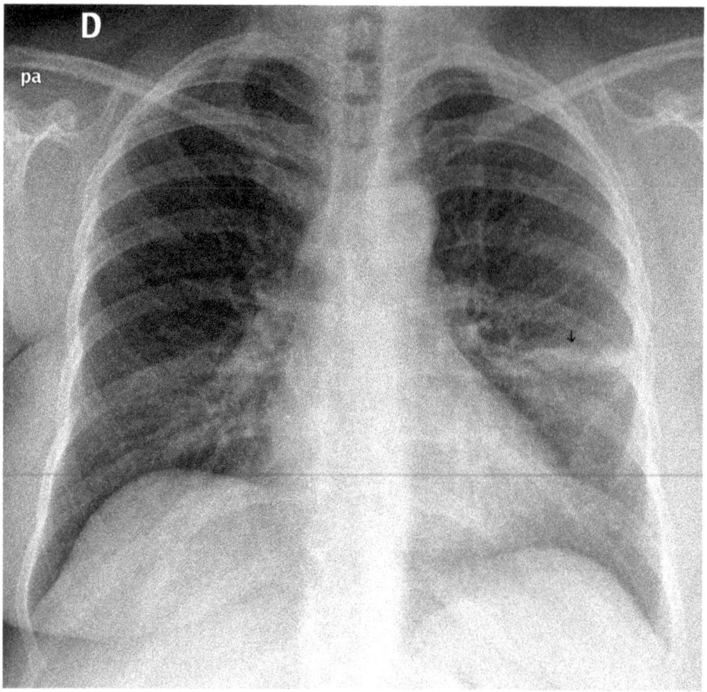

Figure 10. A false negative example of an alveolar opacity (black arrow).

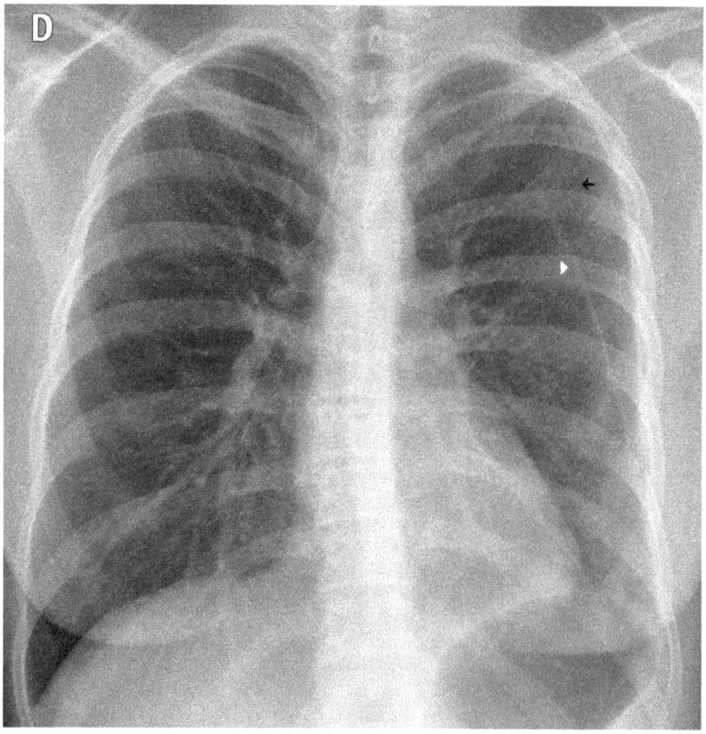

Figure 11. A false negative example of a missed loculated pneumothorax. The presence of pulmonary markings (black arrow) beyond the pleural line (white arrowhead) may have misled the algorithm.

3.4. Clinical Workflow

As previously stated, clinicians implement TRIA in a clinical scenario. Upon image acquisition, CXRs are automatically forwarded from the institution's PACS to the TRIA server. The algorithm processes the study and sends its findings—including the classification derived from the possibility ensemble and visual explainability aids, such as Grad-CAM heatmaps—directly back to the PACS. These results are then displayed to the radiologist within their standard viewer, alongside the original image (Figure 12). This seamless integration embeds the entire analysis within the patient's study, enabling immediate worklist prioritization and concurrent review by the attending physician.

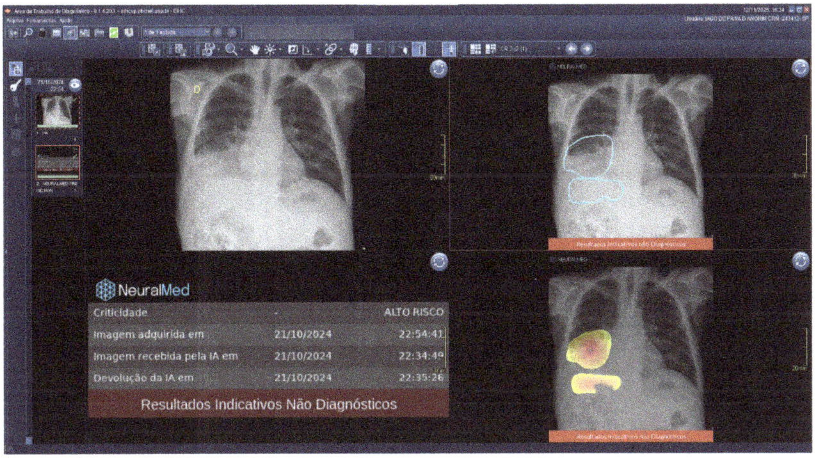

Figure 12. A real-world example of the TRIA system's clinical integration within a commercial Picture Archiving and Communication System (PACS) viewer. The viewer displays the original posterior-anterior CXR (**top left**), the generated external contour image (**top right**), a heatmap visualization (**bottom right**), and the dedicated AI results panel (**bottom left**), which shows the possibility assessment and processing timestamps.

4. Discussion

The intended clinical application for the TRIA system is as a triage tool to prioritize patients, a typical and valuable use case for radiology AI [3,16]. This study provides a necessary external validation of the system for this purpose. The evaluation methodology we used is a standard approach in AI validation, as highlighted in systematic reviews and other external evaluations [16–18].

A key methodological strength of the underlying AI model is the use of a tongue-shaped segmentation mask. By including the mediastinum and hilar regions in the ROI, the model analyzes these diagnostically critical areas, which are often excluded by traditional lung-only segmentation. This approach creates a more clinically relevant area for analysis, which may improve the detection of central pathologies, especially those related to the cardiopulmonary system.

However, a significant trade-off in the model's design is the use of a very low input resolution (75 × 75 pixels) for classification. While this approach allows for computational efficiency, it inherently risks the loss of fine-grained details necessary for detecting subtle pathologies, such as small nodules or early interstitial disease. This was reflected in the error analysis, where false negatives were often subtle cases. The high false-positive rate for conditions like opacity and consolidation suggests the model may be oversensitive to non-specific patterns, highlighting a discrepancy between pure pattern recognition and a radiologist's clinical interpretation, which incorporates a higher threshold for significance.

The set of pathologies chosen to build the tool reflects the importance of critical findings for emergency physicians who are not assisted by radiology specialists. The limited number of specific pathologies favors computational efficiency, while the general normal/abnormal classifier ("yesfinding") provides a safeguard for unlisted pathologies, as depicted by the ensemble results.

In real-world clinical settings, the prevalence of abnormal CXR is substantially lower than that in research datasets, often leading to significant class imbalance. This imbalance tends to skew diagnostic performance toward more common findings such as opacities and cardiomegaly, while less frequent pathologies—such as pleural effusion, pulmonary nodules, and pneumothorax—are underrepresented. For instance, unpublished internal data from various initial deployments of the algorithm at a new client site, typically a survey of 300 consecutive examinations, indicate an abnormal-to-normal ratio of approximately 1:5, with several subsets containing no cases of the three less prevalent conditions mentioned earlier. This observation justified the use of a curated dataset for validation, ensuring adequate representation of all target pathologies. Furthermore, it is essential to note that lower disease prevalence intrinsically reduces the positive predictive value and increases the negative predictive value, even when sensitivity and specificity remain constant [19].

From a methodological standpoint, a consecutive prospective dataset could provide higher distributional validity; however, the low frequency of abnormal findings in such samples can limit the precision and statistical power for estimating algorithm accuracy. Therefore, we opted for a balanced and enriched dataset to ensure adequate representation of clinically relevant abnormalities. This lower proportion of normal cases does not compromise the validity of our evaluation, given that the validation dataset comprising 1045 curated CXR provides a statistically robust sample size. This cohort yields 95% confidence intervals with margins of error of approximately ±3–4% for key performance metrics, surpassing typical requirements for medical imaging validation. Nevertheless, we still acknowledge that this enrichment does not replicate true disease prevalence and differs from studies employing large, consecutive, real-world datasets, which provide a more realistic benchmark of clinical performance [20,21].

We established ground truth through LLM–assisted extraction of findings from reports authored by senior radiologists, a pragmatic strategy for large-scale datasets. A radiologist independently reviewed a subset of 300 reports, yielding an accuracy of 0.9838 (95% CI: 0.9783–0.9883), thereby supporting the reliability of the adopted approach. Nevertheless, more rigorous standards for ground truth determination exist, such as consensus interpretation by a panel of expert radiologists or correlation with reference imaging modalities, including computed tomography [20,22–24].

A comparative analysis reveals a landscape of varied performance among CXR AI tools. Regarding the individual pathologies classification, we compared TRIA's performance with CheXNet [25], a well-established deep learning model trained on the NIH ChestX-ray14 dataset and often used as a benchmark for CXR classification. As shown in Table 6, TRIA achieved higher AUROC values for cardiomegaly and pleural effusion compared to CheXNet, while the consolidation and opacity classifiers demonstrated comparable performance.

In this study, the possibility-based ensemble (used in the commercial product) obtained high sensitivity. In contrast, the weighted sum ensemble demonstrated robust and balanced performance for abnormality stratification, achieving an AUROC of 0.927 with a sensitivity of 84.5% and a specificity of 86.1%. This balanced profile contrasts with other AI triage tools, such as the one evaluated by Blake et al., which was optimized for very high sensitivity (99.6%) at the expense of lower specificity (67.4%) [16]. Another algorithm evaluated in a primary care setting showed excellent specificity (92.0%) but significantly lower sensitivity

(47.0%) [26]. These differences represent fundamental design choices: one prioritizes minimizing missed findings, accepting more false positives, while the other seeks to balance sensitivity and specificity to reduce workload more efficiently. The overall AUROC for TRIA is comparable to that of high-performing algorithms evaluated in other studies, which often achieve AUROCs in the 0.92 to 0.94 range [27,28].

Table 6. Comparison of TRIA Performance with CheXNet [25].

Pathology	CheXNet AUC (95% CI)	TRIA AUROC (95% CI)
Atelectasis	0.862 (0.825–0.895)	–
Consolidation	0.893 (0.859–0.924)	0.775 (0.703–0.835)
Edema (Opacity)	0.924 (0.886–0.955)	0.865 (0.841–0.888)
Pneumonia(Opacity)	0.851 (0.781, 0.911)	0.865 (0.841–0.888)
Effusion	0.901 (0.868–0.930)	0.935 (0.907–0.959)
Cardiomegaly	0.831 (0.790–0.870)	0.968 (0.960–0.977)
Emphysema	0.704 (0.567–0.833)	–
Hernia	0.851 (0.785–0.909)	–

Notes: As pathology mappings of CheXNet and TRIA were different, Edema and Pneumonia in CheXNet were mapped to opacity. In the TRIA training dataset, these two former classes were included in the opacity class. TRIA did not classify atelectasis, Emphysema, and Hernia.

These results demonstrate that TRIA performs on par with or above the level of reference models in the literature, particularly for acute pathologies most relevant to emergency triage workflows. Importantly, TRIA was externally validated using an independent real-world hospital dataset, thereby reinforcing its generalizability of performance across diverse imaging conditions.

The error analysis of TRIA, which noted that false negatives were often subtle or challenging cases, is a consistent finding across the field. For instance, Plesner et al. similarly found that the performance of four different commercial tools declined for smaller-sized findings and on complex radiographs with multiple pathologies [20]. Our study identifies the model's low input resolution as a potential factor contributing to the missing of fine-grained details. Despite this, while the model may misclassify or miss a specific finding, its ability to flag an exam as generally abnormal remains high, ensuring that complex cases are still prioritized for radiologist review. The variability highlighted in Table 7 also shows that algorithm performance is highly dependent on the clinical task and validation setting, suggesting that a single set of metrics may not fully capture an algorithm's utility.

We acknowledge that the primary potential source of conflict in this study is sponsor bias. To minimize this risk, the study was initiated at the request of the participating institution to independently assess the performance of the TRIA algorithm after its clinical deployment. Notably, the validation dataset originated from an external institution, entirely independent from the one involved in TRIA's development. We derived the ground truth from diagnostic reports authored by senior radiologists at this external center, without any involvement from company personnel. Researchers from HCFMUSP exclusively performed case selection and data extraction, ensuring an impartial and methodologically sound process. We predefined the study protocol and analysis plan before data analysis, thereby reinforcing methodological transparency. All patient data were fully anonymized at the source in accordance with institutional policies and data protection regulations. The institutional review board (IRB) approved the study and waived the requirement for informed consent due to its retrospective, observational design. We extracted data directly from the hospital PACS after the AI system had already been integrated into routine clinical workflows, ensuring real-world representativeness of the validation process.

We also recognize that this validation was conducted at a single tertiary academic hospital, which may limit the generalizability of our findings to other clinical contexts, such as primary care or community hospitals, where patient demographics, equipment, and workflow conditions may differ. Future research should include prospective, multicenter evaluations across diverse healthcare settings to confirm the robustness and clinical impact of TRIA under varying operational conditions. Additionally, this study's retrospective design may overestimate algorithmic performance compared to real-time prospective use, as reported in prior work on diagnostic AI translation to practice [17]. Finally, the validation dataset was enriched with clinically significant pathologies, which does not reflect the true prevalence of abnormalities in unselected populations and may influence the apparent predictive performance.

Table 7. Comparative Performance Metrics of some AI Algorithms for CXR Abnormality Detection.

Study/Algorithm	Type	AUROC	Sens. (%)	Spec. (%)
This Study				
TRIA (Possibility)	R	N/A	92.2	68.5
TRIA (Weighted Sum)	R	0.927	84.5	86.1
Blake et al., 2023 [16]				
Qure.ai qXR	R	N/A	99.6	67.4
Vasilev et al., 2023 [17]				
Lunit INSIGHT	R	0.940	90.0	89.0
Lunit INSIGHT	P	0.840	77.0	81.0
Catalina et al., 2024 [26]				
Oxipit ChestEye	P	N/A	47.0	92.0
Arzamasov et al., 2024 [28]				
Qure.ai qXR	R	0.921	N/A	N/A
Lunit INSIGHT	R	0.932	N/A	N/A
de Camargo et al., 2025 [23]				
LAM Algorithm	R	0.938	36.3	99.5
Qin et al., 2019 [27]				
Lunit INSIGHT	R	0.940	95.0 †	80.0 †
Qure.ai qXR	R	0.940	95.0 †	72.0 †

Notes: N/A = Not Available or not reported as a primary endpoint; R = Retrospective; P = Prospective; LAM = Lung Abnormality Model. † Metrics from Qin et al. represent the operating point required to achieve a sensitivity of at least 95%.

Further refinement of the classification model, particularly by adding more pathologies and exploring higher input resolutions, could enhance its ability to detect more subtle findings and improve its clinical utility.

5. Conclusions

This independent retrospective validation demonstrates that the TRIA AI algorithm achieves robust and accurate performance in discriminating between normal and abnormal CXR. The actual commercial version has excellent sensitivity and provides confidence for clinical implementation as a reliable tool for triaging CXRs. The strong and balanced performance of the weighted sum ensemble strategy offers a viable alternative when greater specificity is required. The tool could help manage reporting backlogs, prioritize urgent cases for radiologist review, and potentially support earlier patient intervention. This study provides a foundation for future prospective and comparative research to evaluate the algorithm's clinical utility further.

Author Contributions: Conceptualization, A.M.E. and A.C.C.; Methodology, A.C.C. and M.F.B.W.; Software, M.F.B.W., A.R.Y. and A.C.C.; Validation, I.d.P.D., M.V.Y.S. and M.A.E.; Formal Analysis, M.F.B.W. and A.C.C.; Investigation, A.C.C., I.d.P.D., M.V.Y.S. and M.A.E.; Resources, I.d.P.D., M.V.Y.S. and M.A.E.; Data Curation, M.F.B.W., I.d.P.D., M.V.Y.S. and M.A.E.; Writing—Original Draft Preparation, A.C.C.; Writing—Review and Editing, all authors; Supervision, M.V.Y.S., A.C.C. and A.M.E.; Project Administration, A.C.C.; Funding Acquisition, A.M.E. All authors have read and agreed to the published version of the manuscript.

Funding: This research and the article processing charges were supported by NeuralMed using its regular institutional funds.

Institutional Review Board Statement: The study was conducted in accordance with the Declaration of Helsinki and approved by the Ethics Committee of HCFMUSP (protocol code CAAE: 85444924.9.0000.0068) on 16 January 2025.

Informed Consent Statement: Patient consent was waived due to the retrospective nature of the study, which involved the analysis of fully anonymized pre-existing medical data.

Data Availability Statement: The processed datasets generated and analyzed during the current study are publicly available on https://zenodo.org/records/17401230—accessed on 8 November 2025. However, the images and complete reports, which contain confidential and sensitive health data from HCFMUSP, have not been released.

Acknowledgments: The authors would like to thank the Department of Radiology at HCFMUSP for their support and for providing the data for this validation study.

Conflicts of Interest: A.C.C. and A.M.E. are founders and stakeholders of NeuralMed, the company that manufactures the TRIA system and funded the study. A.C.C., A.M.E., M.F.B.W., and A.R.Y. are employees of NeuralMed. The other authors declare no conflicts of interest. The funder had a role in the design of the study; in the data analysis and interpretation; in the writing of the manuscript, and in the decision to publish the results.

References

1. Smith-Bindman, R.; Miglioretti, D.L.; Johnson, E.; Lee, C.; Feigelson, H.S.; Flynn, M.; Greenlee, R.T.; Kruger, R.L.; Hornbrook, M.C.; Roblin, D.; et al. Use of Diagnostic Imaging Studies and Associated Radiation Exposure for Patients Enrolled in Large Integrated Health Care Systems, 1996–2010. *JAMA* **2012**, *307*, 2400–2409. [CrossRef]
2. Esteva, A.; Kuprel, B.; Novoa, R.A.; Ko, J.; Swetter, S.M.; Blau, H.M.; Thrun, S. Dermatologist-level classification of skin cancer with deep neural networks. *Nature* **2017**, *542*, 115–118. [CrossRef]
3. Annarumma, M.; Withey, S.J.; Bakewell, R.J.; Pesce, E.; Goh, V.; Montana, G. Automated Triaging of Adult Chest Radiographs with Deep Artificial Neural Networks. *Radiology* **2019**, *291*, 196–202. [CrossRef]
4. Anderson, P.G.; Tarder-Stoll, H.; Alpaslan, M.; Keathley, N.; Levin, D.L.; Venkatesh, S.; Bartel, E.; Sicular, S.; Howell, S.; Lindsey, R.V.; et al. Deep learning improves physician accuracy in the comprehensive detection of abnormalities on chest X-rays. *Sci. Rep.* **2024**, *14*, 25151. [CrossRef] [PubMed]
5. Windecker, D.; Baj, G.; Shiri, I.; Kazaj, P.M.; Kaesmacher, J.; Gräni, C.; Siontis, G.C. Generalizability of FDA-Approved AI-Enabled Medical Devices for Clinical Use. *JAMA Netw. Open* **2025**, *8*, e258052. [CrossRef]
6. Agência Nacional de Vigilância Sanitária. Consulta de Registro de Software como Dispositivo Médico-A2 Tecnologia Ltda. 2023. Available online: https://consultas.anvisa.gov.br/#/saude/25351120732202361/?nomeProduto=tria (accessed on 10 October 2025).
7. Agência Nacional de Vigilância Sanitária. Dispõe Sobre as Boas Práticas de Fabricação de Produtos Médicos e Produtos para Diagnóstico de Uso In Vitro e dá Outras Providências. RDC N° 657/2022. Ministério da Saúde. 2022. Available online: https://in.gov.br/pt/web/dou/-/resolucao-de-diretoria-colegiada-rdc-n-657-de-24-de-marco-de-2022-389603457 (accessed on 8 November 2025).
8. Brasil. Lei Geral de Proteção de Dados Pessoais (Lei n° 13.709). Diário Oficial da União. 14 August 2018. Available online: http://www.planalto.gov.br/ccivil_03/_ato2015-2018/2018/lei/l13709.htm (accessed on 5 October 2025).
9. Jaeger, S.; Candemir, S.; Antani, S.; Wang, Y.J.; Lu, P.; Thoma, G. Two public chest X-ray datasets for computer-aided screening of pulmonary diseases. *Quant. Imaging Med. Surg.* **2014**, *4*, 475–477.

10. Demner-Fushman, D.; Kohli, M.D.; Rosenman, M.B.; Shooshan, S.E.; Rodriguez, L.; Antani, S.; Thoma, G.R.; McDonald, C.J. Preparing a collection of radiology examinations for distribution and retrieval. *J. Am. Med. Inform. Assoc.* **2016**, *23*, 304–310. [CrossRef] [PubMed]
11. Shiraishi, J.; Katsuragawa, S.; Ikezoe, J.; Matsumoto, T.; Kobayashi, T.; Komatsu, K.I.; Matsui, M.; Fujita, H.; Kodera, Y.; Doi, K. Development of a digital image database for chest radiographs with and without a lung nodule: Receiver operating characteristic analysis of radiologists' detection of pulmonary nodules. *Am. J. Roentgenol.* **2000**, *174*, 71–74. [CrossRef] [PubMed]
12. Wang, X.; Peng, Y.; Lu, L.; Lu, Z.; Bagheri, M.; Summers, R.M. ChestX-ray8: Hospital-scale chest X-ray database and benchmarks on weakly-supervised classification and localization of common thorax diseases. In Proceedings of the IEEE Conference on Computer Vision and Pattern Recognition (CVPR), Honolulu, HI, USA, 21–26 July 2017; pp. 3462–3471.
13. Bustos, A.; Pertusa, A.; Salinas, J.M.; de la Iglesia-Vayá, M. PadChest: A large chest x-ray image dataset with multi-label annotated reports. *Med. Image Anal.* **2020**, *66*, 101797. [CrossRef]
14. Gemini Team. Gemini 2.5: Pushing the Frontier with Advanced Reasoning, Multimodality, Long Context, and Next Generation Agentic Capabilities. Google, 2025. Available online: https://storage.googleapis.com/deepmind-media/gemini/gemini_v2_5_report.pdf (accessed on 5 October 2025).
15. Youden, W.J. Index for rating diagnostic tests. *Cancer* **1950**, *3*, 32–35. [CrossRef]
16. Blake, S.R.; Das, N.; Tadepalli, M.; Reddy, B.; Singh, A.; Agrawal, R.; Chattoraj, S.; Shah, D.; Putha, P. Using Artificial Intelligence to Stratify Normal versus Abnormal Chest X-rays: External Validation of a Deep Learning Algorithm at East Kent Hospitals University NHS Foundation Trust. *Diagnostics* **2023**, *13*, 3408. [CrossRef] [PubMed]
17. Vasilev, Y.; Vladzymyrskyy, A.; Omelyanskaya, O.; Blokhin, I.; Kirpichev, Y.; Arzamasov, K. AI-Based CXR First Reading: Current Limitations to Ensure Practical Value. *Diagnostics* **2023**, *13*, 1430. [CrossRef]
18. Harris, M.; Qi, A.; Jeagal, L.; Torabi, N.; Menzies, D.; Korobitsyn, A.; Pai, M.; Nathavitharana, R.R.; Ahmad Khan, F. A systematic review of the diagnostic accuracy of artificial intelligence-based computer programs to analyze chest X-rays for pulmonary tuberculosis. *PLoS ONE* **2019**, *14*, e0221339. [CrossRef]
19. Pepe, M.S. *The Statistical Evaluation of Medical Tests for Classification and Prediction*; Oxford University Press: Oxford, UK, 2003.
20. Lind Plesner, L.; Müller, F.C.; Brejnebøl, M.W.; Laustrup, L.C.; Rasmussen, F.; Nielsen, O.W.; Boesen, M.; Brun Andersen, M. Commercially Available Chest Radiograph AI Tools for Detecting Airspace Disease, Pneumothorax, and Pleural Effusion. *Radiology* **2023**, *308*, e231236. [CrossRef]
21. Niehoff, J.H.; Kalaitzidis, J.; Kroeger, J.R.; Schoenbeck, D.; Borggrefe, J.; Michael, A.E. Evaluation of the clinical performance of an AI-based application for the automated analysis of chest X-rays. *Sci. Rep.* **2023**, *13*, 3680. [CrossRef]
22. Khader, F.; Han, T.; Müller-Franzes, G.; Huck, L.; Schad, P.; Keil, S.; Barzakova, E.; Schulze-Hagen, M.; Pedersoli, F.; Schulz, V.; et al. Artificial Intelligence for Clinical Interpretation of Bedside Chest Radiographs. *Radiology* **2023**, *307*, e220510. [CrossRef] [PubMed]
23. de Camargo, T.F.O.; Ribeiro, G.A.S.; da Silva, M.C.B.; da Silva, L.O.; Torres, P.P.T.E.S.; da Silva, D.D.S.R.; de Santos, M.O.N.; Filho, W.S.; Rosa, M.E.E.; Novaes, M.D.A.; et al. Clinical validation of an artificial intelligence algorithm for classifying tuberculosis and pulmonary findings in chest radiographs. *Front. Artif. Intell.* **2025**, *8*, 1512910. [CrossRef]
24. van Leeuwen, K.G.; Schalekamp, S.; Rutten, M.J.; Huisman, M.; Schaefer-Prokop, C.M.; de Rooij, M.; van Ginneken, B.; Maresch, B.; Geurts, B.H.; van Dijke, C.F.; et al. Comparison of Commercial AI Software Performance for Radiograph Lung Nodule Detection and Bone Age Prediction. *Radiology* **2024**, *310*, e230981. [CrossRef] [PubMed]
25. Rajpurkar, P.; Irvin, J.; Ball, R.L.; Zhu, K.; Yang, B.; Mehta, H.; Duan, T.; Dsing, D.; Bagul, A.; Langlotz, C.P.; et al. Deep learning for chest radiograph diagnosis: A retrospective comparison of the CheXNeXt algorithm to practicing radiologists. *PLoS Med.* **2018**, *15*, e1002686. [CrossRef]
26. Catalina, Q.M.; Vidal-Alaball, J.; Fuster-Casanovas, A.; Escalé-Besa, A.; Ruiz Comellas, A.; Solé-Casals, J. Real-world testing of an artificial intelligence algorithm for the analysis of chest X-rays in primary care settings. *Sci. Rep.* **2024**, *14*, 5199. [CrossRef]
27. Qin, Z.Z.; Sander, M.S.; Rai, B.; Titahong, C.N.; Sudrungrot, S.; Laah, S.N.; Adhikari, L.M.; Carter, E.J.; Puri, L.; Codlin, A.J.; et al. Using artificial intelligence to read chest radiographs for tuberculosis detection: A multi-site evaluation of the diagnostic accuracy of three deep learning systems. *Sci. Rep.* **2019**, *9*, 15000. [CrossRef] [PubMed]
28. Arzamasov, K.; Vasilev, Y.; Zelenova, M.; Pestrenin, L.; Busygina, Y.; Bobrovskaya, T.; Chetverikov, S.; Shikhmuradov, D.; Pankratov, A.; Kirpichev, Y.; et al. Independent evaluation of the accuracy of 5 artificial intelligence software for detecting lung nodules on chest X-rays. *Quant. Imaging Med. Surg.* **2024**, *14*, 5288–5303. [CrossRef] [PubMed]

diagnostics

MDPI

Article

Classification Performance of Deep Learning Models for the Assessment of Vertical Dimension on Lateral Cephalometric Radiographs

Mehmet Birol Özel [1,*], Sultan Büşra Ay Kartbak [1] and Muhammet Çakmak [2]

[1] Department of Orthodontics, Faculty of Dentistry, Kocaeli University, Kocaeli 41190, Türkiye; sultanbusraay@gmail.com

[2] Department of Computer Engineering, Faculty of Engineering, Giresun University, Giresun 28200, Türkiye; muhammet.cakmak@giresun.edu.tr

* Correspondence: birol.ozel@kocaeli.edu.tr

Abstract

Background/Objectives: Vertical growth pattern significantly influences facial aesthetics and treatment choices. Lateral cephalograms are routinely used for the evaluation of vertical jaw relationships in orthodontic diagnosis. The aim of this study was to evaluate the performance of deep learning algorithms in classifying cephalometric radiographs according to vertical skeletal growth patterns without the need for anatomical landmark identification. **Methods**: This study was carried out on lateral cephalometric radiographs of 1050 patients. Cephalometric radiographs were divided into 3 subgroups based on FMA, SN-GoGn, and Cant of Occlusal Plane angles. Six deep learning models (ResNet101, DenseNet 201, EfficientNet B0, EfficientNet V2 B0, ConvNetBase, and a hybrid model) were employed for the classification of the dataset. The performances of the well-known deep learning models and the hybrid model were compared for accuracy, precision, F1-Score, mean absolute error, Cohen's Kappa, and Grad-CAM metrics. **Results**: The highest accuracy rates were achieved by the Hybrid Model with 86.67% for FMA groups, 87.29% for SN-GoGn groups, and 82.71% for Cant of Occlusal Plane groups. The lowest accuracy rates were achieved by ConvNet with 79.58% for FMA groups, 65% for SN-GoGn, and 70.21% for Cant of Occlusal Plane groups. **Conclusions**: The six deep learning algorithms employed demonstrated classification success rates ranging from 65% to 87.29%. The highest classification accuracy was observed in the FMA angle, while the lowest accuracy was recorded for the Cant of the Occlusal Plane angle. The proposed DL algorithms showed potential for direct skeletal orthodontic diagnosis without the need for cephalometric landmark detection steps.

Keywords: deep learning; artificial intelligence; cephalometry; vertical discrepancies

1. Introduction

Accurately evaluating a patient's facial skeletal pattern in three dimensions—transverse, vertical, and sagittal—is crucial for orthodontic diagnosis and treatment planning [1]. Variations in vertical growth are frequent and carry particular orthodontic significance. Abnormalities in hard or soft tissues can cause the face to lengthen or shorten. Insufficient lips, an elongated face, and a gummy smile may occur due to an excessive vertical dimension. On the other hand, insufficient vertical growth can lead to inadequate incisor display and a short face [2].

Assessing the vertical jaw relationship is crucial because the vertical growth pattern influences facial balance and treatment choices, such as the need for anchorage, macro aesthetics, extraction or non-extraction treatment/surgical or non-surgical treatment decision, and treatment time [3]. Since the vertical growth of the face ends last, the evaluation of vertical discrepancies is extremely important not only for correct diagnosis and effective treatment planning, but also to prevent relapse after treatment [4].

Cephalometry is one of the radiographic methods that provides morphological and descriptive diagnostic data about skeletal and dentoalveolar malocclusion [5]. Different angular and linear cephalometric techniques have been utilized to evaluate vertical jaw relationships, each with its own set of advantages and disadvantages. However, there is no single extensively studied method in the literature for determining vertical plane discrepancies, as the vertical plane can be affected by a multitude of factors such as age, gender, type of malocclusion, and mandibular plane angle [3,6].

Artificial intelligence (AI) algorithms have demonstrated their effectiveness across multiple medical fields, often exceeding the abilities of seasoned healthcare professionals. These algorithms facilitate the examination, organization, visualization, and classification of healthcare data [7].

Deep learning (DL), a subset of artificial intelligence, allows computers to learn and make decisions without being explicitly programmed. These algorithms, inspired by the neural networks found in the human brain, have diverse applications across various industries, including healthcare [8]. In the field of computer vision, particularly in image classification tasks, deep convolutional neural networks (CNNs) have emerged as the primary algorithms, achieving state-of-the-art performance in many applications. The strength of CNNs lies in their deep architecture, which enables the extraction of a hierarchy of discriminative features at multiple levels of abstraction [9]. In orthodontics, deep learning-based convolutional neural networks (CNNs) are utilized in a wide range of applications, including the prediction of growth and developmental stages, as well as diagnosis and treatment planning [10].

The integration of AI into clinical orthodontic practice enhanced various aspects of patient care, including diagnosis, treatment planning, evaluation of growth and development, monitoring of treatment progress and outcomes, maintenance phase management, remote monitoring, and long-term follow-up [11]. Additionally, chatbot systems developed based on large language models (LLMs) present substantial potential in the field, facilitating broader and more accessible applications of artificial intelligence due to their ease of access via the internet and their ability to perform a wide range of tasks [10]. AI also offers promising opportunities to enhance patient education and the dissemination of medical information [12].

As AI systems advance, numerous research efforts are focused on automatic landmark identification for cephalometric analyses. While there is no universally accepted gold standard for evaluating vertical discrepancies in cephalometric analysis, most clinical and research applications rely on expert-defined criteria or commonly used reference angles such as FMA, SN-GoGn, and Occlusal Plane Inclination. These reference points serve as practical benchmarks despite variability in their application across studies and institutions. A systematic review and meta-analysis investigated the application of DL for cephalometric landmark detection. Applications like WebCeph, OrthoDx, Ceph-X, AudaxCeph, and WeDoCeph have been created to automate the marking of cephalometric points, analysis, and calculations through the use of artificial intelligence technology [13].

Artificial intelligence (AI) algorithms employed for automated landmark identification on lateral cephalometric radiographs are generally characterized by high accuracy. Across most studies, over 80% of landmarks were detected within a 2 mm confidence interval [14].

Since the diagnosis of abnormalities through cephalometric analysis relies on measurements within a narrow range of millimeters or degrees, even minor errors in landmark localization can lead to significant misclassification [15]. Beyond traditional cephalometric radiographs, several studies have demonstrated that skeletal classifications can also be performed by applying cephalometric analysis directly to photographic images [16–18].

The aim of this study was to evaluate the performance of deep learning algorithms in classifying lateral cephalometric radiographs in terms of vertical classifications done using FMA, SN-GoGn, and Occlusal Plane Inclination measurements. Unlike traditional landmark-based diagnostic approaches, the proposed deep learning framework aims to eliminate the dependency on anatomical point identification, which is prone to inter- and intra-observer variability and may introduce cumulative measurement errors. To the best of our knowledge, this is one of the first studies to compare traditional cephalometric angles with landmark-independent deep learning classifiers in the context of vertical discrepancy classification.

The null hypothesis (H_0) of our study is as follows: Deep learning models do not exhibit comparable diagnostic accuracy with landmark-based diagnostic approaches in terms of vertical cephalometric evaluation.

2. Materials and Methods

This is a cross-sectional retrospective study that was carried out in the Department of Orthodontics and Dentofacial Orthopedics, Kocaeli University, after approval from the Institutional Ethics Committee (KU GOKAEK-2025/15/30).

2.1. Data Acquisition and Classification

Lateral cephalograms of 1050 subjects were selected for the study from the department's record archive (mean age = 15.6 years, age range = 8.8 to 47.8 years, 588 females, 462 males). The inclusion criteria were (1) high-quality lateral cephalometric radiographs with fully visible craniofacial landmarks, (2) patients aged 10 to 30 years at the time of imaging, (3) radiographs acquired prior to any orthodontic or surgical intervention, and (4) availability of corresponding vertical cephalometric measurements (FMA, SN-GoGn, and OP angles). Exclusion criteria were (1) radiographs with significant anatomical distortion or motion artifacts, (2) history of craniofacial trauma or syndromic conditions (e.g., cleft lip/palate), (3) incomplete clinical records or missing reference measurements, and (4) presence of orthodontic appliances at the time of imaging. All lateral cephalometric radiographs were taken under standard method with an X Ray device (J. Morita MFG. Corp Veraviewepocs 2D, Kyoto, Japan) with a magnification difference of 1.1 mm as determined by the manufacturer (80 kV, 10 mA, and 7.4 s). Lateral cephalometric radiographs were taken with the patient in neutral head position, teeth in centric occlusion, and lips in a relaxed position.

Webceph AI-based orthodontic and orthognathic online platform (AssembleCircle Corp., Seongnam, Republic of Korea) was used for performing the cephalometric measurements. Digital images of lateral cephalometric radiographs were uploaded to the WebCephTM server. Magnification correction was undertaken based on a known distance of 10 mm between two fixed points on the cephalostat rod in the radiograph. After automatic landmark identification was performed by WebCeph, anatomical landmarks were checked and manually repositioned.

Eleven landmarks were marked on each cephalogram (Or, Po, Go, Gn, Me, S, N, U6, U1, L6, L1), and the following three measurements were made using three planes formed by these landmarks (Figure 1a,b):

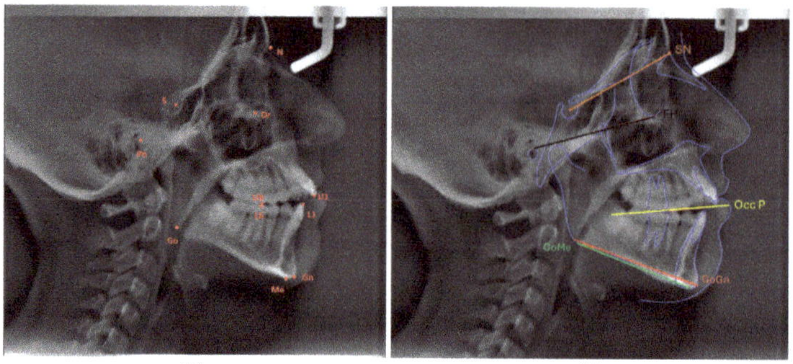

(a) (b)

Figure 1. (**a**) Cephalometric landmarks and their definitions: Or (Orbitale): The most inferior point of the orbital floor, Po (Porion): Superior point of the meatus acusticus exter-nus, Go (Gonion): Posteroinferior point of the angulus mandibula formed by the intersection of posterior border of the mandibular ramus and the inferior border of the mandibular corpus, Gn (Gnathion): The most anteroinferior point of the mandibular symphysis between pogonion and menton, Me (Menton): The most inferior point on the mandibular symphysis, S (Sella): The center point of the sella turcica, N (Nasion): The most anterior point on the nasofrontal suture, U6: Tip of the mesiobuccal cusp of upper permanent first molar, U1: Incisal tip of the maxillary central incisor, L6: Tip of the mesiobuccal cusp of lower permanent first molar, L1: Incisal tip of the mandibular central incisor. (**b**) cephalometric measurements.

FMA: The angle formed between the Frankfort Horizontal Plane (Or-Po) and the mandibular plane (Go-Me).

SN-GoGn (Mandibular plane angle): The angle between the GoGn and SN lines.

Cant of Occlusal Plane: The angle between the occlusal plane (the line bisecting the overlapping cusps of first molars and incisor overbite) and the Frankfort Horizontal Plane.

To assess the reproducibility of the measurements, the same researcher re-evaluated 50 randomly chosen lateral cephalometric radiographs one week after the completion of all four cephalometric measures. The intraclass correlation coefficient, which measures intraobserver agreement, was found to be between 0.89 to 0.98, indicating strong reproducibility of cephalometric measurements.

Each cephalometric parameter—FMA, SN-GoGn, and Occlusal Plane Inclination—was divided into three subgroups representing vertical skeletal patterns: hypodivergent (low angle), normodivergent (average angle), and hyperdivergent (high angle). These groups were formed based on the numerical distribution of the dataset rather than fixed normative thresholds. Classification intervals were derived by dividing the full range of values into three equal-sized quantiles (see Table 1). This approach ensured statistical balance across subgroups for model training.

Table 1. Classification values of cephalometric measurements.

Class	Subclass	Classification Value Range
FMA	FMA 1	8.1–22.49
	FMA 2	22.51–27.79
	FMA 3	27.8–46.68
SN-GoGn	SN-GoGn1	11.81–28.08
	SN-GoGn 2	28.14–33.29
	SN-GoGn 3	33.34–57.09
Cant of Occlusal Plane	Cant of Occlusal Plane 1	−6.97–6.64
	Cant of Occlusal Plane 2	6.65–10.63
	Cant of Occlusal Plane 3	10.7–20.64

2.2. Dataset Formation, DL Algorithms, and Training

The dataset used in this study comprised three classes: FMA, SN-GoGn, and the Cant of the occlusal plane. The original dataset contained 350 images for each subclass. To augment the dataset, several image processing techniques were applied, including horizontal translation, rotation, width shift, height shift, and zoom. As a result of these augmentation techniques, the number of images in each subclass was increased to 800. Following the data augmentation process, the dataset was partitioned into training and testing sets, with labeled examples used for all DL models. In all models, 80% of the dataset was allocated for training, while the remaining 20% was designated for testing.

In this study, six DL models were utilized: ResNet101, DenseNet201, EfficientNet B0, EfficientNet V2 B0, ConvNetBase, and a hybrid model.

This study employed widely used convolutional neural network architectures—ResNet101, DenseNet201, EfficientNet B0, EfficientNet V2 B0, and a hybrid model integrating EfficientNet B0 and DenseNet201. These models were selected due to their proven performance in medical image classification tasks and their architectural advantages: ResNet's residual connections mitigate vanishing gradient problems in deep networks; DenseNet promotes feature reuse through dense connectivity; EfficientNet optimizes accuracy and computational cost via compound scaling; and the proposed hybrid model aims to combine DenseNet's rich feature extraction with EfficientNet's parameter efficiency to improve diagnostic precision.

ResNet101 (Residual Network 101) is a deep convolutional neural network comprising 101 layers, designed to address the vanishing gradient problem in very deep networks through the use of skip (residual) connections. As the depth of a neural network increases, training becomes increasingly difficult due to the degradation of gradient flow, which can hinder the update of model parameters. ResNet101 mitigates this issue by enabling direct information transfer between non-adjacent layers, thereby maintaining efficient gradient propagation and facilitating effective learning even in extremely deep architectures.

DenseNet201 (densely connected convolutional network) is a 201-layer deep neural network that introduces dense connectivity between layers. Unlike conventional CNNs, where each layer receives input only from the preceding layer, in DenseNet201, each layer has direct access to the outputs of all preceding layers. This architecture enhances gradient flow, encourages feature reuse, and reduces the number of parameters required, resulting in more efficient learning and improved model performance.

EfficientNet B0 is a convolutional neural network that prioritizes parameter efficiency while maintaining high accuracy. Traditional CNNs often scale model performance by increasing depth or width independently; in contrast, EfficientNet employs a compound scaling method that jointly optimizes network depth, width, and input resolution. This balanced approach enables EfficientNet B0 to achieve superior accuracy with significantly fewer parameters, making it suitable for deployment in resource-constrained environments such as mobile or edge devices.

EfficientNetV2 B0 is an enhanced version of EfficientNet B0, offering faster training and improved performance. It incorporates a progressive learning strategy, wherein data augmentation is gradually increased throughout training. This method accelerates convergence and enhances generalization. EfficientNetV2 B0 achieves higher accuracy while requiring fewer floating-point operations (FLOPs), thereby improving training efficiency and inference speed.

ConvNetBase is a baseline convolutional neural network model built upon the core principles of traditional CNN architectures. It consists of standard convolutional layers, activation functions (typically ReLU), and pooling operations. While it is more lightweight and computationally less demanding than more complex architectures, its performance in terms of accuracy is generally lower. ConvNetBase is often utilized in scenarios involving small datasets or when rapid model training is a priority.

The hybrid model, a robust classification architecture, was developed by integrating the EfficientNet B0 and DenseNet201 networks. The architecture processes a 224 × 224 × 3 input image, which was simultaneously fed into two distinct deep learning models. EfficientNet B0, known for its parameter efficiency, optimizes the features extracted from deeper layers, generating a feature vector of size 1280. In contrast, DenseNet201 leverages dense connections to extract richer, more detailed features, resulting in a feature vector of size 1920. These two feature vectors were then merged to form a unified feature space of 3200 dimensions. Subsequently, a squeeze-and-excitation (SE) attention block was applied to enhance the model's learning by emphasizing critical information. This attention mechanism refines feature selection through channel-based scaling, enabling the model to focus on more informative features. The final stage of the model consists of a multi-layer perceptron (MLP) classifier. The MLP classifier was designed with a series of layers, starting at 1024 units, gradually reducing to 512 and 256 units, before producing the final class prediction. To promote a more stable and regular learning process, several techniques were employed, including batch normalization, ReLU activation, and dropout between the layers (Figure 2).

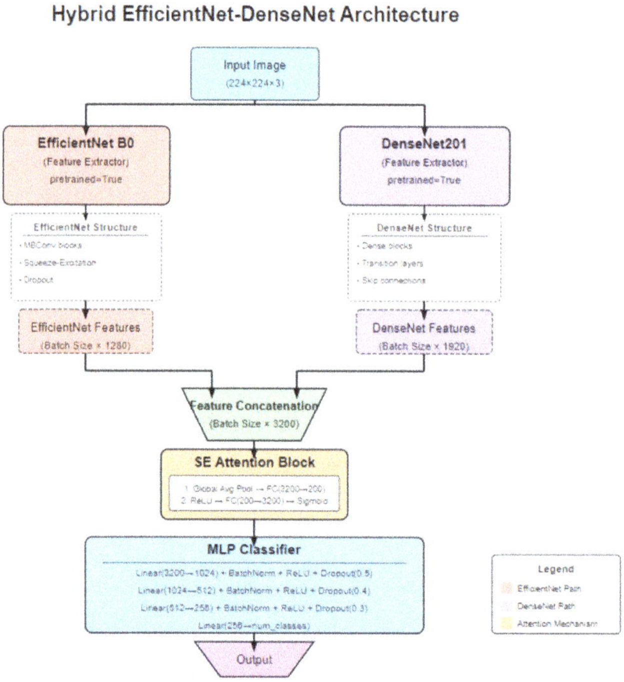

Figure 2. Hybrid model architecture.

All deep learning models were trained using a Google Cloud-based system equipped with an NVIDIA Tesla T4 GPU (16 GB VRAM), Intel Xeon CPU (2.20 GHz), and 16 GB RAM. The average training time per model was approximately 3.8 h. Inference time per image was ~85 milliseconds (0.085 s), enabling near-real-time prediction.

Diagnostic accuracy, sensitivity, specificity, the area under the curve (AUC), Cohen's Kappa metrics among training and test groups, mean absolute error (MAE), and confusion matrices were used to test the performance of DL algorithms among training and test groups.

The Grad-CAM (gradient-weighted class activation mapping) method was used to visualize the decision mechanism of the model and analyze it with explainable artificial intelligence methods.

3. Results

The results according to the parameters used in our study are as follows:

3.1. FMA

The accuracy, MAE, and Cohen's Kappa metric values for six deep learning algorithms applied to the FMA parameter are provided in Table 2.

Table 2. Model performance metrics of FMA.

Model	Accuracy	MAE	Cohen's Kappa
ResNet101	0.8271	0.1958	0.7406
DenseNet201	0.8375	0.1708	0.7562
EfficientNetV2 B0	0.8167	0.1938	0.725
ConvNetBase	0.7958	0.2313	0.6937
EfficientNet B0	0.8375	0.1688	0.7562
Hybrid	0.8667	0.1354	0.8000

The highest accuracy rate for FMA was obtained by the hybrid model (86.67%), with 416 correct classifications out of 480 images. ConvNetBase presented the lowest accuracy rate, at 79.58%, with correct classifications for 382 images out of 480. Evaluation using the MAE and Cohen's Kappa metrics indicates that the hybrid model is the most reliable among the models assessed.

The precision–recall curve and the AUC-ROC curve for FMA using the hybrid model are presented in Figure 3. The lowest precision–recall value across the three subgroups was 0.9149, while the lowest AUC value recorded was 0.9510.

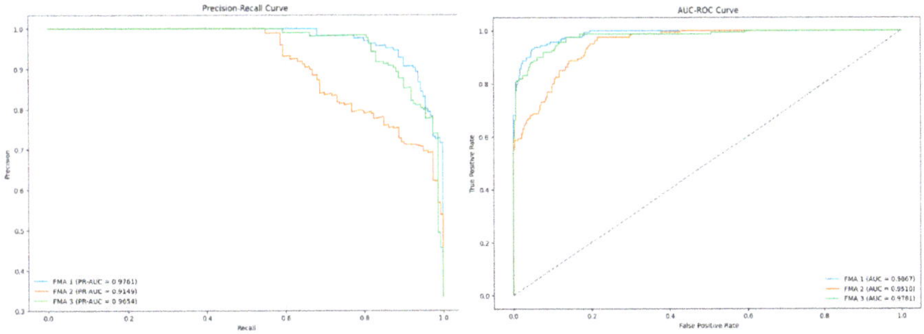

(a) (b)

Figure 3. (**a**) The precision–recall curve of FMA; (**b**) AUC-ROC curve of FMA.

Figure 4 shows an example of heatmap images reflecting the characteristics of the learning and classification behavior of the hybrid model for FMA.

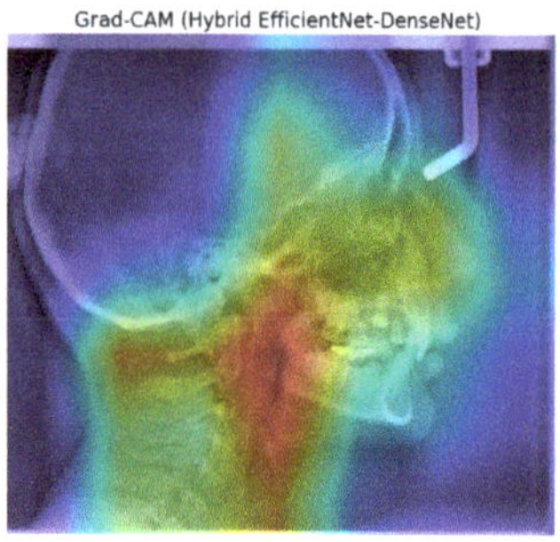

Figure 4. Grad-CAM of the hybrid model for FMA.

3.2. SN-GoGn

The accuracy, MAE, and Cohen's Kappa metric values for six deep learning algorithms applied to the SN-GoGn parameter are provided in Table 3.

Table 3. Model performance metrics of SN-GoGn.

Model	Accuracy	MAE	Cohen's Kappa
ResNet101	0.8042	0.225	0.7063
DenseNet201	0.8208	0.1917	0.7312
EfficientNetV2 B0	0.7917	0.2125	0.6875
ConvNetBase	0.65	0.5021	0.475
EfficientNet B0	0.8583	0.1417	0.7875
Hybrid	0.8729	0.1375	0.8094

The highest accuracy rate for SN-GoGn was obtained by the hybrid model (87.29%), with 419 correct classifications out of 480 images. ConvNetBase presented the lowest accuracy rate, at 65%, with correct classifications for 312 images out of 480. Evaluation using the MAE and Cohen's Kappa metrics indicates that the hybrid model is the most reliable among the models assessed.

The precision–recall curve and the AUC-ROC curve for SN-GoGn using the hybrid model are presented in Figure 5. The lowest precision–recall value across the three subgroups was 0.9176, while the lowest AUC value recorded was 0.9506.

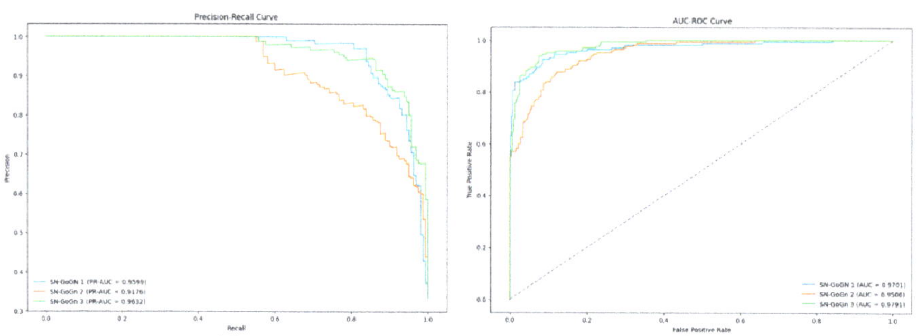

(a) (b)

Figure 5. (**a**) The precision–recall curve of SN-GoGn; (**b**) AUC-ROC curve of SN-GoGn.

Figure 6 shows an example of heatmap images reflecting the characteristics of the learning and classification behavior of the hybrid model for SN-GoGn.

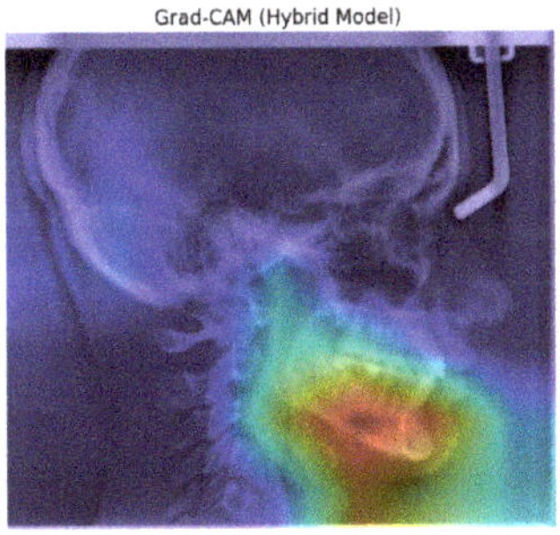

Figure 6. Grad-CAM of the hybrid model for SN-GoGn.

3.3. Cant of Occlusal Plane

The accuracy, MAE, and Cohen's Kappa metric values for six deep learning algorithms applied to the Cant of the Occlusal Plane parameter are provided in Table 4.

Table 4. Model performance metrics of the Cant of the Occlusal Plane.

Model	Accuracy	MAE	Cohen's Kappa
ResNet101	0.7625	0.3521	0.6438
DenseNet201	0.75	0.3688	0.625
EfficientNetV2 B0	0.775	0.3333	0.6625
ConvNetBase	0.7021	0.4104	0.5531
EfficientNet B0	0.7917	0.2979	0.6875
Hybrid	0.8271	0.2521	0.7406

The highest accuracy rate for the Cant of Occlusal Plane was obtained by the Hybrid model (82.71%), with 397 correct classifications out of 480 images. ConvNetBase presented the lowest accuracy rate, at 70.21%, with correct classifications for 337 images out of 480. Evaluation using the MAE and Cohen's Kappa metrics indicates that the hybrid model is the most reliable among the models assessed.

The precision–recall curve and the AUC-ROC curve for the Cant of the Occlusal Plane using the hybrid model are presented in Figure 7. The lowest precision–recall value across the three subgroups was 0.8770, while the lowest AUC value recorded was 0.9178.

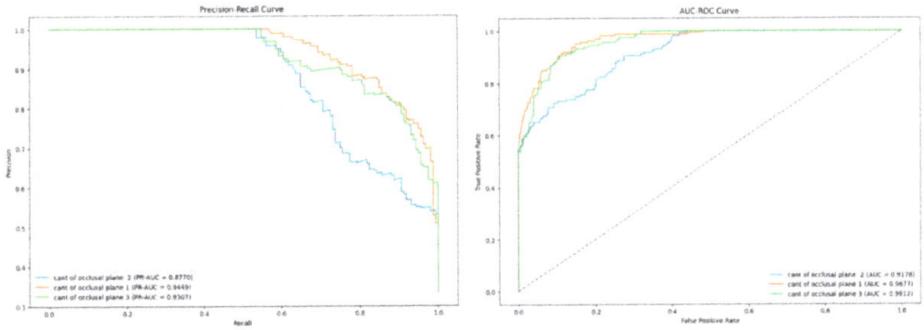

(**a**) (**b**)

Figure 7. (**a**) The precision–recall curve of Cant of the Occlusal Plane; (**b**) AUC-ROC curve of Cant of the Occlusal Plane.

Figure 8 shows an example of heatmap images reflecting the characteristics of the learning and classification behavior of the hybrid model for the Cant of the Occlusal Plane.

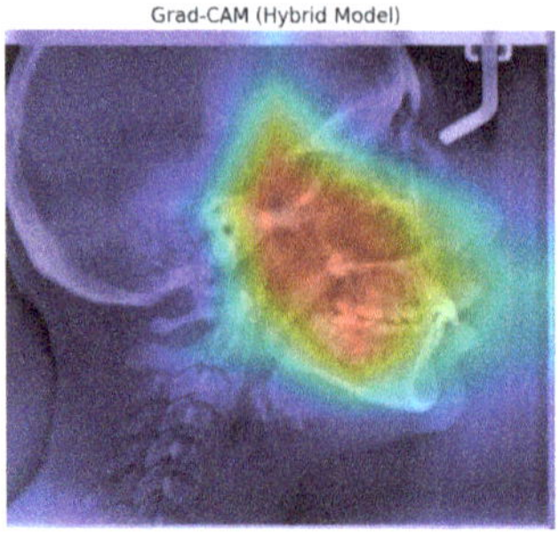

Figure 8. Grad-CAM of the hybrid model for the Cant of the Occlusal Plane.

3.4. Visualization of Localization Results

Grad-CAM analysis of ResNet101, DenseNet201, ConvNetBase, EfficientNet B0, EfficientNet V2 B0, and the hybrid model is given in Figure 9.

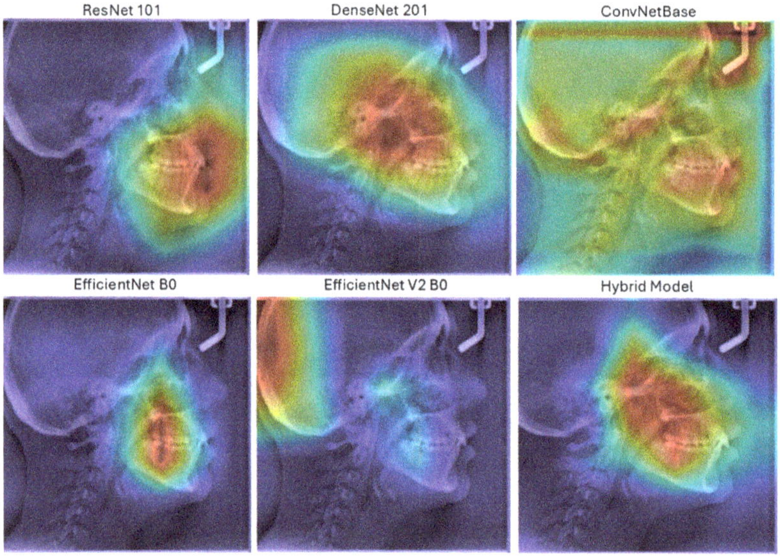

Figure 9. Grad-CAM analysis of DL models used in this study.

The Grad-CAM visualization of the ResNet101 architecture reveals that it typically focuses on the central features of the object, although the focus area is relatively dispersed. In comparison, the DenseNet architecture exhibits a more concentrated activation region. The ConvNetBase model shows a wider and less precise activation area compared to the other architectures. EfficientNet B0 demonstrates a more balanced focus on the object's characteristic features. The improved version, EfficientNet V2, produces more focused and less noisy activation regions than EfficientNet B0. As observed in the Grad-CAM visualizations, the hybrid model generates more accurate, concentrated, and meaningful activation regions than the others.

The whole confusion matrices, tables, and graphs of the DL models used in this study are included in the Supplementary Data.

4. Discussion

Among orthodontic malocclusions, vertical discrepancies are one of the most challenging to diagnose and treat due to their complex nature. The interaction and involvement of different contributing elements and their subsequent effects on the treatment approaches and results become an important priority compared to other types of malocclusions [19].

Numerous cephalometric measurements are employed in the evaluation of vertical discrepancies. For instance, the FMA angle is utilized in Tweed analysis; however, accurately determining the Frankfort Horizontal Plane is not always feasible. In Steiner analysis, the SN-GoGn angle is used to assess the vertical direction. However, the SN plane can be influenced by the inclination of the anterior cranial base, which may reduce its reliability in effectively evaluating growth patterns. Research suggests that SN-GoGn and FMA angles can be measured with greater precision in hyperdivergent and normodivergent patients [2]. Given that there is no single correct parameter for vertical direction assessment, our study incorporated three different parameters, and the classification successes among these parameters were compared and evaluated.

In our study, the classification performance of three different vertical parameters was compared using six different DL algorithms. The highest classification success rates were achieved for the SN-GoGn group, with 87.29%, for the FMA group with 86.67%, and for the Cant of Occlusal Plane group with 82.71% by the hybrid model. While all groups yielded promising classification results, the Cant of the Occlusal Plane group demonstrated relatively lower performance.

AI refers to the ability of a machine to mimic human intelligence in performing specific tasks. In recent years, significant advancements have been made in the field of artificial intelligence. Its applications have also increasingly been integrated into the medical field. In particular, digital radiographs offer a valuable resource for artificial intelligence in both medicine and dentistry. These images can be digitally encoded and easily translated into computational language, making them ideal for creating large datasets that can be analyzed using AI technologies [20]. As in our study, there are many studies in the literature in which deep learning algorithms use cephalometric radiographs as a dataset. Automated anatomical landmark detection, cervical vertebral maturation assessment, evaluation of extraction needs in orthodontic treatments, or determination of the necessity for orthognathic surgery, among other evaluations, have achieved successful results using deep learning algorithms on cephalometric radiographs [21–26].

In recent years, numerous traditional machine learning and deep learning methods have been developed for cephalometric analysis [27]. Recent studies have predominantly focused on unimodal deep learning approaches, which primarily utilize convolutional neural networks (CNNs) to detect anatomical landmarks from lateral cephalograms [28]. High performance has been reported in recent efforts aimed at the accurate identification of these landmarks. For instance, Lee et al. reported a successful detection rate of 82.11%; Zeng et al. reported 81.37% and 70.58% in two different tests; Uğurlu et al. reported 76.2%; and Yao et al. reported 97.3% [29–32]. One of the major limitations in training and testing deep learning models for the cephalometric analysis of radiographs is the complexity of data annotation. There is no single ground-truth localization for a given anthropometric landmark that can be universally accepted as a gold standard. Typically, multiple experts manually annotate a particular landmark, and the aggregated results are used to generate the reference labels for training deep learning algorithms [14]. Our study differs from these anatomical landmark detection approaches in that it does not require the detection of cephalometric landmarks. This characteristic offers a significant advantage by mitigating potential misclassifications that may arise due to incorrectly labeled landmarks.

As such, our method addresses one of the key challenges in current deep learning-based cephalometric analysis.

In the present study, deep learning models were evaluated using vertical direction parameters. Comparable research has been carried out as well, though concentrating on the assessment of sagittal direction parameters. In the sagittal skeletal classification study conducted by Nan L. et al., the classification performance of the DenseNet algorithm was evaluated based on ANB and Wits measurements from cephalometric radiographs. The study reported an accuracy of 90.33% [18]. Zahng JN et al. reported that they achieved 85% accuracy in their study using a deep learning-based convolutional neural network (CNN) model to predict the growth trend of the mandible of a child with anterior crossbite from pretreatment cephalometric radiographs [33].

Similar to our study, Yu HJ et al. researched automatic skeletal classification using lateral cephalometric radiographs with deep learning, as they classified the vertical direction assessment based on the Björk sum and Jarabak ratio. They achieved 96.40% classification accuracy in this study using the Densenet algorithm. They reported that the classification success of hyperdivergent and hypodivergent groups showed a higher rate than the normal group [34]. Similarly, in our study, we observed that the classification accuracy of hyperdivergent and hypodivergent patients was higher.

Kocakaya DNC et al., in their study evaluating the classification performance of profile photographs using deep learning algorithms, reported achieving a classification accuracy of 97% based on the FMA angle [16]. The differing success rates between the photographs and cephalometric radiographs used as the dataset for the same parameter suggest the need for further research.

ConvNet was the model with the lowest classification accuracy in our study. To the best of our knowledge, ConvNet has not been applied to cephalometric radiographs; however, it has been applied to other radiographic data in certain research. He et al. employed ConvNet, DenseNet, and ResNet architectures for the detection of abnormalities in musculoskeletal radiographs, reporting that ConvNet achieved the lowest classification accuracy at 82%, while DenseNet demonstrated the highest accuracy at 90% [35]. Similar to this, Showkhatian et al. evaluated the architectures of ConvNet, DenseNet, VGG16, VGG19, ResNet50, Exception, and Inception V3 on chest radiographs for the detection of tuberculosis. They discovered that ConvNet had the lowest classification accuracy (87%), while Exception, ResNet50, and VGG16 performed the best (90%) [36].

From a methodological standpoint, landmark-based classification relies on first detecting anatomically defined reference points, followed by deterministic geometric calculations. This pipeline offers high diagnostic transparency, as the decision path is grounded in established cephalometric measurements. However, it is susceptible to cumulative error propagation from landmark misplacement, and it typically requires human oversight or post hoc verification, potentially slowing clinical workflows. By contrast, the end-to-end deep learning model proposed in this study eliminates the need for manual or automatic landmark annotation and learns discriminative features directly from raw radiographic input. This enhances classification speed and simplifies deployment, especially in high-throughput or chairside environments. Yet, it reduces interpretability for clinicians accustomed to traditional cephalometric angles and may obscure the basis for individual predictions unless explainable AI techniques are used. In practice, a hybrid strategy may be ideal—leveraging end-to-end models for initial screening while preserving landmark-based tools for transparent clinical auditing. Future research should explore how these approaches can be integrated seamlessly within digital orthodontic workflows.

The proposed landmark-independent deep learning model offers several practical advantages in orthodontic clinical settings. First, by eliminating the need for manual or automated landmark identification, the model significantly reduces the time required for cephalometric analysis—making real-time chairside diagnosis feasible. Second, it mitigates inter- and intra-examiner variability commonly associated with landmark placement, thereby increasing diagnostic consistency. Third, early and reliable classification of vertical skeletal growth patterns facilitates timely intervention planning, such as growth modification therapies in hyperdivergent patients or vertical control strategies in hypodivergent cases. Finally, the model can be integrated into digital orthodontic platforms to support automated pre-screening and triage, improving overall clinic efficiency.

Grad-CAM is a technique used to visualize the interpretability of models and can easily be applied to various CNN architectures for better understanding [37]. In our study, the hybrid model presents a unique approach by combining the strengths of different architectures. As observed from the Grad-CAM visualizations, this model produces activation maps that are more accurate, focused, and meaningful compared to others. This enhances the model's performance in classification tasks. In contrast to other models, where activations are scattered across irrelevant regions, the hybrid model's activation map concentrates more consistently on semantically significant parts of the object.

Recent advancements in artificial intelligence have expanded beyond image classification to include more complex analytical methods such as AI-assisted chaotic functional analysis. This approach leverages nonlinear dynamics and fractal-based pattern recognition to model the complex biological processes underlying craniofacial growth [38]. Integrating metaheuristic optimization techniques into our deep learning framework, where direct image-based classification is complemented by AI-driven chaotic functional models, may have potential for providing a comprehensive tool for individualized orthodontic diagnosis and treatment planning.

There are some limitations to our study. First of all, since this study was conducted at a single center, there is no data that may affect facial features belonging to different ethnic groups. In a multicenter study, the inclusion of radiographic data obtained with different cephalometric devices may allow our findings to be developed more comprehensively. DL algorithms may show more accurate classification performance by increasing the dataset. Although training the proposed models requires GPU acceleration, the final inference phase, once the model is deployed, can be executed on a mid-range CPU-based system with acceptable latency (<0.1 s/image). Therefore, it is technically feasible to implement the model on chair-side computers in clinical environments. However, for large-scale processing or training on new datasets, GPU or cloud resources remain preferable. While our end-to-end classification framework bypasses the landmark annotation step, future work may explore a comparative approach involving CNN-based landmark detection followed by angle-based geometric classification using FMA, SN-GoGn, and Occlusal Plane Inclination. This would allow for a direct evaluation of the performance and practicality trade-offs between fully automated image-to-class networks and semi-automated landmark-dependent systems.

The fact that only vertical parameters were examined in our study is one of the limitations of the study, since other factors that may affect these parameters were excluded. Finally, the use of a dataset consisting of 3D images instead of 2D images may contribute to obtaining more clinically valuable and comprehensive results.

Strengths of the Study

This study presents several methodological and practical strengths: (1) The use of a novel hybrid deep learning architecture combining EfficientNet and DenseNet allows the model to benefit from both efficient scaling and dense feature propagation, resulting in robust classification performance. (2) Advanced data augmentation techniques, including rotation, translation, and brightness normalization, were applied to improve generalization and mitigate overfitting. (3) The inclusion of Grad-CAM–based visualization enhances the interpretability of the model by highlighting the anatomical regions that contribute most to the classification, promoting clinical trust in AI-generated decisions. (4) The model was trained and validated on a balanced and expertly annotated dataset with clearly defined vertical skeletal pattern categories, ensuring both clinical relevance and methodological rigor.

Our results support the alternative hypothesis (H_1): deep learning models—especially the proposed hybrid architecture—can classify vertical skeletal patterns from cephalometric radiographs with high accuracy, surpassing the constraints of traditional landmark-dependent methods. The landmark-free pipeline not only improves diagnostic efficiency but also minimizes error propagation, thereby offering a practical tool for chairside clinical implementation.

5. Conclusions

This study demonstrates the feasibility of using deep learning models, specifically a hybrid CNN architecture, to classify vertical skeletal growth patterns directly from lateral cephalometric radiographs without relying on anatomical landmarks. Achieving high diagnostic performance and a time-efficient solution through bypassing manual or automated landmark detection, our findings support the integration of end-to-end DL models into clinical orthodontic assessment systems, with potential for real-time chairside implementation.

Supplementary Materials: The following supporting information can be downloaded at: https://www.mdpi.com/article/10.3390/diagnostics15172240/s1.

Author Contributions: Conceptualization, M.B.Ö., S.B.A.K. and M.Ç.; methodology, M.B.Ö.; S.B.A.K. and M.Ç.; software, M.Ç.; validation, M.B.Ö.; S.B.A.K. and M.Ç.; formal analysis, M.B.Ö.; investigation, S.B.A.K.; resources, M.B.Ö., S.B.A.K. and M.Ç.; data curation, M.Ç.; writing—original draft preparation, M.B.Ö. and S.B.A.K.; writing—review and editing, M.B.Ö. and S.B.A.K.; visualization, S.B.A.K.; supervision, S.B.A.K.; project administration, M.B.Ö. All authors have read and agreed to the published version of the manuscript.

Funding: This research received no external funding.

Institutional Review Board Statement: Our study was found scientifically and ethically appropriate by the Kocaeli University Non-Interventional Clinical Research Ethics Committee, with decision number KU GOKAEK-2025/15/30 and project number 2025/383 (approval date 3 July 2025).

Informed Consent Statement: Informed consent was obtained from all subjects involved in the study.

Data Availability Statement: The raw data supporting the conclusions of this article will be made available by the authors upon request. The Python (version 3.10.12) and TensorFlow (version 2.12.0) code used to implement and evaluate the deep learning models will be made publicly available on GitHub upon publication of this article.

Conflicts of Interest: The authors declare no conflicts of interest.

Abbreviations

The following abbreviations are used in this manuscript:

AI	Artificial intelligence
DL	Deep learning
MAE	Main absolute error

AUC Area under the curve
CNN Convolutional neural network

References

1. Arnett, G.W.; Bergman, R.T. Facial Keys to Orthodontic Diagnosis and Treatment Planning. Part I. *Am. J. Orthod. Dentofac. Orthop.* **1993**, *103*, 299–312. [CrossRef]
2. Azeez, S.M. Evaluating diagnostic performance of three cephalometric vertical parameters. *Indian J. Dent. Res.* **2023**, *34*, 49–53. [CrossRef] [PubMed]
3. Roy, P.; Roy, P.; Koley, S. Comparative Assessment of Various Cephalometric Parameters Used for Determining Vertical Skeletal Dysplasia. *Cureus J. Med. Sci.* **2024**, *16*, e55101. [CrossRef] [PubMed] [PubMed Central]
4. Ahmed, M.; Shaikh, A.; Fida, M. Diagnostic performance of various cephalometric parameters for the assessment of vertical growth pattern. *Dental Press. J. Orthod.* **2016**, *21*, 41–49. [CrossRef] [PubMed] [PubMed Central]
5. Devereux, L.; Moles, D.; Cunningham, S.J.; McKnight, M. How important are lateral cephalometric radiographs in orthodontic treatment planning? *Am. J. Orthod. Dentofac. Orthop.* **2011**, *139*, e175–e181. [CrossRef] [PubMed]
6. Gandhi, K.K.; Rai, A. Novel cephalometric parameters for the assessment of vertical skeletal dysplasia. *J. Orthod. Sci.* **2022**, *11*, 38. [CrossRef] [PubMed]
7. Kazimierczak, N.; Kazimierczak, W.; Serafin, Z.; Nowicki, P.; Nożewski, J.; Janiszewska-Olszowska, J. AI in Orthodontics: Revolutionizing Diagnostics and Treatment Planning-A Comprehensive Review. *J. Clin. Med.* **2024**, *13*, 344. [CrossRef] [PubMed] [PubMed Central]
8. Surendran, A.; Daigavane, P.; Shrivastav, S.; Kamble, R.; Sanchla, A.D.; Bharti, L.; Shinde, M. The Future of Orthodontics: Deep Learning Technologies. *Cureus J. Med. Sci.* **2024**, *16*, e62045. [CrossRef] [PubMed] [PubMed Central]
9. Makaremi, M.; Lacaule, C.; Mohammad-Djafari, A. Deep Learning and Artificial Intelligence for the Determination of the Cervical Vertebra Maturation Degree from Lateral Radiography. *Entropy* **2019**, *21*, 1222. [CrossRef]
10. Yıldırım, A.; Cicek, O.; Genç, Y.S. Can AI-Based ChatGPT Models Accurately Analyze Hand–Wrist Radiographs? A Comparative Study. *Diagnostics* **2025**, *15*, 1513. [CrossRef]
11. Dipalma, G.; Inchingolo, A.D.; Inchingolo, A.M.; Piras, F.; Carpentiere, V.; Garofoli, G.; Azzollini, D.; Campanelli, M.; Paduanelli, G.; Palermo, A.; et al. Artificial Intelligence and Its Clinical Applications in Orthodontics: A Systematic Review. *Diagnostics* **2023**, *13*, 3677. [CrossRef] [PubMed]
12. Kurt Demirsoy, K.; Buyuk, S.K.; Bicer, T. How Reliable Is the Artificial Intelligence Product Large Language Model ChatGPT in Orthodontics? *Angle Orthod.* **2024**, *94*, 602–607. [CrossRef] [PubMed]
13. Koz, S.; Uslu-Akcam, O. Artificial Intelligence-Supported and App-Aided Cephalometric Analysis: Which One Can We Trust? *Diagnostics* **2025**, *15*, 559. [CrossRef] [PubMed] [PubMed Central]
14. Kiełczykowski, M.; Kamiński, K.; Perkowski, K.; Zadurska, M.; Czochrowska, E. Application of Artificial Intelligence (AI) in a Cephalometric Analysis: A Narrative Review. *Diagnostics* **2023**, *13*, 2640. [CrossRef]
15. Hong, W.; Kim, S.-M.; Choi, J.; Ahn, J.; Paeng, J.-Y.; Kim, H. Automated Cephalometric Landmark Detection Using Deep Reinforcement Learning. *J. Craniofac. Surg.* **2023**, *34*, 2336–2342. [CrossRef]
16. Kocakaya, D.N.C.; Özel, M.B.; Kartbak, S.B.A.; Çakmak, M.; Sinanoğlu, E.A. Profile Photograph Classification Performance of Deep Learning Algorithms Trained Using Cephalometric Measurements: A Preliminary Study. *Diagnostics* **2024**, *14*, 1916. [CrossRef]
17. Kartbak, S.B.A.; Özel, M.B.; Kocakaya, D.N.C.; Çakmak, M.; Sinanoğlu, E.A. Classification of Intraoral Photographs with Deep Learning Algorithms Trained According to Cephalometric Measurements. *Diagnostics* **2025**, *15*, 1059. [CrossRef]
18. Nan, L.; Tang, M.; Liang, B.; Mo, S.; Kang, N.; Song, S.; Zhang, X.; Zeng, X. Automated Sagittal Skeletal Classification of Children Based on Deep Learning. *Diagnostics* **2023**, *13*, 1719. [CrossRef]
19. Akl, H.E.; Mostafa, Y.A. Digitization and validation of the open bite checklist manifesto: A step toward artificial intelligence. *Angle Orthod.* **2024**, *94*, 51–58. [CrossRef] [PubMed] [PubMed Central]
20. Putra, R.H.; Doi, C.; Yoda, N.; Astuti, E.R.; Sasaki, K. Current applications and development of artificial intelligence for digital dental radiography. *Dentomaxillofac. Radiol.* **2022**, *51*, 20210197. [CrossRef] [PubMed] [PubMed Central]
21. Xie, X.; Wang, L.; Wang, A. Artificial neural network modeling for deciding if extractions are necessary prior to orthodontic treatment. *Angle Orthod.* **2010**, *80*, 262–266. [CrossRef] [PubMed] [PubMed Central]
22. Kunz, F.; Stellzig-Eisenhauer, A.; Zeman, F.; Boldt, J. Artificial intelligence in orthodontics: Evaluation of a fully automated cephalometric analysis using a customized convolutional neural network. *J. Orofac. Orthop.* **2020**, *81*, 52–68. (In English) [CrossRef] [PubMed]
23. Hwang, H.W.; Park, J.H.; Moon, J.H.; Yu, Y.; Kim, H.; Her, S.B.; Srinivasan, G.; Aljanabi, M.N.A.; Donatelli, R.E.; Lee, S.J. Automated identification of cephalometric landmarks: Part 2-Might it be better than human? *Angle Orthod.* **2020**, *90*, 69–76. [CrossRef] [PubMed] [PubMed Central]

24. Choi, H.I.; Jung, S.K.; Baek, S.H.; Lim, W.H.; Ahn, S.J.; Yang, I.H.; Kim, T.W. Artificial Intelligent Model With Neural Network Machine Learning for the Diagnosis of Orthognathic Surgery. *J. Craniofac Surg.* **2019**, *30*, 1986–1989. Erratum in *J. Craniofac. Surg.* **2020**, *31*, 1156. https://doi.org/10.1097/SCS.0000000000006531. [CrossRef] [PubMed]
25. Seo, H.; Hwang, J.; Jeong, T.; Shin, J. Comparison of Deep Learning Models for Cervical Vertebral Maturation Stage Classification on Lateral Cephalometric Radiographs. *J. Clin. Med.* **2021**, *10*, 3591. [CrossRef] [PubMed] [PubMed Central]
26. Zhang, Y.; Lu, Z.; Zhou, J.; Sun, Y.; Yi, W.; Wang, J.; Du, T.; Li, D.; Zhao, X.; Xu, Y.; et al. CDSNet: An automated method for assessing growth stages from various anatomical regions in lateral cephalograms based on deep learning. *J. World Fed. Orthod.* **2025**, *14*, 154–160. [CrossRef] [PubMed]
27. Jiang, F.; Guo, Y.; Yang, C.; Zhou, Y.; Lin, Y.; Cheng, F.; Quan, S.; Feng, Q.; Li, J. Artificial Intelligence System for Automated Landmark Localization and Analysis of Cephalometry. *Dentomaxillofac. Radiol.* **2023**, *52*, 20220081. [CrossRef]
28. Gao, F.; Tang, Y. Multimodal Deep Learning for Cephalometric Landmark Detection and Treatment Prediction. *Sci. Rep.* **2025**, *15*, 25205. [CrossRef]
29. Lee, J.-H.; Yu, H.-J.; Kim, M.-J.; Kim, J.-W.; Choi, J. Automated Cephalometric Landmark Detection with Confidence Regions Using Bayesian Convolutional Neural Networks. *BMC Oral Health* **2020**, *20*, 270. [CrossRef]
30. Zeng, M.; Yan, Z.; Liu, S.; Zhou, Y.; Qiu, L. Cascaded Convolutional Networks for Automatic Cephalometric Landmark Detection. *Med. Image Anal.* **2021**, *68*, 101904. [CrossRef]
31. Ugurlu, M. Performance of a Convolutional Neural Network-Based Artificial Intelligence Algorithm for Automatic Cephalometric Landmark Detection. *Turk. J. Orthod.* **2022**, *35*, 94–100. [CrossRef]
32. Yao, J.; Zeng, W.; He, T.; Zhou, S.; Zhang, Y.; Guo, J.; Tang, W. Automatic Localization of Cephalometric Landmarks Based on Convolutional Neural Network. *Am. J. Orthod. Dentofacial Orthop.* **2022**, *161*, e250–e259. [CrossRef]
33. Zhang, J.N.; Lu, H.P.; Hou, J.; Wang, Q.; Yu, F.Y.; Zhong, C.; Huang, C.Y.; Chen, S. Deep learning-based prediction of mandibular growth trend in children with anterior crossbite using cephalometric radiographs. *BMC Oral Health* **2023**, *23*, 28. [CrossRef] [PubMed] [PubMed Central]
34. Yu, H.J.; Cho, S.R.; Kim, M.J.; Kim, W.H.; Kim, J.W.; Choi, J. Automated Skeletal Classification with Lateral Cephalometry Based on Artificial Intelligence. *J. Dent. Res.* **2020**, *99*, 249–256. [CrossRef] [PubMed]
35. He, M.; Wang, X.; Zhao, Y. A calibrated deep learning ensemble for abnormality detection in musculoskeletal radiographs. *Sci. Rep.* **2021**, *11*, 9097. [CrossRef] [PubMed] [PubMed Central]
36. Showkatian, E.; Salehi, M.; Ghaffari, H.; Reiazi, R.; Sadighi, N. Deep learning-based automatic detection of tuberculosis disease in chest X-ray images. *Pol. J. Radiol.* **2022**, *87*, e118–e124. [CrossRef] [PubMed] [PubMed Central]
37. Zhang, H.; Ogasawara, K. Grad-CAM-Based Explainable Artificial Intelligence Related to Medical Text Processing. *Bioengineering* **2023**, *10*, 1070. [CrossRef] [PubMed]
38. Cicek, O.; Özçelik, Y.B.; Altan, A. A New Approach Based on Metaheuristic Optimization Using Chaotic Functional Connectivity Matrices and Fractal Dimension Analysis for AI-Driven Detection of Orthodontic Growth and Development Stage. *Fractal Fract.* **2025**, *9*, 148. [CrossRef]

diagnostics

MDPI

Article

Data Analytics and Machine Learning Models on COVID-19 Medical Reports Enhanced with XAI for Usability

Oliver Lohaj [1,*], Ján Paralič [1], Zuzana Paraličová [2], Daniela Javorská [2] and Elena Zagorová [1]

[1] Department of Cybernetics and Artificial Intelligence, Faculty of Electrical Engineering and Informatics, Technical University of Kosice, Letná 9, 042 00 Košice, Slovakia; jan.paralic@tuke.sk (J.P.); elena.zagorova@student.tuke.sk (E.Z.)
[2] Department of Infectology and Travel Medicine, Faculty of Medicine, L. Pasteur University Hospital, Pavol Jozef Šafárik University, Rastislavova 43, 041 90 Košice, Slovakia; zuzana.paralicova@upjs.sk (Z.P.); daniela.javorska@student.upjs.sk (D.J.)
* Correspondence: oliver.lohaj@tuke.sk

Abstract

Objective—To identify effective data analytics and machine learning solutions that can help in the decision-making process in the medical domain and contribute to the understanding of COVID-19 disease. In this study, we analyze data from anonymized electronic medical records of 4711 patients with COVID-19 disease admitted to hospital in Atlanta. **Methods**—We used random forest, LightGBM, XGBoost, CatBoost, KNN, SVM, logistic regression, and MLP neural network models in this work. The models are evaluated depending on the type of prediction by relevant metrics, especially accuracy, F1-score, and ROC AUC score. Another aim of the work was to find out which factors most affected severity and mortality risk among the patients. To identify the important features, different statistical methods were used, as well as LASSO regression, and explainable artificial intelligence (XAI) method SHAP values for model explainability. The best models were implemented in a web application and tested by medical experts. The model for prediction of mortality risk was tested on a validation cohort of 45 patients from the Department of Infectiology and Travel Medicine, L. Pasteur University Hospital in Košice (UNLP). **Results**—Our study shows that the best model for predicting COVID-19 disease severity was the LightGBM model with accuracy of 88.4% using all features and 89.5% using the eight most important features. The best model for predicting mortality risk was also the LightGBM model, which achieved a ROC AUC score of 83.7% and a classification accuracy of 81.2% using all features. Using a simplified model trained on the 15 most important features, the ROC AUC score was 83.6% and the classification accuracy was 80.5%. We deployed the simplified models for predicting COVID-19 disease severity and for predicting the risk of COVID-19-related death in a web-based application and tested them with medical experts. This test resulted in a ROC AUC score of 83.6% and an overall prediction accuracy of 73.3%.

Keywords: COVID-19 risk factors; COVID-19 severity prediction; COVID-19 mortality; machine learning; model explainability; risk prediction

1. Introduction

The COVID-19 pandemic has significantly impacted nearly every aspect of human life across the globe, presenting profound challenges not only in the medical field but also in social, technological, and economic domains. The causative agent, the SARS-CoV-2 virus, was first identified in December 2019 in patients with severe respiratory disease in Wuhan,

 https://doi.org/10.3390/diagnostics15151981

Hubei Province, China [1]. By 11 March 2020, the World Health Organization (WHO) officially declared COVID-19 a global pandemic, prompting international public health responses and the recommendation to isolate individuals with respiratory symptoms, even in countries that had not yet reported any confirmed cases [2].

Since then, the pandemic has placed immense pressure on healthcare systems worldwide and highlighted the urgent need for effective tools to assist in medical decision making and patient triage. According to the WHO epidemiological update from 15 March 2024 [3], more than 774 million COVID-19 cases and over 7 million related deaths have been recorded globally, underlining the critical importance of continued research and preparedness.

In this work, we aim to explore the potential of machine learning and data analytics in predicting the severity of COVID-19 and the associated mortality risk based on electronic medical records. Our goal is to identify which models are most effective in supporting clinical decision making and to determine the most influential clinical and demographic factors contributing to severe outcomes in patients.

The structure of the article is as follows: the section Related Work provides a brief review of existing studies in this domain. The following section, Data Understanding, describes the dataset used, including its key features and characteristics. In Data Preprocessing, we detail the steps taken for cleaning, transforming, and selecting data. The section Data Modeling and Identifying Important Features is divided into two subsections: Modeling COVID-19 Severity and Modeling COVID-19 Mortality Risk. Each subsection outlines the models used, their performance metrics, and the methods applied for feature importance analysis. Simplified models using the most relevant features are also proposed to enhance practical applicability. Finally, the section Model Deployment and Testing on a New Cohort explains how the models were implemented in a web application and evaluated by medical experts using real-world patient data.

The novelty of our work lies in the combination of broad model comparison, explainability-focused modeling, and practical deployment in a clinical usability context. While earlier studies often limit themselves to a narrow algorithmic focus or lack post-model validation, we go further by (1) evaluating a wide spectrum of ML models, (2) simplifying them based on SHAP and domain expertise to ensure clinical applicability, (3) integrating explainable AI into a web-based tool, and (4) validating the system with real-world patient data and expert feedback. This end-to-end approach ensures not only performance but also usability, transparency, and real-world readiness. While expert consultation played a valuable role in validating feature relevance and interpretability, it was used in conjunction with statistical methods such as chi-square tests, ANOVA, LASSO regression, and SHAP values. As highlighted in Related Work, expert opinion alone is considered among the lowest levels of clinical evidence; robust machine learning in healthcare should integrate statistical modeling with empirical validation [4].

2. Related Work

Multiple studies have explored the use of machine learning (ML) on COVID-19 medical record data. Yu et al. [5] employed logistic regression and XGBoost models to predict mortality risk and assess the added value of respiratory support data. Similarly, Jha et al. [6] used XGBoost to forecast pulmonary fibrosis in COVID-19 patients. Sottile et al. [7] implemented a stacked generalization framework to improve mortality prediction over the SOFA score, using logistic regression with ridge regularization as the top-level model and several established clinical scores (SOFA, qSOFA, CURB-65, CCI, etc.) as component inputs.

Jiang et al. [8] investigated long COVID-19 risk prediction using vital sign time series from the first 7 days of hospitalization, applying PCA, Kolmogorov–Smirnov tests, XGBoost, and deep learning. Rivera et al. [9] explored the impact of statin use on COVID-19 severity using a super learner ensemble that included logistic regression, LASSO, random forest, and gradient-boosted trees.

In another study, Gao et al. [10] used LASSO regression for feature selection followed by Cox analysis to predict mortality at hospital admission, reducing the dataset to 34 key features. Butler et al. [11] employed SHAP values to identify key predictors of infection, ARDS, ICU admission, and mortality from structured EHR data. Zucco et al. [12] extracted over 2700 features from clinical records and selected the 22 most influential ones (e.g., age, BMI, number of diagnoses) using mean absolute SHAP values. A separate study [13] also emphasized the importance of using explainable AI (XAI) when working with sensitive health data.

Collectively, these studies underscore the role of ML in predicting COVID-19 outcomes such as mortality, complications, and long COVID, using techniques like XGBoost, random forest, and SHAP. However, many rely on a limited model set or focus on narrow outcomes. In contrast, our work employs a broader set of models—including LightGBM, CatBoost, KNN, SVM, logistic regression, and MLP—benchmarked using robust metrics (accuracy, F1-score, ROC AUC). We also integrate statistical techniques (e.g., LASSO) and XAI (SHAP) to enhance interpretability and identify risk factors. Most notably, we extend beyond modeling to practical implementation, deploying our best models in a web application tested with real-world patient data and clinical expert feedback. This bridges the gap between prediction performance and clinical usability.

3. Data Understanding

The dataset that was selected for this research consists of anonymized data from 4711 COVID-19-positive patients from a hospital in Atlanta (available at: https://www.kaggle.com/datasets/harshwalia/mortality-risk-clinincal-data-of-covid19-patients/data, accessed on the 15 May 2024). The dataset was made publicly available by Harsh Walia on the Kaggle platform, where it is licensed for unrestricted use in academic and research applications. It consists of anonymized clinical records from hospitalized COVID-19 patients and has been cited in several ML studies. The original dataset contained 85 features, including data from medical reports, clinical laboratory measurements, data about comorbidities, and general patient data. After discussion with the domain expert, we found that the dataset also contained so-called supplementary features, which provide information on whether a given laboratory measurement was performed or not, and other supplementary features indicating whether a given laboratory measurement value of the patient exceeded the normal range. Table 1 lists all the features in the dataset excluding the supplementary features. For each feature there is description completed in collaboration with the expert, as well as the feature type.

Table 1. Description of features in dataset.

Feature	Description	Type
Derivation cohort	Dataset is divided into 2 cohorts—first 3 weeks of the pandemic and second 3 weeks of the pandemic	Binary
LOS	Length of stay = Duration of hospitalization in the hospital in days	Numerical
Death	Patient died during hospitalization	Binary
Severity	Severity of COVID-19 illness, expressed numerically in the range 0 to 11	Categorical
Black	Ethnicity	Binary
White	Ethnicity	Binary
Asian	Ethnicity	Binary
Latino	Ethnicity	Binary
Age.1	Age listed as a number	Numerical
AgeScore	Age category number (1, 2, 3, 4)	Categorical

Table 1. *Cont.*

Feature	Description	Type
MI	Myocardial infarction	Binary
PVD	Peripheral vascular disease	Categorical
CHF	Congestive heart failure	Binary
CVD	Cardiovascular disease	Binary
DEMENT	Dementia	Binary
COPD	Chronic obstructive pulmonary disease	Binary
DM Complicated	Diabetes mellitus complicated	Binary
DM Simple	Diabetes mellitus simple	Binary
Renal Disease	Kidney disease	Binary
All CNS	All diseases of the central nervous system	Binary
Pure CNS	Diseases only of the central nervous system	Binary
Stroke	Stroke	Binary
Seizure	Seizures	Binary
OldSyncope	Syncope (short-term loss of consciousness)	Binary
OldOtherNeuro	Other neurological diseases	Binary
OtherBrnLsn	Brain lesions	Binary
OsSats	Oxygen saturation = oxygen saturation in percentages	Numerical
Temp	Body temperature in degrees Celsius	Numerical
MAP	Mean arterial pressure, in mmHg	Numerical
Ddimer	Level of D-dimer in blood (mg/mL)	Numerical
Plts	Platelets = blood platelets, in thousands per mm^3	Numerical
INR	International normalized ratio = laboratory value informing about the ability of blood to clot	Numerical
BUN	Blood urea nitrogen = blood urea nitrogen level, reflects kidney function (mg/dL)	Numerical
Creatinine	Creatinine level in blood. Reflects kidney function (mg/dL)	Numerical
Sodium	Sodium level in blood (mEq/L)	Numerical
Glucose	Blood glucose (mg/dL)	Numerical
AST	Aspartate aminotransferase in blood, in units/liter, liver tests	Numerical
ALT	Alanine aminotransferase in blood (units/L)	Numerical
WBC	White blood cells, number of white blood cells (in thousands per mm^3)	Numerical
Lympho	Lymphocytes in blood (in thousands per mm^3)	Numerical
IL6	Interleukin-6 in blood (in picogram/mL)	Numerical
Ferritin	Ferritin level in blood—a protein inside cells that stores iron. Indirectly measures iron level (microgram/L)	Numerical
CrctProtein	C-reactive protein level in blood (mg/L)	Numerical
Procalcitonin	Procalcitonin level in blood, ng/mL. Biomarker released in response to bacterial infections	Numerical
Troponin	Troponin level in blood, rises in myocardial infarction (ng/mL)	Numerical

Binary features have a value of 0 or 1 indicating whether the feature applies to the patient or not. mg = milligram, mmHg = millimeter of mercury, mL = milliliter, dL = deciliter.

The age of the patients ranged from 18 to 103 years, and the mean age was 64 years. Figure 1 shows the age distribution of the patients, color-coded into 4 age groups: under 60 years, 61 to 70 years, 71 to 80 years, and over 80 years.

3.1. Data Cleaning

In the original dataset, the missing values were marked with a 0, so it was necessary to first determine in which cases the number 0 is indeed a value of 0 and where it is a missing value. After research, it was determined that all values of the laboratory measurements given as 0 can be considered as missing values. There were also several instances of incorrect values in the original dataset, the most obvious of which was the body temperature listed several times with the number −17.777. Similarly, for the INR, the international normalized ratio, several values were 17.0001, which is also a very unlikely value. In such cases, it was probably an incorrect entry, and these values were also considered as missing. After identifying all the missing values, we analyzed their percentage of occurrence in each feature. Overall, 4.37% of values were missing in the dataset. Features with more than 30% missing values—such as Procalcitonin and Interleukin-6—were excluded to reduce imputation bias. This follows best practices in clinical machine learning, where sparsely populated variables can degrade model performance and introduce instability during training [14,15].

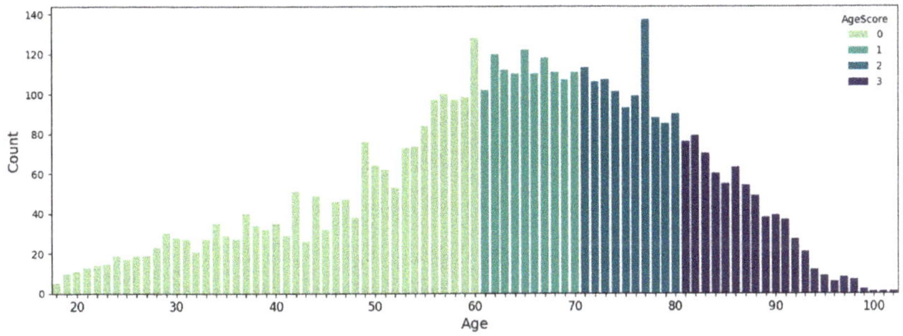

Figure 1. Distribution of patients' ages in dataset.

To maintain data integrity and avoid selection bias, we retained all patient records and imputed missing values using multiple imputation by chained equations (MICE). This approach is recommended for electronic health record datasets in the context of COVID-19, where patient-level deletion may reduce statistical power and introduce bias [16]. Therefore, we used the MICE approach, which is widely adopted for handling missing values in clinical datasets, including COVID-19-related studies [17].

To prevent information leakage during imputation, we ensured that the target variable ("severity" or "death") was excluded from the imputation process.

3.2. Data Transformation and Selection

For statistical analyses where the assumption of normality was required, all continuous numerical features were transformed to approximate a normal distribution using a log transformation. This step was essential for ensuring the validity of parametric tests, which rely on the assumption that data are normally distributed. The log transformation helps reduce skewness, stabilize variance, and improve the symmetry of the data distribution, thereby making the statistical tests more robust and reliable.

In preparation for machine learning modeling, the numerical input features from the original dataset were normalized to a standardized range between 0 and 1 using min–max scaling. This normalization ensures that all features contribute equally to the model and prevents features with larger scales from dominating the learning process. This is particularly important for distance-based algorithms and gradient descent optimization methods, which are sensitive to the scale of input variables.

Categorical variables were also preprocessed to ensure compatibility with machine learning algorithms. Binary categorical variables were encoded as 0 and 1. Categorical features with more than two distinct classes were transformed using one-hot encoding, resulting in the creation of separate binary indicator features for each category. This transformation allows the model to interpret and learn from categorical data without imposing an arbitrary ordinal relationship among the classes.

4. Modeling and Identifying Important Features

4.1. Modeling COVID-19 Severity

COVID-19 severity in the original dataset was on a scale of 0 to 11 (Figure 2), with a mean of 3.6. The x-axis represents the COVID-19 severity, and the y-axis represents the number of patients.

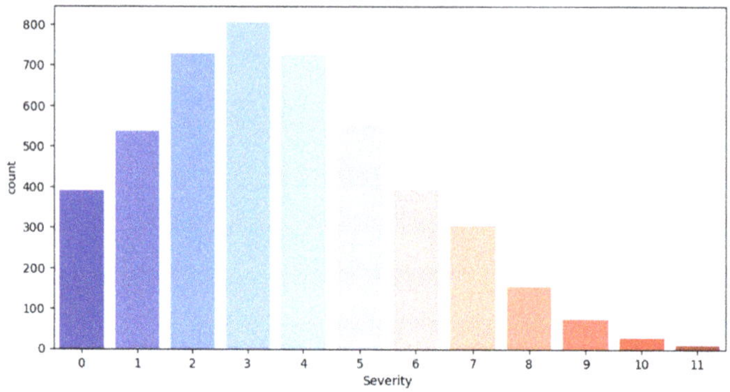

Figure 2. Severity distribution in the dataset, from lowest (0) to highest (11).

4.1.1. Chi-Square

A chi-square test was used to find if there was a statistically significant influence of the categorical independent features on severity. Table 2 shows all categorical features whose p-value was less than 0.05, i.e., they had a statistically significant effect on the severity of COVID-19 disease among patients in dataset. The most significant features were age category (Age_category), and creatinine score (CrtnScore) whose p-values were very close to 0.

Table 2. Chi-square test results of categorical independent features with p-value < 0.05 for Severity modeling.

Feature	p-Value	p-Value Interval
Age_category	0.0	<0.00001
CrtnScore	0.0	<0.00001
Death	1.71×10^{-139}	<0.00001
PltsScore	4.72×10^{-77}	<0.00001
Pure_CNS	3.87×10^{-9}	<0.0001
All_CNS	6.03×10^{-8}	<0.0001
Per_vascular_dis	0.003	<0.01
Derivation cohort	0.030	<0.05

4.1.2. ANOVA

An ANOVA test was performed to find if there was a statistically significant influence of the numeric independent features on severity. Table 3 shows all numerical features whose p-value was less than 0.05. The most significant features were age (Age_number) and blood urea nitrogen (Blood_urea_nitr) whose p-values were very close to 0.

This three-level stratification (low: 0–2, moderate: 3–5, high: 6–11) aligns with typical clinical severity groupings used in COVID-19 case management guidelines, particularly those published by the World Health Organization [18]. As can be seen in the graph (Figure 3), class 0 includes the severity interval 0 to 2 from the original dataset, class 1 includes severity 3 to 5, and the highest class 2 includes severity 6 to 11.

Table 3. ANOVA results of numerical independent features with *p*-value < 0.05.

Feature	*p*-Value	*p*-Value Interval
Age_number	0.0	<0.00001
Blood_urea_nitr	0.0	<0.00001
Creatinine	3.21×10^{-306}	<0.00001
Ddimer	2.61×10^{-271}	<0.00001
CRP	2.15×10^{-226}	<0.00001
Ferritin	1.29×10^{-152}	<0.00001
Inter_norm_ratio	7.27×10^{-150}	<0.00001
Mean_art_press	1.02×10^{-134}	<0.00001
AST	2.27×10^{-114}	<0.00001
Troponin	5.74×10^{-76}	<0.00001
Oxygen_sat	4.46×10^{-59}	<0.00001
Length_of_stay	2.0×10^{-55}	<0.00001
Sodium	2.15×10^{-45}	<0.00001
Lympho	4.78×10^{-37}	<0.00001
Platelets	9.71×10^{-32}	<0.00001
White_blood_cells	3.59×10^{-30}	<0.00001
ALT	1.74×10^{-18}	<0.00001
Glucose	1.07×10^{-13}	<0.0001
Temperature	3.53×10^{-8}	<0.001

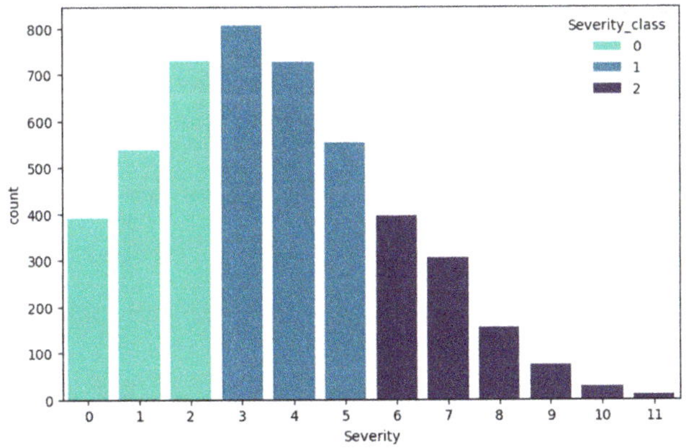

Figure 3. Target feature Severity class.

4.1.3. All Models' Performance

We used the following models to predict COVID-19 disease severity: random forest, LightGBM, XGBoost, KNN, support vector classifier, logistic regression, and MLP neural network. All models were built on a training and testing set split in a ratio of 80:20. In the following Table 4, we report only the accuracy metric, as it was used to establish a baseline comparison across all models. Based on this initial comparison, we identified the model with the highest accuracy and conducted a more detailed analysis of its performance, as seen in the following subsection.

Table 4. Results of models for prediction of severity.

Model	Random Forest	LightGBM	XGB	KNN	SVC	Logistic Regression	MLP
Accuracy	0.855	0.884	0.88	0.631	0.725	0.77	0.792

4.1.4. Best Model for Severity Prediction

The best model was LightGBM, with an accuracy on the test set of 0.884. Table 5 shows the results of each metric when testing this model. The first three rows show the different target feature classes: low, moderate, and high severity, followed by the average of the metrics for all classes (macro_avg) and the weighted average (weighted_avg), which considers the number of examples in each target class. The three columns contain the metrics for measuring model performance, and the last column lists the number of test examples for each class or the total number of examples for the average of the metrics in the last two rows.

Table 5. Results of LightGBM model for Severity prediction trained on all features.

	Precision	Recall	F1-Score	Support
class 0	0.94	0.93	0.93	338
class 1	0.88	0.85	0.87	411
class 2	0.81	0.87	0.84	194
macro_avg	0.88	0.88	0.88	943
weighted_avg	0.89	0.88	0.88	943

As seen in Table 5, the model had the highest precision in predicting low severity (class 0): a precision of 0.94, which means that 94% of the examples predicted as class 0 were actually class 0. For class 1 (moderate severity), precision was 0.88 and for class 2 (high severity) it was 0.81. In terms of recall, for class 0, 93% of the true class 0 examples were also correctly classified, followed by 85% for class 1 and 87% for high severity. The F1-score, i.e., the harmonic mean of the precision and recall metrics, was, for class 0, 0.93; for class 1, it was 0.87; and for class 2, it was 0.84.

4.1.5. SHAP Values for Severity Modeling

Using SHAP values for the LightGBM model, we investigated the importance of features for the prediction. Consistent with current guidance, we did not apply an arbitrary SHAP value cutoff; instead, we prioritized interpretability and clinical consensus, aligning with best practices for explainable AI in healthcare [19]. As the target feature consists of three classes, for simplicity we show a plot of the influence of each feature on only target class 2, the highest COVID-19 severity. The graph (Figure 4) shows the most influential features, with blue representing low values for a given feature and red representing high values. The x-axis shows the SHAP values for each feature. Negative SHAP values (to the left of the vertical axis at point 0) indicate that the given feature values "push" the prediction towards a lower prediction of the target feature—i.e., in our case, a lower severity. Conversely, positive SHAP values (to the right of the vertical axis at point 0) indicate that the given feature values are "pushing" the prediction towards a higher severity. For example, in the case of the feature age (Age_number), we can see that a lower age of patients (purple-blue color) tended towards a lower severity of COVID-19 and a higher age of patients tended towards a higher severity of COVID-19. The opposite is the case for the feature oxygen saturation (Oxygen_sat). The graph clearly shows that high saturation values (red) tended to lower COVID-19 disease severity and lower oxygen saturation (purple and blue) in turn tended to increase severity.

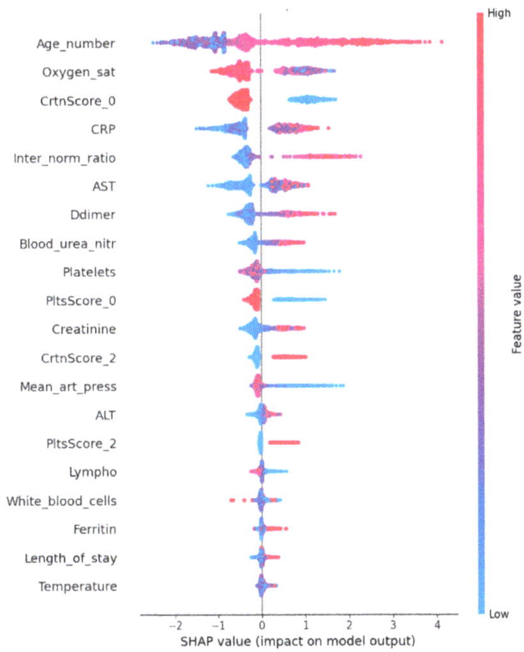

Figure 4. SHAP values for most important features for Severity prediction.

4.1.6. Simplified Model for Severity Modeling

In order to deploy the model in the application and increase usability, it was necessary to create a simplified model that was trained only on the most important features for severity detection. After identifying the most important features for COVID-19 disease severity prediction using the LightGBM model and SHAP values and consulting with a domain expert, te following 8 features were selected: age (Age_number), oxygen saturation (Oxygen_sat), C-reactive protein (CRP), blood aspartate aminotransferase (AST), D-dimer (Ddimer), international normalized ratio (Inter_norm_ratio), creatinine (Creatinine), and platelets (Platelets). We omitted features creatinine score (CrtnScore_0) and platelet score (PltsScore_0) features because it was not clear in the dataset description by which thresholds these scores were given and also the values for both of these measurements are already included in the selected important features.

Through an iterative process of hyperparameter tuning using 5-fold cross-validation, we found that the simplified LightGBM model performed best with the following parameters: learning_rate = 0.1, max_depth = −1, n_estimators = 350, num_leaves = 8.

The simplified model achieved an overall accuracy of 0.895 on the test set, which is higher than the model trained on a larger set of predictors. This result may be because, with a large number of predictors, noise may arise that causes misclassification of some examples in the dataset. Since the target *Severity_class* feature contains 3 classes, we used the accuracy, recall and F1-score metrics for each class to display the results.

Table 6 shows the model results for each target class. As we are able to see, opposed to the previous results mentioned in Table 5, the precision for class 2 has improved. When we look into recall, we can see that two classes, classes 0 and 1, have improved in results. In the F1-score metrics, all classes have seen improvement. Support represents the number of instances from the test set in each target class that were used to calculate these metrics.

Table 6. Results of simplified LightGBM model for severity prediction trained on 8 most important features.

	Precision	Recall	F1-Score	Support
class 0	0.95	0.94	0.94	339
class 1	0.88	0.88	0.88	400
class 2	0.84	0.86	0.85	204
macro_avg	0.89	0.90	0.89	943
weighted_avg	0.90	0,90	0.90	943

Class 0 represents low severity, class 1 medium severity, and class 2 high severity.

Based on the data from the model performance metrics, it can be concluded that the simplified model best predicts class 0 with the highest precision, recall, and F1-score. Classes 1 and 2 have lower values in all metrics, indicating that they are more challenging for the model to predict.

4.2. *Modeling COVID-19 Mortality*

To predict mortality risk of patients, we used the binary target feature "death", which contains the value 0 if the patient did not die and 1 if the patient died during hospitalization. From 4711 COVID-19-positive patients in the dataset, 1148 died and 3563 did not die.

4.2.1. Chi-Square Test

The following Table 7 presents the chi-square test results for the effect of categorical features on patients' mortality risk, showing only features with a p-value less than 0.05.

Table 7. Chi-square test results of categorical independent features with p-value < 0.05 for Mortality modeling.

Feature	p-Value	p-Value Interval
Age_category	2.17×10^{-91}	<0.00001
CrtnScore	3.75×10^{-67}	<0.00001
All_CNS	1.37×10^{-9}	<0.0001
Per_vascular_dis	6.09×10^{-9}	<0.0001
Pure_CNS	3.98×10^{-8}	<0.0001
PltsScore	9.07×10^{-6}	<0.0001
Stroke	2.22×10^{-5}	<0.0001
Renal_dis	0.010	<0.01
Derivation cohort	0.023	<0.05
Chronic_obst_pulm_dis	0.027	<0.05
White	0.027	<0.05

4.2.2. t-Test

We used Student's t-test to determine whether there was a statistically significant difference in the mean value of the features between patients who died versus those who did not. In Table 8, we report the results of Student's t-test for features that have a p-value less than 0.5.

Table 8. Chi-square test results of numerical independent features with p-value < 0.05.

Feature	p-Value	p-Value Interval
Mean_art_press	1.35×10^{-171}	<0.00001
Blood_urea_nitr	1.15×10^{-94}	<0.00001
CRP	8.99×10^{-85}	<0.00001
Age_number	5.93×10^{-66}	<0.00001

Table 8. *Cont.*

Feature	*p*-Value	*p*-Value Interval
Ddimer	1.07×10^{-60}	<0.00001
Creatinine	2.54×10^{-47}	<0.00001
Ferritin	1.38×10^{-37}	<0.00001
Oxygen_sat	2.38×10^{-35}	<0.00001
Troponin	4.35×10^{-31}	<0.00001
AST	7.33×10^{-30}	<0.00001
Inter_norm_ratio	3.58×10^{-25}	<0.00001
Glucose	1.73×10^{-12}	<0.00001
Sodium	8.67×10^{-12}	<0.00001
Lympho	2.15×10^{-10}	<0.00001
White_blood_cells	2.80×10^{-10}	<0.00001
Length_of_stay	3.87×10^{-6}	<0.0001
Platelets	6.07×10^{-6}	<0.0001
ALT	0.02	<0.05

4.2.3. LASSO Logistic Regression

Using LASSO regression, we investigated which features had the greatest impact on patients' mortality. At the top of the graph (Figure 5) are the features with positive coefficients (increasing the mortality risk), and at the bottom are the features with negative coefficients (decreasing mortality risk).

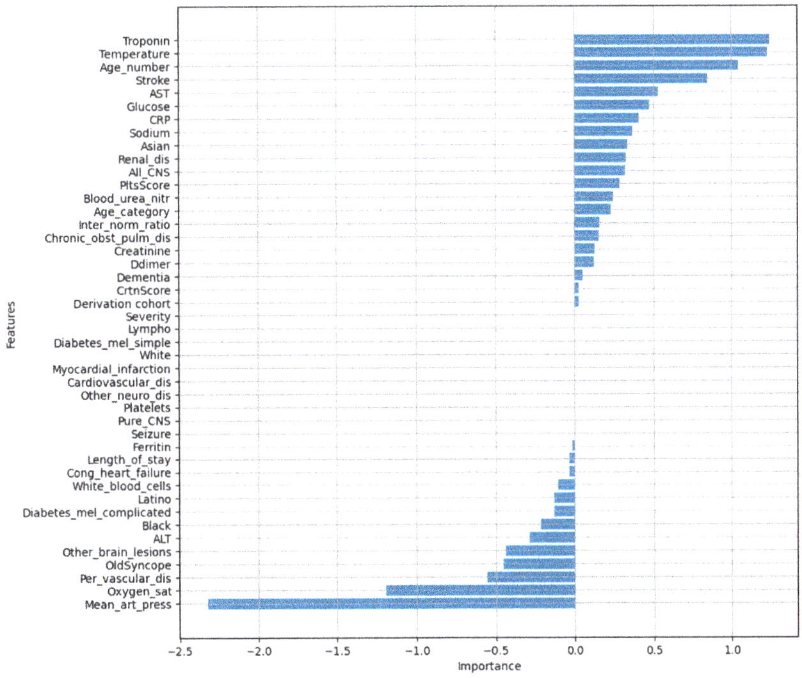

Figure 5. LASSO logistic regression results for Mortality risk.

4.2.4. All Models for Mortality Risk Prediction

Based on the current state analysis and the conclusion of it, we have decided to use the following data analytics and machine learning models to predict the risk of death in COVID-19 patients: random forest, LightGBM, XGBoost, KNN, Naïve Bayes, SVC, logistic regression, and MLP. As this is a binary classification task where target class 1 is underrepresented, it was considerably more difficult for the models to find and correctly classify patients who belonged to this class. Therefore, in addition to the accuracy metric, we used the F1-score metric for class 1 and also the ROC AUC score to evaluate the models. In the following table, we can see the results of the baseline model's performance estimated by cross-validation on the training set, ordered by F1-score of class 1:

As we can see in Table 9, the random forest model had the highest classification accuracy (precision) and ROC AUC scores, but the LightGBM model had a three percent higher F1 class 1 score, with very similar precision metrics and ROC AUC scores. Because the LightGBM model was better able to detect the risk of patient death than the random forest model, we consider the LightGBM model to be the better fit for this problem.

Table 9. Models results for mortality prediction.

Model	Accuracy	F1-Score of Class 1	ROC AUC
Random Forest	0.8272	0.5329	0.837
LGBM	0.8244	0.5682	0.8316
XGB	0.8213	0.5655	0.8253
KNN	0.7519	0.3032	0.6792
Naïve Bayes	0.768	0.5009	0.7898
SVC	0.8007	0.407	0.7952
Logistic Regression	0.8191	0.5344	0.817
MLP	0.7642	0.4976	0.7607

4.2.5. The Best Model for Classification

The overall classification accuracy of the LightGBM model on the test set is 0.812, while the ROC AUC score on the test set was 0.837. Table 10 shows the values of other metrics for the LightGBM model on the test set.

Table 10. Performance of the best model for mortality risk prediction trained on all features.

Model	Precision	Recall	F1-Score	Support
Class 0	0.83	0.93	0.88	699
Class 1	0.71	0.46	0.56	244
Macro Avg	0.77	0.70	0.72	943
Weighted Avg	0.80	0.81	0.80	943

Note: Sensitivity (recall of Class 1) = 0.46; Specificity (recall of Class 0) = 0.93.

In this binary classification task, recall for class 1 corresponds to sensitivity (true positive rate), and recall for class 0 corresponds to specificity (true negative rate). These values are reported in the table above. Table 10 also shows that the LightGBM model trained on all features achieved a precision of 0.83 in classifying examples of target class 0 and also a high recall of 0.93. There were 699 examples in this class from the test set. Regarding the classification of patients into class 1, the model achieved a reasonably good precision of 0.71, but a low recall of 0.46. This means that the model was able to correctly identify 93% of the patients in the test set who did not die and 46% of the patients who died. This may be because there were significantly fewer patients in the target class 1 in the dataset or because the original dataset contained relatively few comorbidities, lacking data on diseases such as obesity or cancer, which have been shown to have an impact on mortality in COVID-19 patients. To provide a clearer picture of model behavior in the context of class imbalance, we also report sensitivity and specificity. The full LightGBM model achieved a sensitivity of 46% and a specificity of 93% on the test set, highlighting its strong performance in identifying non-mortality cases, while still capturing nearly half of the actual mortality cases.

In Figure 6, a visualization of the area under the ROC curve can be seen. The curve is generated by plotting the true positive rate (cases that were in class 1 and correctly identified as being from class 1) against the false positive rate (cases that were in class 0 but classified as class 1 by the model) at different threshold settings.

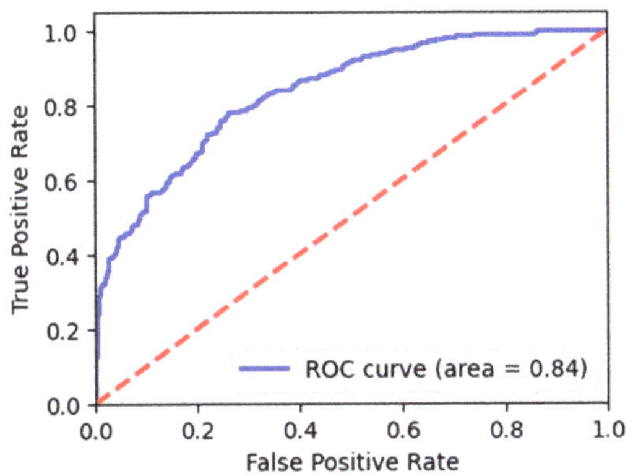

Figure 6. Area under the ROC curve of LightGBM model for mortality risk prediction. The red dotted line represents the line of no-discrimination (AUC = 0.5), indicating random classifier performance.

4.2.6. SHAP Values for Mortality Modeling

Figure 7 shows the most influential features according to SHAP values used for the LightGBM model. For features that are predominantly red to the right of the center axis, this means that a higher value of that feature contributed to a higher risk of death in patients. Conversely, if the values to the right of the center axis are blue, it means that higher values contributed to a lower risk of death. Feature mean arterial pressure (Mean_art_press) had the greatest effect on prediction, and with a lower pressure, the chance of death increased. This may be related to the fact that, as oxygen saturation decreases, blood pressure also decreases. Another important feature was age (Age_number), with the chance of death increasing with age. These findings are consistent with prior studies identifying the same clinical features—such as age, oxygen saturation, CRP, D-dimer, and kidney function markers—as significant predictors of COVID-19 severity and mortality [9,10,12].

4.2.7. Simplified Model for Mortality Modeling

As the original model was trained using 51 predictors, it was necessary to reduce this number for deployment in the application to make it easier to enter new patient data and to increase the usability of the model in practice. The following 15 most important features based on the SHAP values and consultation with medical experts were selected for deploying the model to predict the risk of death in patients:

1. Mean arterial pressure (Mean_art_press);
2. Patient age (Age_number);
3. C-reactive protein level in the blood (CRP);
4. Number of days of hospitalization (Length_of_stay);
5. Creatinine level (Creatinine);
6. Oxygen saturation (Oxygen_sat);
7. Blood urea nitrogen level (Blood_urea_nitr);
8. Blood aspartate aminotransferase (AST);

9. Body temperature (Temperature);
10. Ferritin level (Ferritin);
11. Glucose (Glucose);
12. Troponin (Troponin);
13. Alanine aminotransferase in the blood (ALT);
14. Blood D-dimer level (Ddimer);
15. Platelets (Platelets).

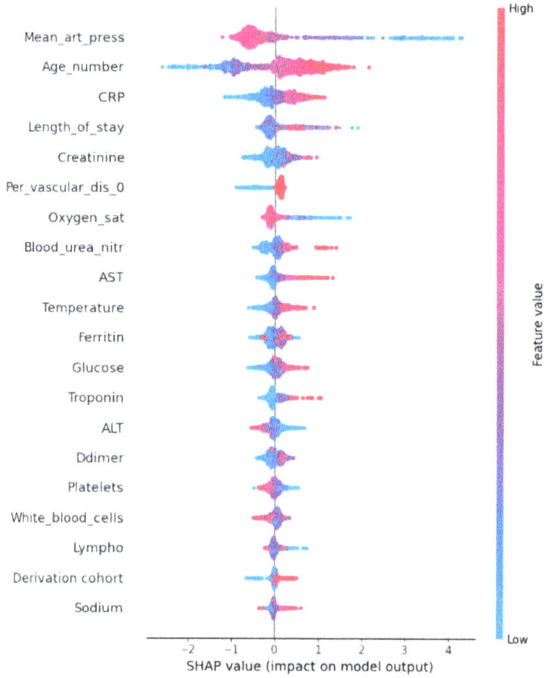

Figure 7. SHAP values for most important features for Mortality risk prediction.

We excluded the feature peripheral vascular disease (Per_vasc_dis_0) because the simplified model will be fitted and tested on a group of patients for whom this was not directly reported in the documentation.

By tuning the hyperparameters, we found that the simplified model performed best in F1-scores at the following settings: reg_alpha = 2, reg_lambda = 1, min_data_in_leaf = 50. This model achieved an overall ROC AUC score on the test set of 0.836, which is almost identical to the model trained on all features (0.837). The overall classification accuracy of the simplified model was 0.805. Table 11 shows that the simplified model has increased the F1-score of the class 1 compared to the model trained on all features, from 0.56 to 0.60.

Table 11. Performance of the simplified model for mortality risk prediction trained on top 15 features.

Model	Precision	Recall	F1-Score	Support
Class 0	0.85	0.89	0.87	699
Class 1	0.64	0.57	0.60	244
Macro Avg	0.75	0.73	0.74	943
Weighted Avg	0.80	0.81	0.80	943

Note: Sensitivity (recall of Class 1) = 0.57; Specificity (recall of Class 0) = 0.89.

The simplified model achieved improved sensitivity of 57% while maintaining specificity of 89%. This increase in sensitivity is particularly important in clinical use, as it indicates better performance in identifying high-risk patients, even with fewer input features.

5. Model Deployment and Testing on New Cohort with Experts

5.1. Model Deployment

To deploy the two simplified models for severity and mortality risk prediction, we created a web application consisting of the following three parts:

1. Machine learning models;
2. Flask application;
3. HTML and CSS for user interface.

The Flask application was implemented using Python's Flask 2.2 library to serve the simplified LightGBM models through a lightweight API. In the application, we used two models that were evaluated and approved by a domain expert who said that the features used in the models and their impact on severity or risk of death correspond to medical practice. The application had two main sections, one for the severity prediction and the other for the mortality risk prediction. In each section, there is a description of the model and form for the patient data. After adding the patient data, a prediction result is shown and, for mortality risk prediction, the risk is displayed as percentual probability of a patient belonging to class 1. For each model there is also shown a SHAP values plot for individual prediction, which displays how features contributed to the prediction result of the patient. The severity prediction section can be seen in Figures 8 and 9. The mortality prediction section is similar, with a different model used.

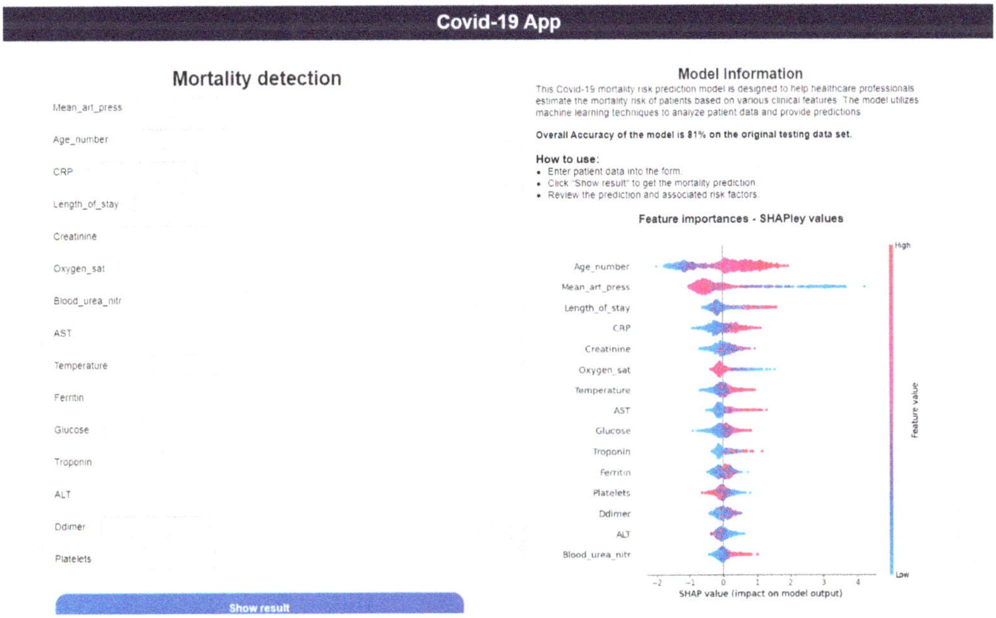

Figure 8. Section for Severity prediction in deployed application.

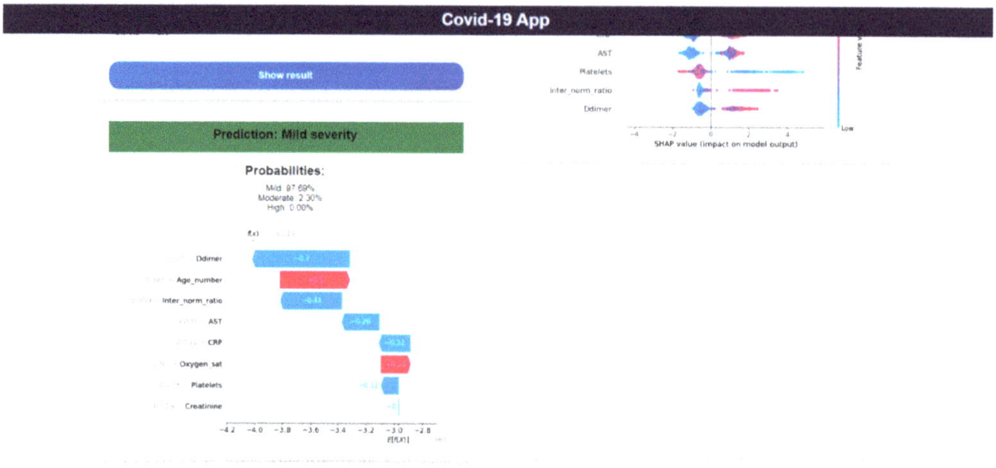

Figure 9. Severity prediction results and explanation in application.

5.2. Model Testing with Experts

The deployed models in the app were tested in person with two experts from medical practice and also using anonymized data of 45 patients with COVID-19 from the Department of Infectiology and Travel Medicine, L. Pasteur University Hospital in Košice (UNLP). This study was approved by the Ethic Committee of the UNLP on 19 February 2024. We used these data to test a model to predict the risk of death. The aim of the testing was to determine whether the developed models were credible and potentially applicable in medical practice.

During testing with two clinical experts from L. Pasteur University Hospital in Košice, no major usability issues were reported. The experts found the interface intuitive and appreciated the integration of SHAP-based explanations for each prediction. They also expressed that the ability to input patient data directly and receive real-time model output enhanced the system's potential for clinical use. Some suggestions were made for future improvements, including clearer labeling of some clinical features (e.g., using standardized medical terminology), the option to export predictions to patient records, and the display of confidence intervals or prediction certainty levels. These suggestions are valuable and will be considered in the next phase of system development.

The overall accuracy of the severity prediction model tested on a group of 45 patients from the UNLP could not be quantified because the patients were not divided into three severity groups in this hospital. The summary severity prediction for the 45 patients was shown to the experts, visually checked, and then the model was tested on several patient data individually using our application, which also displayed the factors influencing a given patient's COVID-19 disease severity. Overall, the model was able to identify the COVID-19 disease severity of individual patients to a high degree of accuracy. The model was also able to identify improvement or worsening of the condition in some of the patients for whom repeated measurements were taken.

The overall ROC AUC score achieved by the model for predicting the risk of death in a group of 45 patients from UNLP was 0.836 (83.6%), and the overall accuracy was 0.733 (73.3%). The lower accuracy rate was probably due to the model failing to identify high risk of death if there were reasons not included in the model or in the original dataset (e.g., muscle bleeding or pulmonary embolism).

5.3. Results

Based on the testing, both experts expressed a positive impression of the models in the application, with higher confidence for the COVID-19 severity prediction model than for the prediction of mortality risk. This corresponds with the performance of the models, as the model for severity prediction already had better results during the modeling phase. As mentioned above, for a more accurate prediction of the risk of death, it is necessary to develop a more comprehensive model and to include as much additional data as possible on comorbidities or other risk factors of patients. Regarding potential use in practice, the experts also expressed that our models have potential for use in medical practice.

After the testing, possible use cases were discussed where such models could be used:

1. In a crisis situation, such as the beginning of the COVID-19 pandemic, the models could assist in identifying the risk of patients' conditions.
2. To investigate changes in patients' condition (continuous display of model results based on repeated patient measurements).
3. To identify possible influential factors using similar models and explainability methods for other diseases.

6. Discussion

In this study, we applied machine learning (ML) and data analytics methods to structured clinical data from 4711 COVID-19 patients treated at a hospital in Atlanta. Our goal was to identify the most effective models for predicting disease severity and mortality and to determine the key clinical features influencing these outcomes.

The original dataset included 85 features, which were refined to 53 through feature selection and preprocessing steps such as MICE-based imputation and categorical encoding. Feature significance was assessed using statistical methods including chi-square tests, ANOVA, *t*-tests, and LASSO regression.

For severity prediction, the LightGBM model performed best, with an accuracy of 88.4%. A simplified version using the top eight features slightly improved accuracy to 89.5%, while enhancing interpretability and clinical usability through SHAP-based explainability.

For mortality risk, LightGBM again achieved the highest performance (ROC AUC 83.7%, accuracy 81.2%). The simplified model using 15 key features achieved nearly identical results (ROC AUC 83.6%, accuracy 80.5%) and showed improved F1-score for the minority class, indicating better handling of class imbalance.

When compared to recent studies in the field, such as those by Moulaei et al. [20], Sun et al. [21], and Baik et al. [22], which achieved AUROC values between 0.86 and 0.99 using advanced ensemble or deep learning methods, our LightGBM model performed slightly worse in terms of AUC. In a different approach, Kim et al. [23] built a mortality prediction model using logistic regression and machine learning techniques, with their linear SVM model reaching an AUC of 0.962 while using only 10 key features. However, our focus was on achieving a balance between predictive performance and interpretability, which is critical for real-world medical application. Unlike many black-box models, our approach offers transparency, ease of understanding, and expert validation—qualities valued in clinical settings.

Importantly, both simplified models were reviewed by clinical experts from L. Pasteur University Hospital (UNLP) in Košice, who confirmed their relevance and practical utility. To further validate the mortality model, we tested it on an external cohort of 45 anonymized patients from UNLP, yielding a ROC AUC of 83.6% and accuracy of 73.3%. These results confirm the robustness and generalizability of the model in real-world conditions.

Despite these promising results, our study has limitations. Our study includes external validation using anonymized patient data from a different hospital and real-world testing with clinical experts. While the size of the validation cohort (45 patients) is modest, it provides valuable insight into the practical usability of our models beyond the original dataset. This type of validation—expert-reviewed and contextually grounded—is an essential step toward real-world clinical deployment. Future work will expand this validation across additional patient populations to further support generalizability. Furthermore, some potentially influential variables—such as viral strain information, socioeconomic status, or vaccination status—were not included. Future research could expand the dataset, integrate multimodal data sources (e.g., imaging, genomics), and evaluate additional model architectures including transformer-based or hybrid deep learning frameworks. Benchmarking against high-performing published models using standardized datasets and protocols is also a planned next step.

7. Conclusions

This research demonstrates the effectiveness of machine learning and data analytics methods in predicting COVID-19 severity and mortality based on structured clinical data. LightGBM models proved to be particularly effective, and through feature selection and explainability techniques (such as SHAP values), we developed simplified models that retain high performance while enhancing interpretability and clinical usability.

Crucially, the models were validated through expert feedback and tested on external patient data, demonstrating real-world applicability. Our work highlights the importance of balancing predictive performance with model transparency—especially in high-stakes domains like healthcare—where usability by medical professionals is essential.

The findings support the potential of explainable ML models to assist clinicians in risk stratification and decision making. Future research should focus on broader validation, integration with clinical workflows, and expanding feature sets to include more diverse patient information. With continued development, such tools could significantly support healthcare systems in managing COVID-19 and similar diseases.

Author Contributions: Conceptualization, O.L. and J.P.; methodology, O.L. and J.P.; software, E.Z., O.L., and J.P.; validation, O.L., Z.P., D.J., and J.P.; formal analysis, O.L.; investigation, D.J. and Z.P.; resources, Z.P.; data curation, O.L., E.Z., and J.P.; writing—original draft preparation O.L. and J.P.; visualization, O.L. and E.Z.; supervision, J.P. and Z.P.; project administration, J.P.; funding acquisition, J.P. and O.L. All authors have read and agreed to the published version of the manuscript.

Funding: This work was partially supported by the Scientific Grant Agency of the Ministry of Education, Research, Development, and Youth of the Slovak Republic and the Slovak Academy of Sciences under grant no. 1/0259/24 and the Slovak Research and Development Agency under grant no. APVV-22-0414.

Institutional Review Board Statement: This study was conducted in accordance with the International Code of Medical Ethics of the World Medical Association Declaration of Helsinki and received approval from the Ethics Committee of the Louis Pasteur University Hospital in Košice on 19 February 2024, under resolution no. 2024/EK/02021.

Informed Consent Statement: Informed consent was obtained from all participants involved in the study. For the use of anonymized patient data from the validation cohort at the L. Pasteur University Hospital in Košice, consent was collected in accordance with the hospital's ethical guidelines and under the approval of the Ethics Committee.

Data Availability Statement: The dataset used in this research for analysis and model training and testing is available at https://www.kaggle.com/datasets/harshwalia/mortality-risk-clinincal-data-of-covid19-patients (accessed on the 15 May 2024). The dataset is published under an open license for academic use, and all data are anonymized. The dataset from UNLP used for validation testing is not available for public sharing at this moment. The source code is available on GitHub at: https://github.com/takemenonemanikto/diagnostics_code (accessed on the 15 May 2024).

Acknowledgments: Special thanks are due to all the participants and staff for their valuable contributions to this work and we also appreciate the support of the University Hospital of L. Pasteur in Košice for their collaboration and access to anonymized patient data.

Conflicts of Interest: The authors declare no conflicts of interest.

Abbreviations

The following abbreviations are used in this manuscript:

KNN	k-Nearest Neighbors
ML	Machine Learning
ROC AUC	Area Under the Curve of the Receiver Operating Characteristic
SHAP	SHapley Additive exPlanations
SVM	Support Vector Machine
XAI	eXplainable Artificial Inteligence
XGBoost	eXtreme Gradient Boosting

References

1. Velavan, T.P.; Meyer, C.G. The COVID-19 epidemic. *Trop. Med. Int. Health* **2020**, *25*, 278–280. [CrossRef] [PubMed] [PubMed Central]
2. Cucinotta, D.; Vanelli, M. WHO Declares COVID-19 a Pandemic. *Acta Biomed.* **2020**, *91*, 157–160. [CrossRef] [PubMed] [PubMed Central]
3. World Health Organization. COVID-19 Epidemiological Update—15 March 2024. 2024. Available online: https://www.who.int/publications/m/item/covid-19-epidemiological-update-15-march-2024 (accessed on 14 April 2024).
4. Smith, G.; Johnson, L.; Nguyen, T. COVID-19 Prognostic Models: A Pro–Con Debate for Machine Learning. *JMIR Public Health Surveill.* **2021**, *7*, e25419. [CrossRef]
5. Yu, S.C.; Hofford, M.R.; Lai, A.M.; Kollef, M.H.; Payne, P.R.O.; Michelson, A.P. Respiratory support status from EHR data for adult population: Classification, heuristics, and usage in predictive modeling. *J. Am. Med. Inform. Assoc.* **2022**, *29*, 813–821. [CrossRef] [PubMed]
6. Jha, M.; Gupta, R.; Saxena, R. A Precise Method to Detect Post-COVID-19 Pulmonary Fibrosis Through Extreme Gradient Boosting. *SN Comput. Sci.* **2023**, *4*, 89. [CrossRef] [PubMed]
7. Sottile, P.D.; Albers, D.; E DeWitt, P.; Russell, S.; Stroh, J.N.; Kao, D.P.; Adrian, B.; E Levine, M.; Mooney, R.; Larchick, L.; et al. Real-time electronic health record mortality prediction during the COVID-19 pandemic: A prospective cohort study. *J. Am. Med. Inform. Assoc.* **2021**, *28*, 2354–2365. [CrossRef] [PubMed]
8. Jiang, S.; Loomba, J.; Sharma, S.; Brown, D. Vital Measurements of Hospitalized COVID-19 Patients as a Predictor of Long COVID: An EHR-based Cohort Study from the RECOVER Program in N3C. In Proceedings of the 2022 IEEE International Conference on Bioinformatics and Biomedicine (BIBM), Las Vegas, NV, USA, 6–8 December 2022; pp. 3023–3030. [CrossRef]
9. Rivera, A.S.; Al-Heeti, O.; Petito, L.C.; Feinstein, M.J.; Achenbach, C.J.; Williams, J.; Taiwo, B. Association of statin use with outcomes of patients admitted with COVID-19: An analysis of electronic health records using superlearner. *BMC Infect. Dis.* **2023**, *23*, 115. [CrossRef] [PubMed]
10. Gao, Y.; Cai, G.-Y.; Fang, W.; Li, H.-Y.; Wang, S.-Y.; Chen, L.; Yu, Y.; Liu, D.; Xu, S.; Cui, P.-F.; et al. Machine learning based early warning system enables accurate mortality risk prediction for COVID-19. *Nat. Commun.* **2020**, *11*, 5033. [CrossRef] [PubMed]
11. Butler, L.; Karabayir, I.; Tootooni, M.S.; Afshar, M.; Goldberg, A.; Akbilgic, O. Image and Structured Data Analysis for Prognostication of Health Outcomes in Patients Presenting to the ED During the COVID-19 Pandemic. *Int. J. Med. Inform.* **2021**, *158*, 104662. [CrossRef] [PubMed]
12. Zucco, A.G.; Agius, R.; Svanberg, R.; Moestrup, K.S.; Marandi, R.Z.; MacPherson, C.R.; Lundgren, J.; Ostrowski, S.R.; Niemann, C.U. Personalized survival probabilities for SARS-CoV-2 positive patients by explainable machine learning. *Sci. Rep.* **2022**, *12*, 13879. [CrossRef] [PubMed]
13. Lohaj, O.; Paralič, J.; Bednár, P.; Paraličová, Z.; Huba, M. Unraveling COVID-19 Dynamics via Machine Learning and XAI: Investigating Variant Influence and Prognostic Classification. *Mach. Learn. Knowl. Extr.* **2023**, *5*, 1266–1281. [CrossRef]
14. Alwateer, M.; Atlam, E.S.; Abd El-Raouf, M.M.; Ghoneim, O.A.; Gad, I. Missing data imputation: A comprehensive review. *J. Comput. Commun.* **2024**, *12*, 53–75. [CrossRef]

15. Mello-Román, J.D.; Martínez-Amarilla, A. COVID-19 Data Analysis: The Impact of Missing Data Imputation on Supervised Learning Model Performance. *Computation* **2025**, *13*, 70. [CrossRef]
16. Zhang, G.; Rose, C.E.; Zhang, Y.; Li, R.; Lee, F.C.; Massetti, G.; Adams, L.E. Multiple imputation of missing race and ethnicity in CDC COVID-19 case-level surveillance data. *Int. J. Stat. Med. Res.* **2022**, *11*, 1. [CrossRef] [PubMed]
17. Bottino, F.; Tagliente, E.; Pasquini, L.; Napoli, A.D.; Lucignani, M.; Figà-Talamanca, L.; Napolitano, A. COVID mortality prediction with machine learning methods: A systematic review and critical appraisal. *J. Pers. Med.* **2021**, *11*, 893. [CrossRef] [PubMed]
18. World Health Organization. Clinical Management of COVID-19: Living Guidance (WHO/2019-nCoV/clinical/2023.1). 2023. Available online: https://www.who.int/publications/i/item/WHO-2019-nCoV-clinical-2023.1 (accessed on 1 June 2025).
19. Salih, A.; Poon, J.; Arrieta, A.B.; Gill, S.S. A Perspective on Explainable AI Methods: SHAP and LIME in Healthcare. *Patterns* **2023**, *4*, 100701. [CrossRef]
20. Moulaei, K.; Iranmanesh, E.; Amiri, P.; Ahmadian, L. Attitudes of COVID-19 patients toward sharing their health data: A survey-based study to understand security and privacy concerns. *Health Sci. Rep.* **2023**, *6*, e1132. [CrossRef] [PubMed] [PubMed Central]
21. Sun, C.; Bai, Y.; Chen, D.; He, L.; Zhu, J.; Ding, X.; Luo, L.; Ren, Y.; Xing, H.; Jin, X.; et al. Accurate classification of COVID-19 patients with different severity via machine learning. *Clin. Transl. Med.* **2021**, *11*, e323. [CrossRef] [PubMed]
22. Baik, S.M.; Hong, K.S.; Park, D.J. Deep learning approach for early prediction of COVID-19 mortality using chest X-ray and electronic health record data. *BMC Bioinform.* **2023**, *24*, 190. [CrossRef] [PubMed]
23. Jee, Y.; Kim, Y.-J.; Oh, J.; Kim, Y.-J.; Ha, E.-H.; Jo, I. A COVID-19 mortality prediction model for Korean patients using nationwide Korean disease control and prevention agency database. *Sci. Rep.* **2022**, *12*, 3311. [CrossRef] [PubMed]

diagnostics

MDPI

Article

A Machine Learning-Based Guide for Repeated Laboratory Testing in Pediatric Emergency Departments

Adi Shuchami [1], Teddy Lazebnik [1,2], Shai Ashkenazi [3,*], Avner Herman Cohen [4,5], Yael Reichenberg [5] and Vered Shkalim Zemer [4,5,*]

1 Department of Mathematics, Ariel University, Ariel 4070000, Israel
2 Department of Cancer Biology, Cancer Institute, University College London, London WC1 9BT, UK
3 Adelson School of Medicine, Ariel University, Ariel 4070000, Israel
4 Faculty of Medical and Health Sciences, Tel Aviv University, Tel Aviv 6997801, Israel
5 Clalit Health Services, Dan-Petach Tikva District, Petach Tikva 4900000, Israel
* Correspondence: shaias@ariel.ac.il (S.A.); shine6@walla.co.il (V.S.Z.)

Abstract

Background/Objectives: Laboratory tests conducted in community settings are occasionally repeated within hours of presentation to pediatric emergency departments (PEDs). Reducing unnecessary repetitions can ease child discomfort and alleviate the healthcare burden without compromising the diagnostic process or quality of care. The aim of this study was to develop a decision tree (DT) model to guide physicians in minimizing unnecessary repeat blood tests in PEDs. The minimal decision tree (MDT) algorithm was selected for its interpretability and capacity to generate optimally pruned classification trees. **Methods:** Children aged 3 months to 18 years with community-based complete blood count (CBC), electrolyte (ELE), and C-reactive protein (CRP) measurements obtained between 2016 and 2023 were included. Repeat tests performed in the pediatric emergency department within 12 h were evaluated by comparing paired measurements, with tests considered justified when values transitioned from normal to abnormal ranges or changed by ≥20%. Additionally, sensitivity analyses were conducted for absolute change thresholds of 10% and 30% and for repeat intervals of 6, 18, and 24 h. **Results:** Among 7813 children visits in this study, 6044, 1941, and 2771 underwent repeated CBC, ELE, and CRP tests, respectively. The mean ages of patients undergoing CRP, ELE, and CBC testing were 6.33 ± 5.38, 7.91 ± 5.71, and 5.08 ± 5.28 years, respectively. The majority were of middle socio-economic class, with 66.61–71.24% living in urban areas. Pain was the predominant presented complaint (83.69–85.99%), and in most cases (83.69–85.99%), the examination was conducted by a pediatrician. The DT model was developed and evaluated on training and validation cohorts, and it demonstrated high accuracy in predicting the need for repeat CBC and ELE tests but not CRP. Performance of the DT model significantly exceeded that of the logistic regression model. **Conclusions:** The data-driven guide derived from the DT model provides clinicians with a practical, interpretable tool to minimize unnecessary repeat laboratory testing, thereby enhancing patient care and optimizing healthcare resource utilization.

Keywords: health economics; quality assurance; pediatric emergency department; laboratory tests; community; children; healthcare; data-driven models

1. Introduction

Repeat laboratory testing is a well-documented and widespread practice in healthcare [1,2], accounting for a substantial proportion of overall laboratory utilization [3–6]. A hospital-based study reported that 20% to 30% of laboratory tests were repeated within a 24 h period [3]. Repeated testing is intended to reduce diagnostic uncertainty, inform therapeutic decision-making, improve patient care [7,8], and acknowledge patients' clinical presentations [2].

Despite these intended benefits, studies indicated that early repeat laboratory testing yielded negligible or clinically insignificant differences and exerted no influence on clinical decision-making, rendering such repeat tests unjustified [3,9,10]. These heighten patient discomfort, raise healthcare costs, delay clinical decision-making, and impair the effectiveness of clinical management [11]. As highlighted in several studies, although clinicians strive to deliver cost-effective care, limited transparency around laboratory testing expenses may inadvertently lead to occasional overutilization of diagnostic tests [3]. The clinical and financial inefficiencies associated with redundant testing have been highlighted [6,7,11].

In line with these observations, laboratory tests conducted in community settings are occasionally repeated within hours of referral to pediatric emergency departments (PEDs) [1,10]. The prevalence of these repeat tests and the factors driving their occurrence remain poorly understood [1,12]. Limited research has investigated repeat testing in PEDs and pediatric intensive care units [1,11,13]. Pageler et al. [13] implemented a computerized physician order entry intervention in a pediatric intensive care unit that restricted select laboratory tests to a single daily order and required daily reassessment of their necessity. This strategy reduced test utilization, shortened both pediatric intensive care unit and overall hospital lengths of stay, and had no adverse effects on mortality. These findings underscore the importance of clear guidelines to minimize unnecessary repeat laboratory testing in clinical decision-making.

Given the lack of clinical benefit and potential harm of unnecessary repeats, multiple interventions have been proposed to reduce the overuse of laboratory testing [7]. Proposed strategies have ranged from physician education and audit-and-feedback programs to electronic health record enhancements that display cost data, financial incentive schemes, and administrative policies limiting specific test orders. While these interventions have been effective in some settings, their availability and applicability in pediatric care remain limited [14,15]. In pediatric settings, decisions to repeat laboratory tests require consideration of additional complexities, including heterogeneous socio-demographic factors [16]. Tailored strategies in pediatric emergency departments must balance the potential risks posed by repeat laboratory testing with the necessity of comprehensive clinical evaluation.

To translate these considerations into a practical solution, this study aims to equip pediatricians with a practical, data-driven guide to minimize unnecessary repeat blood tests in PEDs. To achieve this, a DT model was constructed using routinely available clinical data and initial community laboratory results to predict when repeat testing was warranted. The resulting, user-friendly tool is designed to reduce test repetitions that are unlikely to affect decision-making.

This study constitutes the first comprehensive application of machine learning to assess the necessity of repeat blood testing in pediatric patients across both community and emergency department settings. The model provides a precise, data-driven framework to assist clinicians in minimizing unnecessary repeated laboratory tests, thereby enhancing patient care, improving healthcare quality, and optimizing resource utilization.

2. Materials and Methods

Initially, the study cohort and associated clinical and laboratory data were characterized. Next, a metric to assess the necessity of repeat laboratory tests was established. Finally, the data-driven methodology for developing the clinical decision guide and its statistical validation are presented. Figure 1 demonstrates a schematic view of the methodological flow of this study, including the data collection process and the model development steps.

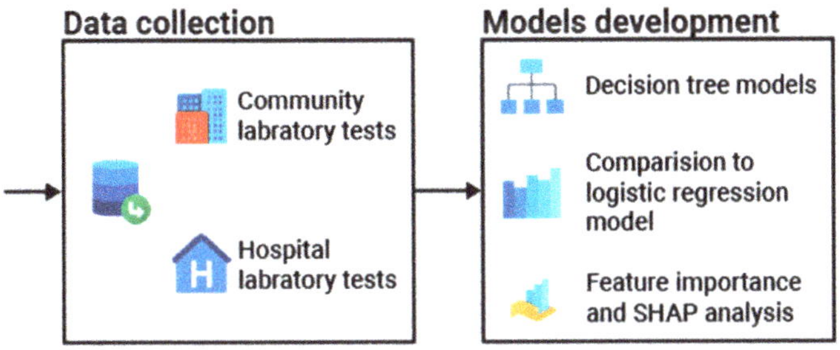

Figure 1. A schematic overview of this study's methodological framework.

The study cohort was assembled from Clalit Health Services (CHS), Israel's largest health maintenance organization, which insures and provides care to approximately 54% of the country's population. CHS maintains a comprehensive electronic database capturing patient demographics, visits to community clinics, emergency departments, and hospitals, laboratory test results, and medication prescriptions and purchases. Each physician visit includes a diagnosis recorded in accordance with the International Classification of Diseases, Ninth Revision (ICD-9). Data were extracted from CHS's electronic medical records via the MDClone© analytics platform. The inclusion criteria comprised medical visits of children aged 3 months to 18 years across Israel's three central administrative districts, between January 1, 2016 and December 31, 2023. Eligible visits included instances in which an initial community laboratory test was repeated in a PED within a 12 h interval.

This study was approved by CHS's Institutional Review Board for Human Studies (approval number: 0099-21-COM). Signed informed consent was waived, as this retrospective cohort analysis of an existing database did not include any clinical intervention or patient contact.

Six laboratory tests were analyzed and grouped into three categories: complete blood count (CBC), including white blood cell count, hemoglobin, and platelet count; serum electrolytes (ELEs), including sodium and potassium; and C-reactive protein (CRP). Data collected from the electronic medical records included socio-demographic information such as age, sex, and socio-economic status (SES), as well as details of the laboratory tests conducted in the community and later in the PED. The patient's SES was based on the Israeli Central Bureau of Statistics classification system, which assigns 10 categories of SES [17]. Categorization was based on multiple variables, including demographic characteristics, educational attainment, employment, income levels, and housing conditions. Complete records were available for every patient in the cohort.

With complete demographic and socio-economic data for all patients, this study then defined criteria for necessary repeat testing. In the absence of a standardized definition in the medical literature, two criteria were applied to classify a repetition as justified. The first criterion deemed tests whose results shifted from within the community's normal reference range to outside the PED's reference limits as clinically necessary. The second criterion employed an absolute difference of $\geq$20% between community and PED to denote clinically significant change. The absolute difference threshold was selected because it has been shown to outperform relative percent change in identifying clinically meaningful variations [18]. Sensitivity analyses were performed for absolute difference thresholds of 10% and 30% and inter-test intervals of 6, 18, and 24 h.

Recent advances in machine learning (ML) model applications in medicine [19–22] highlighted the suitability of decision tree algorithms for clinical decision support. Accordingly, a DT-based model [23], elected for its proven clinical performance and straightforward interpretability [24–26], was developed to translate our established criteria into a practical, data-driven guide. The minimal DT (MDT) algorithm [27] was employed to construct the binary DT model. The MDT algorithm was employed because, unlike conventional machine learning methods that iteratively contract decision tree nodes, it performs a global optimization of the entire tree to produce an optimal classification model [28].

To prepare the data for model development, all continuous variables were converted into discrete categories using a binning approach. To improve the generalization of the results, the k-fold (k = 5) cross-validation method was utilized [29], as well as the SAT post-pruning method [30].

The study population was initially divided into training and validation cohorts for model development and evaluation. Statistical tests were then performed to confirm that age and sex distributions were comparable between the two groups. This step was essential to ensure that the validation set reflected the distribution of the training set, a critical requirement for the generalizability of machine learning models in clinical settings [31]. This balance was achieved using the Directed Bee Colony Optimization algorithm [32]. Model performance was evaluated using the receiver operating characteristic area under the curve (ROC-AUC), along with accuracy, sensitivity, specificity, positive predictive value (PPV), negative predictive value (NPV), Cohen's alpha, and F1 metrics, in accordance with standard practices in medical machine learning [33,34]. For comparison, the widely used logistic regression (LR) model was employed, given its linear structure and interpretability [35].

To explore the decision-making properties of the resulting DT models, two commonly used techniques were applied. First, feature importance was assessed using the standard permutation importance algorithm, which quantifies the average impact of each parameter on the model's final decision [36]. Second, SHapley Additive exPlanations (SHAP) analysis was applied to further interpret the model by quantifying the contribution of each feature to individual predictions [37,38]. The SHAP values provide a unified measure of feature contribution by attributing the effect of each input variable to a specific model prediction. In feature importance analysis, these values quantify the magnitude and direction of each feature's influence, with positive values indicating a positive contribution and negative values indicating a negative impact. All analyses were conducted using Python version 3.9.5, with statistical significance defined as $p < 0.05$.

3. Results

3.1. Study Population

Out of 812,271 pediatric emergency department visits recorded during the study period, 7813 (0.96%) met the inclusion criteria for analysis. Among the included visits, repeated testing was performed in 6044 cases for the complete blood count (CBC), 1941 for electrolytes (ELEs), and 2771 for C-reactive protein (CRP). Some patients underwent more than one type of repeated blood test. The mean ages of patients, stratified by the type of repeated laboratory test, were 5.08 ± 5.28 years for the CBC group, 7.91 ± 5.71 years for the ELE group, and 6.33 ± 5.38 years for the CRP group. The distribution of sexes was balanced, with males comprising 49.43–52.39% across test groups. The majority of patients belonged to the middle SES (66.61–71.24%) and resided in urban areas (66.61–71.24%).

Pain was the most frequently reported complaint across all test groups (83.69–85.99%), and the majority of patients were diagnosed by pediatricians (83.69–85.99%). The detailed description of the study populations is presented in Table 1.

Table 1. Description of the socio-demographic characteristics of the study population *.

Variable	Repeated Complete Blood Count Test (CBC)	Repeated Electrolyte (Na, K) Tests (ELE)	Repeated CRP (CRP)
Visits, *n*	6044	1941	2771
Hospitalization	2924 (48.38%)	1078 (55.56%)	1383 (49.92%)
Age (years), mean (±SD)	5.08 (5.28)	7.91 (5.71)	6.33 (5.38)
Age group			
3 mo–2 years	2758 (45.63%)	434 (22.37%)	1080 (30.96%)
3–10 years	2001 (33.11%)	752 (38.72%)	1175 (42.40%)
11–18 years	1285 (21.29%)	755 (39.91%)	516 (27.64%)
Sex			
Male	2988 (49.43%)	971 (50.05%)	1452 (52.39%)
Female	2056 (50.57%)	969 (49.95%)	1319 (47.61%)
SES			
Low	1692 (27.99%)	615 (31.68%)	914 (32.98%)
Middle	3125 (51.70%)	903 (46.52%)	1306 (47.13%)
High	1227 (20.31%)	423 (21.80%)	551 (19.89%)
Residence type			
City	4219 (69.80%)	1293 (66.61%)	1974 (71.24%)
Village	1458 (24.12%)	495 (25.50%)	638 (23.02%)
Other	367 (6.98%)	152 (7.89%)	159 (5.74%)

* All values are expressed as *N* (%), unless otherwise stated.

3.2. *Repeated Laboratory Testing*

Approximately half of the patients in each blood test group were hospitalized, with rates ranging from 48.38% to 55.56%. Based on the predefined criteria for appropriateness, only 2924 of 6044 (7.32%) CBC tests, 1078 of 1941 (11.85%) ELE tests, and 1383 of 2771 (13.68%) CRP tests were considered appropriate.

3.3. *Models for Predicting the Necessity of Repeated Laboratory Testing*

Table 2 presents the performance metrics of three DT models and three LR models, corresponding to the CBC, ELE, and CRP tests. Model evaluation included accuracy, F1-score, sensitivity, specificity, PPV, NPV, Cohen's alpha, and ROC-AUC. The F1-score, commonly used in classification tasks, represents the harmonic mean of precision and sensitivity.

Table 2. Performance of decision tree and logistic regression models across thresholds of 10%, 20%, and 30% and out-of-normal-range absolute changes for CBC, CHS, and CRP tests. Metrics: accuracy; F1-score; ROC-AUC; sensitivity; specificity; positive predictive value; negative predictive value; and Cohen's κ.

Model	Prediction	Condition	Accuracy	F1-Score	ROC-AUC	Sensitivity	Specificity	PPV	NPV	Cohen's Kappa
Decision tree	CBC	10%	85.81%	78.68%	73.40%	75.48%	89.96%	82.26%	86.97%	68.60%
	ELE	10%	79.78%	75.77%	72.49%	72.57%	82.35%	78.50%	77.01%	56.90%
	CRP	10%	72.46%	70.75%	68.73%	67.55%	75.58%	74.07%	70.36%	44.90%
	CBC	20%	78.72%	72.19%	67.34%	68.99%	85.21%	75.69%	80.46%	55.00%
	ELE	20%	73.18%	69.52%	66.47%	66.32%	77.01%	72.82%	70.81%	45.70%
	CRP	20%	66.48%	64.91%	63.09%	61.71%	70.36%	68.32%	65.04%	33.40%
	CBC	30%	91.70%	84.09%	78.43%	80.89%	93.30%	86.81%	90.76%	79.30%
	ELE	30%	85.24%	81.08%	77.42%	77.88%	87.20%	83.92%	83.18%	68.70%
	CRP	30%	77.44%	75.62%	73.49%	72.42%	80.82%	79.46%	75.62%	56.80%
	CBC	out-of-range	77.15%	70.75%	66.00%	67.55%	84.18%	74.07%	79.16%	52.10%
	ELE	out-of-range	76.84%	72.99%	69.79%	69.79%	80.20%	76.13%	73.80%	51.80%
	CRP	out-of-range	69.80%	68.16%	66.24%	64.96%	73.13%	71.30%	67.92%	39.50%
Logistic regression	CBC	10%	75.57%	73.09%	68.14%	69.89%	78.96%	76.62%	73.71%	49.90%
	ELE	10%	72.87%	70.43%	67.05%	67.23%	76.45%	73.84%	70.93%	44.90%
	CRP	10%	66.00%	65.32%	64.35%	62.12%	70.19%	68.79%	65.55%	34.40%
	CBC	20%	69.33%	67.05%	62.51%	63.85%	72.76%	70.47%	67.57%	38.00%
	ELE	20%	66.85%	64.62%	61.56%	61.42%	70.21%	67.92%	65.05%	33.20%
	CRP	20%	61.48%	59.93%	59.04%	56.73%	65.59%	63.33%	60.19%	23.90%
	CBC	30%	80.76%	78.11%	72.80%	74.91%	84.18%	81.65%	79.16%	60.90%
	ELE	30%	77.85%	75.29%	71.70%	72.09%	81.33%	79.25%	76.44%	54.00%
	CRP	30%	71.62%	70.08%	68.76%	66.88%	74.88%	73.66%	70.76%	44.60%
	CBC	out-of-range	67.94%	65.71%	61.26%	62.51%	71.49%	69.17%	66.27%	35.40%
	ELE	out-of-range	70.19%	67.85%	64.64%	64.65%	73.08%	70.78%	67.92%	38.90%
	CRP	out-of-range	64.55%	62.93%	61.99%	59.73%	68.49%	66.45%	63.36%	29.70%

Focusing on the DT models, the CBC model demonstrates the highest performance, achieving an accuracy of 78.72% and an F1-score of 72.19%. The similarity between these two metrics suggests that the model generalized well without overfitting. Conversely, the CRP model exhibited lower accuracy and performed only slightly better than random classification, indicating limited predictive value. The ELE model achieved an accuracy of 73.18% and an F1-score of 69.52%. Notably, across all three test categories, the DT model outperformed the LR in terms of accuracy, F1-score, and ROC-AUC. The superior performance of the DT model may be attributed to its ability to capture non-linear relationships. Consequently, we did not assume a global linear association between repeat laboratory testing and individual model parameters, such as patient age. The DT model demonstrated a consistent performance across all evaluated criteria, including the 10%, 20%, and 30% absolute difference thresholds and the out-of-range definition, supporting its robustness. Based on this consistency, the 20% threshold was selected for further analysis, as it demonstrated a balanced performance across all evaluation metrics. Sensitivity analyses for 6, 18, and 24 h intervals between repeated tests are presented in Supplementary Table S1.

Supplementary Figure S1 presents the DT models for the CBC, ELE, and CRP laboratory tests, with each node displaying a decision based on a specific model parameter and threshold. The decision path proceeds to the right if the specified condition is met and to the left if it is not, ultimately reaching a leaf node. Each leaf node indicates the model's recommendation regarding the necessity of repeating the laboratory test. Notably, the root node (first row) in all DT models was defined by the corresponding laboratory test result obtained in the community setting. In cases involving multiple laboratory tests, such as the CBC model, additional community-based test results appeared immediately after the root node in the decision path. In higher-order decisions nodes (i.e., the upper levels of the tree structure), the socio-demographic characteristics, such as patient age and sex, played a prominent role.

3.4. Variables Contributing to the Decision Tree Models

Figure 2a–c illustrate the contributions of various clinical and demographic variables to the decision tree models of the CBC, ELE, and CRP laboratory tests. Feature importance reflects the average contribution of each variable to the model's predictions, offering an estimate of which features are most informative in determining the necessity of a repeated laboratory test. The laboratory results obtained in the community emerged as the most influential feature, followed by patient age. In contrast, patient sex (represented by the "Male" variable in Figure 2) had minimal to no impact on the model's predictions, with importance values close to or equal to zero. Furthermore, neither the primary presenting symptom nor the identity of the referring clinician (pediatrician or family physician) demonstrated a measurable predictive value in the models.

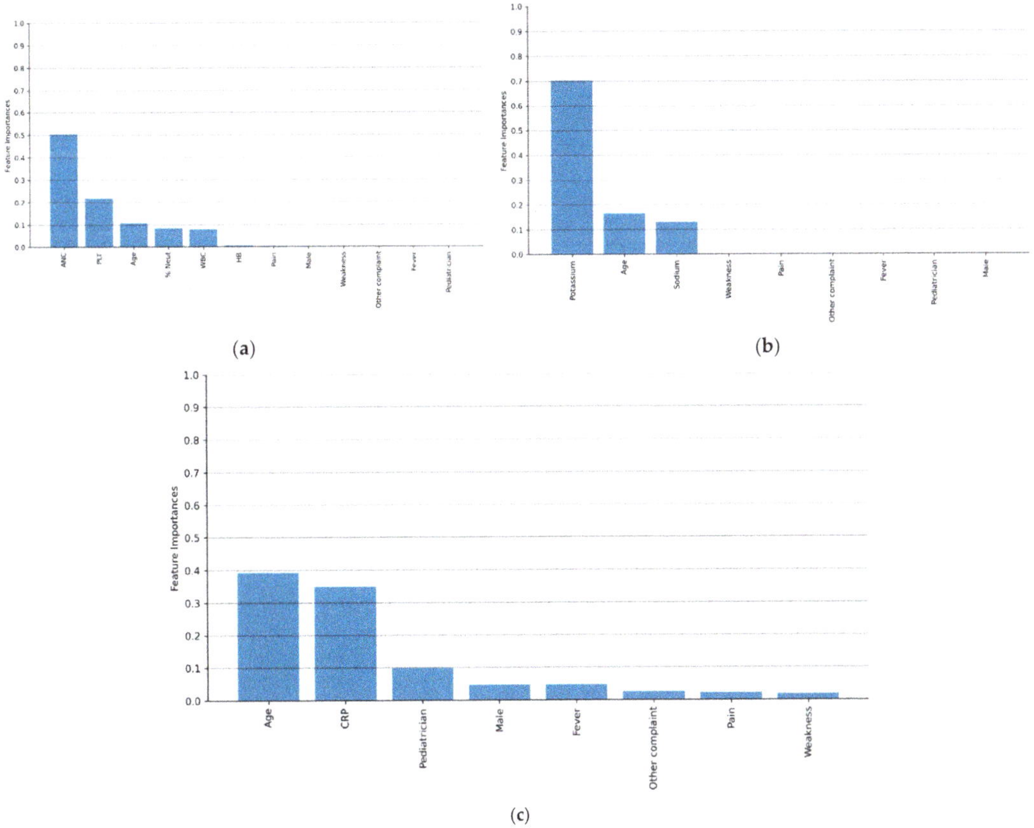

Figure 2. The variables' relative contributions (feature importance) to the justification for repeat blood testing according to the decision tree models (**a**) CBC, (**b**) ELEs, and (**c**) CRP.

Figure 3 presents the SHAP analysis of the three DT models corresponding to the CBC, ELE, and CRP tests. In the CBC model, the absolute neutrophil count (ANC) measured in the community emerged as a key predictor. Higher ANC values were associated with an increased probability of the model recommending repeat testing, as indicated by the concentration of blue points to the right of the central reference line, along with several overlapping purple points. The second most important feature was the platelet count (PLT), which exhibited a pattern similar to that of ANC. The third was patient age, where younger patients had a slightly higher likelihood of requiring repeat testing. As age increased, the predicted need for repetition decreased, as reflected by the red values appearing to the left of the central line. For the ELE model, serum potassium level was the most influential feature, with elevated values associated with an increased likelihood of repeat testing. The second and third most influential features were patients age and serum sodium level, both of which exhibited less distinct patterns in relation to the predicted need for repeat testing. For the CRP model, lower serum values were associated with a higher likelihood of repeat testing. Patient age was the second most important feature. With respect to sex, male patients were more likely than female patients to undergo repeat CRP testing.

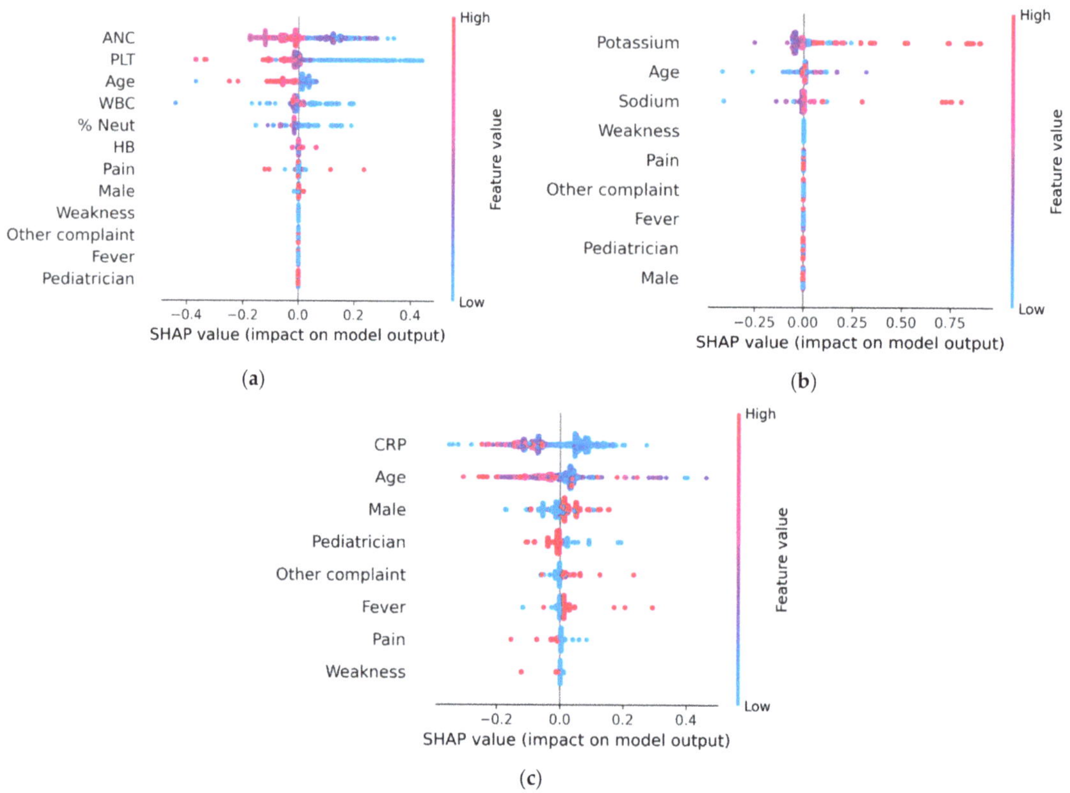

Figure 3. The approximate linear relationship between the decision tree model variables and the predictive need for repeat laboratory testing based on SHAP (Shapley Additive exPlanations) analysis: (**a**) CBC; (**b**) ELEs; (**c**) CRP.

4. Discussion

In this study, data-driven guides were developed to assist physicians in determining whether a repeated laboratory test in the PED is warranted when an identical test was recently performed in the community. The guides were based on widely available data, including socio-demographic characteristics and results from the initial community laboratory tests, supporting both their practicality and generalizability.

Initial findings, as presented in Table 2, indicate that the proportion of repeated laboratory tests classified as appropriate is relatively low (7.32–13.68%). This observation is consistent with previous research in pediatric populations, which also reported high rates of seemingly unjustified laboratory test repetition [12]. These findings underscore the challenges clinicians face in accurately assessing the necessity of repeated laboratory tests. They also highlight the potential value of a decision support tool to reduce unnecessary repeat testing, with implications for improving the patient experience, healthcare quality, and cost efficiency [7,8].

When examining individual laboratory tests, the DT-based data-driven guide demonstrated a strong predictive performance for CBC and ELEs, achieving high accuracy in identifying justified repetitions. However, its performance for CFP was limited, showing only a marginal improvement over random classification (Table 2). The limited performance of the CRP model may be attributed to the relatively long half-life of CRP, approximately 48 h, which reduces the likelihood of observing significant changes within a 12 h retesting period. When examining the DT models under a configuration in which false negatives were set to zero, thereby ensuring that no justified repeat tests were incorrectly dismissed, the models achieved a true positive rate higher than that of random guessing, as shown in Figure 2. This configuration indicates that adopting the proposed guides in this manner does not adversely affect clinical outcomes. When compared to the baseline logistic regression model, the DT demonstrated a marginal improvement in predictive accuracy. This difference may be attributed to the non-linear structure of the DT model, in contrast to the linear nature of LR. The result highlights the importance of models that account for multiple interacting variables, rather than relying on a single factor, such as patient age. It is important to note that these tools are intended to support, not replace, clinical judgment; the pediatrician's assessment and any changes in the patient's condition remain paramount.

The DT models and clinical guides developed in this study are consistent with established clinical understanding. For example, as demonstrated in Figures 2 and 3, patient age plays an important role in decision-making but remains secondary to clinical status, as reflected by the initial community laboratory results. In support of this observation, Desai et al. conducted an electronic survey among 43 pediatric residents and staff physicians to examine perceptions of laboratory stewardship and testing patterns at a tertiary pediatric hospital [16]. The survey revealed a high level of familiarity with laboratory stewardship, with respondents acknowledging that overuse of laboratory testing is a recognized issue both in general medical practice and within their own institution. The majority of survey respondents indicated that increased cost transparency could help reduce laboratory test overuse. However, they reported limited familiarity with key aspects of test utilization, including test costs, specificity and sensitivity, required blood volumes, and existing clinical guidelines for common laboratory tests. The study showed that 53% of laboratory tests were repeated within 7 days, and only half of these repeat tests produced abnormal results [16]. Similar findings were observed in both pediatric and adult populations [39,40]. In addition, previous studies emphasized the importance of cost transparency in reducing the frequency and cost of blood tests and imaging studies [41,42].

This study has several notable strengths, including the large sample size, the real-world, population-based design, and its practical applicability. The analytical tools developed can be adapted to different threshold criteria, applied to additional laboratory tests, and implemented in various clinical settings to support physicians decision-making.

However, several limitations should be acknowledged. First, due to the retrospective design of this study, the proposed analyses and decision guides were simplified, and clinical data such as patients' medical history were not included. This information could have provided additional insight into the patients' medical conditions and potentially influenced the assessment of whether repeat blood testing was warranted. Additionally, this study did not assess the actual impact of repeated testing on clinical decision-making or patient outcomes, which should be addressed in future prospective studies. Furthermore, cases in which a justified repeat test was not performed were not examined. Second, in the absence of an established definition in the literature for justified repeat testing, two criteria were applied: a change from a normal to an out-of-normal range result, and an absolute change of $\geq$20%. Sensitivity analyses were also conducted to support these thresholds. Third, in this analysis, repeat testing was defined as occurring within a 12 h interval. This strict definition captures a specific subset of repeated tests and does not account for those performed over a longer duration, such as during an extended hospital stay or ongoing interactions with the healthcare system. To address this limitation, additional analyses were performed using extended time intervals of 6, 18, and 24 h between repeated tests. The methodology applied in this study can be readily adapted to evaluate other time intervals and alternative definitions for justified repetition thresholds.

5. Conclusions

This study presents a novel, data-driven approach for assessing the necessity of repeated blood testing in pediatric emergency settings, grounded in real-world data from both community and hospital settings. The proposed guide supports clinical decision-making and, when used alongside physician judgment, has the potential to reduce unnecessary repeat testing while maintaining high standards of patient care. The tools presented in this study, which are relatively simple and rely on readily available data, can be adapted for use in clinical settings to help reduce unjustified repetition of laboratory testing. Future prospective studies are recommended to evaluate the effectiveness of the proposed model in reducing unnecessary laboratory testing and in supporting clinical decision-making by pediatricians. Demonstrating effectiveness in real-world settings may lead to an improved quality of care, enhanced patient and family experience, and meaningful reduction in healthcare costs and system burden.

Supplementary Materials: The following supporting information can be downloaded at https://www.mdpi.com/article/10.3390/diagnostics15151885/s1, Figure S1: DT models for the CBC, ELE, and CRP laboratory tests; Table S1. Model performance (decision tree vs. logistic regression) over the time intervals 6, 12, 18, and 24 h.

Author Contributions: Conceptualization, A.S., T.L., S.A., A.H.C. and V.S.Z.; methodology, A.S., T.L., A.H.C. and V.S.Z.; software, T.L. and A.S.; validation, S.A. and A.H.C.; formal analysis, A.S., T.L. and V.S.Z.; data curation, A.H.C., Y.R. and V.S.Z.; visualization, A.S., T.L. and V.S.Z.; supervision, T.L., S.A. and A.H.C.; project administration, Y.R. and V.S.Z. All authors have read and agreed to the published version of the manuscript.

Funding: This research received no external funding.

Institutional Review Board Statement: This study was conducted following the Declaration of Helsinki and approved by the Institutional Review Board of Clalit Health Services (protocol number 0099-21-COM, August 5, 2024).

Informed Consent Statement: Patient consent was waived due to the retrospective nature of this study.

Data Availability Statement: All statistical analyses are available upon reasonable request. Because of ethical and privacy issues, patients' data cannot be shared.

Conflicts of Interest: The authors declare no conflicts of interest.

Abbreviations

The following abbreviations are used in this manuscript:

CBC	Complete blood count
CHS	Clalit Health Services
CRP	C-reactive protein
DT	Decision tree
ELEs	Electrolytes
MDT	Minimal DT
PEDs	Pediatric emergency departments
SES	Socio-economic status

References

1. Adair, A.B.; Dejanovich, B.; Walsh, M. Utilization of transport data to decrease unnecessarily repeated laboratory tests. *Pediatr. Emerg. Care* **2024**, *40*, 218–222. [CrossRef]
2. Jose, A.S.; Srivastav, S.; Mehta, B. Investigating the visit-to-visit repeatability of autonomic neuropathy assessment measures in healthy subjects. *Ann. Neurosci. Online ahead of print.* **2025**, 09727531241310034. [CrossRef]
3. Cadamuro, J.; Gaksch, M.; Wiedemann, H.; Lippi, G.; von Meyer, A.; Pertersmann, A.; Auer, S.; Mrazek, C.; Kipman, U.; Felder, T.K.; et al. Are laboratory tests always needed? Frequency and causes of laboratory overuse in a hospital setting. *Clin. Biochem.* **2018**, *54*, 85–91. [CrossRef] [PubMed]
4. Ahrari, A.; Barrett, S.S.; Basharat, P.; Rohekar, S.; Pope, J.E. Appropriateness of laboratory tests in the diagnosis of inflammatory rheumatic diseases among patients newly referred to rheumatologists. *Jt. Bone Spine* **2020**, *87*, 588–595. [CrossRef]
5. Aichinger, E.; Schleck, C.D.; Harmsen, W.S.; Nyre, L.M.; Patel, R. Nonutility of repeat laboratory testing for detection of Clostridium difficile by use of PCR or enzyme immunoassay. *J. Clin. Microbiol.* **2008**, *46*, 3795–3797. [CrossRef] [PubMed]
6. Hawkins, R.C. Potentially inappropriate repeat laboratory testing in inpatients. *Clin. Chem.* **2006**, *52*, 784–785. [CrossRef]
7. Sedrak, M.S.; Myers, J.S.; Small, D.S.; Nachamkin, I.; Ziemba, J.B.; Murray, D.; Kurtzman, G.W.; Zhu, J.; Wang, W.; Mincarelli, D.; et al. Effect of a price transparency intervention in the electronic health record on clinician ordering of inpatient laboratory tests: The PRICE randomized clinical trial. *JAMA Intern. Med.* **2017**, *177*, 939–945. [CrossRef]
8. Iturrate, E.; Jubelt, L.; Volpicelli, F.; Hochman, K. Optimize your electronic medical record to increase value: Reducing laboratory overutilization. *Am. J. Med.* **2016**, *129*, 215–220. [CrossRef] [PubMed]
9. Kahan, N.R.; Waitman, D.A.; Vardy, D.A. Curtailing laboratory test ordering in a managed care setting through redesign of a computerized order form. *Am. J. Manag. Care* **2009**, *15*, 173–176. [PubMed]
10. Chu, K.H.; Wagholikar, A.S.; Greenslade, J.H.; O'Dwyer, J.A.; Brown, A.F. Sustained reductions in emergency department laboratory test orders: Impact of a simple intervention. *Postgrad. Med. J.* **2013**, *89*, 566–571. [CrossRef]
11. Coon, E.R.; Young, P.C.; Quinonez, R.A.; Morgan, D.J.; Dhruva, S.S.; Schroeder, A.R. Update on pediatric overuse. *Pediatrics* **2017**, *139*, e20162797. [CrossRef]
12. Fieldston, E.S.; Fakeye, O.A.; Friedman, D.F. Repeat laboratory testing in the pediatric emergency department: How often and how important? *Pediatr. Emerg. Care* **2019**, *35*, 190–193. [CrossRef]
13. Pageler, N.M.; Franzon, D.; Longhurst, C.A.; Wood, M.; Shin, A.Y.; Adams, E.S.; Widen, E.; Cornfield, D.N. Embedding time-limited laboratory orders within computerized provider order entry reduces laboratory utilization. *Pediatr. Crit. Care Med.* **2013**, *14*, 413–419. [CrossRef]
14. Chien, A.T.; Ganeshan, S.; Schuster, M.A.; Lehmann, L.S.; Hatfield, L.A.; Koplan, K.E.; Petty, C.R.; Sinaiko, A.D.; Sequist, T.D.; Rosenthal, M.B. The effect of price information on the ordering of images and procedures. *Pediatrics* **2017**, *139*, e20161507. [CrossRef] [PubMed]
15. Johnson, D.P.; Lind, C.; Parker, S.E.; Beuschel, C.; VanVliet, S.; Nichols, J.; Rauch, C.A.; Lee, B.; Muething, S.E. Toward high-value care: A quality improvement initiative to reduce unnecessary repeat complete blood counts and basic metabolic panels on a pediatric hospitalist service. *Hosp. Pediatr.* **2016**, *6*, 1–8. [CrossRef] [PubMed]

16. Desai, T.S.; Tang, K.; Kaul, V.; Blasutig, I.M.; Buba, M. Laboratory stewardship perceptions and testing patterns at a pediatric tertiary care center. *Lab. Med.* **2024**, *55*, 571–579. [CrossRef] [PubMed]
17. Central Bureau of Statistics. Available online: https://www.cbs.gov.il/he/cbsnewbrand/Pages/default.aspx (accessed on 21 July 2025).
18. Wolpern, A.E.; Burgos, D.J.; Janot, J.M.; Dalleck, L.C. Is a threshold-based model a superior method to the relative percent concept for establishing individual exercise intensity? a randomized controlled trial. *BMC Sports Sci. Med. Rehabil.* **2015**, *7*, 16. [CrossRef]
19. Rajkomar, A.; Dean, J.; Kohane, I. Machine learning in medicine. *N. Engl. J. Med.* **2019**, *380*, 1347–1358. [CrossRef]
20. Levi, M.; Lazebnik, T.; Kushnir, S.; Yosef, N.; Shlomi, D. Machine learning computational model to predict lung cancer using electronic medical records. *Cancer Epidemiol.* **2024**, *92*, 102631. [CrossRef]
21. Hasnain, Z.; Mason, J.; Gill, K.; Kuhn, P.; Newton, P.K. Machine learning models for predicting post-cystectomy recurrence and survival in bladder cancer patients. *PLoS ONE* **2019**, *14*, e0210976. [CrossRef]
22. Garg, A.; Mago, V. Role of machine learning in medical research: A survey. *Comput. Sci. Rev.* **2021**, *40*, 100370. [CrossRef]
23. Sokol, K.; Flach, P. Desiderata for interpretability: Explaining decision tree predictions with counterfactuals. In AAAI'19/IAAI'19/EAAI'19. In Proceedings of the Thirty-Third AAAI Conference on Artificial Intelligence (AAAI-19) and Thirty-First Innovative Applications of Artificial Intelligence Conference and Ninth AAAI Symposium on Educational Advances in Artificial Intelligence, Honolulu, HI, USA, 27 January–1 February 2019; Volume 33, pp. 10035–10036. [CrossRef]
24. Deepika, P. Heart disease prediction using classification with different decision tree techniques. *Int. J. Eng. Res. Generic Sci.* **2014**, *2*, 6–11.
25. Didik, M.E.; Rianto, A.; Fernandes Andry, J.; Tannady, H.; Chakir, A. Analysis of big data in healthcare using decision tree algorithm. In Proceedings of the 1st International Conference on Computer Science and Artificial Intelligence (ICCSAI), Jakarta, Indonesia, 28 October 2021; Volume 1, pp. 313–317.
26. Xu, F.; Uszkoreit, H.; Du, Y.; Fan, W.; Zhao, D.; Zhu, J. Explainable AI: A Brief Survey on History, Research Areas, Approaches and Challenges. In *Natural Language Processing and Chinese Computing, Proceedings of the 8th CCF International Conference, NLPCC 2019, Dunhuang, China, 9–14 October 2019*; Tang, J., Kan, M.Y., Zhao, D., Li, S., Zan, H., Eds.; Lecture Notes in Computer Science; Springer: Cham, Switzerland, 2019; Volume 11839, pp. 563–574. [CrossRef]
27. Carrizosa, E.; Molero-Río, C.; Romero Morales, D. Mathematical optimization in classification and regression trees. *Top* **2021**, *29*, 5–33. [CrossRef]
28. Bertsimas, D.; Dunn, J. Optimal classification trees. *Mach. Learn.* **2017**, *106*, 1039–1082. [CrossRef]
29. Normawati, D.; Dewi Pramudi, I. K-fold cross validation for selection of cardiovascular disease diagnosis features by applying rule-based datamining. *Signal Image Process. Lett.* **2019**, *2*, 23–35. [CrossRef]
30. Lazebnik, T.; Bunimovich-Mendrazitsky, S. Decision tree post-pruning without loss of accuracy using the SAT-PP algorithm with an empirical evaluation on clinical data. *Data Knowl. Eng.* **2023**, *145*, 102173. [CrossRef]
31. Doshi-Velez, F.; Perlis, R.H. Evaluating machine learning articles. *JAMA* **2019**, *322*, 1777–1779. [CrossRef] [PubMed]
32. Goodman, M.D.; Dowsland, K.A.; Thompson, J.M. A grasp-knapsack hybrid for a nurse-scheduling problem. *J. Heuristics* **2009**, *15*, 351–379. [CrossRef]
33. Assegie, T.A.; Lakshmi Tulasi, R.; Komal Kumar, N. Breast cancer prediction model with decision tree and adaptive boosting. *IAES Int. J. Artif. Intell.* **2021**, *10*, 184–190. [CrossRef]
34. Lazebnik, T.; Bahouth, Z.; Bunimovich-Mendrazitsky, S.; Halachmi, S. Predicting acute kidney injury following open partial nephrectomy treatment using SAT-pruned explainable machine learning model. *BMC Med. Inform. Decis. Mak.* **2022**, *22*, 133. [CrossRef]
35. Hosmer, D.W., Jr.; Lemeshow, S.; Sturdivant, R.X. *Applied Logistic Regression*, 3rd ed.; John Wiley & Sons: Hoboken, NJ, USA, 2013. [CrossRef]
36. Altmann, A.; Toloşi, L.; Sander, O.; Lengauer, T. Permutation importance: A corrected feature importance measure. *Bioinformatics* **2010**, *26*, 1340–1347. [CrossRef]
37. Lu, S.; Chen, R.; Wei, W.; Belovsky, M.; Lu, X. Understanding heart failure patients EHR clinical features via SHAP interpretation of tree-based machine learning model predictions. *AMIA Annu. Symp. Proc.* **2022**, *2021*, 813–822. [PubMed]
38. Miyakis, S.; Karamanof, G.; Liontos, M.; Mountokalakis, T.D. Factors contributing to inappropriate ordering of tests in an academic medical department and the effect of an educational feedback strategy. *Postgrad. Med. J.* **2006**, *82*, 823–829. [CrossRef] [PubMed]
39. Zhi, M.; Ding, E.L.; Theisen-Toupal, J.; Whelan, J.; Arnaout, R. The landscape of inappropriate laboratory testing: A 15-year meta-analysis. *PLoS ONE* **2013**, *8*, e78962. [CrossRef] [PubMed]
40. Rock, T.A.; Xiao, R.; Fieldston, E. General pediatric attending physicians' and residents' knowledge of inpatient hospital finances. *Pediatrics* **2013**, *131*, 1072–1080. [CrossRef]

41. Feldman, L.S.; Shihab, H.M.; Thiemann, D.; Yeh, H.C.; Ardolino, M.; Mandell, S.; Brotman, D.J. Impact of providing fee data on laboratory test ordering: A controlled clinical trial. *JAMA Intern. Med.* **2013**, *173*, 903–908. [CrossRef]
42. Goetz, C.; Rotman, S.R.; Hartoularos, G.; Bishop, T.F. The effect of charge display on cost of care and physician practice behaviors: A systematic review. *J. Gen. Intern. Med.* **2015**, *30*, 835–842. [CrossRef]

diagnostics

MDPI

Article

Turkish Chest X-Ray Report Generation Model Using the Swin Enhanced Yield Transformer (Model-SEY) Framework

Murat Ucan [1], Buket Kaya [2] and Mehmet Kaya [3,*]

1 Department of Computer Technologies, Vocational School of Technical Sciences, Dicle University, Diyarbakir 21200, Turkey; murat.ucan@dicle.edu.tr
2 Department of Electronics and Automation, Firat University, Elazig 23119, Turkey; bkaya@firat.edu.tr
3 Department of Computer Engineering, Firat University, Elazig 23119, Turkey
* Correspondence: kaya@firat.edu.tr

Abstract

Background/Objectives: Extracting meaningful medical information from chest X-ray images and transcribing it into text is a complex task that requires a high level of expertise and directly affects clinical decision-making processes. Automatic reporting systems for this field in Turkish represent an important gap in scientific research, as they have not been sufficiently addressed in the existing literature. **Methods**: A deep learning-based approach called Model-SEY was developed with the aim of automatically generating Turkish medical reports from chest X-ray images. The Swin Transformer structure was used in the encoder part of the model to extract image features, while the text generation process was carried out using the cosmosGPT architecture, which was adapted specifically for the Turkish language. **Results**: With the permission of the ethics committee, a new dataset was created using image–report pairs obtained from Elazıg Fethi Sekin City Hospital and Indiana University Chest X-Ray dataset and experiments were conducted on this new dataset. In the tests conducted within the scope of the study, scores of 0.6412, 0.5335, 0.4395, 0.4395, 0.3716, and 0.2240 were obtained in BLEU-1, BLEU-2, BLEU-3, BLEU-4, and ROUGE word overlap evaluation metrics, respectively. **Conclusions**: Quantitative and qualitative analyses of medical reports autonomously generated by the proposed model have shown that they are meaningful and consistent. The proposed model is one of the first studies in the field of autonomous reporting using deep learning architectures specific to the Turkish language, representing an important step forward in this field. It will also reduce potential human errors during diagnosis by supporting doctors in their decision-making.

Keywords: medical report generation; chest X-ray; Swin transformer; GPT; Turkish

1. Introduction

Paragraph-level reporting of medical images is a critical and important process for the diagnosis, follow-up, and treatment planning of diseases [1]. In particular, chest X-ray images are a low-cost and rapid acquisition method widely used for the diagnosis of respiratory diseases. However, in traditional methods, chest X-ray images are examined by specialized physicians and medical reports are written. This process is a critical and human error-prone process that requires medical specialists [2]. In addition, the examination of radiology images is a time-limited process that can lead to under-diagnosis in an individual with multiple diseases at the same time.

Recently, with the use of deep learning techniques, researchers have introduced autonomous alternatives to the analysis of images in many medical fields [3]. Promising results have been obtained for deep learning-based disease diagnosis in the fields of classification [4], which focuses only on disease diagnosis and segmentation, which involves the identification of the diseased surface [5,6]. For example, classification, segmentation, and detection-based studies provide only limited information, such as a single word about the presence of the disease or the marking of the diseased surface [7–9]. It is far from providing information about the details of the diagnosis. In the field of medical report generation, images are output as a meaningful report consisting of multiple words and sentences [10]. For this reason, the medical report generation workspace is a good decision support system that can be useful for doctors to make decisions about disease diagnosis [11].

In recent years, studies using deep learning architectures, in particular, have achieved successful results in the generation of meaningful text from images [12]. Studies that generate paragraph-level reports from chest X-ray images generally use the encoder–decoder deep learning architecture, which is a two-stage process [13]. The encoder part involves feature extraction from the images. In the decoder part, the text is generated using the features extracted from the texts and the features extracted from the image in the encoder stage [14]. It is very important that the generated reports are regular and meaningful texts and can be understood by humans when they read them. The main tasks of the decoder stage in this field of study are the generation of correct words, the formation of sentences by ordering the generated words in a regular order, the length of the sentences to maintain the integrity of meaning, and the formation of paragraphs by ordering the sentences correctly.

In the encoder stage, researchers have tried to extract the best possible features from images by choosing convolutional neural networks (CNN) or transformer-based architectures. Liu et al. conducted a study that preferred CNN architectures in the encoder part and RNN architecture in the decoder part [15]. Using the Open-I dataset, the researchers obtained a BLEU-1 score of 0.359 in the methods they named NLG and CCR. In another study using the DenseNet101 architecture on the encoder side, the researchers obtained a word overlap evaluation metric BLEU-1 score of 0.347 with the VSGRU models they used on the decoder side [16]. There are also studies that prefer transformer-based architectures instead of CNN architectures at the encoder stage. In the encoder stage, Ucan et al. used the vision transformer architecture, which was first developed in the visual feature extraction of transformer-based architectures [17]. In the decoder stage, the researchers developed a hybrid encoder–decoder architecture by preferring the bard architecture. The developed architectures achieved an evaluation metric score of 0.274 in the ROUGE metric.

Although there are several studies on medical report generation in English from medical images in the current literature, there are no studies on report generation in Turkish. There are limited studies in the field of image captioning, which is a similar field of study. TasvirEt [18] and TRCaptionNet [19] are pioneering studies on Turkish image captioning. However, these studies focus on datasets created with images taken from everyday life such as Flickr8K, MS COCO, and Flickr30K rather than medical images. Textual reporting of images in medical fields is a new and open area for the Turkish language.

In this paper, we propose a hybrid encoder–decoder-based deep learning architecture for generating Turkish medical reports from chest X-ray images. While features are extracted from chest X-ray images in the encoder stage, the decoder stage aims to generate meaningful and fluent Turkish sentences from these features. In this context, Swin Transformer architecture is used in the encoder part and GPT architecture enriched with Turkish language is used in the decoder part. With the developed encoder–decoder architecture, it is aimed to increase the report generation performance. In addition, a chest X-ray dataset with Turkish descriptions was prepared and made available for training and evaluation of the model. The main contributions of this study can be summarized as follows:

(i) Presentation of one of the first comprehensive approaches to generating medical reports in Turkish from chest X-ray images;

(ii) Designing a novel hybrid encoder–decoder architecture that integrates a Swin Transformer-based model as an image encoder and a Turkish GPT-2-based model as a language decoder, and evaluating its performance effects on medical report production in detail;

(iii) Addressing an important gap in the literature by making the dataset created for use in Turkish medical natural language processing available to the open-access research community.

The rest of the paper is organized as follows: Section 2 summarizes the methodologies used in the research. Section 3 presents the results obtained in the experiments and discussion. Section 4 discusses the conclusions and future work.

2. Materials and Methods

2.1. Turkish Chest X-Ray Images Medical Report Generation Dataset

With the ethics committee permission obtained within the scope of our study, medical images of patients and reports related to the images were obtained from Elazığ Fethi Sekin City Hospital. In addition, the image–report pairs in the Indiana University Chest X-Ray dataset [20], which contains chest X-ray images offered as open access in the literature, were also used in the study. All data obtained by the specialist doctor in the field in our research team were checked and approved. Due to the small number of data obtained from the field within the scope of the study, a hybrid data set was created by translating the data in English open-access data sets into Turkish with expert opinion. All chest X-ray images in the dataset were resized to 224 × 224 to create a standard between the images. Textual report data was cleaned from meaningless texts such as introductory phrases, extra spaces, pause expressions, etc., to ensure a standardized structure. The dataset created within the scope of the study contains 5998 image–report pairs in total. Figure 1 below shows the random images in the dataset. Figure 2 shows randomly selected examples of reports written by doctors who are experts in their field.

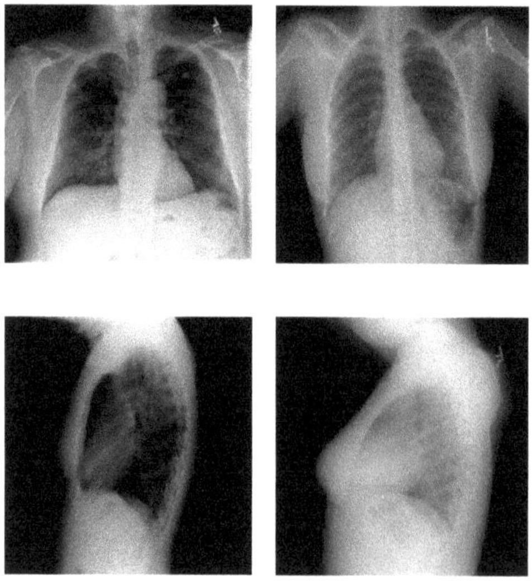

Figure 1. Turkish chest X-ray images reporting dataset randomly selected sample images.

Akciğerler iki taraflı olarak açıktır. Kardiyak ve mediastinal siluetler normaldir. Pulmoner vaskülatür normaldir. Pnömotoraks veya plevral efüzyon yok. Akut kemikli anormallik yok.

Kalp büyüklüğü, mediastinal kontur ve pulmoner vaskülarite normal sınırlar içindedir. Fokal konsolidasyon, plevral efüzyon veya pnömotoraks tanımlanmamıştır.Akut kemik anormalliği tanımlanmadı.

Postoperatif değişiklikler sol beşinci kaburgada bulunur. Sol üst lobda artık radyopak sütürler de bulunur. Akciğerler infiltrat veya kütleler olmadan açıktır. Kalp ve mediastinum normaldir.

Akciğerlerin hiperenflasyonu vardır. Sol kardiyofrenik XXXX bölgesinde küçük bir alan yara izi görülür. Plevral efüzyon veya pnömotoraks yoktur. Kalp önemli ölçüde genişlememiştir. Aortun aterosklerotik değişiklikleri

Figure 2. Turkish chest X-ray images reporting dataset randomly selected sample medical reports.

As part of the study, open-access English image–report matches were translated into Turkish and included in the dataset to address the lack of Turkish chest X-ray report data. This translation process was carried out in multiple stages to ensure both linguistic consistency and medical accuracy. In the first stage, each English report was pre-translated using Google Cloud Translation API, a professional translation tool. These translations were then reviewed in detail by a physician who is a native Turkish speaker and an expert in radiology. The specialist physician, whom we thank in the acknowledgments section of the manuscript, evaluated the medical accuracy of each sentence, corrected any possible meaning shifts, and ensured compliance with Turkish medical reporting terminology. Furthermore, common translation errors identified throughout the process (e.g., ambiguous medical terms, incorrect anatomical expressions) were standardized through a standardized editing process, and the reports were finalized. Thanks to this expert-supported hybrid method, the data generated through translation was structured in accordance with Turkish medical report writing standards, and the reliability of the dataset was ensured.

2.2. *Swin Transformer*

The Swin Transformer architecture, which is effectively used in the field of image processing, was developed by the Microsoft research team [21]. It uses a transformer-based feature extraction mechanism as opposed to convolution operations in traditional CNN-based architectures. The most important point where it differs from other popular transformer-based architectures such as Vision transformer is its shifted window mechanism. In the training phase, the images are processed in progressively smaller claws and features are extracted. One of the most important problems in the analysis of medical images, the problem of identifying fine details while at the same time not losing sight of the overall structure, can be solved thanks to the progressively shrinking window sizes [22]. Swin Transformer architecture was preferred in the encoder part of our encoder–decoder architecture because of its ability to efficiently capture local and global features while reducing computational complexity with the shifted window mechanism in the analysis of medical images.

In the Swin Transformer architecture, the input image is first divided into small non-overlapping patches and transformed into embedding vectors by passing them through a linear layer [23]. These patches are then processed by multiple Swin Transformer layers with hierarchically increasing receptive fields. Each Swin Transformer block contains local window-based self-attention and window shifting operations [24]. After the window shifting step, the architecture continues with a hierarchical fusion step. In the last stage, the obtained features are transmitted to the output layer. This structure contributes to increase the clinical accuracy of reports by better capturing long-range dependencies compared to CNN-based approaches. Figure 3 shows a representative block diagram of the encoder part of the encoder–decoder architecture developed for the Swin Transformer architecture to be used in the Turkish medical reporting task.

2.3. Generative Pre-Training Transformer

Generative pre-training transformer (GPT) is an auto-regressive language model developed by OpenAI [25]. The GPT architecture is transformer-based and powered by multilayer attention mechanisms that can easily capture long-range dependencies [26]. The model, which uses a deep neural network structure with a large number of parameters, works with the working logic of predicting the next word correctly based on previous words. Thanks to the advantage of using masked self-attention in the GPT model, each token can only access the tokens before it, preventing information generated during text generation from leaking and corrupting the trained model. The architecture also has the advantage of a multi-head attention mechanism, which allows the learning of language features to proceed in parallel in a multi-head structure, while preserving the sequential structure of the words.

GPT has been successfully used in many deep learning-based natural language processing applications such as text summarization, text generation, and question–answer systems. GPT is trained using large-scale web text sources such as English language books, articles, and web pages, but since GPT architecture is language-agnostic, it can be used in other languages such as Turkish by fine-tuning. In this study, the Swin Transformer encoder and the cosmosGPT model fine-tuned with the Turkish language are used for Turkish medical report generation; cosmosGPT is a GPT model that has been trained and fine-tuned specifically on Turkish texts [27]. Although this model is quite small compared to other large language models, it gives very successful results in Turkish text generation. Various Turkish sources were used to train the model, and care was taken to minimize possible biases. The use of this cosmosGPT model in our study contributed to both computationally efficient and clinically useful results. The features from the image encoder and the language generation capability of cosmosGPT are combined with the hybrid encoder–decoder architecture developed in our study.

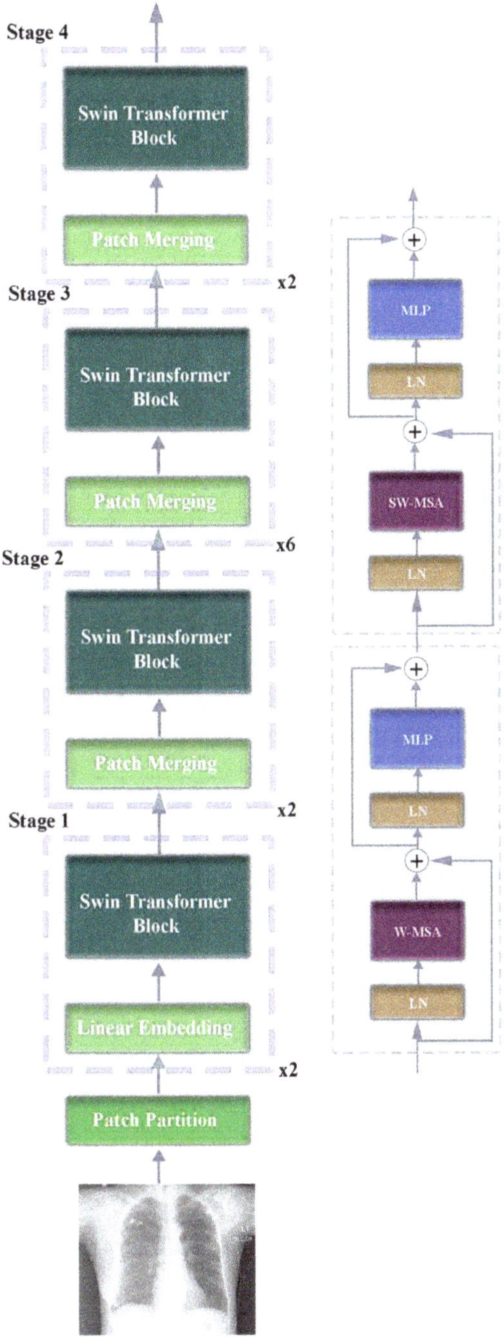

Figure 3. Block diagram of the encoder section of the developed hybrid encoder–decoder model using Swin Transformer architecture.

3. Results and Discussion

In this paper, a hybrid encoder–decoder model is developed to generate Turkish medical reports from chest X-ray images. The encoder part of the proposed model is designed based on Swin Transformer, while the decoder part is based on a fine-tuned Turkish GPT (cosmosGPT) architecture. Our work aims to provide autonomous reporting of diseases that can be detected using chest X-ray images in the Turkish language. Within the scope of our study, a large and comprehensive dataset was obtained by combining medical image–report pairs of patients from Elazığ Fethi Sekin City Hospital located in the Eastern Anatolia region of Turkey and image–report pairs in the Indiana University Chest X-Ray dataset, which is frequently used in the literature. The dataset, which was collected within the scope of the study and planned to be published as open access, was verified by obtaining ethics committee permissions and passing through the controls of the specialist physicians in the field within our research team.

Google Colab Pro+, a paid version that offers high GPU support, was preferred in the training, verification, and testing processes carried out within the scope of the study. NVIDIA A100 GPU and 52 GB RAM were used in all experiments. Equipment such as GPU and RAM were used through a paid membership via a virtual development environment and were not physically sourced. As a result of hyperparameter optimization during model training, the best performance was obtained with batch size 8, learning rate 5×10^{-5}, optimizer AdamW, weight decay 0.01, and epoch 5. Table 1 shows the optimal hyperparameters used in the proposed architecture.

Table 1. Hyperparameter configuration for Model-SEY.

Hyperparameter	Configuration
Learning rate (LR)	5×10^{-5}
Optimizer	AdamW
Weight decay	0.01
Number of epochs	5
Activation function	GELU
Batch size	8

One of the important indicators of model performance is training and validation loss graphs. By examining training and validation loss graphs, the epoch-based performance of models developed in deep learning architectures can be analyzed. Figure 4 shows the training and validation loss graphs of the Model-SEY architecture developed in our study. The model's training time took approximately 3 h and 46 min in the experimental environment created with an NVIDIA A100 GPU and 52 GB RAM.

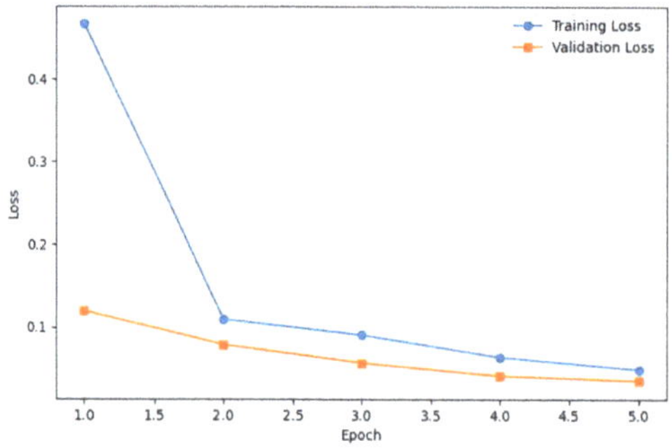

Figure 4. Model-SEY architecture training loss and validation loss graphs.

In order to demonstrate the performance of the model developed within the scope of the study with measurable values, word overlap evaluation metrics widely used in the field of natural language processing were utilized. The BLEU metrics used in this context reveal the similarity of the sentences produced by the model with the reference texts at the n-gram level [28]. BLEU-1 uses n-gram weights (1, 0, 0, 0, 0), considering only single words [29]. The BLEU-2 evaluation metric focuses on the relationships between groups of binary words using (0.5, 0.5, 0, 0) n-gram weights. The BLEU-3 metric is based on (0.33, 0.33, 0.33, 0.33, 0) n-gram weights, while BLEU-4 evaluates all four levels equally and uses (0.25, 0.25, 0.25, 0.25, 0.25) weights. The use of BLEU word overlap evaluation metrics allows us to measure the linguistic accuracy of the developed models at the word level and in word groups. The ROUGE metric, with its recall-based approach, measures the level of overlap between autonomous medical report texts and texts written by doctors with word groups [19]. These metrics can be analyzed by researchers to obtain comprehensive and measurable information about the accuracy and adequacy of the model outputs. Table 2 shows the Turkish medical reporting performance of the hybrid encoder–decoder architecture developed within the scope of this study with word overlap evaluation metrics.

Table 2. Word overlap evaluation metric results of Turkish medical generation hybrid encoder–decoder architecture.

Word Overlap Evaluation Metric	Value	Value (%)
BLEU-1	0.6412	64.12
BLEU-2	0.5335	53.35
BLEU-3	0.4395	43.95
BLEU-4	0.3716	37.16
ROUGE	0.2240	22.40

Upon analysis of the collected results, it is seen that the developed model performs very well in Turkish medical text generation. The high BLEU-1 score of 0.6412 clearly shows that the model is able to use correct and appropriate words. Although BLEU scores tend to decrease as n increases, the BLEU-4 value of 0.3716 shows that the model can produce meaningful outputs even with longer word sequences. The ROUGE score of 0.2240, which is a high value, shows that the model produces outputs that are compatible with the reference texts both at the lexical level and in terms of sentence structure and semantic context. The measurable results obtained show that this model, developed in a field with limited language resources such as Turkish, can make significant contributions to both clinical decision support systems and automatic report generation.

The results obtained with the Model-SEY architecture are the first study in this field in the Turkish language. In order to demonstrate the efficiency of the model with measurable parameters, it was compared with other studies in English found in the literature. Table 3 shares a comparison of the proposed Model-SEY architecture with its major competitors in the field of medical report generation. Table 3 also allows for a comparison of the approaches used in the encoder and decoder sections of the existing models in the literature and the proposed model.

The Model-SEY architecture is optimized for Turkish language report generation by using Swin Transformer on the encoder side and cosmosGPT on the decoder side. When evaluated in terms of BLEU and ROUGE scores, our proposed Model-SEY architecture is particularly effective in BLEU-3 (0.4395) and BLEU-4 (0.3716) scores. It also performs at similar or higher levels than its strong competitors in the literature in terms of BLEU-1 and BLEU-2 scores. However, the relatively low ROUGE score can be attributed to the uniqueness of the Turkish language structure and the differences in preprocessing rules.

In addition, our model stands out not only in terms of success metrics but also in terms of architectural innovation. The Swin Transformer-based encoder structure provides more localized attention regions in the image space. The cosmosGPT-based decoder has the capacity to produce more fluent and contextually consistent sentences. The combined use of these components has increased the model's ability to produce long and detailed Turkish reports.

Table 3. Comparison of architectural details and reporting achievements of previous projects with our Model-SEY architecture.

Method	Year	Target Language	Encoder	Decoder	BLEU-1	BLEU-2	BLEU-3	BLEU-4	ROUGE
CNN-RNN [30]	2015	English	CNN	RNN	0.316	0.211	0.140	0.095	0.267
VSGRU [16]	2021	English	DenseNet	GRU	0.347	0.221	0.156	0.116	0.251
CDGPT2 [16]	2021	English	DenseNet	GPT	0.387	0.245	0.166	0.111	0.289
TieNet [14]	2018	English	CNN	LSTM	0.286	0.159	0.103	0.073	0.226
Gamma Enhancement [2]	2024	English	DenseNet	BERT	0.363	0.371	0.388	0.412	-
Vi-Ba [17]	2024	English	Vision Transformer	BART	-	-	-	0.150	0.274
CNN/RNN and Greedy Search [1]	2023	English	CNN	RNN	0.592	0.422	0.298	0.205	-
G-CNX [10]	2025	English	ConvNeXt	GRU	0.6544	0.5035	0.3682	0.2766	0.4277
(Our) Model-SEY	2025	Turkish	Swin Transformer	CosmosGPT	0.6412	0.5335	0.4395	0.3716	0.2240

The first models in the table use CNN-RNN and TieNet CNN-based encoders and classic sequential processors such as RNN or LSTM. These models show limited success in report generation with low BLEU-3 and BLEU-4 scores. This can be explained by the weakness of classic RNN-based decoders in generating long and context-sensitive medical sentences. Architectures such as VSGRU, CDGPT2, Gamma Enhancement, Vi-Ba, and CNN/RNN with Greedy Search have improved feature extraction success from images with more powerful encoder (DenseNet, Vision Transformer) and transformer-based decoder (GPT, BERT, BART) structures. In particular, the Gamma Enhancement model shows remarkable performance, reaching a BLEU-4 score of 0.412. However, ROUGE scores have either not been reported or have been limited in most models. This indicates that production at the meaning level has not been sufficiently measured, rather than word overlap. Current models such as G-CNX achieve powerful results using a ConvNeXt encoder and a GRU decoder with deeper and more evolved architectural designs. However, the success of this model is specific to the English language, and its generalizability to languages with different structures, such as Turkish, is uncertain.

Model-SEY, on the other hand, proposes a structure optimized for Turkish report generation for the first time in this field, using the Swin Transformer architecture in the encoder part and the cosmosGPT large language model in the decoder part. High scores were obtained in all metrics from BLEU-1 to BLEU-4, with BLEU-2 and BLEU-3 scores being higher than many English models. This demonstrates the model's success in both extracting meaningful visual features from images and converting these features into Turkish natural language output.

In addition to the measurable parameters, the outputs were also checked by observational analysis of the expert doctors in our study team and it was confirmed that medical reports were generated with a success that could support doctors in decision making during the diagnosis phase. Figure 5 shows four randomly selected sample images, reports written by doctors, and medical reports generated by the proposed architecture.

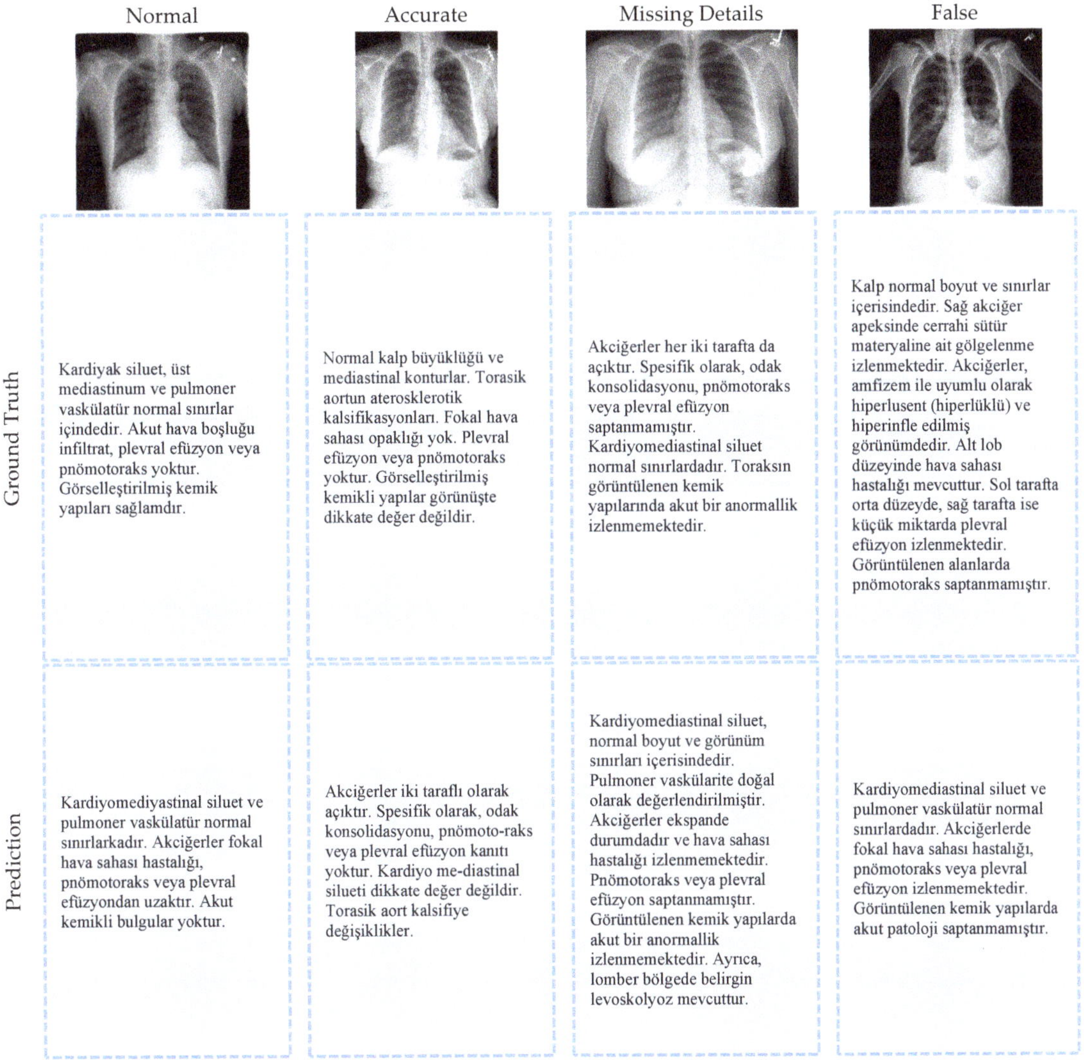

Figure 5. Sample medical reports generated by Model-SEY.

To assess the clinical accuracy of the model outputs, a qualitative analysis was conducted in addition to automatic evaluation metrics like BLEU and ROUGE, which are only based on textual similarity. In this sense, professional radiologists clinically assessed reports produced by Model-SEY for a chosen subset of chest X-rays. Based on the image's findings, each report was categorized into four groups: normal, accurate, missing details, and false. These groups were determined by whether or not the reports contained accurate and comprehensive information. These categories seek to assess the model outputs' clinical reliability, applicability, and linguistic sufficiency. Selected examples from this evaluation process are shown in Figure 5. The original chest X-ray, the reference report, the Model-SEY report, and the expert evaluation category are all included in each example. This analysis shows that the model can produce reliable and clinically appropriate reports in many situations, but it also shows that in certain instances, there may be limited detail deficiencies or incorrect interpretations. Therefore, beyond textual similarity scores, this expert validation offers a more thorough and clinically focused evaluation of model performance.

The clinical impact of this study is to reduce the time and workload of specialized physicians when interpreting chest X-ray images. It will also provide decision-making support in the diagnostic phase, preventing the underdiagnosis or misdiagnosis of diseases. In addition, the proposed architecture accelerates the diagnostic process in regions where healthcare personnel are limited and will contribute to the prevention of possible human errors. In future work, the aim is to integrate this architecture not only into chest X-rays but also into other types of medical imaging such as brain MRI, CT, and mammography. It will also shed light on future work in the field of Turkish medical image captioning and autonomous medical report generation.

4. Conclusions

This study proposes a deep learning architecture framework that produces autonomous reports in Turkish by training image–report pairs. The encoder—decoder-based architecture, named Model-SEY, was developed within the scope of this study. The Swin Transformer architecture was used in the encoder section, while the cosmosGPT architecture, a Turkish architecture, was used in the decoder section. As a result of the training and testing process, a BLEU-1 word overlap evaluation metric score of 0.6412 was obtained. The experimental results show that the proposed model can support doctors in their decision-making processes in the diagnosis and reporting of diseases.

The first limitation of the study is that the model was trained and tested using only transformer-based deep learning architectures. The success of report generation in traditional CNN-based architectures is unknown. In addition, the system was run in a laboratory environment using image–report pairs obtained from hospitals in advance. There is limited information on real-time training and testing processes. Future studies plan to conduct a new study on the detection and reporting of tumorous regions in brain MRI images.

Author Contributions: Conceptualization, M.U. and B.K.; methodology, B.K.; software, M.U.; validation, B.K., M.U. and M.K.; formal analysis, M.U.; investigation, B.K.; resources, M.K.; data curation, B.K.; writing—original draft preparation, M.U.; writing—review and editing, M.K.; visualization, B.K.; supervision, M.K.; project administration, M.K. All authors have read and agreed to the published version of the manuscript.

Funding: This research was supported in part by the Scientific and Technological Research Council of Turkey (TUBITAK) under grant no. 123E171 and in part by the Firat University Scientific Research Projects Unit (FUBAP) under grant MF.24.123.

Institutional Review Board Statement: The study was conducted in accordance with the Declaration of Helsinki, and approved by the Non-Interventional Research Ethics Committee of FIRAT UNIVERSITY (protocol code 17468 and date of approval (27 July 2023)).

Informed Consent Statement: Not applicable.

Data Availability Statement: The data presented in this study are available on request from the corresponding author, due to the fact that this is a new area of research and a very current topic.

Acknowledgments: The authors would like to express their sincere gratitude to Mehtap Çiçekçi for her valuable support in the preparation and validation of the dataset used in this study.

Conflicts of Interest: The authors declare no conflicts of interest.

References

1. Navuduri, A.; Kulkarni, S. Generation of Medical Reports from Chest X-Ray Images Using Multi Modal Learning Approach. *Ind. J. Sci. Technol.* **2023**, *16*, 2703–2708. [CrossRef]
2. Tsaniya, H.; Fatichah, C.; Suciati, N. Automatic Radiology Report Generator Using Transformer With Contrast-Based Image Enhancement. *IEEE Access* **2024**, *12*, 25429–25442. [CrossRef]
3. Ucan, S.; Ucan, M.; Kaya, M. Deep Learning Based Approach with EfficientNet and SE Block Attention Mechanism for Multiclass Alzheimer's Disease Detection. In Proceedings of the 2023 4th International Conference on Data Analytics for Business and Industry (ICDABI), Online, 25–26 October 2023; IEEE: Piscataway, NJ, USA, 2023; pp. 285–289.
4. Sahin, M.E.; Ulutas, H.; Yuce, E.; Erkoc, M.F. Detection and Classification of COVID-19 by Using Faster R-CNN and Mask R-CNN on CT Images. *Neural Comput. Appl.* **2023**, *35*, 13597–13611. [CrossRef] [PubMed]
5. Jiang, H.; Diao, Z.; Shi, T.; Zhou, Y.; Wang, F.; Hu, W.; Zhu, X.; Luo, S.; Tong, G.; Yao, Y.-D. A Review of Deep Learning-Based Multiple-Lesion Recognition from Medical Images: Classification, Detection and Segmentation. *Comput. Biol. Med.* **2023**, *157*, 106726. [CrossRef] [PubMed]
6. Ulutas, H.; Sahin, M.E.; Karakus, M.O. Application of a Novel Deep Learning Technique Using CT Images for COVID-19 Diagnosis on Embedded Systems. *Alex. Eng. J.* **2023**, *74*, 345–358. [CrossRef]
7. Dovganich, A.A.; Khvostikov, A.V.; Pchelintsev, Y.A.; Krylov, A.A.; Ding, Y.; Farias, M.C.Q. Automatic Out-of-Distribution Detection Methods for Improving the Deep Learning Classification of Pulmonary X-Ray Images. *J. Image Graph.* **2022**, *10*, 56–63. [CrossRef]
8. Uysal, E. Statistical Performance Evaluation of the Deep Learning Architectures Over Body Fluid Cytology Images. *IEEE Access* **2025**, *13*, 82540–82553. [CrossRef]
9. Ataş, İ. Comparison of Deep Convolution and Least Squares GANs for Diabetic Retinopathy Image Synthesis. *Neural Comput. Appl.* **2023**, *35*, 14431–14448. [CrossRef]
10. Ucan, M.; Kaya, B.; Kaya, M. Generating Medical Reports With a Novel Deep Learning Architecture. *Int. J. Imaging Syst. Technol.* **2025**, *35*, e70062. [CrossRef]
11. Ahmed, S.B.; Solis-Oba, R.; Ilie, L. Explainable-AI in Automated Medical Report Generation Using Chest X-Ray Images. *Appl. Sci.* **2022**, *12*, 11750. [CrossRef]
12. Shaikh, Z.; Bharti, J. Transformer-Based Chest X-Ray Report Generation Model. In *International Conference on Soft Computing and Signal Processing*; Springer: Singapore, 2024; pp. 227–236.
13. Lin, Z.; Zhang, D.; Shi, D.; Xu, R.; Tao, Q.; Wu, L.; He, M.; Ge, Z. Contrastive Pre-Training and Linear Interaction Attention-Based Transformer for Universal Medical Reports Generation. *J. Biomed. Inf.* **2023**, *138*, 104281. [CrossRef] [PubMed]
14. Wang, X.; Peng, Y.; Lu, L.; Lu, Z.; Summers, R.M. TieNet: Text-Image Embedding Network for Common Thorax Disease Classification and Reporting in Chest X-Rays. *arXiv* **2018**, arXiv:1801.04334. [CrossRef]
15. Liu, G.; Hsu, T.-M.H.; McDermott, M.; Boag, W.; Weng, W.-H.; Szolovits, P.; Ghassemi, M. Clinically Accurate Chest X-Ray Report Generation. In Proceedings of the 4th Machine Learning for Healthcare Conference, Ann Arbor, MI, USA, 9–10 August 2019; Doshi-Velez, F., Fackler, J., Jung, K., Kale, D., Ranganath, R., Wallace, B., Wiens, J., Eds.; PMLR. MLR Press: Philadelphia, PA, USA, 2019; Volume 106, pp. 249–269.
16. Alfarghaly, O.; Khaled, R.; Elkorany, A.; Helal, M.; Fahmy, A. Automated Radiology Report Generation Using Conditioned Transformers. *Inf. Med. Unlocked* **2021**, *24*, 100557. [CrossRef]
17. Ucan, M.; Kaya, B.; Kaya, M.; Alhajj, R. Medical Report Generation from Medical Images Using Vision Transformer and Bart Deep Learning Architectures. In *International Conference on Advances in Social Networks Analysis and Mining*; Springer: Cham, Switzerland, 2025; pp. 257–267.
18. Unal, M.E.; Citamak, B.; Yagcioglu, S.; Erdem, A.; Erdem, E.; Cinbis, N.I.; Cakici, R. TasvirEt: A Benchmark Dataset for Automatic Turkish Description Generation from Images. In Proceedings of the 2016 24th Signal Processing and Communication Application Conference (SIU), Zonguldak, Turkey, 16–19 May 2016; pp. 1977–1980.
19. Yildiz, S.; Memiş, A.; Varli, S. TRCaptionNet: A Novel and Accurate Deep Turkish Image Captioning Model with Vision Transformer Based Image Encoders and Deep Linguistic Text Decoders. *Turk. J. Electr. Eng. Comput. Sci.* **2023**, *31*, 1079–1098. [CrossRef]
20. Demner-Fushman, D.; Kohli, M.D.; Rosenman, M.B.; Shooshan, S.E.; Rodriguez, L.; Antani, S.; Thoma, G.R.; McDonald, C.J. Preparing a Collection of Radiology Examinations for Distribution and Retrieval. *J. Am. Med. Inform. Assoc.* **2016**, *23*, 304–310. [CrossRef] [PubMed]
21. Liu, Z.; Lin, Y.; Cao, Y.; Hu, H.; Wei, Y.; Zhang, Z.; Lin, S.; Guo, B. Swin Transformer: Hierarchical Vision Transformer Using Shifted Windows. In Proceedings of the IEEE/CVF International Conference on Computer Vision, Montreal, BC, Canada, 10–17 October 2021; pp. 10012–10022.
22. Üzen, H.; Firat, H.; Atila, O.; Şengür, A. Swin Transformer-Based Fork Architecture for Automated Breast Tumor Classification. *Expert Syst. Appl.* **2024**, *256*, 125009. [CrossRef]

23. Vuran, S.; Ucan, M.; Akin, M.; Kaya, M. Multi-Classification of Skin Lesion Images Including Mpox Disease Using Transformer-Based Deep Learning Architectures. *Diagnostics* **2025**, *15*, 374. [CrossRef] [PubMed]
24. Ferdous, G.J.; Sathi, K.A.; Hossain, M.A.; Dewan, M.A.A. SPT-Swin: A Shifted Patch Tokenization Swin Transformer for Image Classification. *IEEE Access* **2024**, *12*, 117617–117626. [CrossRef]
25. Radford, A.; Wu, J.; Child, R.; Luan, D.; Amodei, D.; Sutskever, I. Language Models Are Unsupervised Multitask Learners. *OpenAI Blog* **2019**, *1*, 8.
26. Radford, A.; Narasimhan, K.; Salimans, T.; Sutskever, I. Improving Language Understanding by Generative Pre-Training. *OpenAI Blog* **2018**. Available online: https://www.mikecaptain.com/resources/pdf/GPT-1.pdf (accessed on 14 July 2025).
27. Kesgin, H.T.; Yuce, M.K.; Dogan, E.; Uzun, M.E.; Uz, A.; Seyrek, H.E.; Zeer, A.; Amasyali, M.F. Introducing CosmosGPT: Monolingual Training for Turkish Language Models. In Proceedings of the 2024 International Conference on INnovations in Intelligent SysTems and Applications (INISTA), Craiova, Romania, 4–6 September 2024; pp. 1–6.
28. Papineni, K.; Roukos, S.; Ward, T.; Zhu, W.-J. Bleu: A Method for Automatic Evaluation of Machine Translation. In Proceedings of the 40th Annual Meeting of the Association for Computational Linguistics, Philadelphia, PA, USA, 6–12 July 2002; pp. 311–318.
29. Nicolson, A.; Dowling, J.; Koopman, B. Improving Chest X-Ray Report Generation by Leveraging Warm Starting. *Artif. Intell. Med.* **2023**, *144*, 102633. [CrossRef] [PubMed]
30. Vinyals, O.; Toshev, A.; Bengio, S.; Erhan, D. Show and Tell: A Neural Image Caption Generator. In Proceedings of the IEEE Conference on Computer Vision and Pattern Recognition, Boston, MA, USA, 7–12 June 2015; pp. 3156–3164.

diagnostics

MDPI

Article

A Hybrid Artificial Intelligence Approach for Down Syndrome Risk Prediction in First Trimester Screening

Emre Yalçın [1], Serpil Aslan [2,*], Mesut Toğaçar [3] and Süleyman Cansun Demir [1]

1 Department of Obstetrics and Gynecology, Division of Perinatology, Cukurova University School of Medicine, 01330 Adana, Turkey; dremreyalcin23@gmail.com (E.Y.); cansundemir@gmail.com (S.C.D.)

2 Department of Computer Engineering, Faculty of Engineering and Natural Sciences, Malatya Turgut Ozal University, 44210 Malatya, Turkey

3 Department of Management Information Systems, Faculty of Economics and Administrative Sciences, Fırat University, 23119 Elazig, Turkey; mtogacar@firat.edu.tr

* Correspondence: serpil.aslan@ozal.edu.tr

Abstract: Background/Objectives: The aim of this study is to develop a hybrid artificial intelligence (AI) approach to improve the accuracy, efficiency, and reliability of Down Syndrome (DS) risk prediction during first trimester prenatal screening. The proposed method transforms one-dimensional (1D) patient data—including features such as nuchal translucency (NT), human chorionic gonadotropin (hCG), and pregnancy-associated plasma protein A (PAPP-A)—into two-dimensional (2D) Aztec barcode images, enabling advanced feature extraction using transformer-based deep learning models. **Methods**: The dataset consists of 958 anonymous patient records. Each record includes four first trimester screening markers, hCG, PAPP-A, and NT, expressed as multiples of the median. The DS risk outcome was categorized into three classes: high, medium, and low. Three transformer architectures—DeiT3, MaxViT, and Swin—are employed to extract high-level features from the generated barcodes. The extracted features are combined into a unified set, and dimensionality reduction is performed using two feature selection techniques: minimum Redundancy Maximum Relevance (mRMR) and ReliefF. Intersecting features from both selectors are retained to form a compact and informative feature subset. The final features are classified using machine learning algorithms, including Bagged Trees and Naive Bayes. **Results**: The proposed approach achieved up to 100% classification accuracy using the Naive Bayes classifier with 1250 features selected by ReliefF and 527 intersecting features from mRMR. By selecting a smaller but more informative subset of features, the system significantly reduced hardware and processing demands while maintaining strong predictive performance. **Conclusions**: The results suggest that the proposed hybrid AI method offers a promising and resource-efficient solution for DS risk assessment in first trimester screening. However, further comparative studies are recommended to validate its performance in broader clinical contexts.

Keywords: Down syndrome; first trimester prenatal screening; artificial intelligence; risk assessment; feature extraction

1. Introduction

Down Syndrome (DS) is the most common chromosomal abnormality observed at birth, with an incidence rate of about 1 in 1000. This rate increases with maternal age. DS is primarily caused by the presence of an extra copy or partial duplication of the long arm of chromosome 21. This chromosomal abnormality typically occurs due to nondisjunction during meiosis II; however, translocation and mosaicism are also responsible for a smaller number of cases. Clinically, DS is characterized by distinctive facial features, congenital heart defects, and varying degrees of cognitive impairment. These characteristics are largely associated with the q21.1, q22.2, and q22.3 regions of chromosome 21 [1].

A key objective of prenatal care is the early detection of fetal anomalies to enable timely medical intervention during pregnancy or shortly after birth. Although parents have the right to know their unborn child's health status, this right is limited by the available diagnostic technologies and current medical knowledge [2,3]. Because many congenital conditions can only be diagnosed once structural or functional abnormalities reach detectable thresholds, the development of accurate, early screening tools is essential.

Genetic disorders such as DS carry significant social, psychological, and economic burdens. While these conditions are not curable, early detection enables better preparation, counseling, and medical planning. In this context, non-invasive screening methods have become more important. One such method is the first trimester combined screening test, which uses maternal serum markers—free β-human chorionic gonadotropin (β-hCG) and pregnancy-associated plasma protein A (PAPP-A)—along with an ultrasonographic measurement of nuchal translucency (NT). Performed between the 11th and 14th weeks of gestation, this test offers detection rates of up to 90% for DS and other chromosomal anomalies, such as trisomy 13, trisomy 18, and Turner syndrome [4–7].

In pregnancies affected by DS, PAPP-A levels are typically lower and β-hCG levels are higher than expected. These markers are interpreted using "multiple of the median" (MoM) values, which normalize for gestational age [8,9]. Additional risk indicators include NT thickness greater than 2.5 mm, pregnancy-associated plasma protein A (PAPP-A) less than 0.4 MoM, beta-human chorionic gonadotropin (β-hCG) greater than 2.5 MoM, and absence of the nasal bone. Further diagnostic evaluation, such as fetal echocardiography and cell-free DNA (cfDNA) testing, is recommended when NT measurements are $\geq$3 mm or above the 99th percentile [10]. Based on these parameters, risk levels are categorized as high (>1/250), moderate (1/250–1/1000), or low (<1/1000) [11]. Although screening provides valuable risk estimates, a definitive diagnosis still requires invasive procedures, such as chorionic villus sampling (CVS), amniocentesis (AS), or cordocentesis (CS). These methods carry risks, including miscarriage, infection, and membrane rupture. Consequently, many patients hesitate to undergo invasive testing unless it is absolutely necessary. Furthermore, concerns over malpractice may cause healthcare providers to recommend these procedures based solely on screening results, even when ultrasonography reveals no abnormalities. This underscores the need for more reliable, non-invasive tools.

Recent advancements in artificial intelligence (AI) have opened new possibilities in prenatal diagnostics [12]. In countries like China, hundreds of laboratories now apply AI-based statistical models—often combined with ultrasound data—to assess DS risk during the first trimester [13–15]. Machine learning (ML) algorithms are increasingly being used to interpret large-scale screening data and provide individualized risk predictions. Several studies have demonstrated the potential of AI in DS risk estimation. These include approaches based on support vector machines (SVMs), Bayesian classifiers, neural networks, and ensemble learning techniques applied to maternal serum markers and fetal ultrasound measurements [16–22]. Despite these developments, there is still a need for integrated, high-performance models that combine advanced machine learning techniques with clinical screening protocols.

1.1. Related Work

The following are findings from studies similar to the subject of this article: Nguyen-Hoang et al. [23] investigated the ability of AI and ML algorithms to predict pre-eclampsia risk in the first three months of pregnancy in a large pregnancy cohort in Asia. The study found that the AI + ML model developed after calibrating biochemical analysis devices demonstrated higher accuracy in detecting pre-eclampsia compared to the fetal medicine foundation risk prediction model. Verma et al. [24] developed an algorithm called adaptive stochastic gradient descent (ASGIA) to detect structural abnormalities in fetuses and identify potential risks. According to the study's findings, fetal developmental abnormalities could be classified with high accuracy using second-trimester ultrasound scans supported by advanced technology. The results achieved a remarkable success rate of 98.64%. Alonso et al. [25] developed a new screening method to identify women at risk for DS during the first three months of pregnancy. To this end, they trained different ML techniques using a dataset consisting of 90,532 individuals, with less than 1% having a positive case. The models analyzed demographic factors, such as the mother's age, weight, and ethnic origin; and biochemical parameters, such as nuchal translucency, PAPP-A, and B-HCG levels. The results showed that the ROC-AUC values ranged from 0.970 to 0.982, with sensitivity and specificity rates reaching 94%. Chen et al. [26] evaluated multiple ML algorithms to predict the risk of DS in the first trimester of pregnancy among women of East Asian origin. The study utilized a dataset comprising a total of 14 variables, including maternal age, nuchal translucency thickness, and various serum biomarkers. Among the 12 different algorithms applied, the highest sensitivity rate (84%) was achieved with LightGBM, while the highest AUC score (0.939) was obtained using an artificial neural network (ANN) and a long short-term memory (LSTM)-based model.

1.2. Research Question and Contributions

This study seeks to answer the following question: Does converting one-dimensional (1D) patient data into two-dimensional (2D) barcode images and applying transformer-based feature extraction improve the accuracy of DS risk assessment systems? This study introduces a novel, hybrid AI framework designed to improve the prediction of DS risk levels during the first trimester of prenatal screening. The key contributions of this research are summarized below:

- We convert 1D prenatal screening data into 2D Aztec barcode images to improve feature extraction using transformer models.
- We combine multiple transformer architectures (DeiT3, MaxViT, and Swin) to enrich feature representation.
- A dual feature selection process (mRMR and RelieF) reduces dimensionality while maintaining accuracy.
- Provides a practical AI-based tool for reliable and efficient DS risk prediction in the first trimester.

The remainder of this article is organized as follows: Section 2 describes the approaches used in the material and proposed model. Section 3 presents the experimental analysis and results. Section 4 discusses the findings and limitations. Finally, Section 5 summarizes the study's conclusion and outlines future work.

2. Materials and Methods

2.1. Dataset

In order to be used in this study, data from the combined double-screening test applied to 958 women who had a singleton pregnancy in the first trimester between 2020 and 2024 at the Gynecology and Obstetrics Unit of Çukurova University (Adana, Turkey) were collected. The research ethics committee of Çukurova University Faculty of Medicine approved the purpose of the study and the data collection process. Patient records and data were collected from the hospital's gynecology and obstetrics clinic and biochemistry laboratories. Since the patient data were anonymized, no patient identification information was used. DS (Trisomy 21) was diagnosed in 18 of the 958 unique pregnancies included in the study dataset. In addition, four cases with other chromosomal abnormalities, such as Trisomy 18 and Trisomy 13, were identified. The remaining 936 pregnancies, which were considered chromosomally normal, were evaluated as the control group.

The features in the dataset used in the study are given in Table 1. Four features, whose descriptions and data types are given in Table 1, were used as markers that could help infer the risk of DS: "hCH-MoM", "PAPP-A MoM", "NT", and "NT MoM". The "Down Risk" indicator was used to estimate the categorical data. Prenatal screening reports use the features' standard deviations or medians to determine the DS risk [27].

Table 1. The attributes explanation of the collected dataset.

Name	Explanation	Data Type	Range (Min–Max)	Mean	Std Dev
hCG-MoM	Human Chorionic Gonadotropin (hCG), Method of Medians (MoM). hCG is a hormone secreted by the placenta during pregnancy and is found in high levels in the early stages. The MoM value is obtained by dividing the measured value by the average value during the gestational week.	Numeric	0.35–4.81	1.64	0.74
PAPP-AMoM	Pregnancy-Associated Plasma Protein A (PAPP-A). PAPP-A, known as pregnancy-associated plasma protein A, is produced by the placenta during pregnancy.	Numeric	0.18–127	1.20	5.78
NT	Nuchal Translucency (NT). This is the measurement of the nuchal translucency of the fetus by ultrasound.	Numeric	0.45–4.50	1.48	0.52
NT MoM	It is obtained by dividing NT by the mean value during gestational weeks.	Numeric	0.12–4	0.99	0.49
Down Risk	DS is a risk classification. Below 1:250 is considered high risk (High), between 1:250 and 1:1000 is considered medium risk (Medium), and above 1:1000 is considered low risk (Low).	Categorical			

Figure 1 represents the class distributions of the DOWN target variable in the dataset used. After applying the clinically accepted risk thresholds (high: <1:250; medium: 1:250–1:1000; low: >1:1000), the dataset was categorized into three risk groups. Among the 958 records, 196 (~20.5%) were labeled as high risk, 220 (~23%) as medium risk, and 542 (~56.5%) as low risk, as shown in Figure 1.

The sample size used in the study was determined by considering the effect sizes observed in previous, similar studies, as well as statistical power analyses. The primary endpoint is an evaluation of how accurately the model predicts DS risk.

According to standard first trimester prenatal screening (FTS) protocols, DS risk is classified as high, moderate, or low. Those classified as high risk (below the 1:250 threshold) were referred for invasive diagnostic methods, such as amniocentesis or CVS, in accordance with the relevant clinical guidelines. Where such invasive tests were performed, the diagnosis was confirmed through fetal karyotyping. Additionally, postnatal karyotype analysis has been utilized in appropriate cases to enhance diagnostic accuracy. In this context, the classification labels in the dataset are based not only on screening findings, but also on confirmatory clinical diagnoses, particularly in the high-risk group. In particular, the ground truth labels used to train the model for high-risk cases were validated using confirmatory diagnostic procedures, such as amniocentesis or postnatal karyotyping, to ensure clinical validity.

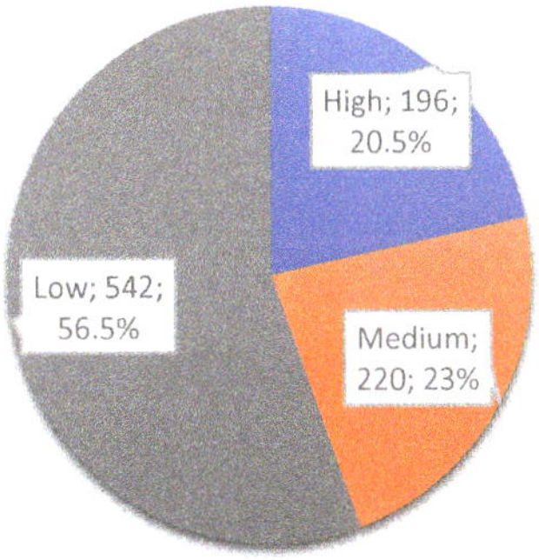

Figure 1. Distribution of Down Risk attribute of dataset.

2.2. Barcode Recognition and 2D Data Generation with Aztec Technique

Barcode scanning refers to the technology of automatically reading data encoded through lines and shapes of varying thicknesses using optical scanning methods [28]. Traditional linear barcodes are categorized as one-dimensional (1D), while advanced formats, such as QR codes, are considered two-dimensional (2D). QR codes, including types such as QR, Data Matrix, and Aztec, have a higher data storage capacity because they encode information both horizontally and vertically. The Aztec code was used in this study. This technique uses a matrix barcode structure organized around a central finder pattern to generate 2D data. This spiral layout allows for more compact encoding of data without requiring a blank margin, making it more efficient than other 2D formats. Aztec codes also use the Reed–Solomon error correction algorithm, which can recover damaged data. Because of these advantages, they are commonly used in fields where data integrity and compact storage are critical, such as healthcare, logistics, and transportation [29,30]. In this study, patient data in CSV format were converted into Aztec barcode images as part of the preprocessing step. The pseudo-code provided in Algorithm 1 outlines the basic algorithm used for this transformation. Each row of the dataset was encoded into a unique Aztec barcode and saved as an image file for subsequent analysis. Figure 2 illustrates an example of how line data were transformed into Aztec barcodes, while Figure 3 shows sample images categorized by DS risk levels: high, medium, and low.

Algorithm 1: Pseudo-code of the Aztec technique

```
function csv_to_aztec_barcode (csv_file): # Read CSV file
    data = read_csv(csv_file)
    aztec_barcodes = [] # Generate AZTEC barcodes
    for row in data:
        barcode = create_aztec(row) # Convert data to AZTEC barcode
        save_image(barcode) # Save 2D barcode
    end
```

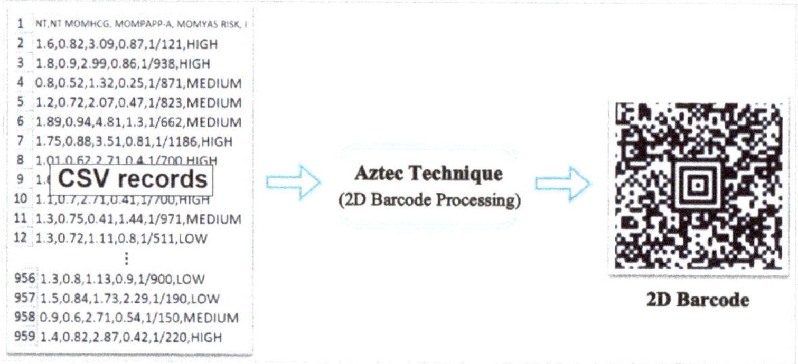

Figure 2. Application of the Aztec barcode technique to raw numerical data from the original dataset. The resulting 2D Aztec code visually encodes structured input features (e.g., hCG-MoM, PAPP-AMoM, NT MoM, etc.) into a fixed-size image representation. This transformation enables the use of vision-based transformers for classification tasks in prenatal DS risk assessment.

Figure 3. Sample Aztec-coded image set generated after pre-processing raw patient data. Each image corresponds to a different risk class used in the classification task: (**a**) high risk, (**b**) low risk, (**c**) medium risk. These visual representations are input to the vision-based transformer models for automated classification in the context of prenatal DS risk evaluation.

2.3. Transformer Models

The concept of Transformer was first developed in 2017 by researchers at the University of Toronto and Google and introduced in the paper "Attention is all you need" [31]. This study selected three different transformer-based models based on their complementary architectural structures and successful performance in visual classification tasks: Data-efficient Image Transformer v3 (DeiT3), Shifted Window Transformer (Swin), and Maximized Vision Transformer (MaxViT). DeiT3 was chosen because of its compact structure and effective performance in scenarios requiring limited data and computational power. This feature makes DeiT3 a suitable option for medical analysis tasks involving small datasets. The Swin transformer features a sliding window-based hierarchical architecture. This structure enables Swin transformer to effectively learn both local and global context, which is advantageous for medical barcode images that have variable structures but maintain a specific order. The MaxViT model combines convolutional layers and self-attention mechanisms within a grid-like structure to provide balanced representations of local details and global relationships. Using these three models together enables the extraction of versatile, rich features from data obtained by converting 1D clinical data into 2D Aztec barcode images. This integrative approach aims to enhance the system's classification accuracy and overall robustness by leveraging the strengths of each model.

2.3.1. DeiT3 Model

DeiT3, the third version of DeiT models, aims to achieve high performance with less data. It accurately classifies images in cases where data constraints exist. It is optimized for applications that require low data usage. Huge indicates that the model has a large parameter size. Patch14 means that the input image is divided into 14 × 14 patches, and 224 means that the model processes 224 × 224 images [32].

2.3.2. MaxViT Model

MaxViT is a model that combines the strengths of Vision Transformers and convolutional neural networks (CNNs). It uses multi-scale attention mechanisms and performs well in visual tasks such as image classification, object detection, and segmentation. The model's name indicates that it is a medium-sized model compatible with TensorFlow that processes images of size 224 × 224 [33].

2.3.3. Swin Model

Swin efficiently processes local and global image features using a sliding attention mechanism within local windows. The model can perform multi-scale image analysis and is used in many areas, including image classification, object detection, and segmentation. Sliding windows provide better visual consistency. In the model, "Base" represents a medium-sized model; "patch4" indicates that the image is divided into 4 × 4 patches; "window7" indicates that 7 × 7 sliding windows are used; and "224" indicates that the model processes 224 × 224 images [34].

2.4. Feature Selection Methods: mRMR and RelieF

Feature selection is creating a subset of a feature vector according to specific criteria. It plays a vital role in reducing the data to be processed and removing unnecessary features [35]. Successful feature selection increases the learning performance of deep neural networks, reduces the learning time, and provides easy learning results. In this study, mRMR [36] and ReliefF [37], which are supervised feature selection algorithms with high performance (Max-Relevance and Min-Redundancy), were used. Supervised feature selection algorithms are frequently used in classification problems. Its basic principle uses the relationship between features and labels. It aims to find the subset of the feature vector that achieves maximum classification performance for a given dataset.

The mRMR method selects features that are highly correlated with the target variable while minimizing redundancy among the selected features. This method typically evaluates the relationship between variables and the target using mutual information (MI). The basic mathematical expression of this approach is as follows:

$$\max_{f_i \in S}[D(f_i, C) - \frac{1}{|S|} \sum_{f_i \in S} R(f_i, f_j)] \tag{1}$$

The meanings of the parameters in Equation (1) are as follows: f_i is a candidate feature; C is the class label. $D(f_i, C)$ quantitatively expresses the information sharing between class labels f_i and C. $R(f_i, f_j)$ indicates the amount of common information between features f_i and f_j, and this value expresses the redundancy between them. S is defined as a subgroup consisting of previously determined characteristics. mRMR establishes a balance between maximum relationship and minimum repetition in order to select features that are highly informative but do not repeat each other. This ensures that the selected features are both meaningful and diverse [36].

RelieF is an example-based feature selection algorithm that evaluates the importance of each feature based on its ability to distinguish between similar examples from different classes. The algorithm determines the following two elements for each randomly selected example X: the closest neighbor example belonging to the same class, X_H (closest match), and the closest neighbor belonging to a different class, X_M (closest divergence).

$$W[f] = W[f] - \text{diff}(f, X, X_H)^2 + \text{diff}(f, X, X_M)^2 \quad (2)$$

This equation calculates the difference among the values of the f feature in the $\text{diff}(f, X_i, X_j)$, X_i, and X_j samples; this distance is usually measured using the absolute value or square difference method. Features that can distinguish more strongly between classes are given higher weights and are therefore evaluated more meaningfully [37].

The reasons for selecting the two methods in this study are as follows: mRMR was chosen because it is successful at identifying features that are highly correlated with the target variable and do not overlap. Relief was selected because it excels at capturing local feature interactions. Together, these methods provide an effective, complementary solution that maintains classification accuracy during dimension reduction.

2.5. Proposed Approach

FTS involves tests designed to evaluate the risk of fetal chromosomal abnormalities, such as DS. Although traditional methods estimate risk levels based on these results, they often overlook important factors. This study proposes a hybrid approach to overcome these limitations and provide accurate risk predictions using FTS data.

The proposed method integrates advanced artificial intelligence techniques and consists of five main stages: data preprocessing, transformer model training, feature extraction, feature fusion, feature selection, and classification.

In the preprocessing stage, 1D patient data stored in CSV format is transformed into 2D barcode images using the Aztec encoding technique. This transformation enables the use of 2D transformer models, which are more efficient at extracting features compared to their 1D counterparts. In the second stage, the Aztec-based images are trained using three transformer models: DeiT3, MaxViT, and Swin. These models were chosen for their relatively simple architecture and lower computational demands. In the third stage, feature sets are extracted from the final layers of each model: DeiT3 (1280 × number of images), MaxViT (768 × number of images), and Swin (1024 × number of images). The fourth stage involves merging feature sets from different models and evaluating their classification performance. Various combinations were tested (e.g., DeiT3 and Swin, DeiT3 and MaxViT, MaxViT and Swin, and all three combined). Machine learning algorithms, including Bagged Trees [38] and Naive Bayes [39], were used to assess the performance of each merged feature set. The combination of all three models (DeiT3, MaxViT, and Swin) yielded the best performance and was selected for further processing. In the final stage, feature selection techniques—mRMR and RelieF—were applied to reduce dimensionality while maintaining classification performance. Each method was tested with varying numbers of selected features (750, 1000, 1250). The most effective feature subsets from both selection methods were identified, and their intersection was used to train new models. This step aimed to enhance performance while reducing computational and hardware costs, ultimately improving the efficiency and practicality of the proposed system. The overall workflow of the proposed hybrid AI system is illustrated in Figure 4.

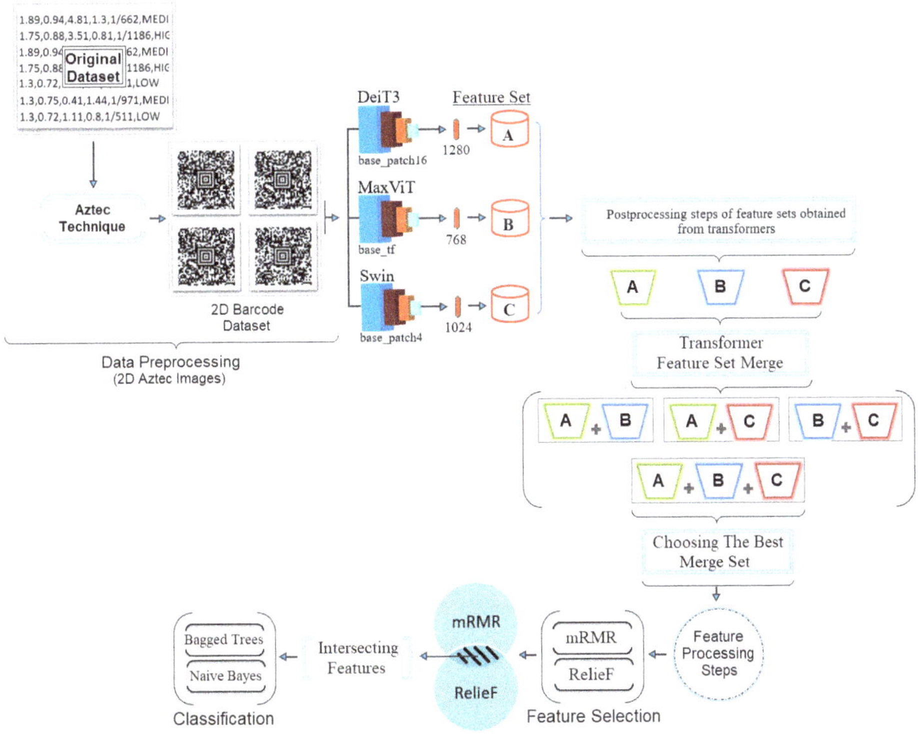

Figure 4. Model design of hybrid approach proposed for this study.

2.6. Experimental Setup and Performance Evaluation

2.6.1. Software and Hardware Environment

Transformer model training and data processing steps were performed in the Jupyter Notebook (7.0.8) environment. This tool enables transparent and repeatable workflows by allowing code to be executed in chunks, visualizations to be presented interactively, and errors to be identified and resolved immediately [40]. Thanks to these features, both model development processes and data preparation tasks have become more accessible and sustainable in clinical research. Subsequent processes, including feature fusion, feature selection, intersection, and classification, were conducted using MATLAB 2023. MATLAB was selected for its robust machine learning and signal processing toolboxes, which facilitated the efficient implementation of feature analysis techniques such as mRMR and ReliefF.

All analyses were conducted on a personal computer equipped with an Intel Core i7 processor (3.40 GHz), 32 GB RAM, and a dedicated GPU with 10 GB memory (NVIDIA Corporation, Santa Clara, CA, USA), ensuring smooth handling of computationally intensive tasks. The system was assembled using components sourced from ASUS (Taipei, Taiwan) and Kingston Technology (Fountain Valley, CA, USA).

2.6.2. Performance Metrics

The confusion matrix is a widely used tool in classification tasks [41], and it was employed in this study to evaluate the accuracy of the proposed models. Performance metrics derived from the confusion matrix were calculated using the equations provided in Equations (3)–(7) [39,41]. These equations involve key terms such as positive (P), negative (N), true (T), and false (F). The corresponding performance metrics include accuracy (Acc), F-score (F-Scr), specificity (Sp), sensitivity (Se), and precision (Pre). Among these, accuracy is frequently used in measurement evaluations and performs well with balanced datasets. The F-score, on the other hand, is particularly valuable in situations where class imbalance is present [42–44].

$$Acc = \frac{TP + TN}{TP + TN + FP + FN} \tag{3}$$

$$F\text{-}Scr = \frac{2 \times TP}{2 \times TP + FP + FN} \tag{4}$$

$$Sp = \frac{TN}{TN + FP} \tag{5}$$

$$Se = \frac{TP}{TP + FN} \tag{6}$$

$$Pre = \frac{TP}{TP + FP} \tag{7}$$

2.6.3. Model Parameters and Configuration

Table 2 provides detailed information on the preferred parameters and their values for the transformer models and machine learning methods used in this study. The preferred parameters for the machine learning methods are the default values. These values were used as the default setting in all steps of the experimental analyses. Five-fold cross-validation was applied in the final experimental steps to evaluate the generalizability and robustness of the proposed model. The dataset was randomly partitioned into five subsets of equal size. Each subset was used once as a validation fold while the remaining four formed the training set. This process was repeated five times, and the resulting metrics were averaged to provide a comprehensive evaluation of performance stability.

Table 2. Parameters and values of transformer models and other methods used in proposed approach.

Model/Method	Parameter	Preference/Value
DeiT3, MaxViT, Swin	Classifier	Linear
	Epoch	15
	Learning rate	10^{-4}
	Loss function	Cross Entropy
	Mini-batch	4
	Optimization	SGD
	Training and testing rate	70–30%
Bagged Trees	Learning rate	0.1
	Number of learners	30
	Number of predictors to sample	All
	Maximum number of splits	670
Naïve Bayes	Misclassification costs	Default
	Preset	Gaussian

3. Results

The experimental analysis of this study consisted of five steps. In the first step of the experimental analysis, data preprocessing was performed. In this step, each patient record was converted into a 2D Aztec-based barcode image. The primary aim of this transformation was to enable training with two-dimensional models, as 2D CNNs and transformer architectures are capable of deeper learning and more effective feature extraction than their one-dimensional counterparts. This preprocessing step laid the groundwork for the second step, where transformer-based training was conducted.

The second step of the experimental analysis involved training the barcode image set using three transformer models. The training accuracy graphs are presented in Figure 5, and the performance results are summarized in Table 3. DeiT3 achieved the highest accuracy at

98.26%, followed by Swin with 96.88% and MaxViT with 94.79%. Among the three, DeiT3 demonstrated superior performance under identical conditions. The high classification accuracy across all three models supports the effectiveness of the barcode-based data representation and validates the model selection for the proposed hybrid approach. In the subsequent step, the feature sets were extracted from the final layer of each transformer model for further processing. The number of features derived from each model is detailed in Table 3.

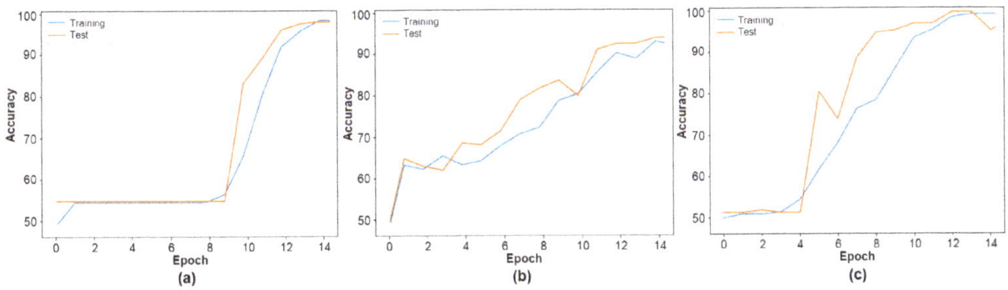

Figure 5. Classification performances of transformers: (**a**) Deit3, (**b**) MaxViT, (**c**) Swin.

Table 3. Test data metric results of transformers (%).

Transformer	Features	Se	Pre	F-Scr	Acc
Deit3	1280	98.26	98.27	98.24	98.26
MaxViT	768	94.79	95.20	94.63	94.79
Swin	1024	96.88	97.27	96.82	96.88

Se: sensitivity; Pre: precision; F-Scr: F1-score; Acc: accuracy.

The third step of the experiment conducted for this study involved combining feature sets. The feature sets obtained from three transformers were merged (DeiT3 and MaxViT, DeiT3 and Swin, MaxViT and Swin, DeiT3 and MaxViT and Swin). In total, four merged feature sets were obtained. Information about the number of features of the merged sets is given in Table 4.

Table 4. The number of features of the models combined using the feature sets and the letter symbols they represent.

Representing Letter Symbol	Models with Combined Features	Feature Counts
W	DeiT3 and MaxViT	2048
V	DeiT3 and Swin	2304
Y	MaxViT and Swin	1792
Z	DeiT3 and MaxViT and Swin	3072

The third step of the experimental analysis involved the use of Bagged Trees and Naive Bayes classifiers. Bagged Trees and Naive Bayes methods classified the combined feature sets. The confusion matrices obtained from the Bagged Trees analysis are shown in Figure 6. The metric results from the Bagged Trees analysis are given in Table 5. Similarly, the confusion matrices obtained from the Naive Bayes analysis are shown in Figure 7. The metric results from the analysis of this method are given in Table 6. Among the combined sets (W, V, Y, Z), the best performance result was obtained by the "DeiT3 & MaxViT & Swin" feature set represented by "Z". The Bagged Trees and Naive Bayes methods preferred in the proposed approach achieved 100% overall accuracy. The performance results obtained on other feature sets also aligned with our expectations. In the analyses performed in this step, the Bagged Trees and Naive Bayes methods gave successful results and were compatible with the proposed approach. This step used a cross-validation technique to verify the success of the best-performing combined feature set "DeiT3, MaxViT, and Swin". Using the cross-validation technique, a k-value of 5 was selected and reclassified using machine learning methods. The confusion matrices obtained by machine learning methods are shown in Figure 8. The metric results of the confusion matrices obtained with the cross-validation technique are given in Table 7. When analyzing Table 7, the Bagged Trees method achieved an overall accuracy of 99.79%, and the Naive Bayes method achieved an overall accuracy of 99.89%. The overall performance obtained with the cross-validation technique confirmed the previous analysis results. In the experimental analyses carried out so far, it was observed that the Naive Bayes method gives better results than the Bagged Trees method. In the next step, considering the time and hardware cost of the proposed approach, the classification process was continued using only the Naive Bayes method.

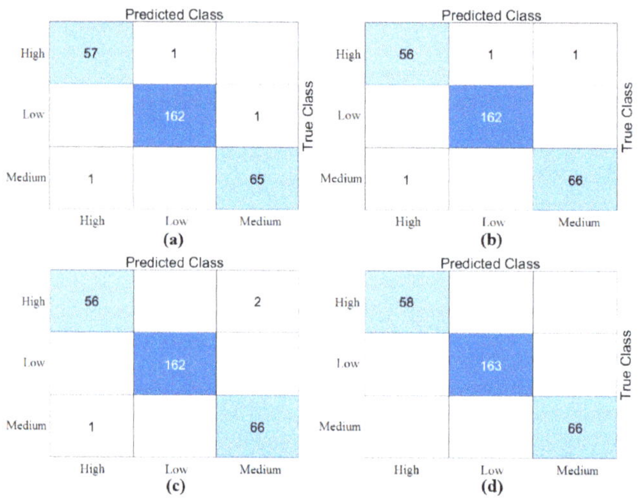

Figure 6. Confusion matrices for combined feature sets using Bagged Trees: (**a**) DeiT3–MaxViT (W), (**b**) DeiT3–Swin (V), (**c**) MaxViT–Swin (Y), (**d**) DeiT3–MaxViT–Swin (Z).

Table 5. Metric results of confusion matrices obtained from analysis of model-based fused feature sets. (classifier: Bagged Trees; training/test rate: 0.7:0.3).

Feature Merging Between Models	Class	Se	Spe	Pre	F-Scr	Acc
W	High	98.27	99.56	98.27	98.27	98.95
	Low	99.38	99.18	99.38	99.38	
	Medium	98.48	99.54	98.48	98.48	
V	High	96.55	99.56	98.24	97.39	98.95
	Low	100	99.18	99.38	99.69	
	Medium	98.50	99.54	98.50	98.50	
Y	High	96.55	99.56	98.24	97.39	98.95
	Low	100	100	100	100	
	Medium	98.50	99.09	97.05	97.77	
Z	High	100	100	100	100	100
	Low	100	100	100	100	
	Medium	100	100	100	100	

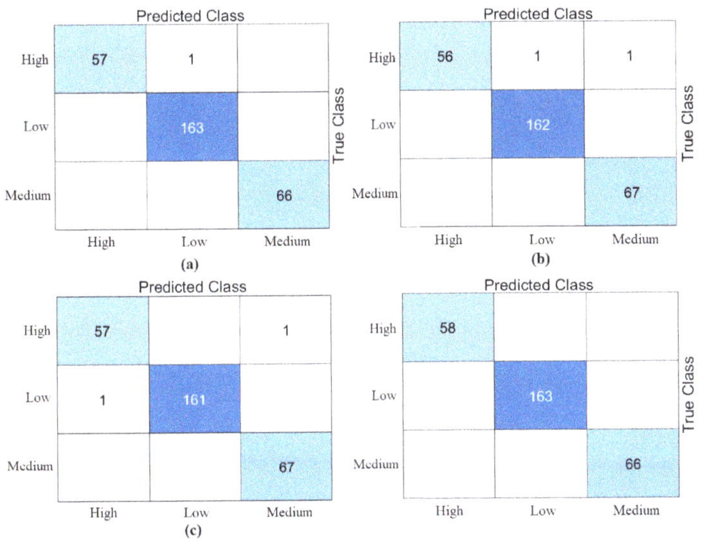

Figure 7. Confusion matrices obtained by combining the feature sets between models (classifier: Naïve Bayes): (**a**) DeiT3 and MaxViT (W), (**b**) DeiT3 and Swin (V), (**c**) MaxViT and Swin (Y), (**d**) DeiT3 and MaxViT and Swin (Z).

Table 6. Metric results of confusion matrices obtained from analysis of model-based fused feature sets. (Classifier: Naïve Bayes; training/test rate: 0.7:0.3).

Feature Merging Between Models	Class	Se	Spe	Pre	F-Scr	Acc
W	High	98.27	100	100	99.13	99.65
	Low	100	99.19	99.39	99.69	
	Medium	100	100	100	100	
V	High	96.55	100	100	98.24	99.30
	Low	100	99.19	99.38	99.69	
	Medium	100	99.54	98.52	99.25	
Y	High	98.27	99.56	98.27	98.27	99.30
	Low	99.38	100	100	99.69	
	Medium	100	99.54	98.52	99.25	
Z	High	100	100	100	100	100
	Low	100	100	100	100	
	Medium	100	100	100	100	

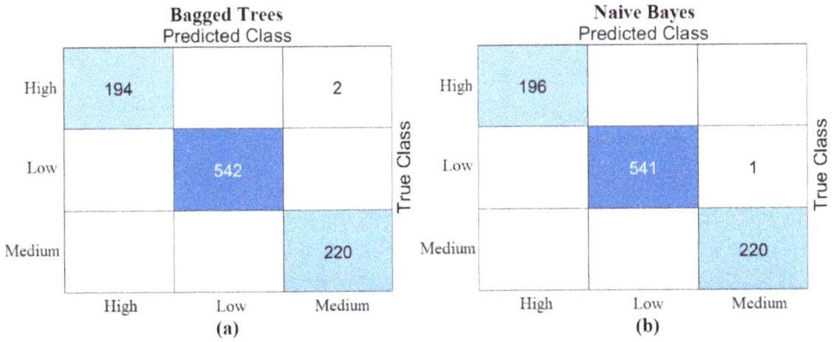

Figure 8. Confusion matrices of best performing feature set "DeiT3 & MaxViT & Swin" analyzed by cross-validation (k = 5 selected): (**a**) Bagged Trees, (**b**) Naïve Bayes.

Table 7. Metric results of the confusion matrices obtained from the analysis of the best performing feature set "Z". (Cross-validation rate/k = 5 was chosen).

Feature Merging Between Models	Classifier	Class	Se	Spe	Pre	F-Scr	Acc
Z 'DeiT3 & MaxViT & Swin'	Bagged Trees	High	98.97	100	100	99.48	99.79
		Low	100	100	100	100	
		Medium	100	99.72	99.09	99.54	
	Naïve Bayes	High	100	100	100	100	99.89
		Low	99.81	100	100	99.90	
		Medium	100	99.86	99.54	99.77	

In the fourth step, the mRMR and ReliefF methods were used as feature selection algorithms. In this step, the operations were performed on the "Z" dataset, which showed the best performance in the previous step. The total number of feature columns in the "Z" dataset was 3072. In this step, feature selection was performed to determine the best 750, best 1000, and best 1250 features among 3072 features. The training data was then classified using the Naive Bayes method, which included 70% of the training data and 30% of the test data. The cross-validation technique was also used to validate the analyses performed on the training data (k = 5 was chosen). The feature columns and score rankings selected by the mRMR and ReliefF methods are presented in Supplementary Materials, Table S1. The "Feature Selection" tool in the MATLAB 2023 interface was used for the feature selection algorithms. The best 750 features, 1000 features, and 1250 features were selected from the "Z" dataset using the mRMR method. These feature sets were then classified as train/test data using the Naive Bayes method. As a result of the classification, the best 1000 features and 1250 feature sets gave 100% overall accuracy. The best 750 features gave an overall accuracy of 98.25%. The confusion matrices of this analysis are shown in Figure 9. The feature sets (750, 1000, 1250) obtained with mRMR were then reclassified with Naive Bayes using cross-validation. An overall accuracy of 99.89% was obtained for all feature sets. The confusion matrices of these classification results are shown in Figure 10.

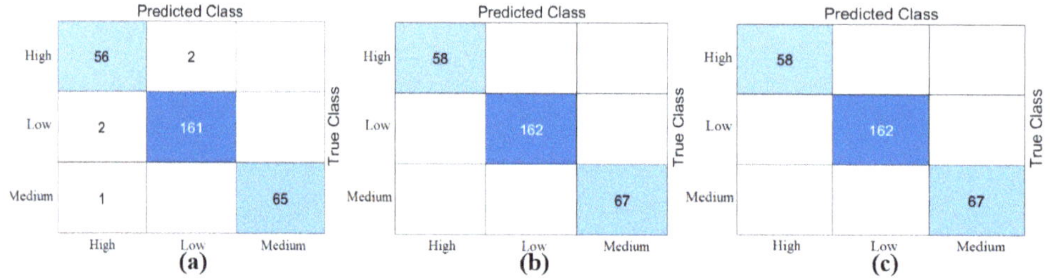

Figure 9. Naive Bayes confusion matrices of the "Z" dataset using the mRMR feature selection method (training/test rate: 0.7/0.3): (**a**) selection of the best 750 features, (**b**) selection of the best 1000 features, (**c**) selection of the best 1250 features.

Continuing with the analysis in the fourth step, the best 750 features, 1000 features, and 1250 features were selected from the "Z" dataset using the ReliefF method. These feature sets were then classified as train/test data using the Naive Bayes method. As a result of the classification, the best 750 features and 1250 feature sets gave 100% overall accuracy. The best 1000 features gave an overall accuracy of 99.65%. The confusion matrices of this analysis are shown in Figure 11. The feature sets (750, 1000, 1250) obtained with ReliefF were then reclassified with Naive Bayes using cross-validation. As a result of the classification, the best 750 and the best 1000 feature sets gave an overall accuracy of 99.89%. The best 1250 feature set achieved an overall accuracy of 100%. The confusion matrices of these classification results are shown in Figure 12. Table 8 shows the overall accuracy of the analyses (training/testing, cross-validation) performed with two feature selection methods (mRMR, RelieF) considering the confusion matrices. When analyzing Table 8, the best performance is the 1250 feature set (with the RelieF method), which gives 100% overall accuracy success considering both the training/test data and the cross-validation technique. The RelieF method gave more effective results than the mRMR method.

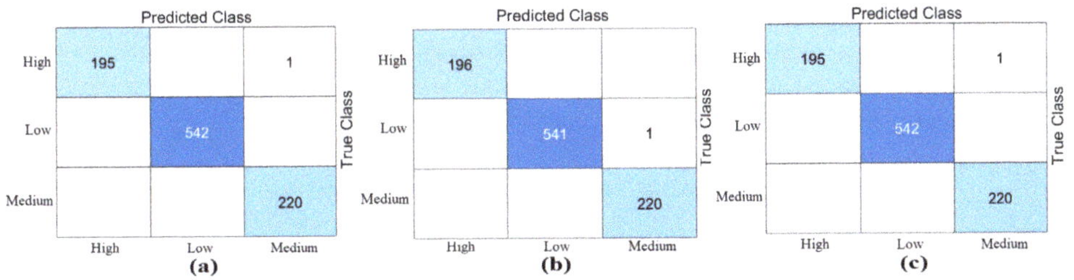

Figure 10. Naive Bayes confusion matrices of the "Z" dataset using the mRMR feature selection method (cross-validation, k = 5): (**a**) selection of the best 750 features, (**b**) selection of the best 1000 features, (**c**) selection of the best 1250 features.

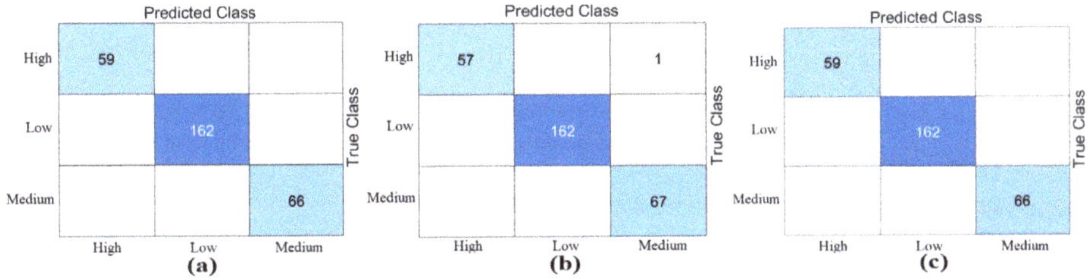

Figure 11. Naive Bayes confusion matrices of the "Z" dataset using the RelieF feature selection method (training/test rate: 0.7/0.3): (**a**) selection of the best 750 features, (**b**) selection of the best 1000 features, (**c**) selection of the best 1250 features.

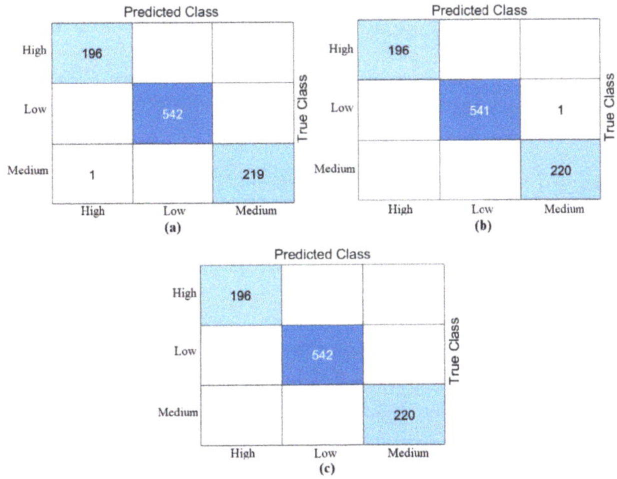

Figure 12. Naive Bayes confusion matrices of the "Z" dataset using the RelieF feature selection method (cross-validation, k = 5): (**a**) selection of the best 750 features, (**b**) selection of the best 1000 features, (**c**) selection of the best 1250 features.

Table 8. Overall accuracy of mRMR and ReliefF for classification of selected features (%).

Feature Set	ML	Feature Selection	Top Features	Acc (Test:0.3)	Acc (Cross Val./k = 5)
'Z' 3072 features	Naïve Bayes	mRMR	750	98.25	99.89
			1000	100	99.89
			1250	100	99.89
		ReliefF	750	100	99.89
			1000	99.65	99.89
			1250	100	100
mRMR top 1250 features in "Z" and ReliefF top 1250 features in "Z"		mRMR and ReliefF intersection	527 *	100	100

* Number of common/intersecting feature columns among top 1250 feature columns determined by mRMR and ReliefF.

In the last step of the experimental analyses (step 5), the feature intersection approach was used. The aim was to identify common feature columns between the best feature columns selected by the two feature methods (mRMR, ReliefF). Since the best performance in the fourth step was based on the first 1250 feature sets, the common/intersecting feature columns between the best 1250 features were identified in this step. In other words, the intersecting feature columns of the best set of 1250 feature columns obtained from the "Z" set by the mRMR method and the best set of 1250 feature columns obtained from the "Z" set by the ReliefF method were determined, and a new feature set containing a total of 527 feature columns was created. This feature set (column set of 527 features) was processed and classified using the Naive Bayes method in both train/test and cross-validation formats. As a result of the classification, 100% overall accuracy was obtained from both the training/testing and cross-validation data. The confusion matrices obtained from the analysis of this step are shown in Figure 13. The results of the analysis are given at the end of Table 8. In the last step of the proposed approach, it was observed that the feature set containing 527 feature columns performed better.

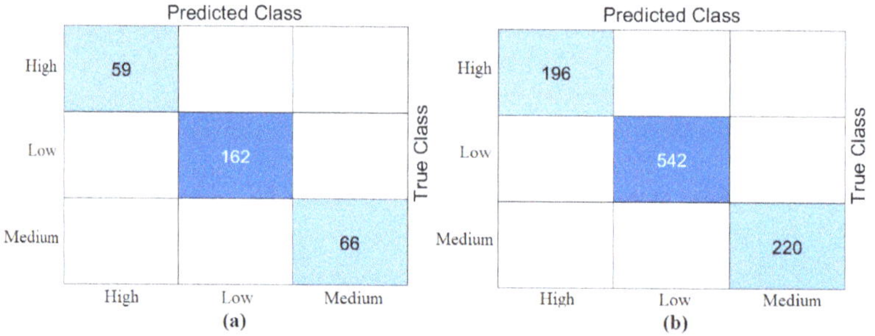

Figure 13. Confusion matrices from Naive Bayes classification using 527 intersecting features from the top 1250 mRMR and ReliefF selections: (**a**) train/test split 0.7/0.3, (**b**) 5-fold cross-validation.

An additional experiment was conducted to compare the proposed transformer-based framework with conventional deep learning models. For this evaluation, Aztec barcode images generated from 1D prenatal screening data were used to train four widely adopted CNN architectures: AlexNet, GoogLeNet, ResNet-18, and VGG-16. These models were then tested on the same dataset, and the resulting confusion matrices are shown in Figure 14. The classification accuracies obtained were 93.03% with AlexNet, 89.54% with GoogLeNet, 90.59% with ResNet-18, and 94.42% with VGG-16. The metric results obtained from the analyses are given in Table 9. While these CNN models demonstrated satisfactory performance, the proposed hybrid transformer-based framework produced superior results, especially in terms of classification accuracy. These results highlight the effectiveness of transformer architectures in extracting discriminative features from barcode-encoded clinical data and affirm the Aztec transformation method's ability to improve model performance across various deep learning paradigms.

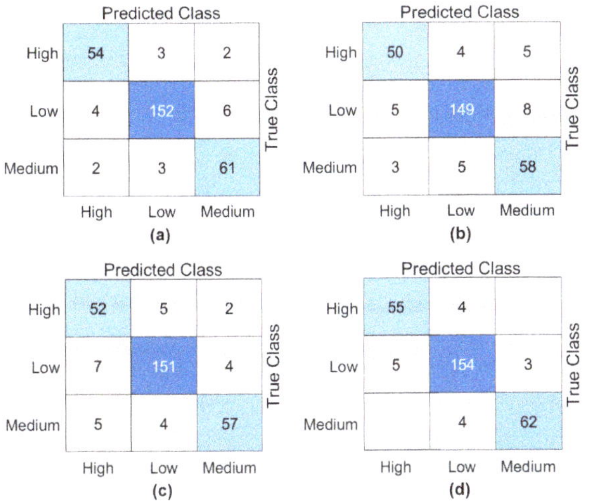

Figure 14. Confusion matrices obtained by training deep learning models using the Aztec-based image set obtained as a result of the experimental analysis of this study (training/test: 0.7/0.3); (**a**) AlexNet, (**b**) GoogLeNet, (**c**) ResNet-18, (**d**) VGG-16.

Table 9. Analysis results (%) of confusion matrices obtained from training deep learning models on Aztec-based image set.

Model	Dataset	Class	Se	Spe	Pre	F-Scr	Acc
AlexNet	Aztec-based image set	High	91.53	97.26	90	90.76	93.03
		Low	93.83	95.04	96.20	95	
		Medium	92.42	96.26	88.41	90.37	
GoogLeNet		High	84.75	96.28	86.21	85.47	89.54
		Low	91.98	92.31	94.30	93.12	
		Medium	87.88	93.87	81.69	84.67	
ResNet-18		High	88.14	94.55	81.25	84.55	90.59
		Low	93.21	92.37	94.38	93.79	
		Medium	86.36	97.13	90.48	88.37	
VGG-16		High	93.22	97.74	91.67	92.44	94.42
		Low	95.06	93.60	95.06	95.06	
		Medium	93.94	98.58	95.38	94.66	

The experimental analysis of the proposed approach in this study consists of five steps, each of which contributes to the performance of the previous step. The cross-validation technique was also used in the analyses to maintain the validity of the proposed approach.

The experimental analyses of this study showed that the proposed approach successfully detects the patient's risk level based on the FTS data. Although the proposed model achieved 100% accuracy in the experimental dataset, this result may not generalize to broader, more diverse populations. Further validation on larger, heterogeneous datasets is necessary to confirm the robustness of the model. This represents a major limitation of the current study.

The proposed hybrid approach consists of the following five key steps: (1) Data preprocessing, in which 1D patient data is converted into 2D Aztec barcode images to enable effective input into 2D transformer models. (2) Transformer model training, in which DeiT3, MaxViT and Swin models are trained on the barcode dataset. (3) Feature extraction and fusion, in which features from the final layers of the models are extracted and combined to form multiple merged feature sets. (4) Feature selection: mRMR and RelieF algorithms are applied to identify the most relevant features, including an intersection set of 527 features. (5) Classification: the refined feature sets are evaluated using machine learning classifiers (particularly Naive Bayes) to achieve high accuracy and efficiency. This multi-stage design provides DS risk estimation with better performance.

4. Discussion

FTS tests are essential for assessing the risk of genetic diseases like DS and other chromosomal disorders in the fetus. In this study, a hybrid AI approach was developed to predict fetal risk levels based on first trimester screening data. The classification results achieved with transformer-based models (e.g., DeiT3: 98.26% accuracy) and selected features demonstrate that the approach can provide high predictive accuracy using a limited number of biomarkers. Early diagnosis, along with timely and appropriate clinical interventions, significantly impacts fetal health. While FTS test accuracy is critical, low sensitivity and false negatives can cause unnecessary anxiety and treatment errors. Improving model accuracy enhances early and precise disease diagnosis. However, several challenges remain for widespread clinical application. The proposed approach developed in this study combines transformer models and advanced data processing techniques to accurately determine fetal risk levels from FTS data. The results showed that this methodology provides high accuracy and efficiency.

Though this study is technical in scope, its findings have significant clinical implications. The proposed AI framework is designed for future clinical applications, especially as a decision support system for first trimester prenatal screenings. Due to its efficient computational design and reduced feature complexity, the model can be integrated with electronic medical records (EMRs) to enable real-time risk evaluation. This would help healthcare providers make more consistent decisions, especially in under-resourced settings. As a proof-of-concept study, future research will focus on clinical validation, usability testing, and practical deployment scenarios in collaboration with obstetric clinics. The developed hybrid AI method contributes to early diagnosis and intervention processes by determining DS risk more accurately and quickly in the first trimester screening. The model's Aztec barcode conversion and transformer-based analysis capabilities can be incorporated into the patient data of clinical laboratories and doctors' decision support systems. This aims to deliver significant time and cost savings in prenatal screening processes.

Table 10 presents a comparison of the proposed approach with similar studies. The studies in Table 10 are analyses of 1D data.

Table 10. Comparison with similar studies in literature.

Article	Year	Model/Method	Acc. (%)
Pi et al. [45]	2025	Multilayer perceptron (MLP)	91
Togunwa et al. [46]	2023	Random forest (RF), ANN	95
Mutlu et al. [47]	2023	Decision tree (DT)	89.16
Jamel et al. [48]	2024	Principal component analysis (PCA), ML	98.25
Saleh et al. [49]	2024	Internet of medical things (IoMT), Explainable artificial intelligence (XAI)	92.60
This paper	2025	Barcode technique, transformers, Feature fusion and intersection	100

Pi et al. [45] compared six machine learning methods that could predict high-risk pregnancies using data collected in Bangladesh. According to their findings, the MLP method produced the most accurate results, achieving an accuracy rate of 91%. Togunwa et al. [46] developed a comprehensive hybrid model that combines ANN and RF methods for classifying risks to maternal health that may arise during pregnancy. The model demonstrated high performance, achieving 95% accuracy on test data. Mutlu et al. [47] evaluated six machine learning algorithms for identifying health threats to mothers with high-risk pregnancies in their study. The DT method achieved the highest accuracy rate of 89.16%. Jamel et al. [48] developed a model that combines PCA with a stacked community classifier method to predict risks to maternal health. This model, which uses attributes obtained through PCA, demonstrated high accuracy with a rate of 98.25%. Saleh et al. [49] proposed a deep learning framework supported by the IoMT and XAI to reduce maternal mortality. The system continuously monitors pregnant individuals' vital signs, evaluates risk factors based on the collected data, and provides regional-level risk predictions with 92.6% accuracy.

As shown in Table 10, previous studies relied on traditional machine learning and preprocessing methods. In contrast, our study paved the way for training 2D transformer models by converting data into barcode images and extracting more efficient features. We combined the feature sets obtained from the models with feature selection and intersection in the final processing step. The proposed approach in this study has achieved a classification accuracy of up to 100% under certain experimental conditions.

This study has several limitations. Firstly, the dataset is relatively small. Secondly, the model was only tested with specific AI approaches. Nevertheless, applying mRMR and RelieF—powerful feature selection techniques—alongside analyzing different transformer-based models has significantly mitigated the impact of these limitations.

Future studies will aim to enhance the model's generalizability by developing it using larger and more diverse datasets. In addition to expanding the dataset, future research could focus on integrating longitudinal data from repeated screenings, exploring ensemble learning methods, and evaluating model performance using multicenter, cross-regional data sources. These steps would strengthen the model's robustness and clinical adaptability. Additionally, future studies should consider incorporating maternal age as a key predictive variable given its well-established association with the risk of having a child with DS. Stratified modeling based on maternal age groups could improve accuracy and clinical relevance.

5. Conclusions

This study presents a hybrid AI approach designed to improve the accuracy, efficiency, and reliability of DS risk prediction during the first trimester of prenatal screening. The method involves converting one-dimensional patient data, including clinically relevant biomarkers such as nuchal translucency, hCG, and PAPP-A, into 2D Aztec barcode representations. This enables more effective feature extraction through transformer-based models such as DeiT3, MaxViT, and Swin.

The results show that combining the proposed pipeline with robust feature selection methods such as mRMR and RelieF can achieve very high classification accuracy. Specifically, integrating 1250 features selected via RelieF and 527 intersecting features from mRMR produced the most successful classification outcome. This method provides promising results in predicting the risk of congenital anomalies and can reduce unnecessary amniocentesis referrals, minimizing stress for patients. The proposed approach offers several advantages, including improved diagnostic accuracy, workload reduction, efficient resource use, and clinical scalability. It demonstrates the potential of AI in healthcare, setting a new standard for FTS data evaluation. Future research could extend this approach to other prenatal screening tests and larger clinical settings.

Although the proposed approach yielded promising results, it is important to note that the findings are based on a limited, ethically approved, private dataset. As such, this study should be considered proof-of-concept. This proof-of-concept study lays the groundwork for future clinical integration of AI-based risk assessment tools in prenatal care, with planned collaborations for real-world validation and usability testing. Future research will focus on validating the proposed method using larger, multicenter, and more diverse datasets to ensure broader clinical applicability and generalizability. Future improvements to the proposed method may include integrating maternal age and other demographic factors to improve predictive performance and ensure greater applicability to diverse populations.

Supplementary Materials: The following supporting information can be downloaded at: https://www.mdpi.com/article/10.3390/diagnostics15121444/s1, Table S1: Feature Selection List.

Author Contributions: Conceptualization, M.T. and S.A.; Methodology, M.T. and S.A.; Software, S.A. and M.T.; Validation, M.T., S.A., E.Y. and S.C.D.; Formal analysis, M.T. and S.A.; Investigation, E.Y., S.C.D. and M.T.; Resources, E.Y. and S.C.D.; Data curation, E.Y. and S.C.D.; Writing—original draft, M.T. and S.A.; Writing—review & editing, M.T. and S.A.; Visualization, S.A. and M.T.; Supervision, M.T. and S.A.; Project administration, S.A. All authors have read and agreed to the published version of the manuscript.

Funding: This research received no external funding.

Institutional Review Board Statement: The ethics committee approval of this study was taken as the 47th decision at the 144th meeting of the Çukurova University Faculty of Medicine Ethics Committee dated 10 May 2024 (10.05.2024-144/7).

Informed Consent Statement: This study does not include any data containing patients' identifiable or personal information; therefore, patient consent was not required.

Data Availability Statement: All data generated or analyzed during this study are available for sharing when appropriate request is directed to the corresponding author. The implementation code used in this study was made publicly available to ensure transparency and reproducibility. Due to ethical concerns, the original patient dataset cannot be shared. However, the code can be accessed at the following GitHub repository: https://github.com/mtogacar/DS_Syndrome_Risk_Prediction- (accessed on 3 June 2025).

Acknowledgments: The authors express their gratitude to the family for granting permission to share this information.

Conflicts of Interest: The authors declare that there is no conflict of interest related to this paper.

References

1. Charlotte, T.N.; Aurore, N.D.; Charlotte, B.; Esther, B.; Eugene, B.P. Prenatal Diagnosis of Congenital Malformations in Douala General Hospital. *Open J. Obstet. Gynecol.* **2015**, *5*, 839–848. [CrossRef]
2. Kiani, A.K.; Paolacci, S.; Scanzano, P.; Michelini, S.; Capodicasa, N.; D'agruma, L.; Notarangelo, A.; Tonini, G.; Piccinelli, D.; Farshid, K.R.; et al. Prenatal Genetic Diagnosis: Fetal Therapy as a Possible Solution to a Positive Test. *Acta Biomed.* **2020**, *91*, e2020021. [CrossRef]
3. Benn, P. Combined Second-Trimester Biochemical and Ultrasound Screening for Down Syndrome. *Obstet. Gynecol.* **2002**, *100*, 1168–1176. [CrossRef]
4. De Biasio, P.; Siccardi, M.; Volpe, G.; Famularo, L.; Santi, F.; Canini, S. First-Trimester Screening for Down Syndrome Using Nuchal Translucency Measurement with Free β-HCG and PAPP-A between 10 and 13 Weeks of Pregnancy—The Combined Test. *Prenat. Diagn.* **1999**, *19*, 360–363. [CrossRef]
5. Bahado-Singh, R.O.; Oz, A.U.; Gomez, K.; Hunter, D.; Copel, J.; Baumgarten, A.; Mahoney, M.J. Combined Ultrasound Biometry, Serum Markers and Age for Down Syndrome Risk Estimation. *Ultrasound Obstet. Gynecol.* **2000**, *15*, 199–204. [CrossRef]
6. Cuckle, H. Biochemical Screening for Down Syndrome. *Eur. J. Obstet. Gynecol. Reprod. Biol.* **2000**, *92*, 97–101. [CrossRef]
7. Orlandi, F.; Damiani, G.; Hallaban, T.W.; Krantz, D.A.; Macri, J.N. First-trimester Screening for Fetal Aneuploidy: Biochemistry and Nuchal Translucency. *Ultrasound Obstet. Gynecol.* **1997**, *10*, 381–386. [CrossRef]
8. Malone, F.D.; Ball, R.H.; Nyberg, D.A.; Comstock, C.H.; Saade, G.R.; Berkowitz, R.L.; Gross, S.J.; Dugoff, L.; Craigo, S.D.; Timor-Tritsch, I.E.; et al. First-Trimester Septated Cystic Hygroma: Prevalence, Natural History, and Pediatric Outcome. *Obstet. Gynecol.* **2005**, *106*, 1415–1416. [CrossRef]
9. Burtis, C.A.; Bruns, D.E. *Tietz Fundamentals of Clinical Chemistry and Molecular Diagnostics-E-Book: Tietz Fundamentals of Clinical Chemistry and Molecular Diagnostics*; Elsevier: Amsterdam, The Netherlands, 2014.
10. Tsakmaki, E.; Ververi, A.; Chatzakis, C.; Cavoretto, P.; Sotiriadis, A. Genomic Abnormalities in Apparently Isolated Polyhydramnios and the Role of Confirmed Fetal Phenotype: A Systematic Review and Meta-Analysis. *Am. J. Obstet. Gynecol. MFM* **2024**, *6*, 101469. [CrossRef]
11. Muñoz-Cortes, M.; Arigita, M.; Falguera, G.; Seres, A.; Guix, D.; Baldrich, E.; Acera, A.; Torrent, A.; Rodriguez-Veret, A.; Lopez-Quesada, E.; et al. Contingent Screening for Down Syndrome Completed in the First Trimester: A Multicenter Study. *Ultrasound Obstet. Gynecol.* **2012**, *39*, 396–400. [CrossRef]
12. Yeganegi, M.; Danaei, M.; Azizi, S.; Jayervand, F.; Bahrami, R.; Dastgheib, S.A.; Rashnavadi, H.; Masoudi, A.; Shiri, A.; Aghili, K.; et al. Research Advancements in the Use of Artificial Intelligence for Prenatal Diagnosis of Neural Tube Defects. *Front. Pediatr.* **2025**, *13*, 1514447. [CrossRef] [PubMed]
13. He, F.; Lin, B.; Mou, K.; Jin, L.; Liu, J. A Machine Learning Model for the Prediction of down Syndrome in Second Trimester Antenatal Screening. *Clin. Chim. Acta* **2021**, *521*, 206–211. [CrossRef] [PubMed]
14. Nix, B.; Wright, D.; Baker, A. The Impact of Bias in MoM Values on Patient Risk and Screening Performance for Down Syndrome. *Prenat. Diagn.* **2007**, *27*, 840–845. [CrossRef]
15. Huang, T.; Meschino, W.S.; Okun, N.; Dennis, A.; Hoffman, B.; Lepage, N.; Rashid, S.; Aul, R.; Farrell, S.A. The Impact of Maternal Weight Discrepancies on Prenatal Screening Results for Down Syndrome. *Prenat. Diagn.* **2013**, *33*, 471–476. [CrossRef]
16. Neocleous, A.C.; Nicolaides, K.H.; Schizas, C.N. First Trimester Noninvasive Prenatal Diagnosis: A Computational Intelligence Approach. *IEEE J. Biomed. Health Inform.* **2016**, *20*, 1427–1438. [CrossRef]
17. Koivu, A.; Korpimäki, T.; Kivelä, P.; Pahikkala, T.; Sairanen, M. Evaluation of Machine Learning Algorithms for Improved Risk Assessment for Down's Syndrome. *Comput. Biol. Med.* **2018**, *98*, 1–7. [CrossRef] [PubMed]
18. Yang, J.; Ding, X.; Zhu, W. Improving the Calling of Non-Invasive Prenatal Testing on 13-/18-/21-Trisomy by Support Vector Machine Discrimination. *PLoS ONE* **2018**, *13*, e0207840. [CrossRef]
19. Alonso, E.; Beristain, A.; Burgos, J.; Gurrutxaga, I. Comparison of Machine Learning Algorithms to Predict Down Syndrome During the Screening of the First Trimester of Pregnancy. *Appl. Sci.* **2025**, *15*, 5401. [CrossRef]
20. Durmuşoğlu, A.; Ay, M.M.; Unutmaz Durmuşoğlu, Z.D. A Classification Model for Predicting Fetus with down Syndrome—A Study from Turkey. *Appl. Artif. Intell.* **2020**, *34*, 898–915. [CrossRef]
21. Uzun, O.; Kaya, H. Prenatal Risk Assessment of Down's Syndrome by Probabilistic Classifiers. In Proceedings of the Signal Processing and Communications Applications Conference (SIU), Haspolat, Turkey, 24–26 April 2013.
22. Catic, A.; Gurbeta, L.; Kurtovic-Kozaric, A.; Mehmedbasic, S.; Badnjevic, A. Application of Neural Networks for Classification of Patau, Edwards, Down, Turner and Klinefelter Syndrome Based on First Trimester Maternal Serum Screening Data, Ultrasonographic Findings and Patient Demographics. *BMC Med. Genom.* **2018**, *11*, 19. [CrossRef]

23. Wøjdemann, K.R.; Shalmi, A.C.; Christiansen, M.; Larsen, S.O.; Sundberg, K.; Brocks, V.; Bang, J.; Nørgaard-Pedersen, B.; Tabor, A. Improved First-trimester Down Syndrome Screening Performance by Lowering the False-positive Rate: A Prospective Study of 9941 Low-risk Women. *Ultrasound Obstet. Gynecol.* **2005**, *25*, 227–233. [CrossRef] [PubMed]
24. Nguyen-Hoang, L.; Sahota, D.S.; Pooh, R.K.; Duan, H.; Chaiyasit, N.; Sekizawa, A.; Shaw, S.W.; Seshadri, S.; Choolani, M.; Yapan, P.; et al. Validation of the First-trimester Machine Learning Model for Predicting Pre-eclampsia in an Asian Population. *Int. J. Gynecol. Obstet.* **2024**, *167*, 350–359. [CrossRef] [PubMed]
25. Verma, D.; Agrawal, S.; Iwendi, C.; Sharma, B.; Bhatia, S.; Basheer, S. A Novel Framework for Abnormal Risk Classification over Fetal Nuchal Translucency Using Adaptive Stochastic Gradient Descent Algorithm. *Diagnostics* **2022**, *12*, 2643. [CrossRef]
26. Chen, Y.-T.; Chen, G.; Lin, Y.-S. Machine Learning-Based Prediction of First Trimester Down Syndrome Risk in East Asian Populations. *Risk Manag. Healthc. Policy* **2025**, *18*, 1109–1120. [CrossRef] [PubMed]
27. Ramanathan, S.; Sangeetha, M.; Talwai, S.; Natarajan, S. Probabilistic Determination Of Down's Syndrome Using Machine Learning Techniques. In Proceedings of the 2018 International Conference on Advances in Computing, Communications and Informatics (ICACCI), Bangalore, India, 19–22 September 2018; IEEE: Piscataway, NJ, USA, 2018; pp. 126–132.
28. Mulac, A.; Mathiesen, L.; Taxis, K.; Gerd Granås, A. Barcode Medication Administration Technology Use in Hospital Practice: A Mixed-Methods Observational Study of Policy Deviations. *BMJ Qual. Saf.* **2021**, *30*, 1021–1030. [CrossRef]
29. Hutchinson, S.A.; Shadid, J.N.; Tuminaro, R.S. *Aztec User's Guide, Version 1.0*; Sandia National Laboratories: Albuquerque, NM, USA; Lawrence Livermore National Laboratory: Livermore, CA, USA, 1995.
30. Aztec Code. Available online: https://en.wikipedia.org/wiki/Aztec_Code (accessed on 23 November 2024).
31. Zhang, Y.; Liu, C.; Liu, M.; Liu, T.; Lin, H.; Huang, C.-B.; Ning, L. Attention Is All You Need: Utilizing Attention in AI-Enabled Drug Discovery. *Brief. Bioinform.* **2023**, *25*, bbad467. [CrossRef]
32. Paçal, İ.; Kunduracıoğlu, İ. Data-Efficient Vision Transformer Models for Robust Classification of Sugarcane. *J. Soft Comput. Decis. Anal.* **2024**, *2*, 258–271. [CrossRef]
33. Lee, S., II; Koo, K.; Lee, J.H.; Lee, G.; Jeong, S.; Seongjun, O.; Kim, H. Vision Transformer Models for Mobile/Edge Devices: A Survey. *Multimed. Syst.* **2024**, *30*, 109. [CrossRef]
34. Agar, M.; Aydin, S.; Cakmak, M.; Koc, M.; Togacar, M. Detection of Thymoma Disease Using MRMR Feature Selection and Transformer Models. *Diagnostics* **2024**, *14*, 2169. [CrossRef]
35. Abed, R.Q.; Dikmen, M.; Aydemir, E.; Barua, P.D.; Dogan, S.; Tuncer, T.; Palmer, E.E.; Ciaccio, E.J.; Acharya, U.R. Automated Reading Level Classification Model Based on Improved Orbital Pattern. *Multimed. Tools Appl.* **2023**, *83*, 52819–52840. [CrossRef]
36. Hanchuan Peng; Fuhui Long; Ding, C. Feature Selection Based on Mutual Information Criteria of Max-Dependency, Max-Relevance, and Min-Redundancy. *IEEE Trans. Pattern Anal. Mach. Intell.* **2005**, *27*, 1226–1238. [CrossRef] [PubMed]
37. Urbanowicz, R.J.; Meeker, M.; La Cava, W.; Olson, R.S.; Moore, J.H. Relief-Based Feature Selection: Introduction and Review. *J. Biomed. Inform.* **2018**, *85*, 189–203. [CrossRef]
38. Dudeja, D.; Noonia, A.; Lavanya, S.; Sharma, V.; Kumar, V.; Rehan, S.; Ramkumar, R. Breast Cancer Diagnosis Using Bagging Decision Trees with Improved Feature Selection. In Proceedings of the RAiSE-2023; MDPI: Basel, Switzerland, 2023; p. 17.
39. Peretz, O.; Koren, M.; Koren, O. Naive Bayes Classifier—An Ensemble Procedure for Recall and Precision Enrichment. *Eng. Appl. Artif. Intell.* **2024**, *136*, 108972. [CrossRef]
40. Ochkov, V.F.; Stevens, A.; Tikhonov, A.I. Jupyter Notebook, JupyterLab—Integrated Environment for STEM Education. In Proceedings of the 2022 VI International Conference on Information Technologies in Engineering Education (Inforino), Moscow, Russia, 12–15 April 2022; IEEE: Piscataway, NJ, USA, 2022; pp. 1–5.
41. Božić, D.; Runje, B.; Lisjak, D.; Kolar, D. Metrics Related to Confusion Matrix as Tools for Conformity Assessment Decisions. *Appl. Sci.* **2023**, *13*, 8187. [CrossRef]
42. Çalışkan, A. Detecting Human Activity Types from 3D Posture Data Using Deep Learning Models. *Biomed. Signal Process. Control* **2023**, *81*, 104479. [CrossRef]
43. Yildirim, M.; Cengil, E.; Eroglu, Y.; Cinar, A. Detection and Classification of Glioma, Meningioma, Pituitary Tumor, and Normal in Brain Magnetic Resonance Imaging Using Deep Learning-Based Hybrid Model. *Iran J. Comput. Sci.* **2023**, *6*, 455–464. [CrossRef]
44. Alaca, Y.; Basaran, E.; Celik, Y. Enhancing Anomaly Detection in Large-Scale Log Data Using Machine Learning: A Comparative Study of SVM and KNN Algorithms with HDFS Dataset. *ADBA Comput. Sci.* **2024**, *1*, 14–18. [CrossRef]
45. Pi, X.; Wang, J.; Chu, L.; Zhang, G.; Zhang, W. Prediction of High-Risk Pregnancy Based on Machine Learning Algorithms. *Sci. Rep.* **2025**, *15*, 15561. [CrossRef] [PubMed]
46. Togunwa, T.O.; Babatunde, A.O.; Abdullah, K.-R. Deep Hybrid Model for Maternal Health Risk Classification in Pregnancy: Synergy of ANN and Random Forest. *Front. Artif. Intell.* **2023**, *6*, 1213436. [CrossRef]
47. Mutlu, H.B.; Durmaz, F.; Yücel, N.; Cengil, E.; Yıldırım, M. Prediction of Maternal Health Risk with Traditional Machine Learning Methods. *NATURENGS MTU J. Eng. Nat. Sci. Mal. Turgut Ozal Univ.* **2023**, *4*, 16–23. [CrossRef]

48. Jamel, L.; Umer, M.; Saidani, O.; Alabduallah, B.; Alsubai, S.; Ishmanov, F.; Kim, T.; Ashraf, I. Improving Prediction of Maternal Health Risks Using PCA Features and TreeNet Model. *PeerJ Comput. Sci.* **2024**, *10*, e1982. [CrossRef] [PubMed]
49. Saleh, S.N.; Elagamy, M.N.; Saleh, Y.N.M.; Osman, R.A. An Explainable Deep Learning-Enhanced IoMT Model for Effective Monitoring and Reduction of Maternal Mortality Risks. *Futur. Internet* **2024**, *16*, 411. [CrossRef]

diagnostics

MDPI

Article

Machine Learning-Based Identification of Phonological Biomarkers for Speech Sound Disorders in Saudi Arabic-Speaking Children

Deema F. Turki [1] and Ahmad F. Turki [2,3,*]

[1] Speech and Hearing Pathology Department, Faculty of Medical Rehabilitation Sciences, King Abdulaziz University, Jeddah 21589, Saudi Arabia; dturki@kau.edu.sa
[2] Electrical and Computer Engineering Department, Faculty of Engineering, King Abdulaziz University, Jeddah 21589, Saudi Arabia
[3] Center of Excellence in Intelligent Engineering Systems (CEIES), King Abdul Aziz University, Jeddah 21589, Saudi Arabia
* Correspondence: aftorke@kau.edu.sa

Abstract: Background/Objectives: This study investigates the application of machine learning (ML) techniques in diagnosing speech sound disorders (SSDs) in Saudi Arabic-speaking children, with a specific focus on phonological biomarkers, particularly Infrequent Variance (InfrVar), to improve diagnostic accuracy. SSDs are a significant concern in pediatric speech pathology, affecting an estimated 10–15% of preschool-aged children worldwide. However, accurate diagnosis remains challenging, especially in linguistically diverse populations. Traditional diagnostic tools, such as the Percentage of Consonants Correct (PCC), often fail to capture subtle phonological variations. This study explores the potential of machine learning models to enhance diagnostic accuracy by incorporating culturally relevant phonological biomarkers like InfrVar, aiming to develop a more effective diagnostic approach for SSDs in Saudi Arabic-speaking children. **Methods:** Data from 235 Saudi Arabic-speaking children aged 2;6 to 5;11 years were analyzed using several machine learning models: Random Forest, Support Vector Machine (SVM), XGBoost, Logistic Regression, K-Nearest Neighbors, and Naïve Bayes. The dataset was used to classify speech patterns into four categories: Atypical, Typical Development (TD), Articulation, and Delay. Phonological features such as Phonological Variance (PhonVar), InfrVar, and Percentage of Consonants Correct (PCC) were used as key variables. SHapley Additive exPlanations (SHAP) analysis was employed to interpret the contributions of individual features to model predictions. **Results:** The XGBoost and Random Forest models demonstrated the highest performance, with an accuracy of 91.49% and an AUC of 99.14%. SHAP analysis revealed that articulation patterns and phonological patterns were the most influential features for distinguishing between Atypical and TD categories. The K-Means clustering approach identified four distinct subgroups based on speech development patterns: TD (46.61%), Articulation (25.42%), Atypical (18.64%), and Delay (9.32%). **Conclusions:** Machine learning models, particularly XGBoost and Random Forest, effectively classified speech development categories in Saudi Arabic-speaking children. This study highlights the importance of incorporating culturally specific phonological biomarkers like InfrVar and PhonVar to improve diagnostic precision for SSDs. These findings lay the groundwork for the development of AI-assisted diagnostic tools tailored to diverse linguistic contexts, enhancing early intervention strategies in pediatric speech pathology.

https://doi.org/10.3390/diagnostics15111401

Keywords: speech sound disorders (SSDs); machine learning (ML); infrequent variance (InfrVar); phonological development; Saudi Arabic-speaking children

1. Introduction

Speech sound disorders (SSDs) affect an estimated 10–15% of preschool-aged children globally and represent a significant challenge in pediatric speech pathology due to their impact on language development, literacy acquisition, and social communication [1,2]. In recent years, machine learning (ML) techniques have emerged as promising tools to enhance the diagnostic process for SSDs by improving accuracy, reducing subjectivity, and enabling the analysis of complex phonological patterns [3].

Despite the clinical importance of SSDs, accurate diagnosis remains challenging, particularly in linguistically diverse populations [4]. Traditional diagnostic tools, such as the Percentage of Consonants Correct (PCC), have long been the gold standard for assessing phonological accuracy [5]. However, PCC and similar phoneme-based measures rely on a binary classification of correct versus incorrect productions, failing to account for subtle yet clinically meaningful phonological variations [6]. These limitations are particularly pronounced in non-English languages, where phonotactic constraints, coarticulatory effects, and dialectal variability influence speech production patterns, potentially leading to under-identification or misdiagnosis of SSDs [7].

Studies in Jordanian Arabic have provided insights into the developmental trajectory of multisyllabic word production, phonological error patterns in children with SSDs, and syllable structure acquisition [8–10]. For instance, research by Amayreh and Dyson showed that Arabic-speaking children tend to acquire plosives (/b, t, d/) and nasals (/m, n/) earlier than fricatives, with voiced fricatives like /z/ and emphatics such as /sˤ/ acquired later [8]. The alveolar /r/ is often substituted with l in early development. Regarding syllable structure, Abdoh reported that open syllables (e.g., CV, CVV) are typically mastered before closed forms (e.g., CVC), with complex structures like word-final CCs or heterosyllabic clusters remaining difficult beyond age four [9]. In terms of phonological processes, Dyson and Amayreh identified fronting, stopping, devoicing, cluster reduction, final consonant deletion, and weak syllable deletion as the most common patterns among Arabic-speaking children, some of which may persist beyond the expected age depending on dialectal influences [10]. These findings highlight important cross-dialectal and language-specific developmental norms that must be considered in culturally valid diagnostic models. However, there remains a critical need to examine these issues within the Saudi Arabic context, particularly given dialectal differences that can impact phoneme realization and phonotactic structure [8–10].

To address these diagnostic limitations, researchers have sought to identify alternative markers that provide a more granular analysis of phonological variation [11]. Phonological Variance (PhonVar), introduced by Albrecht, offers a framework for capturing deviations in speech production beyond traditional binary classification models [11]. This framework includes Type Variance, referring to systematic phoneme substitutions or distortions; Token Variance, which denotes inconsistent phoneme productions within the same phonological context; and Infrequent Variance (InfrVar), a subcategory that represents phonological deviations occurring with low frequency and irregular distribution [11]. Among these subtypes, InfrVar has garnered increasing attention as a potential biomarker for early SSD detection, as it reflects subtle speech inconsistencies that may not be captured by conventional metrics like PCC [11]. Albrecht's findings suggest that a higher incidence of InfrVar is associated with increased phonological instability and a heightened risk of atypical speech development [11]. Expanding on this work, Fox-Boyer conducted a large-scale phonological analysis and reported that more than 50% of phonological variation tokens observed in children with SSDs fell into the InfrVar category [12]. This underscores its diagnostic significance and suggests that phonological irregularities previously dismissed as idiosyncratic or developmentally transient may, in fact, serve as early indicators of speech pathology [12]. InfrVar was selected based on its emerging role as a sensitive marker of phonological instability, particularly in languages with complex phonemic inventories and rich morphophonemic variation such as Arabic. Prior research, including Albrecht and Fox-Boyer et al., has demonstrated that children with SSDs exhibit a disproportionately high number of infrequent phonological variants often overlooked by conventional metrics like PCC [11,12]. InfrVar captures subtle, low-frequency deviations that may reflect unstable or non-systematic speech motor planning [11,12]. In the context of Arabic, which features emphatic consonants, guttural sounds, and dialectal coarticulatory effects, such rare patterns provide a refined lens for detecting atypical development [11,12]. Additionally, by quantifying error patterns that do not cluster under common phonological processes, InfrVar helps clinicians and models identify outlier behavior that may signal diagnostic risk with higher sensitivity [11,12].

Most Arabic studies focus on frequent phonological patterns and exclude rare variants, which limits sensitivity in early SSD detection [13]. In Saudi Hejazi Arabic specifically, features such as emphatics, pharyngeals, and complex syllable structures increase the likelihood of low-frequency, dialect-specific errors [14].

Despite advancements in phonological analysis, clinical speech pathology has remained largely dependent on manual transcription and expert-based classification, a process that is inherently time-consuming, subjective, and susceptible to inter-rater variability [15–17]. The increasing accessibility of machine learning (ML) algorithms in computational linguistics and medical diagnostics has presented an opportunity to overcome these limitations by automating SSD classification, improving diagnostic objectivity, and enhancing predictive accuracy [15]. Machine learning algorithms can process high-dimensional phonetic and phonological data, recognizing complex, non-linear relationships in speech patterns that may be imperceptible through traditional auditory-perceptual analysis [18]. A growing body of research has demonstrated the efficacy of ML-based phonological assessment tools in distinguishing typical from atypical speech production [19]. Such studies highlight the promising role of ML in automating tasks traditionally requiring significant manual effort, such as phonetic transcription and forced alignment for assessing speech sound disorders (SSDs) [19–21]. For example, Li et al. presented a state-of-the-art ML model that utilizes the wav2vec 2.0 acoustic model to automate phonetic transcriptions, achieving an impressive phoneme error rate (PER) of just 0.15, significantly outperforming traditional methods [20]. Additionally, ML applications in the diagnosis and treatment of aphasia, as demonstrated in studies by Cordella et al. and Benway and Preston, show how machine learning models can improve accuracy and reliability, even in complex, heterogeneous conditions [19–21]. These innovations enable new possibilities for integrating ML into clinical practice, from improving diagnostic precision in SSDs and aphasia to offering real-time, data-driven therapeutic recommendations, ultimately enhancing the quality of patient care.

The key advantage of ML in SSD assessment lies in its ability to simultaneously assess multiple phonological markers, identify patterns within speech errors, and classify children based on distinct phonological profiles [15–22]. Unlike conventional statistical models, ML algorithms can adaptively learn from speech datasets, enabling the refinement of diagnostic thresholds for language-specific populations [17]. This is particularly relevant for Arabic-speaking children, where existing diagnostic tools lack linguistic specificity, resulting in potential misdiagnoses [23–25]. However, despite the potential of ML for SSD diagnostics, research remains disproportionately focused on English-speaking populations, with minimal investigation into its applicability within Arabic speech pathology [26–28]. Existing ML-based speech assessment models have yet to incorporate culturally adapted phonological markers such as InfrVar, limiting their generalizability across diverse linguistic contexts. Addressing this gap necessitates the development of ML-driven diagnostic models that integrate phonological biomarkers tailored to the phonetic and phonological characteristics of Arabic.

The ultimate aim of this study is to train and test several machine learning models to classify children's speech into typical versus atypical speech production using phonological markers tailored to Saudi Arabic. This study seeks to bridge this gap by introducing a machine learning-based classification system for SSDs in Saudi Arabic-speaking children, with a specific focus on InfrVar as a novel diagnostic marker. The primary objectives of this research are to evaluate the diagnostic efficacy of Infrequent Variance as a phonological biomarker for SSDs relative to established measures such as PCC and PhonVar, to develop and compare the performance of supervised machine learning models, including Random Forest, Support Vector Machines, and XGBoost, in classifying SSDs based on phonological error patterns, and to assess the interpretability of ML-driven classifications using SHapley Additive exPlanations (SHAP) analysis to ensure model transparency and clinical applicability. Furthermore, this study aims to contribute to the development of culturally adaptive AI-driven diagnostic tools for Arabic-speaking populations, addressing the current linguistic gap in SSD research. By integrating ML methodologies with language-specific phonological analysis, this study advances the field of pediatric speech pathology by establishing an AI-assisted clinical decision support system (CDSS) for SSD diagnosis. The anticipated outcomes will not only enhance the diagnostic accuracy of SSDs in Arabic-speaking children, but also pave the way for broader applications of AI in culturally informed speech pathology research.

This study introduces a novel application of machine learning to the classification of speech sound development in Saudi Hejazi Arabic-speaking children. By incorporating culturally relevant phonological biomarkers such as InfrVar and PhonVar, this study evaluates the performance of established ML models on this unique dataset and uses K-Means clustering to uncover latent developmental subgroups. The inclusion of SHAP analysis further enhances model interpretability, supporting its use in clinical decision-making.

2. Materials and Methods

This section outlines the study design, participant characteristics, data collection procedures, phonological feature coding, and machine learning model training. It separates the materials (i.e., participant information and speech data) from the procedures used in the analysis to comply with reviewer requests.

2.1. Participants

Participants were 235 monolingual children (119 female, 116 male) aged 2 years, 6 months to 5 years, 11 months. They were recruited from public and private preschools in Jeddah, Saudi Arabia, and evenly stratified across seven age groups. To ensure the sample accurately represented typically developing monolingual Saudi-Hejazi Arabic (SHA)-speaking children, specific inclusion and exclusion criteria were applied during participant recruitment and screening, as outlined below:

Inclusion Criteria

- Children aged between 2 years, 6 months and 5 years, 11 months.
- Must be monolingual speakers of Saudi-Hejazi Arabic (SHA).

- The primary language spoken at home must be Hejazi Arabic.
- No history of speech, language, hearing, developmental, or congenital disorders.
- Children must be deemed typically developing based on parent reports.
- Parental consent was obtained through signed forms, and eligibility was verified via a detailed parent questionnaire covering:
    - Linguistic background.
    - Exposure to SHA vs. Modern Standard Arabic (MSA).
    - Early speech and language development.
    - Hearing history.

Exclusion Criteria

- Exposure to another Arabic dialect or a second language at home (e.g., bilingual children).
- Reported concerns about the child's speech, language, or hearing development.
- Presence of any diagnosed or suspected medical or developmental condition.
- Absence on the testing day or failure to complete the phonological assessment.
- Lack of motivation or cooperation during testing sessions.
- Participants were also excluded if their age group had already reached saturation in the sample.

Participants were equitably distributed across seven distinct age groups to ensure comprehensive age-related analysis, as detailed in Table 1. This stratified approach supports age-based comparisons and enhances the generalizability of the study's findings across the early developmental spectrum.

Table 1. Participant distribution by age group and gender.

Age Groups (Year; Month)	*N*	Female	Male	Mean Age (Months)	SD Age (Months)	% of Sample
2; 6–2; 11	30	15	15	32.20	1.86	12.77
3; 0–3; 5	27	14	13	30.00	1.92	11.49
3; 6–3; 11	38	17	21	45.24	1.79	16.17
4; 0–4; 5	39	17	22	50.33	1.63	16.60
4; 6–4; 11	31	16	15	57.19	1.74	13.19
5; 0–5; 5	37	22	15	62.38	1.53	15.74
5; 6–5; 11	33	18	15	68.45	1.79	14.04
Total	235	119	116			

Note: Participants were stratified into 6-month age bands to allow age-specific comparisons of phonological measures.

2.2. Speech Sample Collection

Speech data were collected using a structured single-word naming task consisting of 145 items designed to reflect the phonological structure of Saudi Arabic. This assessment, referred to as the Saudi Hejazi Arabic Phonology Assessment (SHAPA), elicited target productions from each child through picture prompts. Sessions were conducted in quiet school settings, and all productions were audio-recorded using a high-quality digital recorder. The SHAPA word list was carefully constructed to comprehensively represent the phonological system of Saudi Hejazi Arabic and included Modern Standard Arabic (MSA) phonemes. All consonantal phonemes were represented across word-initial, medial, and final positions with balanced distribution. The list also incorporated diverse syllable structures (e.g., CV, CVC, CVCC, CVCCVC), varying word lengths, and stress patterns, ensuring that phonotactic diversity and dialect-specific features were adequately captured. This design supports detailed phonological analysis and reflects both common and diagnostically relevant speech patterns for Arabic-speaking children.

2.3. Phonological Data Analysis

All speech samples were phonetically transcribed using the International Phonetic Alphabet (IPA) by the first author, a certified speech-language pathologist with formal training in phonetic transcription. Phonological variants were classified into two main categories: developmental typical variants, which refer to age-appropriate phonological errors, and infrequent variants, which are those that did not meet the pattern-level threshold criteria (i.e., occurring fewer than 4 or 6 times across the dataset, depending on the variant type). Each child's dataset included token counts, types per child, and standardized scores (e.g., PCC and M–1SD thresholds). Inter- and intra-rater reliability were calculated on 10% of the dataset, yielding agreement scores above 80%.

The dataset used in this study originates from the previous investigation aimed at establishing normative data on the phonological development of Saudi Hejazi Arabic-speaking children [29]. While the original study focused on developmental benchmarks through phonetic accuracy and qualitative phonological patterns, the present analysis repurposes this dataset from a diagnostic perspective. Machine learning techniques are applied to classify speech development profiles, with InfrVar and other phonological measures being key variables to examine their ability to distinguish between typical, delayed, and atypical speech sound development. This reanalysis introduces a novel approach by leveraging culturally specific diagnostic markers and utilizes predictive models for the early identification of speech sound disorders.

By reanalyzing these descriptive developmental data, this study aimed to convert them into actionable diagnostic tools for identifying atypical phonological development. Through this process, this study explored the clinical utility of phonological biomarkers such as PhonVar and InfrVar, contributing valuable insights to the field of speech disorder diagnosis.

Although children included in this study were considered typically developing based on parent report and exclusion of known speech or developmental conditions, no formal diagnostic assessments were conducted to confirm the absence of speech sound disorders (SSDs). Therefore, it is possible that some participants exhibited undiagnosed SSDs. This is supported by our reanalysis, which identified a small number of children in each age group whose phonological profiles (e.g., elevated InfrVar or token counts) deviated markedly from normative trends. These observations underscore the likelihood of subtle, unrecognized atypical patterns within the normative sample and support the utility of using such data for early risk profiling.

The primary phonological measures used in the analysis are:

- **Articulation Patterns (Artic Patterns)**: The number of articulation errors observed.
- **Phonology Patterns (PhonVar)**: The different phonological patterns exhibited by the children.
- **Delay Patterns**: Instances where speech development was delayed compared to age norms.
- **Atypical Patterns**: Patterns that deviate from typical developmental trajectories.
- **InfrVar**: A measure of infrequent phonological variations, recorded both per child and as an average for each age group.
- **Token Counts**: The total number of phonetic tokens produced per child and the average for each age group.
- **Types per Child**: The variety of speech sounds (types) produced by each child.

The dataset also includes several standardized scores, calculated for each child within each age group:

- **PCC (Percentage of Correct Consonants)**: The percentage of correctly produced consonants by each child.
- **Age Group**: Children are classified into age groups (from **2;6 to 5;11 years**) to assess age-related changes in speech development.
- **PCC Adjustments**: PCC scores were calculated both for each child and adjusted by one standard deviation (M–1 SD) for each age group.

Phonological patterns were classified as typical when they occurred in fewer than six instances across an age group and were present in less than 10% of children. InfrVar was defined as phonological variants that occurred fewer than six times in total across the sample, potentially reflecting developmental instability or chance occurrences. Descriptive statistics including mean, standard deviation, and range were computed for all key phonological measures to support classification modeling.

Children's speech was classified into typical versus atypical speech production according to the mean number of the following measurements: PhonVar, including InfrVar and phonological patterns (Tokens) as counted per child, as well as the PCC, which was used for comparability purposes. First, the overall number of phonologically variants from adult-like speech were counted per child. All phonological variants per child were analyzed by hand. Second, these variations were differentiated into infrequent variants and phonological patterns depending on their frequency of occurrence, since a single instance of a variation may be due to developmental fluctuation or occur by chance.

To define the nature of the patterns used in this research, the following criteria are presented, and subsequently the rationale for the decisions made are provided.

- A pattern was considered to be age-appropriate if it was produced by 10% or more of the Saudi Arabic-speaking monolingual children in this age group.
- A pattern was considered to be delayed if it occurred in less than 10% of the Saudi Arabic-speaking monolingual children in an age group, but was evident in at least 10% of the children in at least six months younger age group.
- A pattern was considered to be deviant if it was not produced by at least 10% of the children in any age group in the Saudi Arabic-speaking monolingual children.

Additionally, the total number of articulation errors (reflecting distortion patterns), as well as developmental, delayed, and atypical phonological patterns, were calculated based on previously established normative benchmarks. Using these benchmarks, accepted performance thresholds for each age group were set for the three key measures: PCC, PhonVar, and InfrVar. The threshold for typical performance was defined as the mean minus one standard deviation (M–1SD) for each measure, which provided a clear guideline for distinguishing typical from atypical phonological development.

Each child's phonological performance was compared to the established normative thresholds to determine whether their development was typical or atypical. Patterns were classified as typical if they fell within the expected age range for that particular measure. If a pattern persisted beyond the typical age range, the child was classified as exhibiting a phonological delay. Conversely, if the observed patterns were not present in the normative dataset at all, the child was identified as having atypical phonological development. This classification process allowed for a clear distinction between children with typical developmental trajectories, those experiencing delays, and those with atypical phonological patterns, providing valuable insights into speech development and potential areas for intervention.

The thresholds used in this study, including the 10% criterion for defining typical, delayed, and atypical patterns and the M–1SD cutoff for measures such as PCC and PhonVar, are consistent with established practices in developmental phonology and clinical speech pathology [30–33]. Prior studies and diagnostic tools have used similar benchmarks to distinguish normative from disordered speech patterns [30–33]. For example, Dodd et al. and McLeod and Baker describe the 10% occurrence rule as a reliable indicator of developmental appropriateness [30,31]. Likewise, the M–1SD threshold aligns with the use of statistical cutoffs proposed by Shriberg et al. (1997) in the development of the Percentage of Consonants Correct (PCC) metric [32]. These standards, also reflected in widely used diagnostic tools like the DEAP (Dodd et al., 2002), support the validity of our classification framework [33].

2.4. Machine Learning Procedure

This study utilized machine learning techniques to analyze the phonological development of Saudi Arabic-speaking children, with a focus on classifying speech patterns into typical or atypical development using Python version 3.11.5 (Python Software Foundation, Wilmington, DE, USA). The dataset, collected from 235 monolingual children aged 3 to 6 years, was preprocessed by addressing missing values and standardizing numerical features using the StandardScaler to ensure consistent scaling and enhance the model's performance. The target variable, representing speech development categories such as Atypical Phonological Development, Typical Development (TD), Articulation Disorder, and Phonological Delay, was mapped to numerical labels. The dataset was split into training and testing sets (80% for training and 20% for testing) to ensure an unbiased evaluation of model performance.

Cross-validation techniques (e.g., k-fold) were not implemented in this study, as the objective was to establish baseline performance using default model settings on a held-out test set. Future research will incorporate cross-validation and hyperparameter tuning to further optimize classification accuracy and generalizability.

To address potential class imbalance across the four diagnostic categories Atypical, Typical Development, Articulation, and Delay, a stratified train–test split was implemented to preserve class distribution across subsets. This ensured each class was proportionally represented in both training and testing datasets, reducing the risk of biased model learning. The dataset consisted of 235 children, categorized into four diagnostic groups: Atypical (n = 22), Typical Development (n = 79), Articulation (n = 97), and Delay (n = 37). To ensure balanced representation of each class in both training and testing phases, stratified sampling was employed. Specifically, 80% of the data from each category was allocated to the training set, and the remaining 20% to the test set. This approach preserved the original class distribution across the splits and minimized the risk of biased model performance due to class imbalance.

Additionally, macro-averaged evaluation metrics, including precision, recall, and F1-score, were computed to provide a balanced assessment of performance across all classes, especially for those with lower frequencies.

2.4.1. Feature Preprocessing

Before model training, several preprocessing steps were applied to the dataset to ensure data quality and consistency:

Missing Values Handling: Missing data were handled using median imputation to reduce bias and preserve central tendency without being influenced by outliers.

Label Encoding: The target variable, representing speech development categories (Atypical, Typical Development, Articulation, and Delay), was encoded numerically using a mapping scheme (1–4 mapped to 0–3) to enable compatibility with classification algorithms.

Feature Standardization: All numerical features were standardized using StandardScaler, which transforms each feature to have zero mean and unit variance. This step was crucial for ensuring that features with larger numeric ranges did not dominate distance-based models like KNN or influence optimization in gradient-based algorithms.

2.4.2. Model Development and Validation Strategy

To ensure rigorous development and evaluation of the classification models, we implemented the following procedures:

Feature Selection

Phonological features were selected based on theoretical and clinical relevance, including Infrequent Variance (InfrVar), Percentage of Correct Consonants (PCC), phonological patterns (PhonVar), and articulation error counts. These features are well-established in the literature as indicators of speech sound development. No automatic feature elimination or correlation pruning was applied to preserve interpretability and clinical transparency.

Cross-Validation

To enhance generalizability, we used stratified 5-fold cross-validation on the training set. This approach ensured that each fold contained representative proportions of all four diagnostic categories (Atypical, TD, Articulation, Delay). Performance metrics were averaged across folds before final evaluation on the test set.

Model Optimization Strategy

We intentionally used default hyperparameters for all models to establish baseline performance and evaluate the predictive value of phonological features without overfitting. While no grid search or hyperparameter tuning was conducted in this phase, we acknowledge this as a limitation and outline it as a direction for future work. Exploratory performance enhancement was achieved by incorporating unsupervised K-Means cluster labels as new features and applying Principal Component Analysis (PCA) to reduce noise and dimensionality.

2.4.3. Theoretical Foundation of Analytical Models

To classify speech sound disorder (SSD) subtypes and uncover underlying phonological patterns, this study applied both supervised and unsupervised machine learning techniques grounded in established computational frameworks.

Supervised Machine Learning Models:
Six supervised classifiers were employed to predict SSD subtype labels based on phonological, articulatory, and acoustic features:
Random Forest Classifier: An ensemble method that builds multiple decision trees and aggregates their predictions to enhance accuracy and control overfitting. It is particularly effective for handling high-dimensional data with complex feature interactions.
Support Vector Machine (SVM): A powerful classifier that finds the optimal hyperplane to separate classes in a high-dimensional space, well-suited for datasets with clear margins between categories.
XGBoost: A scalable gradient boosting framework that builds additive predictive models in a sequential manner. It is known for its speed and performance in structured data classification tasks.
Logistic Regression: A linear model used for binary and multi-class classification that estimates the probability of class membership using a logistic function.
K-Nearest Neighbors (KNN): A non-parametric method that classifies new data points based on the majority vote of their K-Nearest Neighbors in the feature space.
Naïve Bayes: A probabilistic classifier based on Bayes' theorem with the assumption of feature independence, suitable for baseline performance comparison.

Model performance was evaluated using standard metrics including accuracy, precision, recall, F1-score, and area under the receiver operating characteristic curve (AUC), ensuring a robust comparison across classifiers.

Each model was trained using the training subset and evaluated on the testing set using the following performance metrics; these metrics were used to assess the ability of each model to distinguish between typical and atypical speech development.

Accuracy: This metric evaluates the overall correctness of the model by calculating the ratio of correctly classified instances (both true positives and true negatives) to the total number of instances [34]. In this study, accuracy provides a general measure of the model's effectiveness in classifying speech development patterns into the categories of Atypical, Typical Development (TD), Articulation, and Delay. It helps to determine how well the model can correctly distinguish between typical and atypical phonological development across all age groups and features.

$$Accuracy = \frac{(TP + TN)}{(TP + TN + FP + FN)} \times 100 \tag{1}$$

where

TP (True Positive): The number of instances where the model correctly predicted the Atypical or Typical Development (TD) or Articulation or Delay category (i.e., the model correctly identified a child's speech as typical or atypical).

TN (True Negative): The number of instances where the model correctly predicted that the speech did not belong to a specific category.

FP (False Positive): The number of instances where the model incorrectly predicted that a child's speech belonged to a particular category (e.g., a child classified as Atypical when they are actually Typical Development (TD)).

FN (False Negative): The number of instances where the model failed to predict the correct speech category (e.g., a child classified as Typical Development (TD) when they actually have Atypical speech).

Precision: In this study, precision is used to measure the accuracy of the model's positive predictions, specifically for each speech development category (Atypical, Typical Development (TD), Articulation, and Delay). It is calculated by determining the proportion of true positives among all instances predicted as positive by the model [34].

$$Precision = \frac{TP}{(TP + FP)} \times 100 \tag{2}$$

Recall (or sensitivity): In this study, recall is used to measure the model's ability to identify all relevant instances of a particular speech development category (Atypical, Typical Development (TD), Articulation, and Delay). It calculates the proportion of true positives among all actual positive instances in the dataset, providing an indication of how effectively the model captures true positives and minimizes false negatives [34].

$$Recall = \frac{TP}{(TP + FN)} \times 100 \tag{3}$$

F1-Score: In this study, the *F1-score* is used to provide a balanced evaluation of the model's performance across the different speech development categories, including Atypical, Typical Development (TD), Articulation, and Delay. The *F1-score* combines both precision and recall, calculating their harmonic mean to deliver a single metric that accounts for both false positive (*FP*) and false negative (*FN*) occurrences [34].

$$F1\ Score = 2 \times \frac{Precision \times Recall}{(Precision + Recall)} \times 100 \tag{4}$$

Area Under the Receiver Operating Characteristic Curve (*AUC*): The *AUC* evaluates the overall performance of a classification model by quantifying its ability to distinguish between different classes [34]. It is computed by measuring the area under the Receiver Operating Characteristic (*ROC*) curve, which plots the True Positive Rate (TPR) or sensitivity against the False Positive Rate (FPR), calculated as 1−Specificity; mathematically, *AUC* can be expressed as [34]:

$$AUC = \int_0^1 ROC\ curve(TP)\ d(FP) \times 100 \tag{5}$$

To improve model performance, we implemented a feature engineering strategy that included Principal Component Analysis (PCA) for dimensionality reduction and K-Means clustering to identify latent subgroups in the phonological profiles. The resulting cluster labels were incorporated as additional features, and models were re-evaluated accordingly. This process led to a noticeable improvement in classification accuracy. However, no explicit hyperparameter tuning (e.g., grid search or random search) was conducted, as the goal was to establish baseline performance using default model parameters. Future research will incorporate advanced optimization techniques to refine model performance further.

SHAP analysis was applied to interpret the contributions of individual features in the model's predictions [34]. SHAP values quantify the impact of each feature on the model's output, providing insights into the most influential features for distinguishing between speech categories (Atypical, Typical Development (TD), Articulation, and Delay).

The SHAP value for a feature is calculated as:

$$\phi(f) = \phi_0 + \sum_{j=1}^{M} \frac{f(x_i) - E[f(x_i)]}{M} \tag{6}$$

where

$\phi(f)$: Represents the SHAP values for a particular feature.
ϕ_0: Is the expected value of the model's prediction.
M: Is the total number of features.
$f(x_i)$: Is the model's prediction when feature i is included.
$E[f(x_i)]$: Is the expected prediction when feature i is excluded.

For this study, SHAP values were calculated using TreeExplainer for Random Forest and XGBoost models, and KernelExplainer for the SVM model. The analysis highlighted features like Percentage of Consonants Correct (PCC) and Phonological Variance (PhonVar) as the most critical for distinguishing between Atypical and Typical Development (TD) speech patterns. PCC was linked to TD speech, while PhonVar was more indicative of Atypical speech, providing clear insights into which phonological features influenced the model's predictions.

Unsupervised Clustering with K-Means

To uncover natural groupings in the phonological profiles, K-Means clustering was implemented. This algorithm partitions data into k clusters by minimizing intra-cluster variance, making it useful for identifying developmental subtypes based on error patterns [35].

The Elbow Method and Silhouette Score were used to determine the optimal number of clusters, enhancing the validity of the groupings [35].

Additionally, Principal Component Analysis (PCA) was applied to reduce dimensionality for visualization purposes, aiding in the interpretation of cluster structure and the relationship between features and developmental trends [35].

To classify speech development patterns into distinct groups based on phonological features, an unsupervised clustering approach using K-Means clustering was used. This method allowed for the identification of natural subgroups within the dataset based on phonological characteristics such as Phonological Variance (PhonVar), Infrequent Variance (InfrVar), and Percentage of Consonants Correct (PCC). Children were categorized into phonological subgroups using the K-Means clustering algorithm, which minimizes the within-cluster variance [35]:

$$J = \sum_{k=1}^{K} \sum_{i \epsilon C_k} \left|\left| x_i - \mu_k \right|\right|^2 \quad (7)$$

where

J: Cost function (Within-Cluster Sum of Squares, WCSS).
K: Number of clusters.
x_i: Phonological feature vector of child i.
C_k: Set of children assigned to cluster k.
μ_k: Centroid (mean feature vector) of cluster k.
$||x_i - \mu_k||^2$: Squared Euclidean distance between child i and the centroid of its cluster.

The clustering process was applied with K = 4, corresponding to the four speech categories: Atypical, Typical Development (TD), Articulation, and Delay. The choice of four clusters was based on the categorization criteria of the study.

To ensure robust clustering results, missing data were addressed systematically. Missing values, primarily due to occasional data recording errors, were handled through listwise deletion to exclude any incomplete records. This approach prevented biased or distorted cluster formation, as clustering algorithms rely on complete datasets to effectively differentiate subgroups. Additionally, Z-score standardization was applied to all phonological features to ensure that differences in the scale of these features did not disproportionately affect clustering outcomes. This transformation standardized each feature to have a mean of zero and a standard deviation of one, ensuring equitable contribution of all phonological features in the clustering analysis.

To determine the optimal number of clusters, the Elbow Method was applied by analyzing the Within-Cluster Sum of Squares (WCSS) across a range of cluster values (k = 2 to 10). The Silhouette Score was also used to evaluate the quality of cluster separation. The results indicated that k = 4 provided the best balance between distinct subgrouping and meaningful separation. Following this, K-Means clustering (k = 4) was applied to the standardized dataset, and each child was assigned to one of the four clusters.

For visualization, Principal Component Analysis (PCA) was conducted to reduce the high-dimensional phonological dataset to two principal components (PC1 and PC2). The first component (PC1) captured the majority of the variance in phonological features, reflecting overall speech development patterns. The second component (PC2) accounted for additional variability, particularly changes in specific phonological patterns. A PCA scatter plot was generated to visually distinguish the child subgroups based on clustering results, providing a clear representation of how speech development varied among the children in the study.

Ethical approval for this study was obtained from the Institutional Review Board (IRB) of the Center of Excellence in Intelligent Engineering Systems (CEIES) at King Abdulaziz

University, Jeddah, Saudi Arabia (Protocol Code: 20-CEIES-Bioeth-2024; Approval Date: 12 February 2024). Prior to data collection, all parents received a detailed information sheet outlining the study procedures and provided written informed consent for their children's participation.

3. Results

The performance of six machine learning models, Random Forest, SVM, XGBoost, Logistic Regression, K-Nearest Neighbors, and Naïve Bayes, was evaluated using several metrics: accuracy, precision, recall, F1-score, and AUC. These models were trained and tested on the phonological dataset to classify children into different speech development categories. The results are summarized in Table 2.

Table 2. Model evaluation results.

Model	Accuracy	Precision	Recall	F1-Score	AUC
XGBoost	91.49%	92.73%	91.49%	91.32%	99.14%
Random Forest	91.49%	91.71%	91.49%	91.38%	98.17%
Logistic Regression	89.36%	90.66%	89.36%	89.31%	98.44%
SVM	85.11%	89.64%	85.11%	84.76%	98.70%
K-Nearest Neighbors	85.11%	86.10%	85.11%	85.06%	95.47%
Naïve Bayes	55.32%	41.09%	55.32%	44.46%	90.23%

The XGBoost model outperformed the other models with the highest accuracy (91.49%), precision (92.73%), recall (91.49%), F1-score (91.32%), and AUC (99.14%). This indicates that XGBoost was the most effective in classifying speech patterns, followed by Random Forest, which also showed strong performance across all metrics, including an accuracy of 91.49% and an AUC of 98.17%.

The SVM model achieved a solid performance, with an accuracy of 85.11% and an AUC of 98.70%, while the Logistic Regression model showed a slightly lower performance, with an accuracy of 89.36% and an AUC of 98.44%. K-Nearest Neighbors and Naïve Bayes were less effective, particularly Naïve Bayes, which had the lowest performance across all metrics, with an accuracy of 55.32%, precision of 41.09%, and AUC of 90.23%.

These results highlight the varying performance of different machine learning models in classifying phonological features, with XGBoost demonstrating the best overall performance, closely followed by Random Forest and SVM.

To further interpret the performance of the machine learning models, SHAP (SHapley Additive exPlanations) analysis was conducted on the highest-performing models: Random Forest, Logistic Regression, and XGBoost. SHAP values were calculated to understand the contribution of each feature to the model's decision-making process and to identify the most influential phonological features used for classifying the speech development categories: Atypical, Typical Development (TD), Articulation, and Delay.

Figure 1 illustrates the SHAP feature importance results for the XGBoost model. The figure shows the relative influence of different phonological features on the model's predictions across the four speech categories.

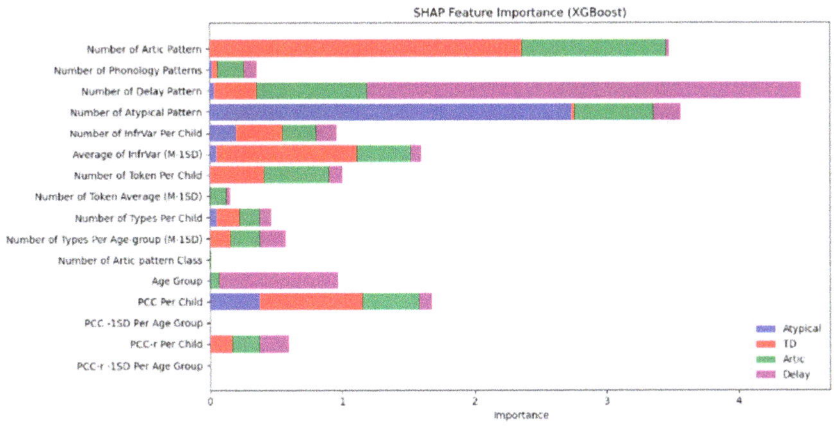

Figure 1. SHAP feature importance (XGBoost).

Number of Artic Pattern emerged as the most important feature for distinguishing between the Atypical (blue) and Delay (purple) categories, as shown by the longest bars for these categories.

Number of Phonology Patterns was another highly influential feature, contributing significantly to the identification of Atypical and Delay speech patterns.

Number of Delay Pattern had a strong impact on classifying Delay (purple), while Number of Atypical Pattern contributed notably to identifying the Atypical (blue) group.

Other features, such as InfrVar (Infrequent Variance) and PCC (Percentage of Consonants Correct), played a role in distinguishing Articulation (red) and Delay (purple), but with less significance than the primary phonological features.

These findings provide insights into the phonological patterns that are most influential in differentiating speech development categories, further supporting the development of targeted diagnostic models for children with speech disorders. In Figure 1, the color bars represent different speech categories, with each bar's length corresponding to the importance of that feature in predicting the class. Longer bars indicate greater influence on the classification decision, providing a clear understanding of which phonological features are most critical in differentiating between the four categories.

This SHAP analysis reinforces the role of phonological patterns, particularly Artic Pattern and Phonology Patterns, in speech classification and can guide future diagnostic and therapeutic approaches for children exhibiting speech delays.

In Figure 2, Number of Artic Pattern and Number of Phonology Patterns were the most influential features, particularly in distinguishing between Atypical and Delay categories, with a higher contribution from Atypical (red) and Delay (purple) classes.

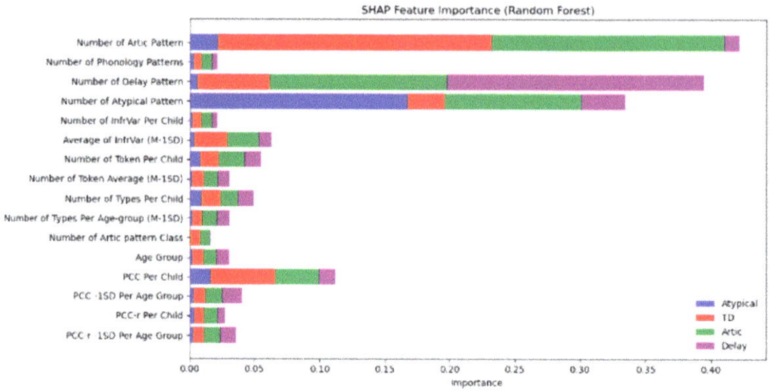

Figure 2. SHAP feature importance (Random Forest).

Number of Delay Pattern and Number of Atypical Pattern were critical in identifying Atypical speech (red) and Delay (purple).

Other features such as PCC (Percentage of Consonants Correct), InfrVar (Infrequent Variance), and Number of Types Per Age-group also contributed to the model's classification decisions, but with lower significance compared to the primary phonological patterns.

Figure 2 visually demonstrates the feature importance based on SHAP values, where the red bars represent the Atypical category, blue bars indicate Typical Development (TD), green bars represent Articulation, and purple bars reflect Delay. By analyzing these results, we gain deeper insights into the phonological features that most effectively differentiate between the speech categories, supporting the development of more targeted diagnostic and intervention strategies.

In addition to the Random Forest model, SHAP (SHapley Additive exPlanations) analysis was also conducted on the Logistic Regression model to further understand the influence of each phonological feature on the classification of speech development categories. The SHAP values for the Logistic Regression model are shown in Figure 3.

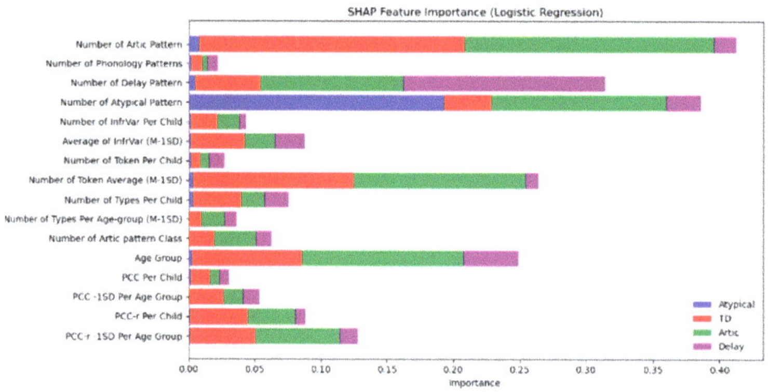

Figure 3. SHAP feature importance (Logistic Regression).

Key findings from the Logistic Regression SHAP analysis:

Number of Artic Pattern and Number of Phonology Patterns are again the most influential features, with a particularly strong impact on distinguishing between Atypical (blue) and Delay (purple) categories.

Number of Delay Pattern and Number of Atypical Pattern are the most important features for classifying Atypical (blue) and Delay (purple) groups.

PCC (Percentage of Consonants Correct) and InfrVar (Infrequent Variance) also play significant roles, particularly in differentiating Articulation (red) from Atypical (blue) and Delay (purple) categories. Similar to the Random Forest model, Figure 3 demonstrates that phonological patterns such as Number of Artic Pattern and Number of Phonology Patterns stand out as the most influential in determining the speech category, emphasizing the relevance of phonological features in diagnosing typical and atypical speech development.

To determine the optimal number of clusters for the K-Means clustering analysis, the Elbow Method was applied. Figure 4 shows the plot of the Within-Cluster Sum of Squares (WCSS) as a function of the number of clusters, ranging from 1 to 10.

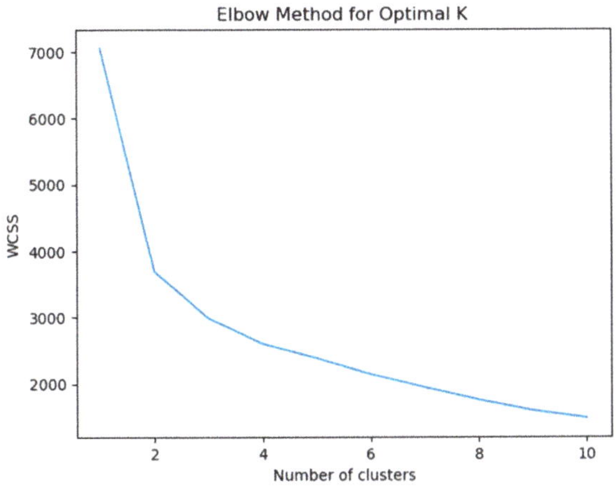

Figure 4. Elbow method for optimal K.

The Elbow Method identifies the optimal number of clusters by looking for the point at which the rate of decrease in WCSS slows significantly, forming an "elbow." In Figure 4, the sharp drop in WCSS from 1 to 2 clusters is followed by a more gradual decline as the number of clusters increases. Although the most significant change occurs between 1 and 2 clusters, the plot indicates that adding more clusters (particularly 4 clusters) still provides meaningful reduction in variance, and the improvement starts to plateau after that.

Therefore, the 4 clusters chosen in the study represent a reasonable balance between minimizing WCSS and ensuring meaningful segmentation. These four clusters correspond to the key speech categories, Atypical, Typical Development (TD), Articulation, and Delay, each of which was identified as an important factor in classifying speech development patterns. Figure 4 demonstrates the trade-off between cluster number and WCSS, helping justify the choice of four clusters as the optimal solution for analyzing speech development trends in this study. The four clusters provide the necessary granularity to distinguish different speech patterns effectively while maintaining model simplicity and interpretability.

To further explore the data and visualize the distribution of the clusters, Principal Component Analysis (PCA) was applied to reduce the dimensionality of the dataset. Figure 5 shows the 2D representation of the phonological data, with the four identified clusters color-coded: Atypical (yellow), Typical Development (TD) (blue), Articulation (green), and Delay (purple).

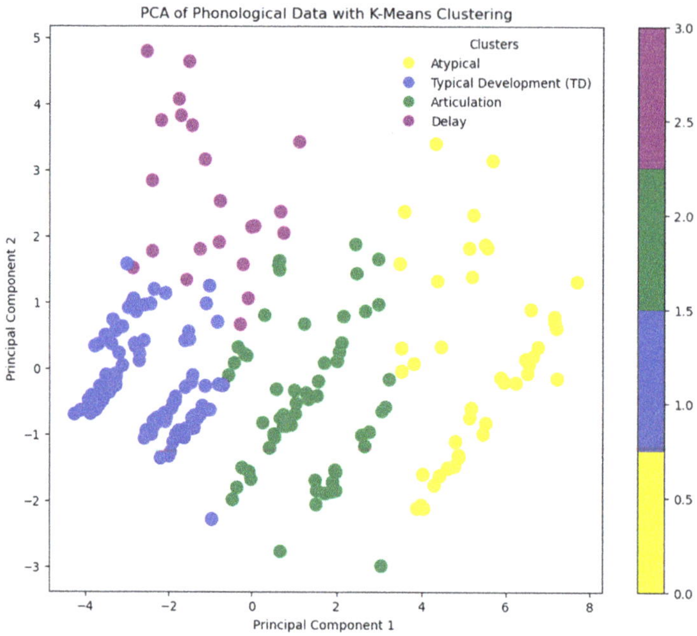

Figure 5. PCA of phonological data with K-Means clustering.

The plot effectively captures the variation in speech development across the four clusters. The clusters are well-separated along Principal Component 1 (PC1), with each category clearly grouped based on its phonological features.

Atypical (yellow): This group, representing atypical speech development, is positioned distinctly towards the top-right of the plot, indicating that children in this group show phonological characteristics that are significantly different from the other groups.

Typical Development (TD) (blue): The TD group appears in the lower half of the plot, suggesting that their phonological patterns align with expected developmental milestones for their age.

Articulation (green): This cluster is positioned between the TD and Delay groups, indicating that children in this category exhibit some atypical features, but are closer to the TD group than the Delay group.

Delay (purple): Children in this cluster exhibit the most distinct phonological patterns, with this group being positioned separately from the other three clusters.

The color-coded scatter plot provides an intuitive understanding of how phonological features relate to each group, making it easier to differentiate between typical and atypical speech patterns. The plot illustrates that clustering based on these phonological features effectively identifies distinct subgroups in the dataset, which is valuable for further analysis of speech development in Saudi Arabic-speaking children.

Following the application of PCA for dimensionality reduction and K-Means clustering to identify distinct subgroups based on phonological data, the performance of the machine learning models was re-evaluated. The integration of cluster labels as additional features improved the models' ability to classify speech development patterns more effectively.

Table 3 shows the updated evaluation results after incorporating the clustering features into the models:

Table 3. Updated models evaluation.

Model	Accuracy	Precision	Recall	F1-Score	AUC
Random Forest	93.62%	93.88%	93.62%	93.57%	98.80%
XGBoost	93.62%	93.88%	93.62%	93.57%	98.63%
SVM	86.17%	86.69%	86.17%	86.14%	95.40%
Logistic Regression	85.11%	85.11%	85.11%	85.06%	93.06%
K-Nearest Neighbors	78.72%	79.03%	78.72%	78.57%	91.94%
Naïve Bayes	59.57%	69.04%	59.57%	52.48%	91.39%

After incorporating the clustering features, both Random Forest and XGBoost demonstrated the best performance, with Accuracy, Precision, Recall, F1-score, and AUC all significantly higher than those of the other models. Both models achieved an AUC greater than 0.98, indicating their strong ability to distinguish between different speech development categories. SVM, while also performing well, fell behind the ensemble methods, with a slightly lower AUC and F1-score. Logistic Regression showed reasonable performance, but displayed a slight drop in metrics compared to the tree-based models. On the other hand, K-Nearest Neighbors (KNN) and Naïve Bayes exhibited the lowest performance, particularly in terms of F1-score and AUC, suggesting that these models had more difficulty in accurately classifying the speech development categories.

Integrating the PCA-derived cluster labels into the models significantly enhanced their ability to differentiate between typical and atypical speech development patterns. Random Forest and XGBoost, both ensemble methods, were the most effective, likely due to their superior capability in handling complex feature interactions and utilizing the additional cluster information. These findings underscore the importance of combining dimensionality reduction and clustering techniques with machine learning models to improve their performance in analyzing speech development.

The clustering results revealed four distinct subgroups based on the speech development patterns observed in the dataset. Typical Development (TD) was the largest subgroup, comprising 110 children, representing 46.61% of the total sample. This group displayed characteristics consistent with typical speech development patterns.

The second-largest subgroup, Articulation Issues, consisted of 60 children, or 25.42% of the sample. These children exhibited speech patterns that indicated specific articulation difficulties, but did not fall into the category of atypical development.

The third group, Atypical Speech Development, included 44 children, accounting for 18.64% of the sample. This subgroup showed significant deviations from typical speech patterns, suggesting atypical developmental trajectories.

Finally, the Speech Delay group, which represented 9.32% of the total sample (22 children), exhibited delays in speech development compared to age-appropriate norms, but did not necessarily show atypical phonological patterns.

These findings, illustrated in Table 4, highlight the heterogeneity in speech development within the study population, with a significant proportion of children exhibiting either articulation issues or delayed speech development. The cluster labels derived from the analysis provide valuable insights into these distinct developmental categories, offering a basis for targeted intervention strategies in speech therapy.

Table 4. Distribution of Speech Development Subgroups Identified Through Clustering.

Cluster	Subgroup Name	Number of Children	Percentage%
0	Atypical Speech Development	44	18.64
1	Typical Development (TD)	110	46.61
2	Articulation Issues	60	25.42
3	Speech Delay	22	9.32

4. Discussion

The results of this study offer critical insights into the classification of speech development patterns among monolingual Saudi Arabic-speaking children. By leveraging machine learning models, including Random Forest, XGBoost, SVM, Logistic Regression, K-Nearest Neighbors, and Naïve Bayes, this research aimed to distinguish between four key speech categories: Atypical, Typical Development (TD), Articulation Issues, and Speech Delay. The performance of these models was assessed based on standard metrics, including accuracy, precision, recall, F1-score, and AUC. The Random Forest and XGBoost models emerged as the most effective classifiers, demonstrating their superior capacity to differentiate between these speech categories.

4.1. Strengths of Random Forest and XGBoost Models

The remarkable performance of the Random Forest and XGBoost models can be attributed to their ensemble nature, which allows them to combine multiple decision trees to make more robust predictions. These models are particularly adept at capturing complex, non-linear relationships between the features, making them best for this study where phonological features exhibit intricate patterns. Moreover, these algorithms can model interactions between features effectively, which is crucial when working with speech data that involves high-dimensional features such as Phonology Patterns, InfrVar, and PCC.

The significant improvement in model performance after incorporating cluster labels derived from PCA and K-Means clustering further reinforces the importance of this approach. By adding cluster information to the models, we were able to enhance the differentiation between Atypical and TD children, leading to improved accuracy and higher AUC scores. This suggests that the clustering approach helped capture additional structure in the data, allowing the models to classify speech patterns with greater precision.

4.2. Support Vector Machine (SVM) Performance

While SVM also performed relatively well, its metrics were slightly lower than those of Random Forest and XGBoost. The AUC and F1-score for SVM were lower, indicating that this model struggled more in distinguishing between some of the subtler differences in speech development patterns. SVM is a powerful algorithm when the data have clear linear decision boundaries, but it may not perform as well when the relationships between features are highly non-linear, as is the case with the phonological features in this study. This may explain why SVM showed slightly reduced performance compared to the tree-based methods.

4.3. Logistic Regression and Its Limitations

Logistic Regression exhibited reasonable performance, but showed a noticeable drop in accuracy and AUC compared to Random Forest and XGBoost. Logistic regression is a relatively straightforward model that assumes a linear relationship between the features and the outcome. However, this assumption may not hold true in complex classification tasks, such as those involving speech development, where the relationships between features are often non-linear and multifactorial. Consequently, relying on logistic regression in such contexts may limit the model's ability to accurately capture the intricate and dynamic nature of speech development. The AUC score of 0.930 suggests that while it provides a decent classification model, it does not capture the complexities of phonological variations as effectively as the ensemble methods. This could be due to its inability to model feature interactions and non-linearities, as well as tree-based algorithms.

4.4. K-Nearest Neighbors (KNN) and Naïve Bayes

Both K-Nearest Neighbors (KNN) and Naïve Bayes exhibited the lowest performance among the models tested. KNN, despite being a simple and effective algorithm for some tasks, struggles with high-dimensional data, which often leads to reduced classification accuracy. The F1-score and AUC for KNN were significantly lower, suggesting that it was unable to accurately capture the subtle distinctions between speech development categories. Naïve Bayes, with its assumption of feature independence, is also less suitable for this type of task. Phonological features are likely correlated with each other, and the Naïve Bayes model's inability to account for these dependencies likely explains its poor performance in this context.

4.5. SHAP Analysis: Interpreting Feature Importance

The SHAP (SHapley Additive exPlanations) analysis provided valuable insights into which phonological features were most influential in the classification decisions of the Random Forest, Logistic Regression, and XGBoost models. The Number of Articulation Patterns and Number of Phonology Patterns were identified as the most important features for distinguishing between the Atypical and TD groups, with these features showing the highest impact on model predictions. The prominence of these features aligns with the existing literature, which emphasizes the importance of phonological variations in speech development, especially when identifying atypical patterns.

Other significant features identified in the SHAP analysis, such as PCC (Percentage of Consonants Correct) and InfrVar (Infrequent Variance), further highlighted the critical role of specific phonological measures in distinguishing between Articulation Issues and Speech Delay. The SHAP results confirm that PCC and InfrVar are effective markers for identifying phonological difficulties and delays, with SHAP values ranking these features consistently within the top five across all models. This reinforces their clinical utility, especially when used alongside Articulation and Phonology Pattern counts, which demonstrated the highest SHAP contributions overall. Across all models, the top five features by SHAP importance were (1) Number of Articulation Patterns, (2) Number of Phonology Patterns, (3) Number of Delay Patterns, (4) Percentage of Consonants Correct (PCC), and (5) Infrequent Variance (InfrVar), demonstrating their strong predictive influence on classification decisions

These SHAP-based insights align with our empirical findings regarding Infrequent Variance (InfrVar). In this study, a high incidence of InfrVar was interpreted as a potential red flag for atypical phonological development. While not diagnostic in isolation, elevated InfrVar values, particularly when combined with low PCC or a high number of atypical patterns, served as strong indicators of SSD risk or presence. This rationale is supported by prior phonological research, and our analysis of 235 monolingual Saudi Hejazi Arabic-speaking children further substantiates it [11,12]. InfrVar accounted for a substantial portion of phonological variation, and its progressive reduction with age corresponded with developmental stabilization. This trend reinforces InfrVar's value as a sensitive diagnostic marker. Unlike earlier studies that often excluded rare phonological errors, our approach integrates InfrVar to model phonological variability that may otherwise be dismissed, thereby enhancing early identification efforts in culturally specific speech assessment.

4.6. K-Means Clustering and Subgroup Identification

The K-Means clustering approach identified four distinct subgroups within the dataset, representing different speech development patterns: Typical Development (TD), Articulation Issues, Atypical Speech Development, and Speech Delay. The largest group, TD, comprised 46.6% of the sample, reflecting typical speech development characteristics. Articulation Issues (25.4%) and Atypical Speech Development (18.6%) represented a significant proportion of children, indicating that a large segment of the population exhibited some level of phonological variation that warranted attention. The smallest group, Speech Delay (9.3%), highlighted the presence of children who exhibited delays in speech development, although they did not show atypical phonological patterns.

These results emphasize the heterogeneity of speech development and the need for targeted interventions based on the specific challenges children face. The clustering approach allowed us to uncover subgroups that may have been overlooked using traditional methods, providing a clearer picture of the diverse developmental trajectories in the sample. Although this study focused on Saudi Hejazi Arabic, the classification model was trained on abstracted phonological features rather than raw speech, allowing for potential generalization to other Arabic dialects. Provided that dialect-specific normative data are available and processed using the same analytic framework, the model could be retrained or adapted for broader use across diverse Arabic-speaking populations.

Additionally, this study did not compare the results to non-machine learning methods such as expert-derived scoring or rule-based classification frameworks. This was due to the exploratory nature of the analysis and the focus on evaluating the diagnostic utility of machine learning algorithms. Future research should include comparative benchmarks against traditional clinical or statistical approaches to more comprehensively assess the added value of ML-based tools in speech disorder diagnostics.

The classification criteria employed in this study, specifically the use of a 10% occurrence threshold for phonological pattern classification and the application of the M–1SD cutoff for PCC and other measures, were based on well-established practices in speech-language pathology. These thresholds are commonly used in clinical phonological assessments to differentiate between age-appropriate, delayed, and deviant patterns [30–33]. For instance, the DEAP diagnostic framework adopts similar thresholds for determining clinical significance [33], while normative studies such as Dodd et al. support the use of frequency-based criteria for distinguishing typical and atypical speech development [30]. Additionally, Shriberg et al. provided empirical validation for the use of PCC and its standard deviation adjustments in identifying children at risk for speech sound disorders [32]. Although the dataset used here was originally normative, our application of these thresholds allowed for meaningful identification of phonological profiles consistent with atypical development. Nonetheless, these thresholds serve as heuristic tools, and future studies should validate their diagnostic sensitivity and specificity against clinical evaluations in diverse populations.

4.7. Limitations

This study has several limitations that should be acknowledged. First, the dataset used was originally collected as part of a normative study and did not include formally diagnosed cases of speech sound disorders (SSDs). As such, while the classification models identified patterns consistent with atypical development, these findings require validation against clinically confirmed data. Second, the machine learning models were trained using default hyperparameters without extensive tuning or optimization, which may limit their performance relative to fully optimized models. Third, the speech data were based on structured single-word naming tasks rather than spontaneous speech samples, which may restrict the generalizability of the findings to naturalistic settings.

Fourth, while the study focused on Saudi Hejazi Arabic, broader generalization to other dialects of Arabic would require retraining the models using dialect-specific phonological norms. Fifth, the use of principal component analysis (PCA) prior to K-Means clustering, while effective for linear dimensionality reduction, may not capture non-linear relationships in the data as well as alternatives like t-SNE or UMAP. Sixth, some diagnostic subgroups, such as Atypical ($n = 22$) and Delay ($n = 37$), were underrepresented compared to others, which may reduce the statistical power and generalizability of findings for these categories. Seventh, model performance was evaluated only on internal train–test splits; no external validation dataset was used, which may limit generalizability across populations or settings.

Eighth, although phonological transcriptions were performed by a certified speech-language pathologist with high inter- and intra-rater reliability, manual transcription inherently carries the risk of subjectivity and perceptual bias. Future studies may benefit from incorporating semi-automated transcription tools to enhance objectivity and reproducibility. Finally, the study design was cross-sectional, limiting the ability to evaluate the longitudinal predictive validity of measures like InfrVar. Prospective, longitudinal studies are needed to determine whether these phonological markers reliably predict persistent SSD outcomes over time.

Future work should address these limitations by including clinical samples, conducting hyperparameter optimization, incorporating spontaneous speech data, applying advanced dimensionality reduction techniques, expanding to additional dialects, validating models with external datasets, and exploring longitudinal developmental trajectories.

5. Conclusions

In conclusion, the combination of machine learning models, dimensionality reduction (PCA), and clustering techniques has proven to be effective in analyzing speech development in Saudi Arabic-speaking children. The Random Forest and XGBoost models performed exceptionally well, with AUC scores above 0.98, indicating their high capacity to distinguish between different speech development patterns. The integration of cluster labels derived from PCA and K-Means clustering further improved the models' performance, highlighting the value of clustering in capturing latent patterns in the data. Additionally, the SHAP analysis provided critical insights into the key phonological features, such as Number of Articulation Patterns and PCC, which were instrumental in classifying speech development categories. These findings underscore the importance of using advanced machine learning techniques to analyze and interpret complex speech data, providing a foundation for more targeted and effective interventions for children with speech delays or disorders.

Author Contributions: Conceptualization, D.F.T.; methodology, A.F.T.; software, A.F.T.; validation, A.F.T.; writing—original draft, A.F.T. and D.F.T.; visualization, A.F.T.; Supervision, D.F.T.; project administration, D.F.T. All authors have read and agreed to the published version of the manuscript.

Funding: This project was funded by the Deanship of Scientific Research (DSR) at King Abdulaziz University, Jeddah, Saudi Arabia, under grant no. (GPIP: 1018-883-2024). The authors gratefully acknowledge the DSR for its technical and financial support.

Institutional Review Board Statement: This study was conducted in accordance with the Declaration of Helsinki and was approved by the Institutional Review Board (IRB) of the Center of Excellence in Intelligent Engineering Systems (CEIES) at King Abdulaziz University, Jeddah, Saudi Arabia (protocol code 20-CEIES-Bioeth-2024, approved on 12 February 2024).

Informed Consent Statement: Informed consent was obtained from all subjects involved in the study.

Data Availability Statement: Data supporting the results reported in this study are available upon reasonable request. Due to privacy and ethical considerations, the dataset generated and analyze during this study is not publicly available. Requests for access to the data can be directed to the corresponding author and will be evaluated in accordance with institutional and ethical guidelines.

Acknowledgments: We would like to express our gratitude to our colleagues from the Center of Excellence in Intelligent Engineering Systems (CEIES) at King Abdulaziz University for their valuable contributions.

Conflicts of Interest: The authors declare no conflicts of interest.

References

1. Brahmi, Z.; Mahyoob, M.; Al-Sarem, M.; Algaraady, J.; Bousselmi, K.; Alblwi, A. Exploring the Role of Machine Learning in Diagnosing and Treating Speech Disorders: A Systematic Literature Review. *Psychol. Res. Behav. Manag.* **2024**, *17*, 2205–2232. [CrossRef] [PubMed] [PubMed Central]
2. Hitchcock, E.R.; Harel, D.; Byun, T.M. Social, Emotional, and Academic Impact of Residual Speech Errors in School-Aged Children: A Survey Study. *Semin. Speech Lang.* **2015**, *36*, 283–294. [CrossRef] [PubMed] [PubMed Central]
3. American Speech-Language-Hearing Association. Speech Sound Disorders: Articulation and Phonology [Practice Portal]. Available online: https://www.asha.org/practice-portal/clinical-topics/articulation-and-phonology/ (accessed on 17 April 2025).
4. Preston, J.L.; Seki, A. Identifying Residual Speech Sound Disorders in Bilingual Children: A Japanese-English Case Study. *Am. J. Speech Lang. Pathol.* **2011**, *20*, 73–85. [CrossRef] [PubMed] [PubMed Central]
5. Fabiano-Smith, L.; Hoffman, K. Diagnostic Accuracy of Traditional Measures of Phonological Ability for Bilingual Preschoolers and Kindergarteners. *Lang. Speech Hear. Serv. Sch.* **2018**, *49*, 121–134. [CrossRef] [PubMed] [PubMed Central]
6. Preston, J.L.; Ramsdell, H.L.; Oller, D.K.; Edwards, M.L.; Tobin, S.J. Developing a Weighted Measure of Speech Sound Accuracy. *J. Speech Lang. Hear. Res.* **2011**, *54*, 1–18. [CrossRef] [PubMed] [PubMed Central]
7. SLP Now. The SLP's Guide to Speech Sound Disorders: Articulation & Phonological Development [Blog post]. Available online: https://slpnow.com/the-slps-guide-to-speech-sound-disorders-articulation-phonological-development/ (accessed on 17 April 2025).
8. Amayreh, M.M.; Dyson, A.T. The Acquisition of Arabic Consonants. *J. Speech Hear. Res.* **1998**, *41*, 642–653. [CrossRef]
9. Abdoh, E. The Acquisition of Syllable Structure in the Speech of Typically Developing Saudi Arabic-Speaking Children. Ph.D. Thesis, University of Leeds, Leeds, UK, 2010.
10. Dyson, A.T.; Amayreh, M.M. Phonological errors and sound changes in Arabic-speaking children. *Clin. Linguist. Phon.* **2000**, *14*, 79–109. [CrossRef]
11. Albrecht, K.M. The Identification of Typical and Atypical Phonological Acquisition in Turkish-German Bilingual Children. Ph.D. Thesis, University of Sheffield, Sheffield, UK, 2017.
12. Fox-Boyer, A.; Lavaggi, S.; Fricke, S. Phonological variations in typically-developing Italian-speaking children aged 3; 0–4; 11. *Clin. Linguist. Phon.* **2021**, *0–19*, 241–259. [CrossRef]
13. Elrefaie, D.A.; Hegazi, M.A.E.F.; El-Mahallawi, M.M.; Hegab, M.H.; El-Attar, Y.M. Descriptive Analysis of the Development of the Arabic Speech Sounds among Typically Developing Colloquial Egyptian Arabic-Speaking Children. *Egypt. J. Otolaryngol.* **2021**, *37*, 38. [CrossRef]
14. Al-Solami, M. Arabic Emphatics: Phonetic and Phonological Remarks. *Open J. Mod. Linguist.* **2013**, *3*, 432–440. [CrossRef]
15. Suthar, K.; Yousefi Zowj, F.; Speights Atkins, M.; He, Q.P. Feature engineering and machine learning for computer-assisted screening of children with speech disorders. *PLOS Digit. Health* **2022**, *1*, e0000041. [CrossRef] [PubMed] [PubMed Central]
16. Kuo, Y.M.; Ruan, S.J.; Chen, Y.C.; Tu, Y.W. Deep-Learning-Based Automated Classification of Chinese Speech Sound Disorders. *Children* **2022**, *9*, 996. [CrossRef] [PubMed] [PubMed Central]
17. Aljarallah, N.A.; Dutta, A.K.; Sait, A.R.W. Image classification-driven speech disorder detection using deep learning technique. *SLAS Technol.* **2025**, *32*, 100261. [CrossRef]
18. Zhang, J.; Wu, J.; Qiu, Y.; Song, A.; Li, W.; Li, X.; Liu, Y. Intelligent speech technologies for transcription, disease diagnosis, and medical equipment interactive control in smart hospitals: A review. *Comput Biol Med.* **2023**, *153*, 106517. [CrossRef] [PubMed] [PubMed Central]
19. Cordella, C.; Marte, M.J.; Liu, H.; Kiran, S. An introduction to machine learning for speech-language pathologists: Concepts, terminology, and emerging applications. *Perspect. ASHA Spec. Interest Groups* **2025**, *10*, 432–450. [CrossRef]
20. Li, Y.; Pham, D.-S.; Ward, R.; Hennessey, N.; Tan, T. Using AI to automate phonetic transcription and perform forced alignment for clinical application in the assessment of speech sound disorders. In Proceedings of the 39th Annual AAAI Conference on Artificial Intelligence, GenAI4Health Workshop. Philadelphia, PA, USA, 25 February–4 March, 2025; Available online: https://openreview.net/forum?id=WDEf1pTFwE (accessed on 16 April 2025).

21. Benway, N.R.; Preston, J.L. Artificial intelligence–assisted speech therapy for /ɹ/: A single-case experimental study. *Am. J. Speech-Lang. Pathol.* **2024**, *33*, 2461–2486. [CrossRef]
22. Han, G.R.; Goncharov, A.; Eryilmaz, M.; Ye, S.; Palanisamy, B.; Ghosh, R.; Lisi, F.; Rogers, E.; Guzman, D.; Yigci, D.; et al. Machine learning in point-of-care testing: Innovations, challenges, and opportunities. *Nat. Commun.* **2025**, *16*, 3165. [CrossRef]
23. Al Huneety, A.; Al-Omari, M.A.K.; Mashaqba, B.; Abu Guba, M.N. Assessing the Phonological Abilities of Jordanian Arabic-speaking Children with Phonological Disorders. *Commun. Sci. Disord.* **2024**, *29*, 127–144. [CrossRef]
24. Alyahya, R.S.W. The Development of a Novel, Standardized, Norm-Referenced Arabic Discourse Assessment Tool (ADAT), Including an Examination of Psychometric Properties of Discourse Measures in Aphasia. *Int. J. Lang. Commun. Disord.* **2024**, *59*, 2103–2117. [CrossRef]
25. Taha, J.; Stojanovik, V.; Pagnamenta, E. Nonword Repetition Performance of Arabic-Speaking Children with and without Developmental Language Disorder: A Study on Diagnostic Accuracy. *J. Speech Lang. Hear. Res.* **2021**, *64*, 2750–2765. [CrossRef]
26. Mesallam, T.A.; Farahat, M.; Malki, K.H.; Alsulaiman, M.; Ali, Z.; Al-Nasheri, A.; Muhammad, G. Development of the Arabic Voice Pathology Database and Its Evaluation by Using Speech Features and Machine Learning Algorithms. *J. Healthc. Eng.* **2017**, *2017*, 8783751. [CrossRef]
27. Hanani, A.; Attari, M.; Farakhna, A.; Joma'a, A.; Hussein, M.; Taylor, S. Automatic Identification of Speech Disorders for Arabic Children Speakers. In Proceedings of the 5th Workshop on Child Computer Interaction (WOCCI 2016), San Francisco, CA, USA, 6–7 September 2016.
28. Shareef, S.R.; Al-Irhayim, Y.F. Towards Developing Impairments Arabic Speech Dataset Using Deep Learning. *Indones. J. Electr. Eng. Comput. Sci.* **2022**, *25*, 1400–1405. [CrossRef]
29. Turki, D.F. Phonological Development of Typically Developing Monolingual Saudi Hejazi Arabic-speaking Children Aged 2; 6–5; 11. Ph.D. Thesis, The University of Sheffield, Sheffield, UK, September 2022.
30. Dodd, B.; Holm, A.; Hua, Z.; Crosbie, S. Phonological development: A normative study of British English-speaking children. *Clin. Linguist. Phon.* **2003**, *17*, 617–643. [CrossRef]
31. McLeod, S.; Baker, E. *Children's Speech: An Evidence-Based Approach to Assessment and Intervention*; Pearson Education: London, UK, 2017.
32. Shriberg, L.D.; Austin, D.; Lewis, B.A.; McSweeny, J.L.; Wilson, D.L. The Percentage of Consonants Correct (PCC) metric: Extensions and reliability data. *J. Speech Lang. Hear. Res.* **1997**, *40*, 708–722. [CrossRef]
33. Dodd, B.; Zhu, H.; Crosbie, S.; Holm, A.; Ozanne, A. *Diagnostic Evaluation of Articulation and Phonology (DEAP)*; Pearson Clinical Assessment: London, UK, 2002.
34. Turki, A.; Raml, E. Enhancing pediatric adnexal torsion diagnosis: Prediction method utilizing machine learning techniques. *Children* **2023**, *10*, 1612. [CrossRef] [PubMed] [PubMed Central]
35. Basri, A.M.; Turki, A.F. Evaluating Heart Rate Variability as a Biomarker for Autonomic Function in Parkinson's Disease Rehabilitation: A Clustering-Based Analysis of Exercise-Induced Changes. *Medicina* **2025**, *61*, 527. [CrossRef]

diagnostics

MDPI

Article

Predicting Early Outcomes of Prostatic Artery Embolization Using *n*-Butyl Cyanoacrylate Liquid Embolic Agent: A Machine Learning Study

Burak Berksu Ozkara [1], David Bamshad [1], Ramita Gowda [2], Mert Karabacak [3], Vivian Bishay [1], Kirema Garcia-Reyes [1], Ardeshir R. Rastinehad [4], Dan Shilo [1] and Aaron Fischman [1,*]

1 Department of Diagnostic, Molecular and Interventional Radiology, Icahn School of Medicine at Mount Sinai, New York, NY 10029, USA
2 School of Medicine, St. George's University, True Blue, Grenada
3 Department of Neurosurgery, Mount Sinai Health System, New York, NY 10029, USA
4 Department of Urology, Lenox Hill Hospital, New York, NY 10075, USA
* Correspondence: aaron.fischman@mountsinai.org

Abstract: Background/Objectives: Prostatic artery embolization (PAE) has been increasingly recognized, especially with recent progress in embolization techniques for the management of lower urinary tract symptoms due to benign prostatic hyperplasia. Nevertheless, a proportion of patients undergoing PAE fail to demonstrate clinical improvement. Machine learning models have the potential to provide valuable prognostic insights for patients undergoing PAE. **Methods**: A retrospective cohort study was performed utilizing a modified prior-data fitted network architecture to predict short-term (7 weeks) favorable outcomes, defined as a reduction greater than 9 points in the International Prostate Symptom Score (IPSS), in patients who underwent PAE with *n*BCA glue. Patients were stratified into two groups based on the median IPSS reduction value, and a binary classification model was developed to predict the outcome of interest. The model was developed using clinical tabular data, including both pre-procedural and intra-procedural variables. SHapley Additive ExPlanations (SHAP) were used to uncover the relative importance of features. **Results**: The final cohort included 109 patients. The model achieved an accuracy of 0.676, an MCC of 0.363, a precision of 0.666, a recall of 0.856, an F1-score of 0.731, and a Brier score of 0.203, with an AUPRC of 0.851 and an AUROC of 0.821. SHAP analysis identified pre-PAE IPSS, prior therapy, right embolization volume, preoperative quality of life, and age as the top five most influential features. **Conclusions**: Our model showed promising discrimination and calibration in predicting early outcomes of PAE with *n*BCA glue, highlighting the potential of precision medicine to deliver interpretable, individualized risk assessments.

Keywords: prostate artery embolization; machine learning; IPSS; artificial intelligence

1. Introduction

Prostatic artery embolization (PAE) is gaining prominence, particularly with recent advancements in embolization techniques for managing lower urinary tract symptoms associated with benign prostatic hyperplasia [1,2]. However, a subset of patients treated with PAE do not experience any improvement, and a notable proportion faces symptom recurrence [3–5]. Carnevale et al. reported symptom recurrence in 23% of patients at a median follow-up of 72 months, while Xu et al. observed cumulative recurrence rates of 6.8%, 12.7%, and 60.4% after 1, 2, and 5 years, respectively [3,4].

Several novel embolic agents, such as ethylene–vinyl alcohol copolymers, shear-thinning hydrogels, and on-demand degradable microspheres, are being developed to improve precision and safety in embolization procedures, with *n*-butyl cyanoacrylate (*n*BCA) emerging as one of the promising options in this evolving landscape. The use of *n*BCA glue for PAE represents a potentially significant advancement as an alternative to embolization with traditional microspheres, as demonstrated in recent studies showing improvements in patient outcome metrics such as the International Prostate Symptom Score (IPSS) and quality of life (QoL), along with potentially decreased recanalization rates [6–8]. While technical advancements are crucial for improving patient outcomes, optimizing patient selection through advanced interpretable machine learning (ML)/artificial intelligence (AI) models using pre-procedural data may also play a critical role, especially considering the risks inherent to any medical procedure [9,10]. With refinements and further improvements, such models may help determine whether to perform the procedure, foster informed discussions with patients about likely outcomes, and serve as a quality assessment tool when results fall below expectations [11].

The literature on the prognostic prediction of PAE outcomes using ML/AI is extremely limited, with most studies focusing on identifying individual parameters that influence outcomes [2,12–14]. While revealing singular parameters affecting outcomes is essential, by analyzing the combined effects of multiple variables and their interactions, ML/AI models may uncover hidden patterns and capture complex relationships, potentially aiding in prognostication and selecting suitable candidate patients. Martin et al. explored MRI radiomics but unfortunately provided limited benefit, while Vigneswaran et al. successfully utilized tabular pre-treatment data and applied traditional regression-based algorithms in their important study, such as linear regression, to predict the baseline IPSS and the change in IPSS 1 year after PAE [2,15].

In our study, we employed TabPFN, an advanced and novel ML model based on a modified prior-data fitted network (PFN) architecture, to predict IPSS reduction at a 6-week follow-up appointment of PAE performed with *n*BCA using pre-procedural and intra-procedural tabular data. The model was designed for binary classification of the outcome, distinguishing between favorable (IPSS reduction > 9) and unfavorable results. Unlike traditional techniques, our model incorporates interpretable tools, offering actionable insights into feature importance on outcomes. However, this study did not involve computer vision or imaging-derived features, focusing instead on clinical and procedural tabular data. All code has been made publicly available to enhance transparency and foster collaboration.

2. Materials and Methods

This retrospective cohort study used ML to predict a short-term (7 weeks) favorable outcome ([Pre-IPSS] − [Post-IPSS] = IPSS reduction > 9) in patients who underwent PAE. Patients were divided into two groups based on the median value and a binary classifier was created to predict the outcome of interest. Our study followed the Transparent Reporting of Multivariable Prediction Models for Individual Prognosis or Diagnosis–Artificial Intelligence statement [16].

2.1. Patient Selection

This study used a patient cohort from a previous publication by our group [8]. A retrospective review was conducted on 244 consecutive patients who underwent PAE with *n*BCA and ethiodized oil from June 2022 to May 2024 (Figure 1). The study excluded patients who underwent secondary microsphere embolization (n = 5) or returned for contralateral embolization after initial unilateral embolization (n = 8), due to potential confounding effects. In addition, 43 patients missing pre-PAE IPSS, 69 patients missing post-PAE IPSS, and 10 patients missing pre-PAE QoL were excluded from the current study. The final cohort included 109 patients, with data sourced from a Health Insurance Portability and Accountability Act-compliant database under a retrospective protocol approved by the institutional review board at Mount Sinai Hospital (Study number: 21-01756). Due to this study's retrospective nature, individual informed consent was not required.

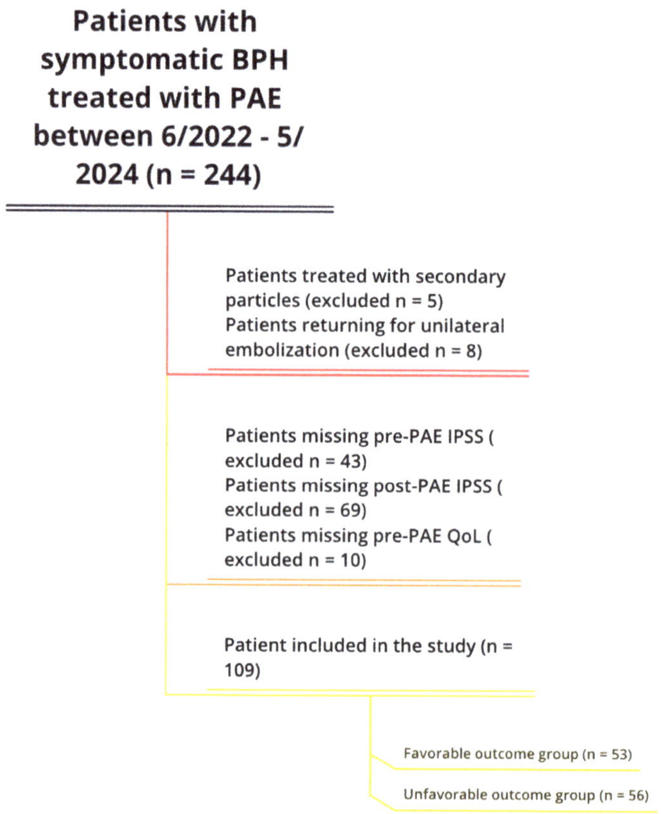

Figure 1. Patient selection.

2.2. Data Collection

The severity of clinical manifestations was evaluated using the 7-item IPSS and the single-item QoL scale, following the AUA Practice Guidelines Committee recommendations [17]. Baseline data were collected for age, pre-PAE IPSS and QoL, uroflowmetry parameters (Qmax and Qavg), prostate gland volume (PGV), pre-operative post-void residual (PVR), pre-operative hematuria, prior therapies, and history of intermittent catheterization or indwelling catheter use. Procedural details, including right and left embolization volumes, the dilution ratio of the embolization material, and the treatment approach (bilateral glue embolization versus unilateral glue embolization with contralateral coil embolization), were documented. The primary outcome, IPSS reduction, was assessed at the 6-week follow-up appointment post PAE. The details of the PAE procedure are explained in the prior study [8].

2.3. Data Preprocessing

To minimize exclusion bias, imputation methods were applied to handle missing data. Among the continuous variables, six had at least one missing value. Variables with over 30% missing data (Qavg, Qmax, and PVR) were excluded. For the remaining variables, the k-nearest neighbor (kNN) algorithm (k = 5) was used to impute missing values by drawing on data from the entire dataset [18]. The kNN method fills in missing values using data from the five most similar cases. For categorical variables, two had missing values, but none were excluded since no variable had more than 30% missing data. Missing values in categorical variables were imputed using the mode. After these steps, all variables were included in the model without feature selection.

2.4. Model Development and Assessment

A modified PFN architecture (TabPFN) was employed for model development. The model was developed to perform binary classification, differentiating between favorable outcomes (IPSS reduction > 9) and unfavorable outcomes (IPSS reduction $\leq$ 9). The >9-point threshold was chosen based on the median IPSS reduction in our cohort to enable a balanced binary classification for model training. TabPFN leverages a meta-learning framework to adapt to novel, unseen data by drawing on insights from various dataset. Prior-data fitted networks are pre-trained on synthetic datasets to approximate Bayesian inference for real-world scenarios, enabling TabPFN to recognize complex patterns in tabular data and adapt well to new datasets, making it especially valuable for small to medium-sized tabular datasets due to its ability to generalize without extensive hyperparameter tuning [19].

Model performance assessment was performed with a 10-repeat, 10-fold stratified cross-validation technique. The dataset was divided into ten nearly equal parts for each repetition with a different random split, ensuring that the outcome class proportions remained consistent across all parts. For each fold in every repetition, the data were divided into a training subset (70% of the total data), a validation subset (10%), and a test set (20%). The validation sets were used for sigmoid calibration to tune predicted risks to observed outcomes. Predictions and probability estimates were generated by the calibrated TabPFN model on each test fold across the ten cross-validation repetitions. Results from all folds and repeats were combined to assess overall performance. Implementing ten repeats enhances the robustness of performance evaluations, minimizes the influence of particular random splits, reduces the risk of overfitting to specific data partitions, and offers a more thorough analysis of model stability. Overall, cross-validation provides a dependable evaluation of the model's generalizable predictive capabilities [11].

Model performance was visually assessed using a receiver operating characteristic (ROC) curve, a precision–recall curve (PRC), and a calibration plot to evaluate the alignment between predicted probabilities and actual outcomes. Furthermore, the area under the ROC curve (AUROC), the area under the PRC (AUPRC), the Brier score, precision, recall, F1-score, and Matthews Correlation Coefficient (MCC) were calculated. For each metric, a 95% confidence interval (CI) was calculated using bootstrapping with 1000 resampled datasets, determined by the 2.5th and 97.5th percentiles of the bootstrapped metric mean values.

To enhance interpretability, SHapley Additive ExPlanations (SHAP) were used to uncover the relative importance of features. The SHAP plot ranked the features in descending order, displaying the most impactful feature at the top. The study's GitHub repository (https://github.com/mertkarabacak/PAE-ML [accessed on 22 May 2025]) provides access to the model code, ensuring complete transparency.

3. Results

As shown on Figure 1, the final cohort included 109 patients in our study. Table 1 presents the patient characteristics for the unfavorable outcome group, the favorable outcome group, and the overall cohort. The mean short-term follow-up period was 7 weeks. All patients underwent PAE with *n*BCA, and all were technically successful. The favorable outcome group (IPSS reduction > 9) consisted of 53 patients, whereas the unfavorable outcome group (IPSS reduction ≤ 9) included 56 patients. The median age was 73.5 (interquartile range [IQR] = 13.5) years in the unfavorable outcome group, 70 (IQR = 12.5) in the favorable outcome group, and 72 (IQR = 13) in the entire cohort.

Table 1. Patient characteristics. IQR = interquartile range, SD = standard deviation, PAE = prostate artery embolization, IPSS = International Prostate Symptom Score, QoL = quality of life, Qmax = maximum flow rate, Qavg = average flow rate, PGV = prostate gland volume, and PVR = post-void residual.

Variables		**Unfavorable Outcome Group (*n* = 56)**	**Favorable Outcome Group (*n* = 53)**	**Combined (*n* = 109)**
		Baseline Characteristics		
Age	Median (IQR), *n*	73.5 (13.5), 56	70 (12.5), 53	72 (13), 109
	Mean ± SD, *n*	73.7 ± 9.7, 56	70 ± 8, 53	71.9 ± 9.1, 109
Pre-PAE IPSS	Median (IQR), *n*	16 (7), 56	25 (8.5), 53	20 (9.5), 109
	Mean ± SD, *n*	16.1 ± 5, 56	24.5 ± 5.2, 53	20.2 ± 6.6, 109
Pre-PAE QoL	Median (IQR), *n*	4 (1), 56	5 (1.5), 53	4 (2), 109
	Mean ± SD, *n*	3.6 ± 1.2, 56	4.2 ± 1.1, 53	3.9 ± 1.2, 109
Pre-PAE Qmax	Median (IQR), *n*	7 (5.5), 33	6.9 (4.4), 29	7 (4), 62
	Mean ± SD, *n*	8.7 ± 6.9, 33	12.7 ± 33.5, 29	10.6 ± 23.3, 62
Pre-PAE Qavg	Median (IQR), *n*	4.05 (4), 6	4.5 (1.55), 12	4.4 (1.9), 18
	Mean ± SD, *n*	5 ± 2, 6	4.5 ± 1.8, 12	4.6 ± 1.8, 18
Pre-PAE PGV	Median (IQR), *n*	86.5 (94), 38	135 (106.85), 40	109 (117.6), 78
	Mean ± SD, *n*	118.9 ± 85.6, 38	143.8 ± 82.1, 40	131.7 ± 84.2, 78
Pre-PAE PVR	Median (IQR), *n*	133.2 (181.5), 20	100 (257.5), 21	120 (235.5), 41
	Mean ± SD, *n*	217 ± 266, 20	167.5 ± 166.7, 21	191.6 ± 219.4, 41
Pre-PAE Hematuria	Yes	20 (35.7%)	21 (39.6%)	41 (37.6%)
	No	27 (48.2%)	29 (54.7%)	56 (51.4%)
	N/A	9 (16.1%)	3 (5.7%)	12 (11.0%)
Prior Therapy	Yes	14 (25%)	4 (7.5%)	18 (16.5%)
	No	42 (75%)	49 (92.5%)	91 (83.5%)
	N/A	0 (0%)	0 (0%)	0 (0%)
Prior Catheterization	Yes	10 (17.9%)	11 (20.8%)	21 (19.3%)
	No	45 (80.3%)	42 (79.2%)	87 (79.8%)
	N/A	1 (1.8%)	0 (0%)	1 (0.9%)
		Procedural Characteristics		
Left Embolization Volume	Median (IQR), *n*	1 (0.3), 49	1 (0.4), 49	1 (0.3), 98
	Mean ± SD, *n*	0.91 ± 0.34, 49	0.90 ± 0.37, 49	0.90 ± 0.35, 98
Right Embolization Volume	Median (IQR), *n*	1 (0.3), 49	1 (0.4), 48	1 (0.3), 97
	Mean ± SD, *n*	0.98 ± 0.47, 49	0.91 ± 0.4, 48	0.95 ± 0.43, 97
Dilution Ratio	Median (IQR), *n*	0.1 (0), 54	0.1 (0), 52	0.1 (0), 106
	Mean ± SD, *n*	0.098 ± 0.006, 54	0.097 ± 0.007, 52	0.098 ± 0.007, 106
Treatment Approach	BGE	52 (92.9%)	52 (98.1%)	104 (95.4%)
	UGE with CCE	4 (7.1%)	1 (1.9%)	5 (4.6%)
		Outcome		
IPSS Reduction	Median (IQR), *n*	4.5 (5), 56	16.5 (7), 53	9 (11.8), 109
	Mean ± SD, *n*	3.7 ± 4.6, 56	17.1 ± 5, 53	10.2 ± 8.2, 109

The mean pre-PAE IPSS was 16.1 (standard deviation [SD] = 5) in the unfavorable outcome group, 24.5 (SD = 5.2) in the favorable outcome group, and 20.2 (SD = 6.6) across all participants. The median pre-PAE QoL score was 4 (IQR = 1) in the unfavorable outcome group, 5 (IQR = 1.5) in the favorable outcome group, and 4 (IQR = 2) in the overall cohort. The median pre-PAE PGV was 86.5 mL (IQR = 94) in the unfavorable outcome group, 135 mL (IQR = 106.85) in the favorable outcome group, and 109 mL (IQR = 117.6) in the overall cohort. History of prior therapy was reported in 25% (n = 14) of the unfavorable outcome group and 7.5% (n = 4) of the favorable outcome group. Unilateral glue embolization with contralateral coil embolization was performed in 7.1% (n = 4) of the unfavorable outcome group and 1.9% (n = 1) of the favorable outcome group, with the remaining patients receiving bilateral glue embolization. The median IPSS reduction was 4.5 (IQR = 5) in the unfavorable outcome group, 16.5 (IQR = 7) in the favorable outcome group, and 9 (IQR = 11.8) in the full cohort.

Table 2 summarizes the model evaluation results. The predictive capabilities of the model were demonstrated by an accuracy of 0.676 (95% CI: 0.647–0.705), an MCC of 0.363 (95% CI: 0.302–0.423), a precision of 0.666 (95% CI: 0.640–0.698), a recall of 0.856 (95% CI: 0.825–0.885), an F1-score of 0.731 (95% CI: 0.709–0.752), and a Brier score of 0.203 (95% CI: 0.196–0.210). The AUPRC was 0.851 (95% CI: 0.824–0.874), while the AUROC was 0.821 (95% CI: 0.790–0.848), reflecting excellent discriminatory ability [20]. The ROC curve, PRC, and calibration curve for the model's performance are shown in Figure 2A–C, respectively.

Table 2. Model evaluation results. AUROC = area under the receiver operating characteristic curve; AUPRC = area under the precision–recall curve.

Performance Metric	Metric Value (95% Confidence Interval)
Precision	0.666 (0.640, 0.698)
Recall	0.856 (0.825, 0.885)
F1 Score	0.731 (0.709, 0.752)
Accuracy	0.676 (0.647, 0.705)
Matthews Correlation Coefficient	0.363 (0.302, 0.423)
AUROC	0.821 (0.790, 0.848)
AUPRC	0.851 (0.824, 0.874)
Brier Score	0.203 (0.196, 0.210)

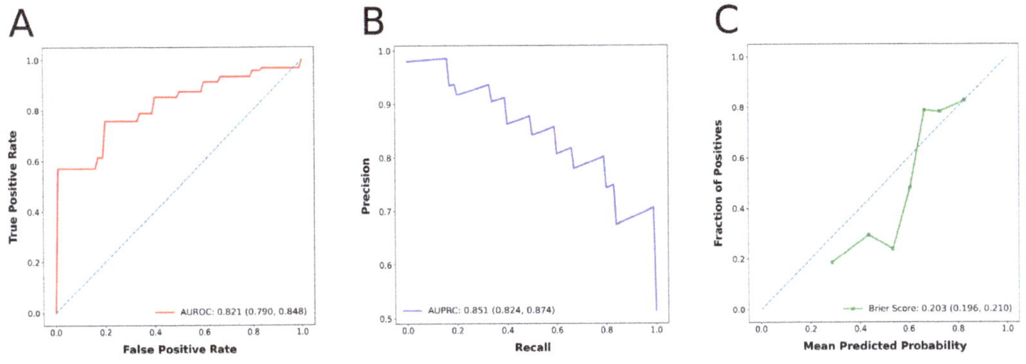

Figure 2. The receiver operating characteristic curve (**A**), precision–recall curve (**B**), and calibration curve (**C**) for the model's performance.

Figure 3 illustrates the relative feature importance based on SHAP values, revealing pre-PAE IPSS, prior therapy, right embolization volume, pre-op QoL, and age as the top five most important features.

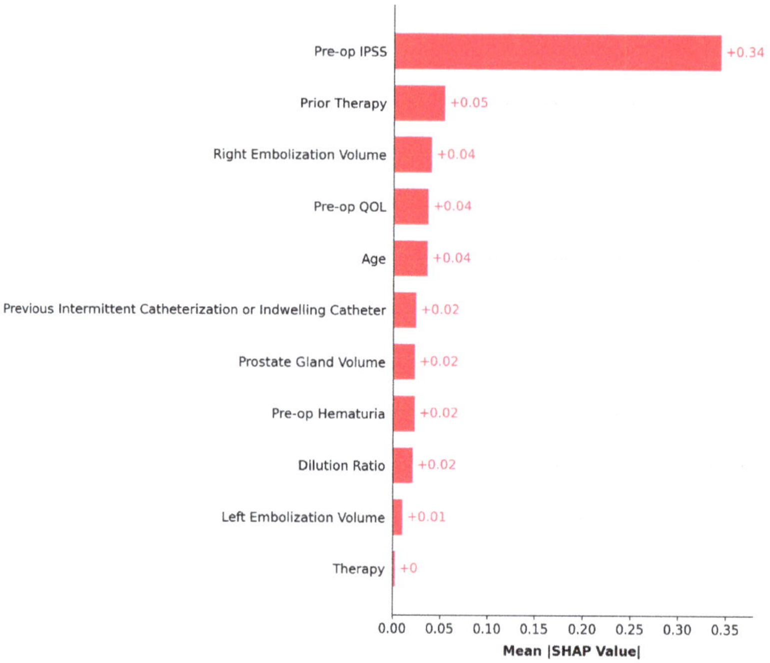

Figure 3. SHapley Additive exPlanations. IPSS = International Prostate Symptom Score; QoL = quality of life.

4. Discussion

Although trial results will be critical for determining the efficacy of *n*BCA glue in PAE and improving patient selection, reliable ML/AI-based prognostic tools can also play an important role in facilitating informed discussions with patients about their expected outcomes. Our study demonstrates the potential of ML/AI models to improve prognostic predictions for patients undergoing PAE with *n*BCA glue by developing a valuable tool for predicting the early favorable outcome. Our model achieved an AUROC of 0.821 and a Brier score of 0.203, demonstrating promising discriminatory ability and calibration for predicting the early favorable outcome. These results highlight the potential of ML/AI to enable individualized prognostication for PAE with *n*BCA glue by leveraging key clinical parameters. To the best of our knowledge, this is the first prognostic ML model specifically developed to predict IPSS reduction outcomes in PAE procedures using *n*BCA glue.

A key strength of our approach lies in the inclusion of the SHAP feature importance plot, which offers a detailed overview of how critical features influence predicted outcomes across the entire dataset, thereby revealing the underlying behavior of the model. This approach provides a level of transparency that is not seen in previous studies, allowing for a deeper understanding of the factors driving each prediction [11]. This feature enhances the model's interpretability and bolsters its credibility, helping researchers to evaluate the key influences on predictions.

In our study, global SHAP analysis revealed that the five most influential features in predicting outcomes were pre-PAE IPSS, prior therapy, right embolization volume, pre-PAE QoL, and age. Bilhim et al. identified older age and higher pre-PAE IPSS as predictors of clinical failure following PAE, findings that are consistent with our study, where these features also emerged as key features in our model's predictions [14]. Given that higher pre-PAE IPSS predicts clinical failure following PAE, it suggests that baseline QoL, often correlated with IPSS, may predict clinical success, emphasizing its role as a key feature in our model [21]. Right embolization volume was another critical feature in our study. Although its significance may not be immediately apparent, one possible explanation is that Zhang et al. found that 67.3% of their study population had a prostate primarily supplied by a unilateral prostatic artery, and in our cohort, the right side may be the dominant supply in some patients, which could have influenced the outcomes and predictions [22]. The inclusion of such procedural factors highlights the potential utility of ML models not only for pre-procedural prognostication but also as tools to inform and adapt intra-procedural decision-making in real time.

As stated earlier, to our knowledge, this is the first study exploring a prognostic ML model to predict outcomes in PAE procedures using *n*BCA glue. Meanwhile, Vigneswaran et al. recently published an impressive study on predicting exact IPSS changes 1 year after PAE (the exact embolization techniques are not mentioned) using traditional models such as linear regression and random forests [2]. It is worth noting the differences between the two studies. Firstly, our study focused on predicting binary outcomes based on IPSS change, categorizing patients into those with favorable and unfavorable outcomes rather than predicting the exact change in IPSS. Predicting binary outcomes may simplify the interpretation of results for clinicians, providing straightforward classifications that are easier to apply in practice, similar to urologic literature, which defines clinical success as an improvement in IPSS of >25%, a binary outcome structure [23]. Meanwhile, detailed predictions such as exact IPSS changes may also be beneficial for clinical decision-making, as even a modest advancement in IPSS might be deemed adequate to prefer PAE over more invasive techniques [12]. Moreover, we predicted early outcomes, in contrast to their 1-year follow-up, where long-term outcomes may be more clinically meaningful. To accurately evaluate the lasting benefits of PAE, a prolonged follow-up period is necessary, as clinical improvements may emerge gradually. Furthermore, we implemented sophisticated imputation methods for missing data, in contrast to including only patients with complete records, which could lead to potential bias [24]. Moreover, we employed TabPFN, an advanced meta-learning model, which enhances model adaptability and generalization to unseen data, providing a robust approach for predicting patient outcomes, particularly when dealing with small datasets [25]. Another important advantage of our study is using the advanced explainability method SHAP. SHAP values provide a clear and quantitative understanding of how each feature influences the model's predictions by showing their importance values. This approach allows for increased transparency, making it easier for clinicians to understand the rationale behind the predictions. This is especially important, as it is well known that black box models cause interpretability issues, making clinicians hesitant [10]. By identifying the most impactful features, SHAP analysis not only improves model interpretability but also provides actionable insights that may help guide clinical decision-making, ensuring that the model's outputs are both reliable and clinically relevant. While the two studies have differences, we believe both are important foundational studies, serving as pioneering contributions to the field.

Despite our rigorous methods, our study has limitations. Firstly, our study has the inherent limitations of retrospective research. The modest sample size limits the generalizability of our findings. The lack of an independent test set further restricts our ability to evaluate the model's generalizability. Furthermore, the data were sourced from a high-volume tertiary center, which may not reflect the broader range of clinical settings where PAEs are performed. Another limitation of our study is that we focused on short-term outcomes, which may not necessarily predict long-term outcomes. The clinical effects of PAE may evolve over time, and a longer follow-up period would be needed to capture sustained efficacy [26]. Also, using kNN for imputing missing data has limitations when handling non-random missingness, which could potentially introduce bias. Moreover, the distribution of outcomes reflects a methodological decision to dichotomize patients based on the median IPSS reduction, enabling a balanced dataset for binary classification modeling. Consequently, patients with an IPSS reduction of $\leq$9 were labeled as having "unfavorable" outcomes purely for statistical modeling purposes; this categorization does not imply procedural failure in a clinical sense. Rather, it serves as a pragmatic framework to facilitate the development and validation of machine learning models. Another limitation of this study is the strong influence of baseline IPSS on model performance. Although the model integrated a variety of clinical and procedural features, its predictive capacity may still be partially driven by the baseline symptom burden, which differed significantly between outcome groups. This may limit the incremental benefit of using complex models over simpler heuristics in certain scenarios. Future work using continuous outcome measures or longer follow-up intervals may help clarify the added value of ML/AI approaches beyond dominant single predictors. It is important to note that although certain variables show prognostic relationships with outcomes, these associations should not be interpreted as causal without further investigation. The model predicts outcomes based on patterns and correlations, not on establishing causality. Therefore, model outputs should be regarded as prognostic predictions rather than confirmations of causal mechanisms or treatment effectiveness. This model should not be used in clinical settings.

5. Conclusions

In conclusion, our ML approach demonstrated promising discrimination and calibration in predicting early outcomes for PAE with *n*BCA glue. By converting predictive modeling into transparent and interpretable risk assessments, our method highlights the potential of precision medicine to provide detailed prognostic insights for PAEs. However, the current model should be regarded as a proof-of-concept and a research tool for risk stratification rather than a clinically deployable decision-support system. Larger multicenter datasets, external validation, and long-term follow-up are essential next steps to assess generalizability. Prospective studies, the evaluation of real-world clinical impact, and model calibration across diverse patient populations will be necessary before such a tool can be safely and effectively integrated into clinical decision-making.

Author Contributions: Conceptualization, B.B.O., M.K. and A.F.; methodology, B.B.O., M.K. and A.F.; software, B.B.O. and M.K.; validation, D.B. and R.G.; formal analysis, B.B.O. and M.K.; investigation, B.B.O. and M.K.; resources, V.B., K.G.-R., A.R.R., D.S. and A.F.; data curation, D.B. and R.G.; writing—original draft preparation, B.B.O.; writing—review and editing, B.B.O., D.B. and A.F.; visualization, B.B.O. and M.K.; supervision, V.B., K.G.-R., A.R.R., D.S. and A.F; project administration, V.B., K.G.-R., A.R.R., D.S. and A.F. All authors have read and agreed to the published version of the manuscript.

Funding: This research received no external funding.

Institutional Review Board Statement: A retrospective protocol approved by the institutional review board at Mount Sinai Hospital (Study number: 21-01756; date of approval: 17 March 2022).

Informed Consent Statement: Patient consent was waived due to this study's retrospective nature.

Data Availability Statement: The data are unavailable due to privacy and ethical restrictions.

Conflicts of Interest: The authors declare no conflicts of interest.

Abbreviations

The following abbreviations are used in this manuscript:

PAE	Prostatic artery embolization
*n*BCA	*n*-butyl cyanoacrylate
IPSS	International Prostate Symptom Score
QoL	Quality of life
ML	Machine learning
AI	Artificial intelligence
PFN	Prior-data fitted network
Qmax	Maximum flow rate
Qavg	Average flow rate
PGV	Prostate gland volume
PVR	Post-void residual
kNN	K-nearest neighbor
ROC	Receiver operating characteristic
PRC	Precision–recall curve
AUROC	Area under the ROC curve
AUPRC	Area under the PRC
MCC	Matthews Correlation Coefficient
CI	Confidence interval
SHAP	SHapley Additive ExPlanations
IQR	Interquartile range
SD	Standard deviation

References

1. Checcucci, E.; Veccia, A.; De Cillis, S.; Piramide, F.; Volpi, G.; Amparore, D.; Pecoraro, A.; Piana, A.; Granato, S.; Verri, P.; et al. New Ultra-minimally Invasive Surgical Treatment for Benign Prostatic Hyperplasia: A Systematic Review and Analysis of Comparative Outcomes. *Eur. Urol. Open Sci.* **2021**, *33*, 28–41. [CrossRef] [PubMed]
2. Vigneswaran, G.; Doshi, N.; Maclean, D.; Bryant, T.; Harris, M.; Hacking, N.; Farrahi, K.; Niranjan, M.; Modi, S. Machine Learning to Predict Prostate Artery Embolization Outcomes. *Cardiovasc. Interv. Radiol.* **2024**, *47*, 1248–1254. [CrossRef] [PubMed]
3. Carnevale, F.C.; Moreira, A.M.; de Assis, A.M.; Antunes, A.A.; Cristina de Paula Rodrigues, V.; Srougi, M.; Cerri, G.G. Prostatic Artery Embolization for the Treatment of Lower Urinary Tract Symptoms Due to Benign Prostatic Hyperplasia: 10 Years' Experience. *Radiology* **2020**, *296*, 444–451. [CrossRef] [PubMed]
4. Xu, Z.-W.; Zhou, C.-G.; Tian, W.; Shi, H.-B.; Liu, S. Long-Term Efficacy and Recurrence Prediction of Prostatic Artery Embolization for Lower Urinary Tract Symptoms Secondary to Benign Prostatic Hyperplasia. *Cardiovasc. Interv. Radiol.* **2022**, *45*, 1801–1809. [CrossRef]
5. Bilhim, T.; Costa, N.V.; Torres, D.; Pinheiro, L.C.; Spaepen, E. Long-Term Outcome of Prostatic Artery Embolization for Patients with Benign Prostatic Hyperplasia: Single-Centre Retrospective Study in 1072 Patients Over a 10-Year Period. *Cardiovasc. Interv. Radiol.* **2022**, *45*, 1324–1336. [CrossRef]
6. Loffroy, R.; Guillen, K.; Salet, E.; Marcelin, C.; Comby, P.-O.; Midulla, M.; Grenier, N.; Chevallier, O.; Petitpierre, F. Prostate Artery Embolization Using N-Butyl Cyanoacrylate Glue for Urinary Tract Symptoms Due to Benign Prostatic Hyperplasia: A Valid Alternative to Microparticles? *J. Clin. Med.* **2021**, *10*, 3161. [CrossRef]
7. Loffroy, R.; Quirantes, A.; Guillen, K.; Mazit, A.; Comby, P.-O.; Aho-Glélé, L.S.; Chevallier, O. Prostate artery embolization using n-butyl cyanoacrylate glue for symptomatic benign prostatic hyperplasia: A six-month outcome analysis in 103 patients. *Diagn. Interv. Imaging* **2024**, *105*, 129–136. [CrossRef]
8. Bamshad, D.; Sanghvi, J.; Galla, N.; Geffner, A.; Menon, K.; Bishay, V.; Shilo, D.; Garcia-Reyes, K.; Lookstein, R.; Rastinehad, A.; et al. Early Outcomes of Prostatic Artery Embolization using n-Butyl Cyanoacrylate Liquid Embolic Agent: A Safety and Feasibility Study. *J. Vasc. Interv. Radiol.* **2024**, *35*, 1855–1861. [CrossRef]
9. Boeken, T. Commentary on Machine Learning to Predict Prostate Artery Embolization Outcomes? Patient Selection for Prostatic Artery Embolization: Why it Matters. *Cardiovasc. Interv. Radiol.* **2024**, *47*, 1255–1256. [CrossRef]
10. Rudin, C. Stop Explaining Black Box Machine Learning Models for High Stakes Decisions and Use Interpretable Models Instead. *Nat. Mach. Intell.* **2019**, *1*, 206–215. [CrossRef]

11. Karabacak, M.; Ozkara, B.B.; Faizy, T.D.; Hardigan, T.; Heit, J.J.; Lakhani, D.A.; Margetis, K.; Mocco, J.; Nael, K.; Wintermark, M.; et al. Data-Driven Prognostication in Distal Medium Vessel Occlusions Using Explainable Machine Learning. *AJNR Am. J. Neuroradiol.* **2025**, *46*, 725–732. [CrossRef] [PubMed]
12. Vigneswaran, G.; Maclean, D.; Doshi, N.; Harris, M.; Bryant, T.J.C.; Hacking, N.C.; Somani, B.; Modi, S. Cardiovascular Comorbidities Do Not Impact Prostate Artery Embolisation (PAE) Outcomes: Retrospective Analysis of the National UK-ROPE Registry. *Cardiovasc. Interv. Radiol.* **2024**, *47*, 115–120. [CrossRef] [PubMed]
13. Wise, R.; Fu, H.; Tapping, C.R. Prostate volume: Does it predict patient outcomes following prostate artery embolisation? A retrospective cohort study. *CVIR Endovasc.* **2024**, *7*, 51. [CrossRef] [PubMed]
14. Bilhim, T.; Pisco, J.; Pereira, J.A.; Costa, N.V.; Fernandes, L.; Campos Pinheiro, L.; Duarte, M.; Oliveira, A.G. Predictors of Clinical Outcome after Prostate Artery Embolization with Spherical and Nonspherical Polyvinyl Alcohol Particles in Patients with Benign Prostatic Hyperplasia. *Radiology* **2016**, *281*, 289–300. [CrossRef]
15. Martin, A.; Marcelin, C.; Petitpierre, F.; Jambon, E.; Maaloum, R.; Grenier, N.; Le Bras, Y.; Crombé, A. Clinical, Technical, and MRI Features Associated with Patients' Outcome at 3 Months and 2 Years following Prostate Artery Embolization: Is There an Added Value of Radiomics? *J. Pers. Med.* **2024**, *14*, 67. [CrossRef]
16. Collins, G.S.; Moons, K.G.M.; Dhiman, P.; Riley, R.D.; Beam, A.L.; Van Calster, B.; Ghassemi, M.; Liu, X.; Reitsma, J.B.; Van Smeden, M.; et al. TRIPOD+AI Statement: Updated Guidance for Reporting Clinical Prediction Models That Use Regression or Machine Learning Methods. *BMJ* **2024**, *385*, e078378. [CrossRef]
17. AUA PRACTICE GUIDELINES COMMITTEE. AUA Guideline on Management of Benign Prostatic Hyperplasia (2003). Chapter 1: Diagnosis and Treatment Recommendations. *J. Urol.* **2003**, *170*, 530–547. [CrossRef]
18. Beretta, L.; Santaniello, A. Nearest neighbor imputation algorithms: A critical evaluation. *BMC Med. Inform. Decis. Mak.* **2016**, *16*, 74. [CrossRef]
19. Hollmann, N.; Müller, S.; Eggensperger, K.; Hutter, F. TabPFN: A Transformer That Solves Small Tabular Classification Problems in a Second. *arXiv* **2022**, arXiv:2207.01848. [CrossRef]
20. Mandrekar, J.N. Receiver Operating Characteristic Curve in Diagnostic Test Assessment. *J. Thorac. Oncol.* **2010**, *5*, 1315–1316. [CrossRef]
21. Vela-Navarrete, R.; Alfaro, V.; Badiella, L.L.; Fernández-Hernando, N. Age-stratified analysis of I-PSS and QoL values in spanish patients with symptoms potentially related to BPH. *Eur. Urol.* **2000**, *38*, 199–207. [CrossRef] [PubMed]
22. Zhang, G.; Wang, M.; Duan, F.; Yuan, K.; Li, K.; Yan, J.; Chang, Z.; Wang, Y. Radiological Findings of Prostatic Arterial Anatomy for Prostatic Arterial Embolization: Preliminary Study in 55 Chinese Patients with Benign Prostatic Hyperplasia. *PLoS ONE* **2015**, *10*, e0132678. [CrossRef] [PubMed]
23. Uflacker, A.B.; Haskal, Z.J.; Baerlocher, M.O.; Bhatia, S.S.; Carnevale, F.C.; Dariushnia, S.R.; Faintuch, S.; Gaba, R.C.; Golzarian, J.; Midia, M.; et al. Society of Interventional Radiology Research Reporting Standards for Prostatic Artery Embolization. *J. Vasc. Interv. Radiol.* **2020**, *31*, 891–898.e1. [CrossRef] [PubMed]
24. Weber, G.M.; Adams, W.G.; Bernstam, E.V.; Bickel, J.P.; Fox, K.P.; Marsolo, K.; Raghavan, V.A.; Turchin, A.; Zhou, X.; Murphy, S.N.; et al. Biases introduced by filtering electronic health records for patients with "complete data". *J. Am. Med. Inform. Assoc.* **2017**, *24*, 1134–1141. [CrossRef]
25. Liu, Q.; Yang, W.; Liang, C.; Pang, L.; Zou, Z. Tokenize features, enhancing tables: The FT-TABPFN model for tabular classification. *arXiv* **2024**, arXiv:2406.06891. [CrossRef]
26. Sandhu, J.S.; Bixler, B.R.; Dahm, P.; Goueli, R.; Kirkby, E.; Stoffel, J.T.; Wilt, T.J. Management of Lower Urinary Tract Symptoms Attributed to Benign Prostatic Hyperplasia (BPH): AUA Guideline Amendment 2023. *J. Urol.* **2024**, *211*, 11–19. [CrossRef]

diagnostics

MDPI

Article

Bringing AI to Clinicians: Simplifying Pleural Effusion Cytology Diagnosis with User-Friendly Models

Enrico Giarnieri [1,*], Elisabetta Carico [1], Stefania Scarpino [2], Alberto Ricci [3], Pierdonato Bruno [3], Simone Scardapane [4] and Daniele Giansanti [5,*]

1 Cytopathology Unit, Department of Clinical and Molecular Medicine, Sant'Andrea University Hospital, Sapienza University of Rome, Via di Grottarossa 1035, 00189 Rome, Italy; elisabetta.carico@uniroma1.it

2 Morphologic and Molecular Pathology Unit, Department of Clinical and Molecular Medicine, Sant' Andrea University Hospital, Sapienza University of Rome, Via di Grottarossa 1035, 00189 Rome, Italy; stefania.scarpino@uniroma1.it

3 Respiratory Disease Unit, Sant'Andrea University Hospital, Sapienza University of Rome, Via di Grottarossa 1035, 00189 Rome, Italy; alberto.ricci@uniroma1.it (A.R.); pierdo.bruno@gmail.com (P.B.)

4 Department of Information Engineering, Electronics and Telecommunications, Sapienza University of Rome, Via Eudossiana 18, 00196 Rome, Italy; simone.scardapane@uniroma1.it

5 Centre Tisp, ISS, 00161 Rome, Italy

* Correspondence: enrico.giarnieri@uniroma1.it (E.G.); daniele.giansanti@iss.it (D.G.)

Abstract: Background: Malignant pleural effusions (MPEs) are common in advanced lung cancer patients. Cytological examination of pleural fluid is essential for identifying cell types but presents diagnostic challenges, particularly when reactive mesothelial cells mimic neoplastic cells. AI-powered diagnostic systems have emerged as valuable tools in digital cytopathology. This study explores the applicability of machine-learning (ML) models and highlights the importance of accessible tools for clinicians, enabling them to develop AI solutions and make advanced diagnostic tools available even in resource-limited settings. The focus is on differentiating normal/reactive cells from neoplastic cells in pleural effusions linked to lung adenocarcinoma. **Methods:** A dataset from the Cytopathology Unit at the Sant'Andrea University Hospital comprising 969 raw images, annotated with 3130 single mesothelial cells and 3260 adenocarcinoma cells, was categorized into two classes based on morphological features. Object-detection models were developed using YOLOv8 and the latest YOLOv11 instance segmentation models. **Results:** The models achieved an Intersection over Union (IoU) score of 0.72, demonstrating robust performance in class prediction for both categories, with YOLOv11 showing performance improvements over YOLOv8 in different metrics. **Conclusions:** The application of machine learning in cytopathology offers clinicians valuable support in differential diagnosis while also expanding their ability to engage with AI tools and methodologies. The diagnosis of MPEs is marked by substantial morphological and technical variability, underscoring the need for high-quality datasets and advanced deep-learning models. These technologies have the potential to enhance data interpretation and support more effective clinical treatment strategies in the era of precision medicine.

Keywords: cytopathology; cytology; pleural effusion; lung adenocarcinoma; machine learning; YOLOv8; YOLOv11; CNN; prediction; precision medicine

1. Introduction

1.1. Challenges in Diagnostic Pleural Effusion Cytopathology

Malignant pleural effusion (MPE) refers to a paramalignant condition characterized by the presence of neoplastic cells in the pleural fluid. MPE is often associated with the advanced stages of cancers such as lung, breast, and lymphoma [1,2]. Notably, metastasis to the parietal pleura is common in lung adenocarcinoma, which accounts for 45–65% of all lung cancer cases [3]. The onset of pleural effusion in these advanced stages is typically linked to a poor prognosis, with a median survival time (MST) of four months or less. Therefore, early and accurate detection of MPE is essential for determining the most effective treatment strategies.

Therapeutic Strategies and Prognosis

The primary treatment for MPE involves thoracentesis, a procedure used to remove pleural fluid and relieve symptoms. However, thoracentesis does not provide a long-term solution, and its effectiveness can be limited. While some patients may not experience recurrence, others face rapid relapse, sometimes within a month of the procedure [4–9]. Recurrence signals the need for more aggressive treatment options. Hence, a swift and accurate identification of the origin of pleural effusion is crucial to customize individualized treatment plans, including interventions to manage fluid production and improve symptom control.

Diagnostic Obstacles and Methods

Diagnosing MPE typically begins with laboratory tests, including pleural fluid cytology. Although this traditional method remains crucial for distinguishing malignant cells from reactive mesothelial cells, which are commonly seen in non-neoplastic effusions, it can be challenging when the origin of the primary tumor is unclear. The expertise of pathologists plays a key role in increasing the reliability of this diagnostic method. Additionally, collaboration with clinicians provides essential context to help interpret the cytology more accurately [10].

However, cytopathology of pleural effusion can be prone to errors, including false positives and false negatives. These inaccuracies are often due to the complex morphology of cells in effusion fluid, which can resemble malignant cells. Reactive changes in mesothelial cells, such as hyperchromatic nuclei, cytoplasmic vacuolization, binucleation, multinucleation, phagocytic activity, and cell-in-cell configurations, can mimic the appearance of malignant cells, particularly those found in adenocarcinoma or mesothelioma. These morphological similarities pose a risk for false-positive diagnoses (Figure 1). This challenge highlights the need for supplementary diagnostic methods to complement traditional morphological analysis.

The Growing Role of Artificial Intelligence

In recent years, artificial intelligence (AI) has garnered attention for its potential to improve diagnostic accuracy in cytopathology. Machine-learning (ML) and deep-learning (DL) algorithms, particularly Convolutional Neural Networks (CNNs), have shown promise in analyzing medical images.

Machine learning is transforming healthcare [11] by enhancing diagnostic accuracy and treatment personalization. It enables the analysis of vast medical datasets to uncover patterns and insights beyond human capability.

By supporting clinical decision-making, it helps reduce errors and improve patient outcomes. ML-driven tools can detect diseases earlier and suggest the most effective interventions. Predictive models assist in identifying at-risk individuals before symptoms appear. Automation through ML also streamlines workflows, saving time and resources.

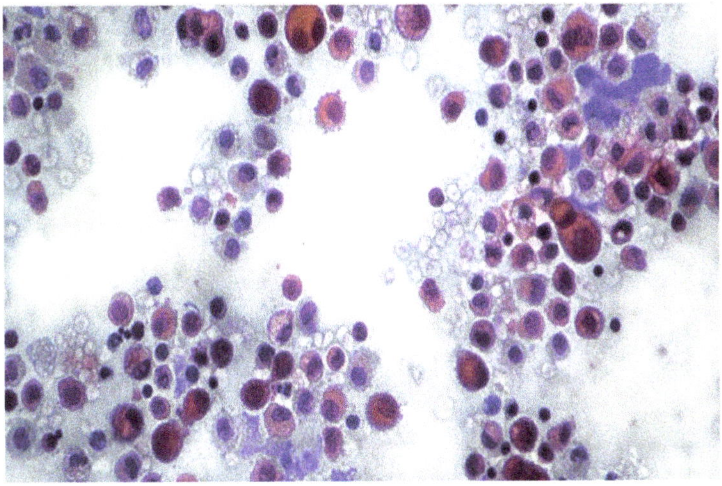

(a)

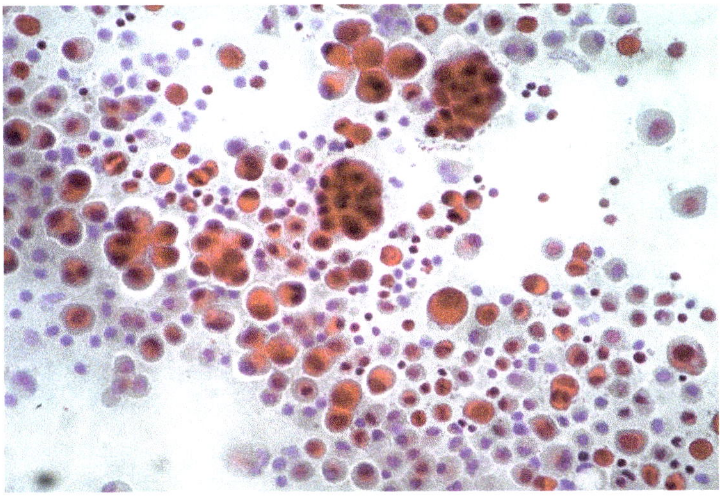

(b)

Figure 1. (**a**) Reactive pleural effusion showing mesothelial cells exhibiting degenerative and reactive features (Papanicolaou staining, ×10). (**b**) Adenocarcinoma pleural effusion showing coexistence of mesothelial and neoplastic cells organized in single and cluster aggregates (Papanicolaou staining, ×10). Neoplastic clusters are easily recognizable, whereas single neoplastic cells may resemble mesothelial cells.

It facilitates real-time monitoring and adaptive care, especially in chronic disease management. Ultimately, machine learning contributes to a more proactive, precise, and patient-centered healthcare system.

AI models have demonstrated diagnostic accuracy comparable to, or even surpassing, that of human experts [12–14]. Initially, these AI models were applied to gynecological cytology, such as Pap smear tests, yielding promising results. However, AI applications have expanded beyond gynecological cytology to include non-gynecological samples, such as those from the urinary tract, breast, thyroid, lung, and pleural metastatic cytopathology [15–21]. In parallel, the literature is exploring the genetic basis of reproductive health and fertility issues [22]. These studies aim to identify and characterize genes that predispose individuals to both syndromic and non-syndromic forms of infertility, thereby contributing to a better understanding of the molecular mechanisms underlying reproductive disorders. Such insights are not only valuable for diagnostic purposes but also for the development of targeted therapeutic strategies and personalized medicine approaches in reproductive care. Separately, despite the growing application of AI in various areas of cytopathology, research focused specifically on pleural effusion cytology remains limited.

A few studies have applied AI models to distinguish between normal and malignant cells in pleural effusions. These studies have focused on cells from various tumor types, including lung, gastric, and breast adenocarcinoma, using different deep-learning architectures. The results suggest that deep-learning models could enhance the accuracy and efficiency of MPE diagnosis, offering new possibilities for clinical practice.

Overview of Literature and AI in Pleural Effusion Diagnosis

Table 1 summarizes the literature on deep-learning-based models aimed at differentiating neoplastic from non-neoplastic pleural effusions in cytopathology. These studies demonstrate the use of AI techniques, such as CNNs, to improve diagnostic accuracy, particularly in distinguishing malignant from benign cells. The success of these studies highlights AI's potential to assist pathologists in diagnosing MPE more accurately and efficiently [18,21,23–31].

Table 1. Deep-learning literature overview in neoplastic and non-neoplastic pleural effusion cytology.

Reference	Pleural Effusion Data Set	Cell Detection Approaches	Metrics
Xie et al. [23]	Lung adenocarcinoma	ResNet-18	AUC 0.67–0.83
Park et al. [18]	Breast cancer	Inception-ResNet-V2	Sensitivity 95% Specificity 98.6% Accuracy 81.1%
Wang et al. [24]	Malignant/nonmalignant cells	ViT vision transformer ResNet-50 Vgg-16 Fundus-DeepNet	Accuracy 96.8 Accuracy 87.3 Accuracy 83.9 Accuracy 88.7
Ren et al. [25]	Lung adenocarcinoma Breast cancer Gastric adenocarcinoma	ResNet-2	AUC 0.807 AUC 0.737 AUC 0.955
Chen et al. [29]	Lung adenocarcinoma	Inception v3 Yolov4	mAP 20% Accuracy 98%
Baykal et al. [30]	Pleural effusion Nuclear detection	Faster R-CNN with ResNet-101	Precision 99.34% Recall 96.93%
Mavropoulos et al. [31]	Breast cancer	Inception v3	AUC 0.96

1.2. Artificial Intelligence in Cytopathology: Enhancing Diagnostic Accuracy Through Cell and Nuclei Segmentation

As cytopathological diagnostic methods continue to advance, particularly with the integration of artificial intelligence (AI), cell and nuclei segmentation in microscopic images has become a critical component of the analysis process. This involves essential tasks like annotating, counting, and tracking cells, which are fundamental for precise diagnoses, especially in the case of pleural effusions. While earlier sections addressed the challenges of identifying malignant pleural effusions, recent developments in AI-driven image analysis are now facilitating more accurate and automated segmentation of cells in pleural fluid samples, further improving diagnostic reliability.

Numerous studies have introduced methods for cell segmentation, which can generally be divided into two main categories: semantic segmentation and instance segmentation. Semantic segmentation involves assigning image pixels to specific objects or regions of interest, such as cells or nuclei, effectively separating these elements from the surrounding background. Some prominent deep-learning models used for semantic segmentation include Fully Convolutional Networks (FCN) and U-Net, which have proven successful in segmenting cell structures in microscopic images [32–34].

Instance segmentation, on the other hand, takes segmentation a step further by distinguishing between individual objects within the same class, such as differentiating between multiple cells or nuclei even within the same image. This method generates bounding boxes and corresponding masks, enabling both detection and segmentation in one step. A well-known instance segmentation model is Mask-RCNN, developed by Facebook AI Research (FAIR), which has become one of the leading algorithms for segmenting objects in complex images [35,36]. Various iterations of Mask-RCNN have been created to enhance its performance in cell and nuclei segmentation in biological imaging [37–39].

More recently, a transformer-based model called Segment Anything (SAM) has shown outstanding success in image segmentation tasks, setting new performance standards across numerous applications, including cell imaging [40]. SAM's effectiveness has led to the development of a hybrid approach, CellsSAM, which combines SAM with CellFinder, another transformer-based object-detection model. This hybrid method has yielded improved results for cell image segmentation, offering an innovative solution for the automatic analysis of microscopic images with diverse cellular features.

YOLO: A Real-Time Solution for Microscopic Image Segmentation

An important development in the field of AI is also driven by You Only Look Once (YOLO), a family of algorithms originally developed for instance segmentation in natural images (https://medium.com/tag/yolo-object-detection, accessed on 5 April 2025; https://pjreddie.com/darknet/yolo/, accessed on 5 April 2025). YOLO is increasingly being used in medical image analysis (https://github.com/sevdaimany/YOLOv8-Medical-Imaging, accessed on 5 April 2025), due to its speed and accuracy. One of YOLO's key advantages over traditional models like R-CNN is its ability to detect multiple objects in a single pass. This makes it especially useful for real-time applications that require rapid and efficient analysis of large data sets. Unlike multi-stage models, YOLO performs detection in one unified step, making it particularly valuable for real-time decision-making scenarios, such as in surgical procedures or emergency diagnostics.

The speed and accuracy of YOLO's object-detection capabilities make it a promising application in analysing pleural effusion samples, the focus of this investigation. By quickly segmenting cells and distinguishing between malignant and benign cells, YOLO algorithms can significantly improve the diagnostic workflow, delivering faster and more reliable results to clinicians. Additionally, YOLO's capacity to handle a variety of image types and complexities ensures its adaptability to different clinical applications, including the segmentation of cells in microscopic imaging.

1.3. Advancing Medical Diagnostics with YOLO: AI-Powered Object Detection in Healthcare

YOLO (You Only Look Once) is an object-detection algorithm that divides input images into a grid system to identify and classify objects within the image. Its architecture comprises three main components: (i) the backbone, (ii) the neck, and (iii) the head [41,42].

1. Backbone: The backbone is responsible for feature extraction. It processes the input image and generates feature maps, which are representations of important patterns and objects in the image [41]. Essentially, the backbone functions as the algorithm's "eyes", capturing key elements in the visual data.

2. Neck: The neck acts as an intermediary between the backbone and the head. It aggregates the features extracted by the backbone and refines them through networks like the Feature Pyramid Network (FPN). This component is crucial in improving the resolution and accuracy of object detection, especially in cases with complex object structures [42].
3. Head: The head is responsible for generating the final predictions, such as the coordinates of bounding boxes (the rectangular areas that contain detected objects), objectness scores (indicating the likelihood that an area contains an object), and classification scores (identifying the type of object detected) [42].

YOLO was first introduced in 2015 with the release of YOLOv1 [42], and it quickly gained attention for its ability to perform real-time object detection. Over the years, the algorithm has gone through several updates, with each new version offering improved accuracy, speed, and versatility. These updates culminated in the release of YOLOv11 in 2024 by Ultralytics, which represents the latest iteration of the YOLO algorithm [42].

One of the most significant versions is YOLOv8, which comes in five scaled versions to meet different performance needs: YOLOv8n (nano), YOLOv8s (small), YOLOv8m (medium), YOLOv8l (large), and YOLOv8x (extra-large) [43]. These variations support a range of vision tasks, including the following:

- Object detection: identifying and localizing objects within images.
- Segmentation: dividing images into segments for more detailed analysis.
- Pose estimation: determining the orientation and position of objects, especially human figures.
- Tracking: monitoring the movement of objects across frames in video data.
- Classification: categorizing objects into predefined classes (e.g., car, dog, person) [43].

YOLO in Medical Applications

One of the key advantages of YOLO is its versatility, making it highly applicable in fields such as healthcare, where image analysis is critical. In the medical domain, YOLO is used to detect and localize abnormalities in diagnostic images. For example, in cytopathology, where detecting abnormal cells is crucial for accurate diagnosis, YOLO's object-detection capabilities allow for fast and reliable identification of cancerous cells in tissue samples. This capability can significantly improve the speed and accuracy of diagnoses, particularly in settings with large volumes of medical images that need to be analyzed quickly [44,45].

A summary of various YOLO applications in cytopathology can be found in Table 2, showcasing studies that have used different versions of YOLO, including the latest YOLOv8 and YOLOv11 models [29,45–53]. YOLOv11 offers further advancements in computer vision. Like YOLOv8, it supports tasks such as object detection, instance segmentation, classification, keypoint detection, and oriented bounding box (OBB) detection. YOLOv11's improvements in accuracy and processing speed [54] make it particularly useful in applications requiring high precision and fast analysis, such as medical diagnostics. These advancements make YOLOv11 ideal for real-time applications where quick, accurate results are needed, such as in detecting abnormalities in medical images or identifying tumors in radiographs.

YOLOv11 and the Future of AI in Healthcare

Despite being relatively new, YOLOv11 has already demonstrated promising applications in medical fields, although the number of studies specifically in cytopathology is still limited [53]. The ongoing development of YOLO's design, especially with YOLOv11, is paving the way for even more efficient and accurate AI-driven solutions in healthcare. In cytopathology, where the speed and precision of image analysis are crucial, these advancements can have a significant impact, ensuring faster, more accurate diagnoses and ultimately improving patient outcomes.

By enhancing object-detection capabilities and enabling fast processing, YOLO and its subsequent versions, like YOLOv11, are transforming the landscape of AI in medical diagnostics, making it more accessible, efficient, and effective in clinical settings.

Table 2. Summary of YOLO models application in cytopathology.

Reference	YOLO Model	Cytopathology Application
Chen et al. [29]	YOLOv4	Pleural effusion cytology
Nambu et al. [45]	YOLOv4	Cervical cytology
Wu et al. [46]	YOLOv5	Bronchoalveolar lavage cells
Shi et al. [47]	YOLOv4	Cervical cytology
Tarimo et al. [48]	YOLOv5	Blood cells
Wijaya et al. [49]	YOLOv8	Cervical cytology
Wang et al. [50]	YOLOv7	Lung cancer cytology (biopsy)
Terasaki et al. [51]	YOLOv5	Endometrial cytology
Rumpf et al. [52]	YOLOv7	Bronchoalveolar lavage cells
Awad et al. [53]	YOLOv8-YOLOv11	Blood cells (ALL)

1.4. Expanding Access to Artificial Intelligence: Empowering Professionals with Accessible AI Tools for Practical Applications

In every sector where AI is used, there is a growing need to enable broader participation in its development, rather than limiting involvement to passive use of applications. This represents a real and concrete opportunity for progress. Platforms that contribute to this direction are essential. In every sector where AI is applied, there is an increasing need to promote active involvement in its development, rather than limiting professionals to passive use of existing applications.

One of the major barriers to the adoption of AI, especially in healthcare and diagnostics, is the technical complexity of training and deploying models. Roboflow, for instance, offers an intuitive platform for building and applying computer vision models, making AI more accessible even to users without programming or data science expertise. This capability is particularly valuable in fields like healthcare, where professionals such as doctors, biologists, and lab technicians, who may lack technical backgrounds, can still benefit from AI support in tasks like image detection and classification.

By allowing users to upload, annotate, and train models on visual datasets, the platform dramatically simplifies the implementation process. This reduces development time and effort and allows users to focus on clinical interpretation rather than algorithmic details.

For example, in digital cytology, object-detection models like YOLO (You Only Look Once) trained on this platform can accurately identify malignant cells in tissue samples, supporting faster and more accurate diagnoses. Integrating such tools into daily workflows enhances efficiency and reduces error margins.

1.5. Rationale for the Study and Purpose

This study aims to explore the integration of artificial intelligence (AI) into the diagnostic process of pleural effusion, a medical condition where fluid accumulates in the pleural cavity. Specifically, it focuses on the use of advanced object-detection algorithms like YOLO, particularly its latest versions, YOLOv8 and YOLOv11, to enhance diagnostic accuracy and efficiency in analyzing pleural effusion cell samples. The purpose is to investigate how AI can support cytologists in detecting and classifying abnormalities in pleural effusion samples, providing a solution that requires no deep expertise in data science, thus making AI accessible to all cytopathologists.

AI for Cytopathologists: Making It Accessible

The main motivation behind this study is to bridge the gap between complex AI technologies and the needs of cytopathologists working with pleural effusion samples. Cytologists, while experts in their field, often lack the specialized knowledge required to use advanced AI models effectively. AI applications such as YOLO are designed to be user-friendly, enabling cytologists to leverage AI without needing in-depth technical knowledge. This allows professionals to enhance diagnostic processes by utilizing AI-powered models for image analysis, improving accuracy and workflow efficiency.

The integration of AI in pleural effusion diagnostics is especially beneficial because it helps cytologists quickly and reliably distinguish between different cell types, such as malignant and benign cells. This support can play a crucial role in reducing human error, expediting diagnoses, and improving patient outcomes. The adoption of AI in pleural effusion analysis ultimately democratizes the use of advanced technology in medical diagnostics, providing a valuable application for all cytologists.

YOLO: Key Innovations

YOLO, which stands for "You Only Look Once," is an object-detection algorithm designed to process images quickly and accurately. Over the years, YOLO has been updated, and the most recent versions—YOLOv8 and YOLOv11—offer significant improvements in speed, precision, and recall, making them highly suitable for medical applications such as cytology.

YOLOv11 introduces optimizations that enhance the accuracy and speed of object detection, classification, and segmentation tasks. These capabilities are particularly valuable in cytopathology, where precision is key to correctly identifying cell types and abnormalities in pleural effusion samples. The model can help cytologists automate the process of identifying and classifying malignant cells, thus improving diagnostic accuracy.

In this study, we focus on evaluating the performance of YOLOv8 and YOLOv11 in detecting and classifying cells from pleural effusion samples. The results show that both models perform well, with YOLOv11 slightly outperforming YOLOv8 in terms of precision and mean Average Precision (mAP). This demonstrates that YOLOv11 can be a powerful application in the analysis of pleural effusion samples, with the potential to aid cytologists in differentiating between malignant and benign cells more effectively.

The Purpose of This Study

The primary purpose of this study is to assess the effectiveness of YOLO-based AI models in analyzing pleural effusion samples. By evaluating the latest versions of YOLO, particularly YOLOv8 and YOLOv11, this research aims to determine how these models can enhance the diagnostic capabilities of cytopathologists, improving both the accuracy and efficiency of pleural effusion analysis. The study highlights how AI, specifically YOLO, can be used as an application to support cytologists in identifying and classifying cells without requiring specialized expertise in machine learning.

This research contributes to the broader field of AI in medical diagnostics by demonstrating how AI can be applied to the specific context of pleural effusion analysis. It explores the benefits of using AI models to detect subtle differences between malignant and benign cells, potentially reducing diagnostic errors and aiding early detection of serious conditions.

Overall, the rationale behind this study is to explore the integration of AI in the diagnosis of pleural effusion, focusing on the use of YOLO-based models. These models can help cytologists analyze pleural effusion samples with greater precision, making AI a valuable application for improving diagnostic workflows. The study underscores the potential for AI to support cytologists in detecting abnormalities in pleural effusion samples, ultimately enhancing the accuracy and efficiency of diagnoses, improving patient care, and making AI accessible to all cytopathologists.

2. Materials and Methods

This study utilized advanced computer vision techniques, powered by the YOLO family of deep-learning models, to segment and analyze cells in pleural effusion images. The primary objective was to develop a robust method for distinguishing malignant cells from benign cells in pleural effusions, particularly focusing on lung adenocarcinoma and mesothelial cells.

The YOLO architecture, known for its efficiency in object detection, was particularly suited for this task as it can perform real-time segmentation, providing both speed and precision in detecting cell structures within microscopic images. This method ensures accurate identification and segmentation of cells and nuclei, critical for diagnosing pleural effusion samples in cytopathology. Below, we describe the process of image collection, dataset preparation, and the specific steps taken in the training and evaluation of the models.

2.1. Collection of Images, Dataset Preparation, and Morphological Criteria for Cells

This pilot study retrospectively analyzed cases of benign and lung adenocarcinoma pleural effusions collected at Sant'Andrea Hospital in Rome between January 2022 and December 2023. The dataset comprises 78 cases with pleural effusions, split into 40 cases of lung adenocarcinoma pleural effusions and 38 benign pleural effusions. The slides were selected by senior cytopathologists (EG, EC), and diagnoses were based on cytological features. Immunohistochemical testing (including Calretinin, TTF-1, and Napsin A antibodies) was utilized to confirm or rule out malignant pleural effusions of lung adenocarcinoma origin. Clinical follow-up information was excluded, and all slides were anonymized for evaluation. The samples were prepared using standard methods and stained using Papanicolaou staining. A digital camera DP27 (Olympus) mounted on a BX45 microscope (Olympus, Tokyo, Japan) was employed to capture up to 100 images per slide. The magnification was set at $\times 200$, focus was manually adjusted, and the depth of focus was optimized to capture the entire area of each cell. Color normalization was applied post-capture for consistency. Some images were excluded due to issues such as preparation defects, blurry photos, overlapping cells, pseudopapillary structures, excessive cytoplasm, or disorganized cell clusters. Mesothelial cells selected for the study exhibited features such as nuclear enlargement, a high nucleus-to-cytoplasm ratio, prominent nucleoli, and bi/multinucleation. Adenocarcinoma cells appeared as isolated atypical cells with enlarged, round nuclei, binucleation or multinucleation, and dense cytoplasm, occasionally containing vacuolization.

2.2. Annotation, Data Augmentation, Model Training, and Metrics Evaluation

The dataset, including image parameters and annotations for each class, is outlined in Table 3. From the collected images, a computer vision dataset was constructed, consisting of 969 manual annotated images showing mesothelial cells (3130) and adenocarcinoma cells (3260) (Figure 2). After annotation, the images were resized to 640×640 pixels.

Table 3. Dataset analytics and overview of the number of annotations of each class.

Images	Annotations	Average size	Median image ratio
969	6390	3.92 mp	2288 × 1712
All splits	**Training set**	**Validation set**	**Test set**
adk cells 3260	adk 2573	adk 345	adk 342
ms cells 3130	ms 2468	ms 309	ms 353

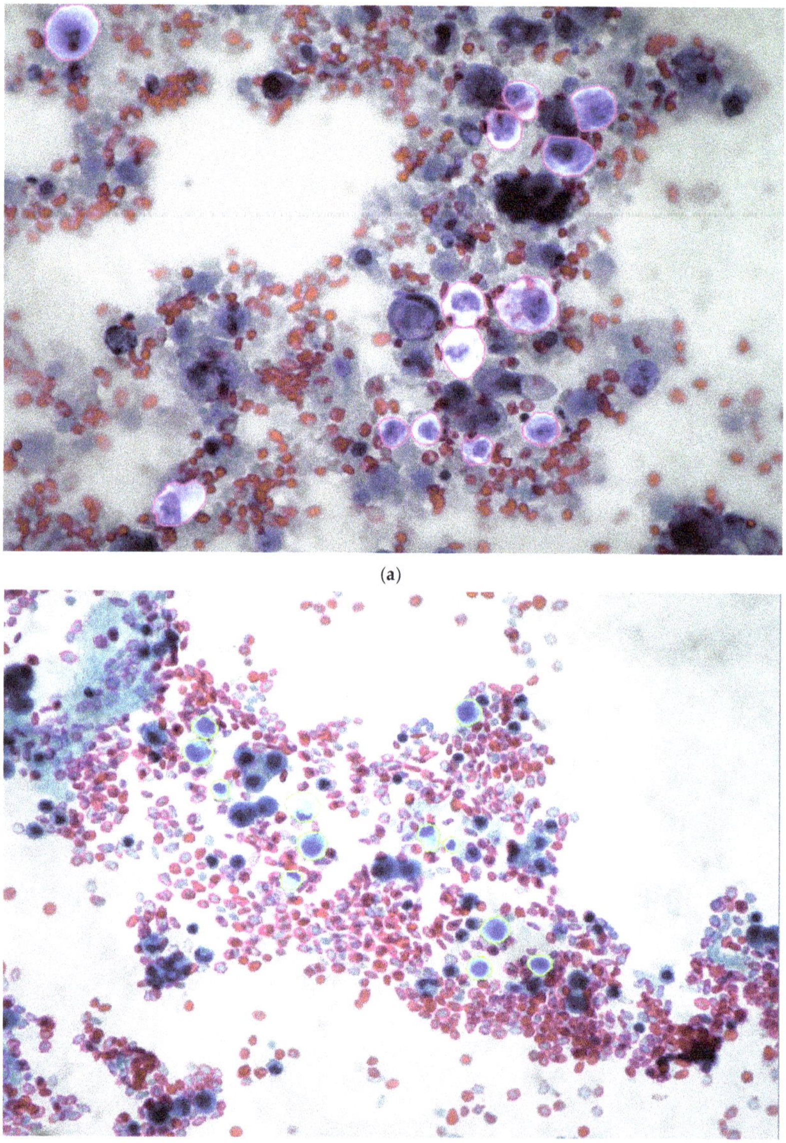

(**a**)

(**b**)

Figure 2. Different cases showing reactive/normal and neoplastic pleural effusion cells were divided into two classes and manually annotated. (**a**) Single adenocarcinoma cells (adk) with violet annotations (Papanicolaou staining). (**b**) Single mesothelial cells (ms) with green annotation (Papanicolaou staining).

The dataset was divided into 80% training, 10% validation, and 10% testing subsets, following a commonly adopted convention in biomedical image classification tasks. This split balances the need for sufficient training data with reliable evaluation through separate validation and testing sets. The 80-10-10 ratio has been shown to yield superior performance in several studies. For instance, Golchubian et al. demonstrated that this split achieved higher accuracy (81.6%) compared to a 60-20-20 configuration in a deep-learning model for photo quality classification [55]. Similarly, in cytological image analysis, Boussel et al. employed the same ratio to ensure balanced class distribution across all subsets in the classification of Pap smear cell images [56]. Given the pilot nature of our study and the limited dataset size, the 80-10-10 split was considered both appropriate and methodologically sound to support robust model development and evaluation.

Roboflow technology was used to facilitate the export of the dataset to Google Colab, enabling custom training and evaluation of model performance. Data augmentation techniques were employed to enhance model performance and mitigate overfitting. The images were horizontally and vertically flipped to increase the model's ability to recognize symmetrical objects. Random cropping allowed the model to identify partially visible objects, and 90-degree rotations were applied to facilitate recognition of cells in various orientations. Following training, performance metrics such as mean Average Precision (mAP) and Precision-Recall (PR) curves were calculated to evaluate the model's efficacy. mAP, which is used to measure model performance across different thresholds, considers both precision (correctness of predictions) and recall (the model's ability to identify all relevant instances). Following data augmentation, instance segmentation was performed using YOLOv8 and YOLOv11 models, trained on a Tesla T4 GPU with NVIDIA driver version 535.104.05 and CUDA 12.2.

3. Results

In this section, we present the evaluation results of two deep-learning models, YOLOv8 and YOLOv11, applied to the task of classifying pleural effusion cells. The goal of this study is to assess the models' ability to distinguish between malignant adenocarcinoma cells (adk) and benign mesothelial cells (ms) in pleural fluid samples. The results presented here include a detailed comparison of both models' performance based on a range of metrics, including precision, recall, F1 score, and mean Average Precision (mAP).

We also examine the models' performance through a confusion matrix, which provides insight into the classification accuracy for each cell type. Furthermore, we conduct external validation using a public dataset of malignant and benign cells derived from body cavity fluid. This additional validation serves to evaluate the generalization ability of the models when applied to new, unseen data.

The following sections present a breakdown of the quantitative performance of YOLOv8 and YOLOv11, as well as visual examples of the models' predictions on both the training and external datasets. By evaluating both models' strengths and weaknesses, we aim to determine which model offers the most reliable classification of pleural effusion cells and explore the potential applications of these models in clinical diagnostics.

3.1. Model Training Results: YOLOv8 vs. YOLOv11

The training results from the pleural effusion cell evaluation dataset revealed key performance metrics for both YOLOv8 and YOLOv11, summarized in Table 4. These results highlight the precision, recall, and overall classification performance of both models across two cell classes: mesothelial cells (ms) and adenocarcinoma cells (adk).

Table 4. Comparison of YOLOv8 and YOLOv11 metrics for all classes.

Models	F1 Score	Precision	Recall	mAP50	mAP50-95
YOLOv8	0.72	0.673	0.784	0.777	0.662
YOLOv11	0.72	0.701	0.756	0.796	0.681

The training results obtained from the pleural effusion cell evaluation dataset showed values and metrics categorized by class (Table 4). YOLOv8 demonstrated a precision of 0.673 for all cells, with 0.672 for mesothelial cells (ms) and 0.674 for adenocarcinoma cells (adk), while recall values were 0.784 overall, 0.806 for ms, and 0.761 for adk. The overall performance, measured by the mean Average Precision (mAP), was 0.777. According to the normalized confusion matrix, classification accuracy reached 0.80 for adk and 0.77 for ms, indicating solid model performance in distinguishing between the two cell types.

Compared to YOLOv8, YOLOv11 achieved slightly better results in terms of precision, mAP50, and mAP50-95, reflecting improvements in average classification accuracy across varying thresholds. However, it performed slightly worse in terms of class-specific accuracy, as shown in the confusion matrix (Figure 3A,B), suggesting a possible trade-off between precision and overall class discrimination.

Overall, YOLOv11 emerges as the more favorable model when considering its consistent performance across multiple key metrics. While both models achieved the same F1 score, YOLOv11 demonstrated higher overall precision (0.701 vs. 0.673), indicating a better ability to reduce false positives across classes. Moreover, it outperformed YOLOv8 in both mAP50 (0.796 vs. 0.777) and mAP50-95 (0.681 vs. 0.662), which reflect not only its superior detection accuracy at a standard threshold but also its robustness across varying levels of IoU. These enhancements are especially relevant in clinical contexts, where precision and reliability are essential for supporting diagnostic decisions. Although YOLOv11 showed a slightly lower class-specific accuracy in the confusion matrix, its overall performance profile—particularly in metrics that better capture generalization and model quality—suggests it may be better suited for practical implementation in AI-assisted cytological analysis.

Figure 3A,B provides a visual comparison of the models' performance metrics.

Precision-Recall (PR) curves provide a valuable tool to evaluate model performance, especially in datasets with class imbalance, as they focus on the trade-off between precision and recall. This is particularly relevant in medical applications, where detecting true positives (recall) without generating excessive false positives (precision) is critical.

The figures show the performance of the YOLOv8 and YOLOv11 models in classifying mesothelial (MS) and adenocarcinoma (ADK) cells, along with their respective performance curves. The thick, dark blue line indicates the average performance across all classes, while the green and orange lines represent ADK and MS cells, respectively. Both models demonstrated reliable discrimination capabilities, as evidenced by the Precision-Recall (PR) curves that tend to approach the top-right corner of the plot—a typical indicator of a favorable balance between precision and recall, especially in datasets where class distribution and label ambiguity can affect performance.

The F1-confidence curves provide further insights into the interplay between precision and recall across a range of confidence thresholds. These curves help visualize how the models' predictions behave as the classification threshold changes, particularly in complex scenarios such as those involving overlapping cell boundaries, subtle morphological features, or heterogeneous staining patterns. A decline in the F1 score at specific thresholds can reflect real-world challenges like class imbalance, ambiguous cell features, inconsistent annotations, or the presence of inflammatory or necrotic cells that may confound classification. The presence of such elements in cytological samples is common and underscores the importance of evaluating performance not only at a fixed threshold but across the entire confidence spectrum.

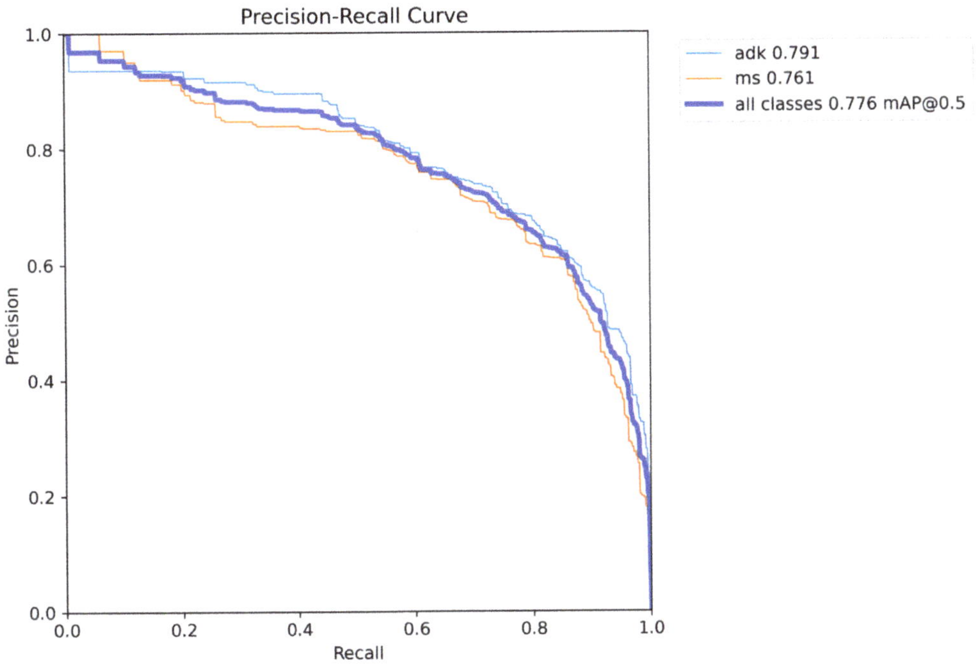

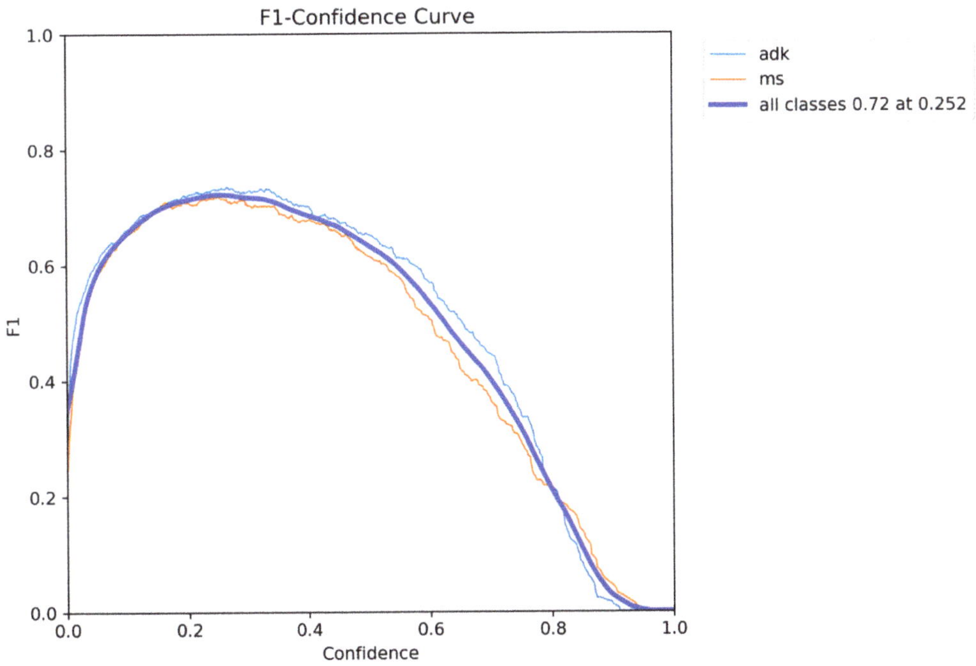

Figure 3. *Cont.*

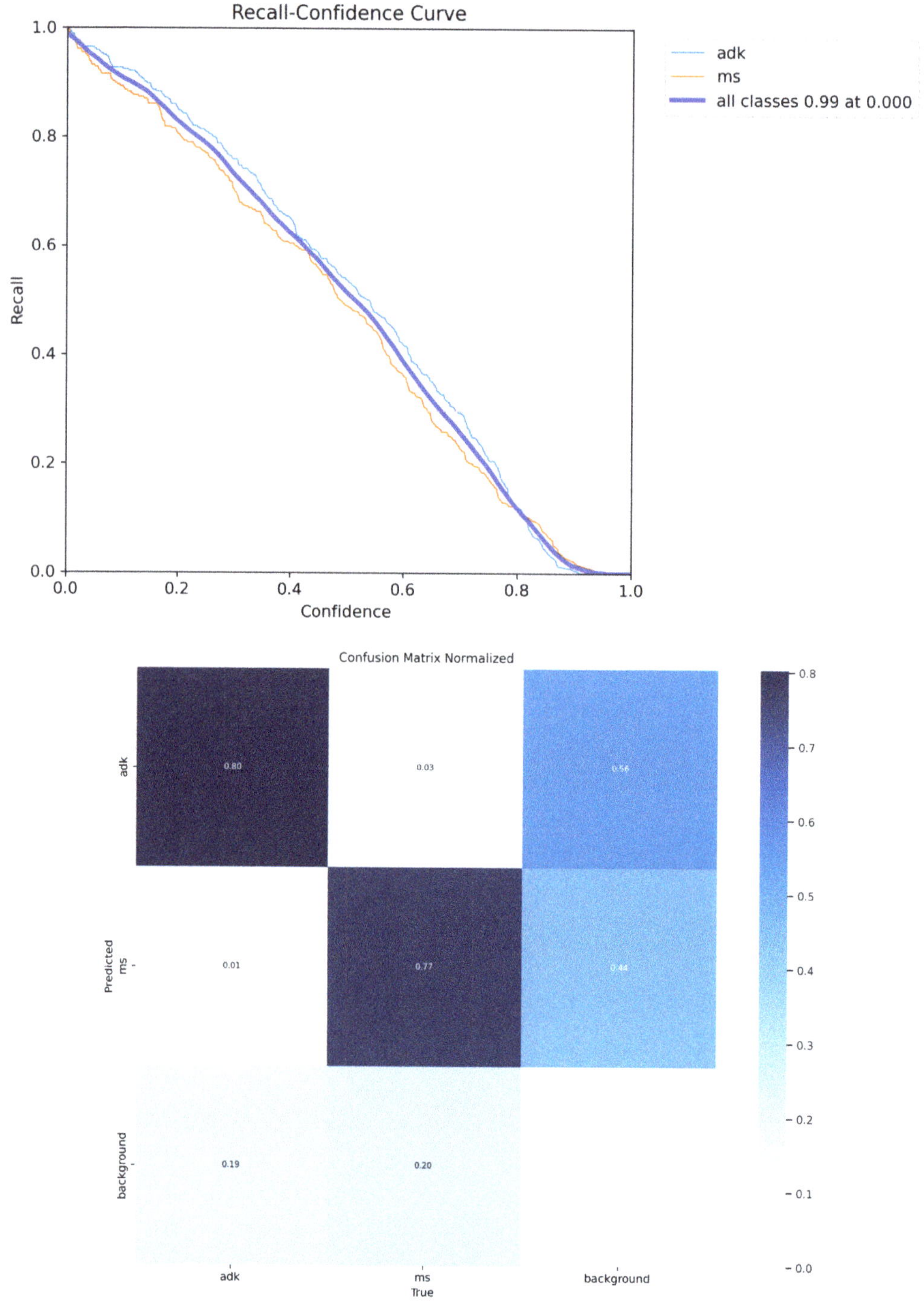

(A)

Figure 3. *Cont.*

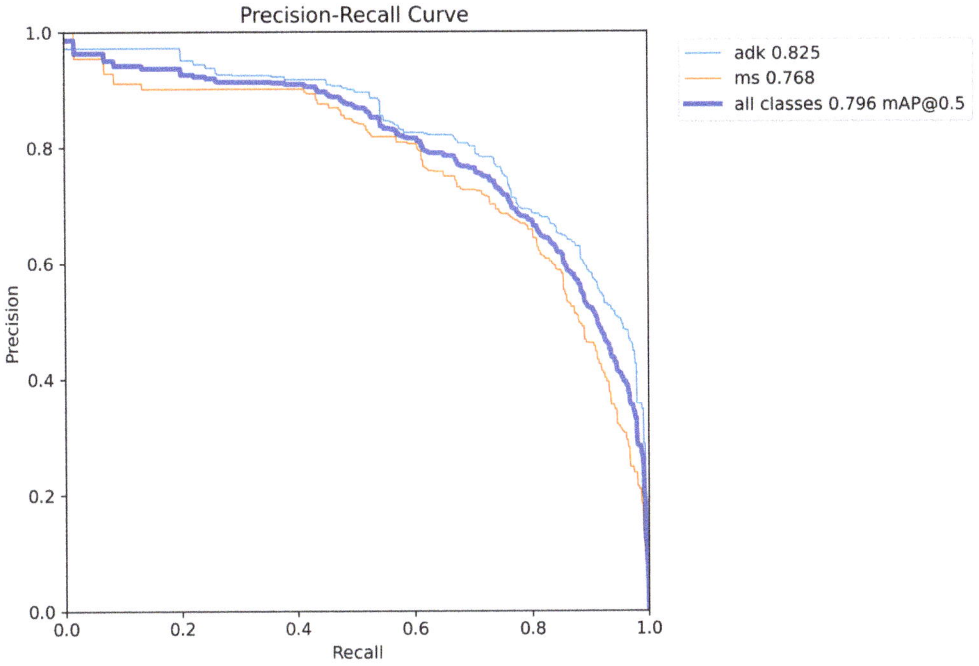

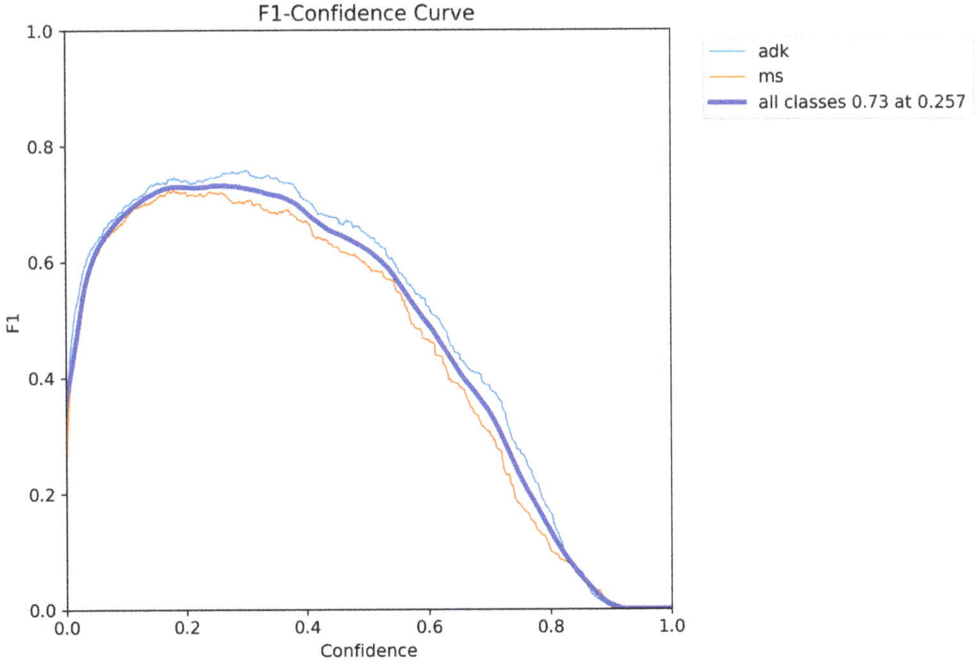

Figure 3. *Cont.*

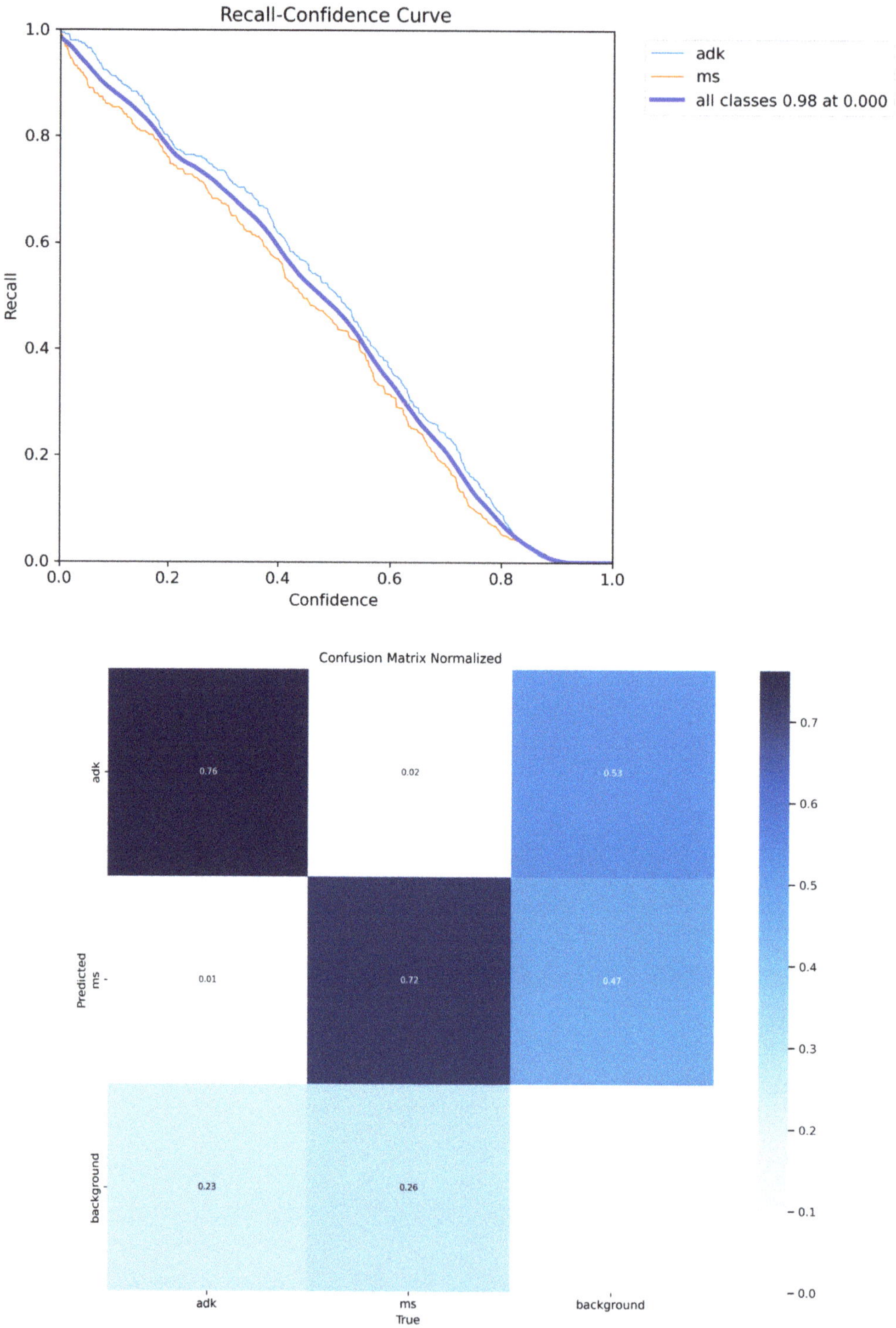

(**B**)

Figure 3. (**A**) YOLOv8 performance metrics. (**B**) YOLOv11 performance metrics.

The recall–confidence curves highlight each model's sensitivity to positive cases, particularly under lower certainty levels. A higher recall at lower thresholds can indicate the model's capacity to flag potentially relevant detections, which can be beneficial in clinical screening workflows where sensitivity is often prioritized. In this context, one of the models, YOLOv8, shows a slightly higher recall for adenocarcinoma cells compared to the other, suggesting a potential advantage in detecting malignant features, particularly in challenging or ambiguous cases.

Complementing these performance curves, the confusion matrix offers a more granular look at the models' classification behavior. It includes three categories—adenocarcinoma (ADK), mesothelial (MS), and background—and has been normalized to reflect proportional performance across classes. This normalization accounts for the varying frequencies of each class in the dataset, allowing a fairer assessment of the models' robustness. The matrix reveals that both models are capable of distinguishing the target cell types with satisfactory accuracy, maintaining low misclassification rates even in challenging conditions. These results support the models' applicability in real-world cytological analysis, where a balanced trade-off between sensitivity and specificity is crucial.

3.2. Evaluation and Validation with External Datasets

To further validate the models' generalization capabilities, external validation was conducted using a public dataset that contained images of malignant and benign cells derived from body cavity fluid. This validation aimed to test the models' ability to classify cells accurately when faced with new, unseen data.

A random selection of images from both the training and external datasets was utilized to assess the models' performance in distinguishing between malignant adenocarcinoma cells (adk) and benign mesothelial cells (ms). These images presented additional challenges, such as overlapping cells and poor image quality, but the models were still able to perform reliably. Figure 4 showcases a random selection of test images used to evaluate the models' performance at a 50% confidence threshold. The images, which specifically assess the ability to distinguish between adenocarcinoma (adk) and mesothelial (ms) cells, include

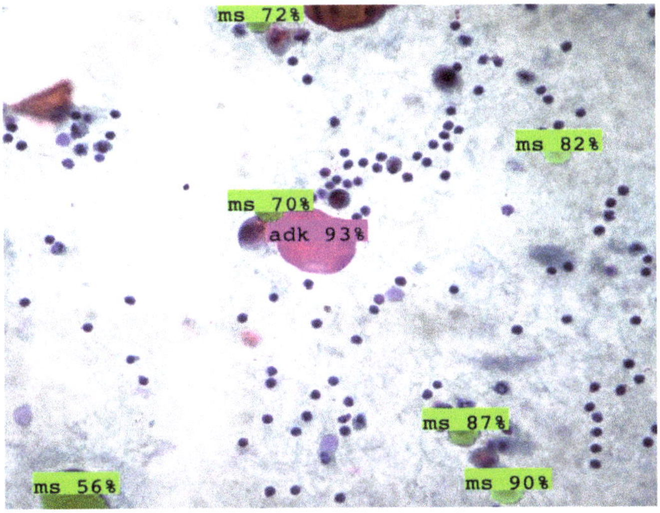

(a)

Figure 4. *Cont.*

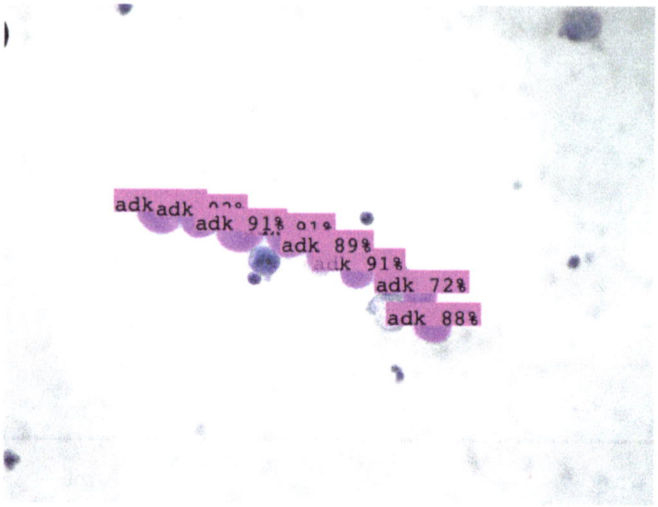

(b)

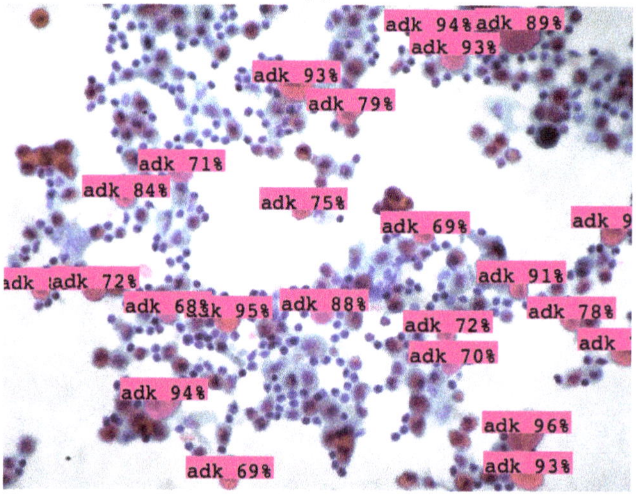

(c)

Figure 4. A random selection of images from the test set to verify prediction performance on the two classes of cells at a 50% confidence threshold. (**a**) Isolated adenocarcinoma cells (adk) among mesothelial cells (ms). (**b**) Cluster of adenocarcinoma cells. (**c**) Isolated adenocarcinoma cells in a context of marked inflammation.

- (a) Isolated adenocarcinoma (adk) cells among mesothelial (ms) cells.
- (b) A cluster of adenocarcinoma cells.
- (c) Adenocarcinoma cells within an area of marked inflammation.

These images highlight the challenges that the models face, such as identifying adenocarcinoma cells in inflammatory conditions. However, they also demonstrate that both models are capable of identifying and classifying these cells effectively, even under these complex circumstances.

Figure 5 presents results from the external dataset, which includes malignant and benign cells derived from body cavity fluid. The external validation confirmed that both

YOLOv8 and YOLOv11 were able to accurately classify the cells, even when faced with new images not included in the training dataset. The validation results include

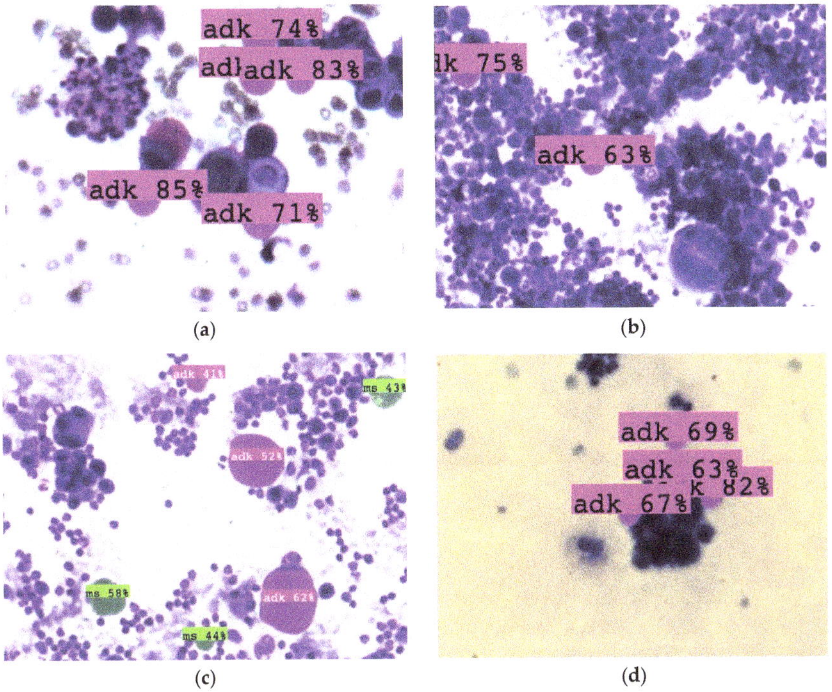

Figure 5. Additional validation was conducted using an external dataset obtained from Kaggle.com containing images of malignant and benign cells derived from body cavity fluid [57]. (**a**–**d**) The results demonstrated predictions consistent with our dataset, even with different staining and magnification. This model could be used in the preliminary observation of and screening to determine whether the sample should be submitted for immunohistochemical evaluation.

- (a) to (d): Images from the external dataset that were correctly classified by both models, demonstrating consistency with the training dataset.

These results underscore the models' ability to generalize to new data, which is essential for their deployment in clinical settings. The accurate classification of cells, even when they are not clearly visible or appear in challenging conditions, suggests that the models could be valuable applications for preliminary screening of pleural effusion samples before submitting them for more detailed immunohistochemical evaluation.

3.3. *Final Performance Summary*

In summary, the comparison between YOLOv8 and YOLOv11 reveals that while YOLOv11 marginally outperformed YOLOv8 in precision, mAP, both models demonstrated strong performance in classifying pleural effusion cells. External validation using both test images and an external dataset further supports the models' ability to generalize to new, unseen data. Figures 3A,B, 4 and 5 provide visual evidence of the models' robust performance in various real-world scenarios, indicating their potential use in clinical practice for early detection and screening of pleural effusion samples. While both YOLOv8 and YOLOv11 achieved the same F1 score (0.72), a closer analysis of the individual metrics reveals nuanced differences in their performance. YOLOv11 demonstrated higher precision (0.701 vs. 0.673) and superior mean Average Precision values, both at the standard IoU threshold of 50% (mAP50: 0.796 vs. 0.777) and across the full IoU range from 50% to 95% (mAP50-95: 0.681 vs. 0.662). These results indicate that YOLOv11 provides slightly more accurate and consistent predictions overall. Conversely, YOLOv8 achieved a marginally higher recall (0.784 vs. 0.756), suggesting it may be more sensitive in detecting relevant instances, albeit at the cost of a few more false positives. Overall, YOLOv11 appears to strike a more favorable balance between detection precision and localization accuracy, making it a compelling choice for clinical applications where reducing false positives and ensuring consistent classification are key.

4. Discussion

4.1. Summary and Added Values

This study investigates the application of YOLOv8 and YOLOv11 object-detection models in pleural effusion cytology, focusing on the challenging task of distinguishing between reactive mesothelial and adenocarcinoma cells. YOLOv11 showed slightly better performance in terms of precision and mAP metrics, likely due to architectural improvements. The feasibility of deploying such models in user-friendly environments, such as web-based applications, was explored. This study provides several contributions to the evolving landscape of AI-assisted cytopathology.

First, it offers a focused comparative assessment of two advanced deep-learning architectures applied to a diagnostically demanding context. The subtle morphological differences between reactive mesothelial cells and adenocarcinoma cells in pleural effusions often pose difficulties even to experienced professionals; this study evaluates how state-of-the-art object-detection models address this challenge through both metric-based and visual assessments.

Second, the research emphasizes practical issues around dataset creation and enrichment in cytology. By discussing the application of YOLO-based object-detection models and suggesting inter-laboratory collaborations, it highlights important strategies for enhancing the development and implementation of AI systems in healthcare.

A third contribution lies in the discussion around expanding access to AI development. The study highlights how user-oriented applications can support data annotation, model training, and integration processes, particularly in fields such as cytology, where dedicated AI development infrastructure is often lacking.

This opens the door to wider participation in AI model development from healthcare professionals without specific computational backgrounds.

Finally, by framing the diagnostic model as a potential decision support application in low-cellularity settings such as malignant pleural effusions, the study contributes to the conversation around precision oncology.

4.2. Discussion on the Contribution of the Study to Advancing Diagnostic Techniques in Pleural Effusion

4.2.1. Recent Advances in AI for Pleural Effusion Diagnosis

In recent years, the focus on the diagnostic approach to pleural effusions has shifted, not only within the laboratory but also among clinicians requiring more information beyond the cytomorphological diagnosis. In patients with advanced neoplastic disease, particularly from lung adenocarcinoma, the cells in the effusion represent a valuable resource for determining the most appropriate therapeutic strategies. Tumor cells may be discovered at the initial diagnosis and provide insights into their molecular profile. In some cases, these effusions tend to reaccumulate during or after the course of treatment. In such instances, neoplastic cells become essential, especially for the changes in their genetic profile. Accurate identification and characterization of these cells represent the first challenge even for experienced cytopathologists [58–60].

Although artificial intelligence (AI) is mostly used in histopathology, the advancement of deep learning has greatly accelerated the development of computational cytology. In recent years, there has been a booming trend in applying deep learning to screening and classification tasks, localization, identification, and segmentation of different cellular compartments. Most deep-learning-based cytology initially focused on the cervix and later expanded into non-gynecological lesions [61–64].

In 1995, Truong et al. built an artificial neural network (ANN) model based on densitometric and morphometric data of effusion cells, reporting 95.3% and 85.7% sensitivity and specificity, respectively [65]. In 2012, Barwad et al. applied ANN to effusion cytology using a supervised learning model for network training, identifying both benign and malignant cases [21]. More recently, Xie et al. used a supervised deep-learning method for classifying benign and malignant pleural effusion cells through a deep convolutional neural network (DCNN), achieving accuracy, sensitivity, and specificity of 91.67%, 87.50%, and 94.44%, respectively. They observed that deep-learning methods could assist pathologists, regardless of their experience, in diagnosing cancer cells in pleural effusions [23]. Park et al. applied deep learning to support the diagnosis of metastatic breast carcinoma in pleural effusions, demonstrating that the deep convolutional neural network (DCNN) model outperforms pathologists by showing higher accuracy, sensitivity, and specificity [18].

4.2.2. YOLO Algorithm in Cytopathology

The object-detection algorithm is an important task in computer vision. Traditionally, manual annotation and segmentation of the region of interest (ROI) were time-consuming and error-prone processes. The YOLO (You Only Look Once) algorithm has gained significant attention in the computer vision community. It is a single-stage detector that identifies all objects in an image in a single forward pass through a convolutional neural network (CNN), predicting bounding boxes and class probabilities of objects in an image [66]. YOLO's application in the medical domain has generated interest due to its ability to enable early diagnosis and detection of various pathologies, including retinal diseases, brain atrophy, abnormal protein deposits, and cardiovascular conditions [67–70].

Regarding digital pathology, Rong et al. applied YOLO (HD-Yolo) for lung, liver, and breast cancer histology-based detection, accelerating nucleus segmentation and tumor microenvironment quantification [71]. Elazab et al. developed a hybrid model combining the extraction and classification capabilities of ResNet50 with YOLOv5 for glioma tumor diagnosis, demonstrating improved accuracy [72]. Nambu et al. used YOLOv4 in combination with ResNet for detecting atypical cells of the cervix, achieving average accuracy and F-measure values of 90.5% and 70%, respectively [45]. Recently, Ultralytics introduced YOLOv8, a significant advancement for object detection and semantic segmentation, with promising results in various applications. Topuz et al. demonstrated YOLOv7 and YOLOv8's ability to detect mitotic cells, a critical indicator of cancer aggressiveness [73].

Ikeda et al. used YOLOv8 applied to 11 human cancer cell lines with different staining methods, observing its efficacy in screening and cell classification in clinical settings [74]. YOLOv8 and YOLOv11 have been shown to be highly effective in detecting malignant and benign cells, with recent studies reporting exceptional performance. For example, Awad et al. used YOLOv8 and YOLOv11 to distinguish between malignant and benign white blood cells, achieving an accuracy of 98.8% [53].

4.2.3. Study Contribution and Comparison to the Literature

In our proposed study, we compared the performance of YOLOv8 and YOLOv11 in the diagnostic challenge presented by the strong inter-class similarity between reactive mesothelial and adenocarcinoma cells, particularly when these cells occur singly. The models were validated using both the training dataset and an external dataset, which demonstrated their ability to generalize to unseen data. We also demonstrated the feasibility of integrating these models into a web application for the cell detection process. The metrics results from YOLOv8 and YOLOv11 both showed a good ability to predict the correct class, with YOLOv11 slightly outperforming YOLOv8 in terms of precision, mean Average Precision (mAP50), and mAP50-95 *.

(Note * mAP50 measures the model's average precision with a minimum overlap threshold of 50%, while mAP50-95 evaluates average precision over a range of overlap thresholds from 50% to 95%, providing a more comprehensive and stringent assessment of model performance. It is important to remember that both average precision (mAP50) and mAP50-95 offer valuable insights into the model's ability to detect and classify objects, with mAP50 focusing on a specific threshold and mAP50-95 providing a broader evaluation across multiple thresholds).

The improved performance of YOLOv11 can be attributed to its enhanced architecture, which includes modifications such as better backbone design and more refined feature extraction, making it more effective in distinguishing subtle differences in cell morphology [75].

Additionally, the prediction visualization on individual images derived from a public dataset (Figure 5) showed comparable outcomes. Both YOLOv8 and YOLOv11 achieved accurate cell detection, with YOLOv11 demonstrating a slight edge in robustness, particularly in distinguishing cells with overlapping structures, which is a common issue in pleural effusion samples [76]. Despite the diagnostic challenges and limited dataset, the results obtained are promising. However, several considerations must be made. The drawbacks of the YOLO model include its requirement for a large dataset to train robust AI models and its difficulty in detecting smaller objects, which could lead to potential false positives or false negatives [77]. Furthermore, while YOLOv11 offers a more accurate and reliable prediction, it may still struggle with certain pathological variations that are less frequent or harder to classify due to the complexity of cellular morphology and staining methods used in cytology [78].

Our results align with the growing body of research supporting the integration of deep learning in cytopathology workflows. Notably, previous studies have shown that YOLO-based models can effectively manage the challenges of morphological heterogeneity and overlapping structures in digital cytology, especially in fluid-based preparations such as pleural effusions. For instance, Nambu et al. demonstrated how YOLOv4 combined with ResNet enhanced the detection of atypical cervical cells, reporting substantial gains in accuracy when compared to conventional CNN-based approaches [45]. Similarly, Topuz et al. highlighted YOLOv7's capacity to identify mitotic figures, a critical feature in cytological assessment of tumor aggressiveness [73]. These studies underscore the suitability of YOLO architectures for tasks that require fine-grained discrimination between cellular subtypes. Moreover, Ikeda et al. applied YOLOv8 to a diverse set of human cancer cell lines and staining conditions, supporting its robustness and transferability across cytological domains [74]. Building on these insights, our study confirms that more recent YOLO iterations, such as YOLOv11, offer concrete advantages in terms of generalization and precision when applied to diagnostically challenging contexts like mesothelial versus adenocarcinoma cell discrimination.

Our findings indicate that YOLOv11 exhibited notable performance improvements over YOLOv8 in metrics particularly relevant to the application of AI models in variable and complex clinical datasets. These enhancements suggest that YOLOv11 may provide a more robust foundation for integrating AI-assisted cytology into routine diagnostic workflows, where consistency, adaptability, and reliable detection are essential.

This aligns with the comparative insights reported by Ultralytics (https://docs.ultralytics.com, accessed on 5 April 2025), supporting the notion that newer YOLO architectures are increasingly refined for deployment in real-world medical contexts.

These findings suggest a potential pathway for the future integration of AI-assisted cytology into clinical settings, where real-time diagnostic support could become a valuable resource, particularly in environments with limited resources or high patient volumes.

However, while larger models such as YOLOv11 and YOLOv8 do require significant computational power, which may not be readily available in many healthcare centers involved in the diagnosis of pleural effusion samples, it is important to note that hospital computational capabilities are advancing rapidly. In recent years, there have been significant improvements in hardware, including the increased availability of GPUs and specialized processing units (e.g., TPUs), as well as the growing use of cloud-based computing solutions. These developments are gradually addressing the challenges related to the high computational demands of deep-learning models.

Moreover, innovations in model optimization, such as quantization and pruning, are making it possible to reduce the size and computational requirements of models like YOLOv11 and YOLOv8, without sacrificing performance. These optimizations could further facilitate the deployment of these models in clinical environments, even in hospitals with more limited computing infrastructure.

As a result, the practical adoption of these models is becoming increasingly feasible, and their potential to enhance diagnostic workflows should not be underestimated. The ability to process large volumes of medical images quickly and accurately can substantially improve the efficiency of diagnoses, enabling healthcare professionals to make more informed decisions in a timely manner. Furthermore, the growing computational capacity within healthcare institutions will likely accelerate the integration of advanced models into routine clinical practice, helping to streamline the diagnostic process and improve accuracy in pleural effusion analysis.

Overall, although computational limitations still represent a challenge, the continuous advancements in hardware and software are progressively mitigating these barriers. As a result, the integration of advanced AI models into clinical practice is becoming increasingly attainable. In particular, such systems have the potential to enhance diagnostic workflows by the following methods:

- Assisting cytopathologists in the preliminary evaluation of cytological samples, effectively acting as a virtual second opinion during the screening phase;
- Reducing the number of cases requiring additional investigations, such as immunohistochemical analyses;
- Lowering overall diagnostic costs and minimizing turnaround times.

4.3. *Challenges and Future Directions*

The increasing availability of user-friendly AI tools is enabling more laboratories and clinical centers to explore deep-learning-based cytology.

This approach not only accelerates AI prototyping but also promotes transparency and data sharing through open repositories. These developments foster the emergence of community-based models and collaborative frameworks that could play a central role in standardizing diagnostic workflows, especially in low-resource or decentralized health networks.

While challenges in collaboration, such as data privacy concerns, geographical barriers, and differences in infrastructure, may arise, these can be addressed through strategic partnerships and innovative solutions. For example, inter-laboratory agreements and consortia can be established to share anonymized data and collectively develop robust datasets. Leveraging cloud platforms and federated learning models can also facilitate the secure and efficient exchange of data across centers, allowing for collaborative efforts without compromising patient privacy.

Looking to the future, Generative Adversarial Networks (GANs) present an exciting opportunity to complement existing methods, particularly in addressing issues like data scarcity and class imbalance. GANs can generate synthetic images that closely resemble real cellular structures, potentially expanding training datasets and improving model performance. For instance, GANs have been used successfully in medical applications, such as generating synthetic histological images [79,80]. In one study, Teramoto et al. employed progressive growing GANs (PGGAN) to classify both real and synthesized lung cytological images, finding that the generated images closely resemble real ones [81]. When integrated with AI models such as YOLO, GANs could enhance the recognition of rare or underrepresented cell types, further improving diagnostic accuracy.

In addition, AI's integration with molecular biology data offers significant potential for advancing precision medicine. By analyzing tumor cell environments alongside traditional cytological images, machine-learning models could enable more personalized cancer treatment strategies, improving both diagnosis and prognosis, particularly in complex cases like malignant pleural effusions (MPEs), where cell numbers are limited.

As the field progresses, AI is expected to play an increasingly vital role in supporting both diagnostic and therapeutic decisions, providing more accurate, efficient, and personalized approaches to cancer care. Overcoming collaboration barriers through technological solutions and inter-center partnerships will be key to ensuring that AI technologies are implemented effectively and that their benefits are realized across diverse healthcare systems.

4.4. Limitation of the Study

This study presents some limitations that should be considered when interpreting the results. The dataset was collected from a single center, the Cytopathology Unit at the Sant'Andrea University Hospital; however, it included a relatively large number of annotated cells for a cytological study, supporting the robustness of the training process. Nonetheless, incorporating multi-center data could enhance morphological diversity and further improve model generalizability.

The analysis focused on cropped and annotated cell images rather than whole-slide images (WSIs). While this approach allowed for accurate object-detection training, future studies could explore how these models perform in real-world diagnostic settings, including WSIs and clinical workflows, where slide quality and imaging variability are important factors. Additionally, although YOLOv11 outperformed YOLOv8 in key metrics, benchmarking against other AI architectures, such as transformer-based or multi-modal models, could offer valuable insights into their comparative diagnostic performance.

Finally, the study did not include explainable AI (XAI) methods. Integrating XAI into future implementations could increase clinical trust and facilitate the adoption of AI-assisted applications in cytopathological practice.

5. Conclusions

This study aimed to explore the potential of machine learning, particularly object-detection models, in enhancing the diagnostic process in cytopathology, specifically for distinguishing between mesothelial and adenocarcinoma cells in malignant pleural effusions (MPEs). One of the key objectives was to explore how AI can help make cytopathology more accessible, bringing advanced diagnostic applications within reach of cytopathologists across a wide range of healthcare settings, including those with limited resources. By offering scalable and user-friendly AI solutions, this approach enables clinicians—even those without extensive expertise in data science—to adopt and contribute to the development of AI-based diagnostic tools. This could significantly reduce the technical barriers and empower healthcare professionals worldwide to improve diagnostic efficiency and accuracy, regardless of their technological expertise.

The results demonstrated that both YOLOv8 and YOLOv11 models were effective in detecting mesothelial and adenocarcinoma cells, with YOLOv11 showing slightly better performance in terms of precision and mAP metrics. These findings highlight the potential of machine-learning models to complement human expertise by assisting pathologists in making more accurate and efficient diagnoses. While the final decision will always require human expertise, the integration of machine learning offers significant advantages, such as reducing diagnostic time and potentially enhancing accuracy by revealing subtle morphological differences that may be difficult to detect manually.

Moreover, this study emphasizes the importance of expanding datasets, particularly in fields like cytopathology, where data availability can be a limiting factor. Strategies such as synthetic image generation through Generative Adversarial Networks (GANs) and fostering collaboration between laboratories to share datasets are crucial to overcoming this challenge and improving model robustness.

Additionally, this study suggests that as future steps, integrating molecular biology data with machine-learning models could further improve diagnostic accuracy. By incorporating biological insights, AI models could enhance the interpretation of cellular features, paving the way for more effective and personalized treatment strategies in the era of precision medicine.

Overall, while AI in cytopathology is still in its early stages, its potential to support diagnostic decision-making, democratize access to advanced applications, and integrate with molecular data offers promising opportunities for improving patient outcomes. The future of AI in healthcare depends on overcoming current challenges, such as dataset limitations and model interpretability, but the progress achieved thus far signals a transformative shift in clinical diagnostics and treatment planning. Looking towards the future, the continued development and integration of AI models in cytopathology offer significant promise for enhancing diagnostic workflows. With platforms empowering clinicians to create and deploy machine-learning models without deep technical expertise, AI has the potential to make advanced diagnostic applications more accessible, even in resource-limited settings. As the field evolves, overcoming challenges such as data limitations and model interpretability will be essential for realizing the full potential of AI in transforming diagnostic practices and improving patient care.

Author Contributions: Conceptualization, E.G., S.S. (Simone Scardapane) and D.G.; methodology, E.G. and S.S. (Simone Scardapane); software, All authors; validation, E.G., S.S. (Simone Scardapane), E.C. and D.G.; formal analysis, E.G., D.G., S.S. (Simone Scardapane), E.C., P.B., S.S. (Stefania Scarpino) and A.R.; investigation, All authors; resources, All authors; data curation E.G., S.S. (Simone Scardapane) and D.G.; writing—original draft preparation, E.G., S.S. (Simone Scardapane), and D.G.; writing—review and editing, E.G., D.G., S.S. (Simone Scardapane), E.C., P.B., S.S. (Stefania Scarpino), and A.R.; visualization, All authors; supervision, E.G. and D.G.; project administration, E.G. All authors have read and agreed to the published version of the manuscript.

Funding: This research received no external funding.

Institutional Review Board Statement: Written informed consent was obtained from participants in the study. This study was approved by the Institutional Ethical Committee of University Sapienza of Rome, Italy (ID: Rif. CE 6098_2020, Prot. Number 210 SA_2020), on 23 September 2020, on the basis that it complied with the Declaration of Helsinki and that the protocol followed existing good clinical practice guidelines.

Informed Consent Statement: Informed consent was obtained from all subjects involved in the study.

Data Availability Statement: The datasets of images used to support the findings of this study are available from the corresponding author upon reasonable request.

Conflicts of Interest: The authors declare no conflicts of interest.

References

1. Gompelmann, D.; Eberhardt, R.; Herth, F.J. Advanced malignant lung disease: What the specialist can offer. *Respiration* **2011**, *82*, 111–123. [CrossRef] [PubMed]
2. Kastelik, J.A. Management of malignant pleural effusion. *Lung* **2013**, *191*, 165–175. [CrossRef] [PubMed]
3. De Andrade, F.M. The role of Indwelling pleural catheter in management of malignant pleural effusion: A creative new technique for an old method. *Lung India* **2015**, *32*, 81–82. [CrossRef]
4. Bibby, A.C.; Clive, A.O.; Slade, G.C.; Morley, A.J.; Fallon, J.; Psallidas, I.; Pepperell, J.C.T.; Slade, M.G.; Stanton, A.E.; Rahman, N.M.; et al. Survival in patients with malignant pleural effusions who developed pleural infection: A retrospective case review from six UK centers. *Chest* **2015**, *148*, 235–241. [CrossRef]
5. Terra, R.M.; Dela Vega, A. Treatment of malignant pleural effusion. *J. Vis. Surg.* **2018**, *4*, 110. [CrossRef]
6. Ryu, J.-S.; Ryu, H.J.; Lee, S.-N.; Memon, A.; Lee, S.-K.; Nam, H.-S.; Kim, H.-J.; Lee, K.-H.; Cho, J.-H.; Hwang, S.-S. Prognostic impact of minimal pleural effusion in non-small-cell lung cancer. *J. Clin. Oncol.* **2014**, *32*, 960–967. [CrossRef]
7. Eberhardt, W.E.; Mitchell, A.; Crowley, J.; Kondo, H.; Kim, Y.T.; Turrisi, A.; Goldstraw, P.; Rami-Porta, R. The IASLC lung cancer staging project: Proposals for the revision of the M descriptors in the forthcoming eighth edition of the TNM classification of lung cancer. *J. Thorac. Oncol.* **2015**, *10*, 1515–1522. [CrossRef]
8. Heffner, J.E.; Klein, J.S. Recent advances in the diagnosis and management of malignant pleural effusions. *Mayo Clin. Proc.* **2008**, *83*, 235–250. [CrossRef]
9. Shaw, P.; Agarwal, R. Pleurodesis for malignant pleural effusions. *Cochrane Database Syst. Rev.* **2004**, *1*, CD002916.
10. Giarnieri, E.; Bellipanni, G.; Macaluso, M.; Mancini, R.; Holstein, A.C.; Milanese, C.; Giovagnoli, M.R.; Giordano, A.; Russo, G. Review: Cell Dynamics in Malignant Pleural Effusions. *J. Cell. Physiol.* **2015**, *230*, 272–277. [CrossRef]
11. Rahmani, A.M.; Yousefpoor, E.; Yousefpoor, M.S.; Mehmood, Z.; Haider, A.; Hosseinzadeh, M.; Ali Naqvi, R. Machine Learning (ML) in Medicine: Review, Applications, and Challenges. *Mathematics* **2021**, *9*, 2970. [CrossRef]
12. Dermawan, J.K.T.; Policarpio-Nicolas, M.L. Malignancies in Pleural, Peritoneal, and Pericardial Effusions. A 17-Year Single-Institution review from 30085 Specimens. *Arch. Pathol. Lab. Med.* **2020**, *144*, 1086–1091. [CrossRef] [PubMed]
13. Layfield, L.J.; Yang, Z.; Vazmitsel, M.; Zhang, T.; Esebua, M.; Schmidt, R. The international system for serous fluid cytopathology: Interobserver agreement. *Diagn. Cytopathol.* **2022**, *50*, 3–7. [CrossRef] [PubMed]
14. Kassirian, S.; Hinton, S.N.; Cuninghame, S.; Chaudhary, R.; Iansavitchene, A.; Amjadi, K.; Dhaliwal, I.; Zeman-Pocrnich, C.; Mitchell, M.A. Diagnostic sensitivity of pleural fluid cytology in malignant pleural effusions: Systematic review and meta-analysis. *Thorax* **2023**, *78*, 32–40. [CrossRef]
15. Wentzensen, N.; Lahrmann, B.; Clarke, M.A.; Kinney, W.; Tokugawa, D.; Poitras, N.; Locke, A.; Bartels, L.; Krauthoff, A.; Walker, J. Accuracy and efficiency of deep-learning–based automation of dual stain cytology in cervical Cancer screening. *JNCI J. Natl. Cancer Inst.* **2021**, *113*, 72–79. [CrossRef]
16. Koss, L.G.; Lin, E.; Schreiber, K.; Elgert, P.; Mango, L. Evaluation of the Papnet cytologic screening system for quality control of cervical smears. *Am. J. Clin. Pathol.* **1994**, *101*, 220–229. [CrossRef]
17. Lilli, L.; Giarnieri, E.; Scardapane, S. A Calibrated Multiexit Neural Network for Detecting Urothelial Cancer Cells. *Comput. Math. Methods Med.* **2021**, *13*, 5569458. [CrossRef]
18. Park, H.S.; Chong, Y.; Lee, Y.; Yim, K.; Seo, K.J.; Hwang, G.; Kim, D.; Gong, G.; Cho, N.H.; Yoo, C.W.; et al. Deep Learning-Based Computational Cytopathologic Diagnosis of Metastatic Breast Carcinoma in Pleural Fluid. *Cells* **2023**, *12*, 1847. [CrossRef]

19. Sanyal, P.; Mukherjee, T.; Barui, S.; Das, A.; Gangopadhyay, P. Artificial intelligence in cytopathology: A neural network to identify papillary carcinoma on thyroid fine-needle aspiration cytology smears. *J. Pathol. Inform.* **2018**, *9*, 43. [CrossRef]
20. Coudray, N.; Ocampo, P.S.; Sakellaropoulos, T.; Narula, N.; Snuderl, M.; Fenyö, D.; Moreira, A.L.; Razavian, N.; Tsirigos, A. Classification and mutation prediction from non–small cell lung cancer histopathology images using deep learning. *Nat. Med.* **2018**, *24*, 1559–1567. [CrossRef]
21. Barwad, A.; Dey, P.; Susheilia, S. Artificial neural network in diagnosis of metastatic carcinoma in effusion cytology. *Cytometry* **2012**, *82*, 107–111. [CrossRef] [PubMed]
22. Yahaya, T.O.; Liman, U.U.; Abdullahi, H.; Koko, Y.S.; Ribah, S.S.; Adamu, Z.; Abubakar, S. Genes predisposing to syndromic and nonsyndromic infertility: A narrative review. *Egypt J. Med. Hum. Genet.* **2020**, *22*, 46. [CrossRef]
23. Xie, X.; Fu, C.-C.; Lv, L.; Ye, Q.; Yu, Y.; Fang, Q.; Zhang, L.; Hou, L.; Wu, C. Deep convolutional neural network-based classification of cancer cells on cytological pleural effusion images. *Mod. Pathol.* **2022**, *35*, 609–614. [CrossRef] [PubMed]
24. Wang, C.; Wang, X.; Gao, Z.; Ran, C.; Li, C.; Ding, C. Multiple serous cavity effusion screening based on smear images using vision transformer. *Sci. Rep.* **2024**, *14*, 7395. [CrossRef]
25. Ren, W.; Zhu, Y.; Wang, Q.; Jin, H.; Guo, Y.; Lin, D. Deep Learning-Based Classification and Targeted Gene Alteration Prediction from Pleural Effusion Cell Block Whole-Slide Images. *Cancers* **2023**, *15*, 752. [CrossRef]
26. Thakur, N.; Alam, M.R.; Abdul-Ghafar, J.; Chong, Y. Recent Application of Artificial Intelligence in Non-Gynecological Cancer Cytopathology: A Systematic Review. *Cancers* **2022**, *14*, 3529. [CrossRef]
27. Jiang, H.; Zhou, Y.; Lin, Y.; Chan, R.; Liu, J.; Chen, H. Deep learning for computational cytology: A survey. *Med. Image Anal.* **2023**, *84*, 102691. [CrossRef]
28. Dey, P. The emerging role of deep learning in cytology. *Cytopathology* **2021**, *32*, 154–160. [CrossRef]
29. Chen, Y.-Y.; Kong, W.; Wu, H.-Q.; Ji, J.-L. Deep learning for artificial intelligence aided cytological diagnosis on exfoliated adenocarcinoma cells of lung in pleural effusion. *Chin. J. Clin. Med.* **2022**, *29*, 396–400.
30. Baykal, E.-D.; Hulya, E.-D.; Mustafa, E.-E.; Safak, E.; Murat, E. Modern convolutional object detectors for nuclei detection on pleural effusion cytology images. *Multimed. Tools Appl.* **2020**, *79*, 15417–15436. [CrossRef]
31. Mavropoulos, A.; Johnson, C.; Lu, V.; Nieto, J.; Schneider, E.-C.; Saini, K.; Phelan, M.L.; Hsie, L.-X.; Wang, M.-J.; Cruz, J.; et al. Artificial intelligence-driven morphology-based enrichment of malignant cells from body fluid. *Mod. Pathol.* **2023**, *36*, 100195. [CrossRef] [PubMed]
32. Zhu, R.; Sui, D.; Qin, H.; Hao, A. An Extended Type Cell Detection and Counting Method based on FCN. In Proceedings of the 2017 IEEE 17th International Conference on Bioinformatics and Bioengineering, Washington, DC, USA, 23–25 October 2017; pp. 51–56.
33. Zhao, T.; Yin, Z. Pyramid-Based Fully Convolutional Networks for Cell Segmentation. In Proceedings of the Medical Image Computing and Computer Assisted Intervention—MICCAI 2018, Granada, Spain, 16–20 September 2018; Lecture Notes in Computer Science. Frangi, A., Schnabel, J., Davatzikos, C., Alberola-López, C., Fichtinger, G., Eds.; Springer: Cham, Switzerland, 2018; p. 11073.
34. Ronneberger, O.; Fischer, P.; Brox, T. U-Net: Convolutional Networks for Biomedical Image Segmentation. Available online: https://arxiv.org/abs/1505.04597 (accessed on 5 April 2025).
35. Tingxi, W.; Tong, B.; Liu, Y.; Pan, T.; Du, Y.; Chen, Y.; Zhang, S. Review of research on the instance segmentation of cell images. *Comput. Methods Programs Biomed.* **2022**, *227*, 107211.
36. He, K.; Gkioxari, G.; Dollár, P.; Girshick, R. Mask R-CNN. Available online: https://arxiv.org/abs/1703.06870v3 (accessed on 5 April 2025).
37. Schwendy, M.; Unger, R.E.; Parekh, S.H. EVICAN—A balanced dataset for algorithm development in cell and nucleus segmentation. *Bioinformatics* **2020**, *36*, 3863–3870. [CrossRef]
38. Fujita, S.; Han, X.H. Cell Detection and Segmentation in Microscopy Images with Improved Mask R-CNN. In Proceedings of the Computer Vision—ACCV 2020 Workshops. ACCV 2020, Kyoto, Japan, 30 November–4 December 2020; Lecture Notes in Computer Science. Sato, I., Han, B., Eds.; Springer: Cham, Switzerland, 2021; p. 12628.
39. Khalid, N.; Munir, M.; Edlund, C.; Jackson, T.R.; Trygg, J.; Sjögren, R. DeepCeNS: An end-to-end Pipeline for Cell and Nucleus Segmentation in Microscopic Images. In Proceedings of the 2021 International Joint Conference on Neural Networks (IJCNN), Shenzhen, China, 18–22 July 2021; pp. 1–8.
40. Kirillov, A.; Mintun, E.; Ravi, N.; Mao, H.; Rolland, C.; Gustafson, L.; Xiao, T.; Whitehead, S.; Berg, A.-C.; Lo, W.-Y.; et al. Segment Anything. Available online: https://arxiv.org/abs/2304.02643 (accessed on 5 April 2025).
41. YOLOv8. Ultralytics YOLOv8. 2023. Available online: https://docs.ultralytics.com/it/models/yolov8/ (accessed on 5 April 2025).
42. Brown, T.; Mann, B.; Ryder, N.; Subbiah, M.; Kaplan, J.-D.; Dhariwal, P.; Neelakantan, A.; Shyam, P.; Sastry, G.; Askell, A.; et al. Language models are few-shot learners. *Adv. Neural Inf. Process. systems* **2020**, *33*, 1877–1901.

43. Pandey, S.; Chen, K.F.; Dam, B.-E. Comprensive Multimodal Segmentation in Medical Imaging: Combining YOLOv8 with SAM and HQ-SAM Models. Available online: https://arxiv.org/abs/2310.12995 (accessed on 5 April 2025).
44. OpenAI. Gpt-4 Technical Report. 2023. Available online: https://arxiv.org/abs/2303.08774 (accessed on 5 April 2025).
45. Nambu, Y.; Mariya, T.; Shinkai, S.; Umemoto, M.; Asanuma, H.; Sato, I.; Hirohashi, Y.; Torigoe, T.; Fujino, Y.; Saito, T. A screening assistance system for cervical cytology of squamous cell atypia based on a two-step combined CNN algorithm with label smoothing. *Cancer Med.* **2022**, *11*, 520–529. [CrossRef]
46. Wu, P.; Weng, H.; Luo, W.; Zhan, Y.; Xiong, L.; Zhang, H.; Yan, H. An improved yolov5s based on transformer back-bone network for detection and classification of bronchoalveolar lavage cells. *Comput. Struct. Biotechnol. J.* **2023**, *2*, 2985–3001. [CrossRef]
47. Shi, J.; Wu, K.; Zheng, Y.; He, Y.; Li, J.; Jiang, Z.; Yu, L. Global-local attention network for weakly supervised cervical cytology roi analysis. In Proceedings of the 2022 IEEE 19th International Symposium on Biomedical Imaging (ISBI), Kolkata, India, 28–31 March 2022; pp. 1–5.
48. Tarimo, S.-A.; Mi-Ae Jang, M.-A.; Ngasa, E.-E.; Shin, H.-B.; Shin, H.; Woo, J. Wbc yolo-vit: 2 way—2 stage white blood cell detection and classification with a combination of yolov5 and vision transformer. *Comput. Biol. Med.* **2024**, *169*, 107875. [CrossRef]
49. Wijaya, H.; Ryanto, T.; Sidhik, S.-C.; Liawatimena, S.; Riana, D. Cervical Cancer Cells Detection Using Yolov8 Algorithm. Available online: https://papers.ssrn.com/sol3/papers.cfm?abstract_id=4779266 (accessed on 5 April 2025).
50. Wang, H.-H.; Guo, M.-X.; Sun, Y.-N.; Zhang, C.-Y.; Long, L.; Liang, Z.-X. Development and diagnostic value of artificial intelligence cytopathological diagnosis system for lung cancer. *Acad. J. Chin. PLA Med. Sch.* **2024**, *45*, 463–468.
51. Mika, T.; Tanaka, S.; Ichito, S.; Etsuko, T.; Takakuma, S.; Tabata, R.; Sakae, K.; Kajimoto, Y.; Shinobu, K.; Akira, S.; et al. From Microscope to AI: Developing an Integrated Diagnostic System with Real-Time Object Detection for Endometrial Cytology. *Res. Sq.* **2024**, *45*, 463–468. [CrossRef]
52. Rumpf, S.; Zufall, N. Is the use of Adam optimiser and label smoothing adequate for optimizing YOLOv7 and YOLOv7-E6E to attain a high-quality automated analysis and differential diagnostic evaluation of bronchoalveolar lavage fluid? *Res. Sq.* **2024**. Available online: https://sciprofiles.com/publication/view/b0b32e213deba6f61689ccc58b1fec88 (accessed on 5 April 2025).
53. Awad, A.; Hegazy, M.; Aly, S.-A. Early Diagnosis of Acute Lymphoblastic Leukemia Using YOLOv8 and YOLOv11 Deep Learning Models. Available online: https://arxiv.org/abs/2410.10701 (accessed on 5 April 2025).
54. Available online: https://roboflow.com/ (accessed on 5 April 2025).
55. Golchubian, A.; Marques, O.; Nojoumian, M. Photo quality classification using deep learning. In *Multimedia Tools and Applications (MTAP)*; Springer: Berlin/Heidelberg, Germany, 2021; Volume 80, pp. 22193–22208.
56. Di Piazza, T.; Boussel, L. An Ensemble-Based Two-Step Framework for Classification of Pap Smear Cell Images. Available online: https://arxiv.org/abs/2503.10312 (accessed on 5 April 2025).
57. Level Up with the Largest AI & ML Community. Available online: https://www.kaggle.com (accessed on 5 April 2025).
58. Lin, R.; Li, Y.; Lin, Y.; Tian, W.; Jiang, L.; Li, J. Role of molecular testing for malignant pleural effusion in targeted therapy for advanced non-small cell lung cancer. *Diagn. Cytopathol.* **2023**, *51*, 397–405. [CrossRef] [PubMed]
59. Scarpino, S.; Leone, A.; Galafate, D.; Pepe, F.; Malapelle, U.; Villani, S.; Giarnieri, E.; Maurizi, G.; De Vitis, C.; Mancini, R.; et al. Integrating the Idylla™ System Alongside a Real-Time Polymerase Chain Reaction and Next-Generation Sequencing for Investigating Gene Fusions in Pleural Effusions from Non-Small-Cell Lung Cancer Patients: A Pilot Study. *Int. J. Mol. Sci.* **2024**, *25*, 7594. [CrossRef] [PubMed]
60. Orlandi, R.; Cara, A.; Cassina, E.M.; Degiovanni, S.; Libretti, L.; Pirondini, E.; Raveglia, F.; Tuoro, A.; Vaquer, S.; Rizzo, S.; et al. Malignant Pleural Effusion: Diagnosis and Treatment—Up-to-Date Perspective. *Curr. Oncol.* **2024**, *31*, 6867–6878. [CrossRef]
61. Pirovano, A.; Almeida, L.-G.; Ladjal, S.; Bloch, I.; Berlemont, S. Computer-aided diagnosis tool for cervical cancer screening with weakly supervised localization and detection of abnormalities using adaptable and explainable classifier. *Med. Image Anal.* **2021**, *73*, 102167. [CrossRef]
62. Zhang, L.; Lu, L.; Nogues, I.; Summers, R.M.; Liu, S.; Yao, J. DeepPap: Deep Convolutional Networks for Cervical Cell Classification. *IEEE J. Biomed. Health Inform.* **2017**, *21*, 633–1643. [CrossRef]
63. Zhou, Y.; Chen, H.; Lin, H.; Heng, P.A. Deep Semi-supervised Knowledge Distillation for Overlapping Cervical Cell Instance Segmentation. In Proceedings of the Medical Image Computing and Computer Assisted Intervention—MICCAI 2020, Lima, Peru, 4–8 October 2020; Lecture Notes in Computer Science; Springer: Cham, Switzerland, 2020; p. 12261.
64. Dey, P. Artificial neural network in diagnostic cytology. *Cytojournal* **2022**, *2*, 19–27. [CrossRef]
65. Truong, H.; Morimoto, R.; Walts, A.E.; Erler, B.; Marchevsky, A. Neural networks as an aid in the diagnosis of lymphocyte-rich effusions. *Anal. Quant. Cytol. Histol.* **1995**, *17*, 48–54.
66. Fang, W.; Wang, L.; Ren, P. Tinier-yolo: A real-time object detection method for constrained environments. *IEEE Access* **2019**, *8*, 1935–1944. [CrossRef]
67. Ali, H.M.; El Abbadi, N.K. Optic disc localization in retinal fundus images based on you only look once network (yolo). *Int. J. Intell. Eng. Syst.* **2023**, *16*, 2.

68. Liang, L.; Wang, Z.; Ye, X. Application of deep learning in imaging diagnosis of brain diseases. In Proceedings of the 2021 3rd International Conference on Machine Learning, Big Data and Business Intelligence (MLBDBI), Taiyuan, China, 3–5 December 2021; IEEE: Piscataway, NJ, USA, 2021; pp. 166–175.
69. Honda, H.; Mori, S.; Watanabe, A.; Sasagasako, N.; Sadashima, S.; Đồng, T.; Satoh, K.; Nishida, N.; Iwaki, T. Abnormal prion protein deposits with high seeding activities in the skeletal muscle, femoral nerve, and scalp of an autopsied case of sporadic Creutzfeldt–Jakob disease. *Neuropathology* **2021**, *41*, 152–158. [CrossRef]
70. Zhuang, Z.; Liu, G.; Ding, W.; Sasagasako, N.; Sadashima, S.; Đồng, T.; Satoh, K.; Nishida, N.; Iwaki, T. Cardiac vfm visualization and analysis based on yolo deep learning model and modified 2d continuity equation. *Comput. Med. Imaging Graph.* **2020**, *82*, 101732. [CrossRef] [PubMed]
71. Rong, R.; Sheng, H.; Jin, K.W.; Wu, F.; Luo, D.; Wen, Z.; Tang, C.; Donghan, M.; Yang, D.; Jia, L.; et al. A deep learning approach for histology-based nuclei segmentation and tumor microenvironment characterization. *bioRxiv* **2022**, *12*, 519641.
72. Elazab, N.; Gab-Allah, W.-A.; Elmogy, M. A multi-class brain tumor grading system based on histopathological images using a hybrid YOLO and RESNET networks. *Sci. Rep.* **2024**, *14*, 4584. [CrossRef]
73. Topuz, Y.; Yildiz, S.; Varli, S. Performance analysis of the YOLO series for object detection: Detection of mitosis cells in histopathology images. In Proceedings of the 2023 Medical Technologies Congress, Famagusta, Cyprus, 10–12 November 2023; pp. 1–4.
74. Ikeda, K.; Sakabe, N.; Ito, C.; Shimoyama, Y.; Toda, K.; Fukuda, K.; Yoshizaki, Y.; Sato, S.; Nagata, K. Staining, magnification, and algorithmic conditions for highly accurate cell detection and cell classification by deep learning. *Am. J. Clin. Pathol.* **2024**, *16*, 399–441. [CrossRef]
75. Wang, S.; Rong, R.; Yang, D.M.; Fujimoto, J.; Yan, S.; Cai, L.; Yang, L.; Luo, D.; Behrens, C.; Parra, E.R.; et al. Computational Staining of Pathology Images to Study the Tumor Microenvironment in Lung Cancer. *Cancer Res.* **2020**, *80*, 2056–2066. [CrossRef]
76. Tomita, N.; Tafe, L.J.; Suriawinata, A.A.; Tsongalis, G.J.; Nasir-Moin, M.; Dragnev, K.; Hassanpour, S. Predicting Oncogene Mutations of Lung Cancer Using Deep Learning and Histopathologic Features on Whole-Slide Images. *Transl. Oncol.* **2022**, *24*, 101494. [CrossRef]
77. Ragab, M.G.; Abdulkadir, S.G.; Muneer, A.; Alqushaibi, A.; Sumiea, E.H.; Qureshi, R.; Al-Selwi, S.M.; Alhussian, H. A Comprehensive Systematic Review of YOLO for Medical Object Detection (2018 to 2023). *IEEE Access* **2024**, *12*, 57815–57836. [CrossRef]
78. Pao, J.J.; Biggs, M.; Duncan, D.; Lin, D.I.; Davis, R.; Huang, R.S.P.; Ferguson, D.; Janovitz, T.; Hiemenz, M.C.; Eddy, N.R.; et al. Predicting EGFR Mutational Status from Pathology Images Using a Real-World Dataset. *Sci. Rep.* **2023**, *13*, 4404. [CrossRef]
79. McAlpine, E.; Michelow, P.; Liebenberg, E.; Turgay Celik, T. Are synthetic cytology images ready for prime time? A comparative assessment of real and synthetic urine cytology images. *J. Am. Soc. Cytopathol.* **2023**, *12*, 126–135. [CrossRef]
80. Sabnam, S.; Rajagopal, S. Application of generative adversarial networks in image, face reconstruction and medical imaging: Challenges and the current progress. *Comput. Methods Biomech. Biomed. Eng. Imaging Vis.* **2024**, *12*, 126–135. [CrossRef]
81. Teramoto, A.; Tsukamoto, T.; Yamada, A.; Kiriyama, Y.; Imaizumi, K.; Saito, K.; Fujita, H. Deep Learning Approach to Classification of Lung Cytological Images: Two-Step Training Using Actual and Synthesized Images by Progressive Growing of Generative Adversarial Networks. *PLoS ONE* **2020**, *15*, 229951. [CrossRef] [PubMed]

diagnostics

MDPI

Article

Deep Learning Approaches to Forecast Physical and Mental Deterioration During Chemotherapy in Patients with Cancer

Joseph Finkelstein [1], Aref Smiley [1,*], Christina Echeverria [2] and Kathi Mooney [2]

[1] Department of Biomedical Informatics, The University of Utah, Salt Lake City, UT 84108, USA; joseph.finkelstein@utah.edu
[2] College of Nursing, The University of Utah, Salt Lake City, UT 84108, USA; christina.echeverria@nurs.utah.edu (C.E.); kathi.mooney@nurs.utah.edu (K.M.)
* Correspondence: aref.smiley@utah.edu; Tel.: +1-(801)-581-4080

Abstract: Background/Objectives: Predicting symptom escalation during chemotherapy is crucial for timely interventions and improved patient outcomes. This study employs deep learning models to predict the deterioration of 12 self-reported symptoms, categorized into physical (e.g., nausea, fatigue, pain) and mental (e.g., feeling blue, trouble thinking) groups. **Methods**: The analytical dataset comprises daily self-reported symptom logs from individuals undergoing chemotherapy. To address class imbalance—where 84% of cases showed no escalation—symptoms were grouped into intervals of 3 to 7 days. Convolutional Neural Networks (CNNs), Long Short-Term Memory (LSTM), and Gated Recurrent Unit (GRU) models were trained on 80% of the data and evaluated on the remaining 20%. **Results**: Results showed that 3-day intervals yielded the best predictive performance. CNNs excelled in predicting physical symptoms, achieving 79.2% accuracy, 84.1% precision, 78.8% recall, and an F1 score of 81.4%. For mental symptoms, GRU outperformed other models, with an accuracy of 77.2%, precision of 71.6%, recall of 62.2%, and an F1 score of 66.6%. Performance declined for longer intervals due to reduced temporal resolution and fewer training samples, though CNNs and GRU remained relatively stable. **Conclusions**: The findings emphasize the advantage of categorizing symptoms for more tailored predictions and demonstrate the potential of deep learning in forecasting symptom escalation. Integrating these predictive models into clinical workflows could facilitate proactive symptom management, allowing timely interventions and enhanced patient care during chemotherapy.

Keywords: chemotherapy symptom prediction; LSTM; CNN; GRU models; AI-driven symptom monitoring; oncology symptom management; digital health; AI

1. Introduction

Effective symptom management is a critical component of oncology care, directly influencing quality of life and treatment adherence. Individuals undergoing chemotherapy often experience a range of symptoms, including pain, fatigue, nausea, vomiting, and cognitive disturbances, which vary based on cancer type, disease stage, and treatment regimen [1]. According to the National Cancer Institute, between 20% and 50% of those receiving treatment experience pain, while fatigue is reported in 14% to 96% of cases [2]. Addressing these symptoms requires a multidisciplinary approach integrating evidence-based strategies, digital health technologies, and machine learning techniques [3].

Studies have demonstrated that proactive symptom monitoring improves outcomes by enabling early interventions and reducing the severity of treatment-related side effects [4–6].

Chemotherapy, while a cornerstone of cancer treatment, often leads to severe adverse effects that compromise well-being, including extreme fatigue, gastrointestinal issues, immune suppression, and neurotoxicity [7]. These side effects frequently contribute to treatment nonadherence, which impacts overall survival and disease progression [1]. Recent studies indicate that integrating self-reported symptoms into clinical workflows enhances symptom detection, extends survival, and improves overall care [8].

The rapid advancement of digital health technologies has facilitated real-time symptom monitoring, allowing automated symptom tracking and timely clinical interventions [9]. Telemonitoring systems have gained widespread acceptance among individuals with chronic conditions and seniors [10–12], providing a structured means for tracking symptom deterioration and alerting healthcare providers to potential complications [13,14]. The implementation of these digital systems has demonstrated significant potential in addressing the evolving and complex needs of individuals undergoing treatment, their caregivers, and healthcare providers [15]. However, a major challenge remains in utilizing self-reported outcomes to predict symptom escalation and determine the optimal timing for clinical intervention [16]. Traditional symptom management protocols often lack specificity, making it difficult for healthcare providers to decide when interventions are necessary [17,18].

Literature Review

There is a crucial demand for novel approaches that provide seamless and ongoing support to improve symptom oversight in patients with cancer. To address these limitations, machine learning (ML) and deep learning (DL) models have emerged as powerful tools for predicting symptom escalation [19,20]. Among these, Long Short-Term Memory (LSTM) networks and Convolutional Neural Networks (CNNs) have demonstrated substantial promise in analyzing longitudinal self-reported data [21–24]. LSTM models effectively capture temporal dependencies in sequential symptom data, identifying early patterns indicative of impending deterioration [25–28]. In contrast, CNNs leverage spatial feature extraction to identify patterns within structured symptom datasets, offering an alternative approach to symptom trajectory modeling [29–31].

Several studies have explored the potential of deep learning to predict symptom progression based on self-reported outcomes [32–34]. This study builds on prior research by investigating the predictive capabilities of CNN, LSTM, and Gated Recurrent Unit (GRU) models in forecasting chemotherapy-related symptom escalation. By analyzing self-reported symptom data across varying time intervals (3 to 7 days), this study evaluates the effectiveness of each model in detecting significant symptom escalation. The findings aim to enhance symptom prediction accuracy, allowing healthcare providers to intervene earlier and personalize treatment strategies.

By integrating deep learning models into digital health systems, clinicians can receive real-time alerts on symptom escalation, enabling proactive management and potentially improving overall treatment outcomes. This study makes several key contributions to the growing field of AI-driven healthcare: (1) it evaluates and compares the performance of three deep learning models—CNN, LSTM, and GRU—using high-frequency, real-world symptom data from chemotherapy patients; (2) it explores varying time intervals and a sliding-window approach to optimize temporal prediction; and (3) it distinguishes between physical and mental symptoms to support more targeted interventions. This research contributes to the growing field of AI-driven healthcare by demonstrating how predictive models can be leveraged to optimize symptom monitoring, reduce distress, and improve adherence to therapy.

2. Methods

Data Collection and Preprocessing

This study utilized data from the Symptom Care at Home Study [35], comprising a total of 26,599 symptom records collected from individuals undergoing chemotherapy. The dataset included a diverse range of participants with variations in age, gender, ethnicity, and socioeconomic status. Table 1 presents a comprehensive demographic summary of the study population. The most common diagnoses are breast cancer (156 participants), lung cancer (61 participants), and ovarian cancer (36 participants), followed by other conditions such as colorectal (26), pancreatic (21), and head and neck cancers (13).

To ensure consistent and reliable data collection, participants were instructed to record their symptoms daily using a technology-based system. This allows continuous tracking of symptom progression. The dataset included 12 key symptoms, categorized into two primary groups:

1. Physical Symptoms: Nausea/vomiting, sore mouth, diarrhea, fatigue, hair loss/weight change, pain/discomfort, numbness/tingling, and fever-related distress. These symptoms reflect physiological responses to chemotherapy and cancer-related effects.
2. Mental Symptoms: Trouble thinking, feeling blue or nervous/anxious, and trouble sleeping. These symptoms represent cognitive and emotional challenges associated with treatment.

For each symptom, two quantitative metrics were recorded:

1. Severity (rated from 1 to 10, where 10 represents the most intense experience).
2. Distress (rated from 1 to 10, indicating the level of emotional burden associated with the symptom).

If a symptom was not reported on a given day, both metrics were recorded as zero. Fever was an exception, where only distress values were recorded. A daily symptom burden score was computed by summing all severity and distress values, resulting in a total possible score range of 0 to 230 per day.

The dataset included 349 participants, each undergoing an average of three chemotherapy cycles, with a median participation period of 81 days. Missing values in the dataset, particularly for symptom severity and distress, were addressed using linear interpolation, which estimated values based on adjacent days' records. This approach ensured the continuity and reliability of data without introducing artificial fluctuations.

Due to the highly imbalanced nature of the dataset, where 84% of recorded instances indicated no symptom escalation, we implemented a resampling strategy to enhance the model's ability to detect meaningful symptom variations. Symptom data were aggregated into multi-day intervals (3 to 7 days), thereby reducing the number of zero scores while preserving temporal progression. This interval-based approach enabled a more balanced distribution of data, allowing for improved model training and detection of symptom escalation trends.

Table 1. This table provides an overview of the demographic characteristics of the 349 participants included in the study.

Category	Count	Percentage
Total Participants	349.0	100%
Gender—Female	263.0	75.4%
Gender—Male	86.0	24.6%
Age—Mean	55.8	-
Age—Median	56.6	-

Table 1. *Cont.*

Category	Count	Percentage
Age—Min	24.0	-
Age—Max	85.0	-
Race—White	290.0	82.96%
Race—Black	40.0	11.45%
Race—Asian	5.0	1.4%
Race—Unknown/Other	5.0	1.4%
Marital Status—Married	184.0	52.7%
Marital Status—Single	112.0	32.1%
Marital Status—Other	53.0	15.2%
Education—Some College/Technical	125.0	35.8%
Education—High School Graduate	87.0	24.9%
Education—Bachelor's Degree	66.0	18.9%
Education—Graduate/Professional Degree	22.0	6.3%
Education—Less than High School	49.0	14.1%
Employment—Full-time (31+ h)	73.0	20.9%
Employment—Part-time (11–30 h)	55.0	15.8%
Employment—Minimal (1–10 h)	18.0	5.2%
Employment—Unemployed/Retired	203.0	58.1%
Income—USD 10,000-USD 19,999	82.0	23.5%
Income—USD 30,000-USD 39,999	64.0	18.2%
Income—USD 40,000-USD 49,999	54.0	15.4%
Income—USD 50,000-USD 69,999	47.0	13.5%
Income—Below USD 10,000 or Above USD 70,000	102.0	29.4%
Insurance—Medicaid/Medicare	165.0	47.3%
Insurance—Private	133.0	38.2%
Insurance—Uninsured	51.0	14.5%
Diagnosis—Breast Cancer	109.0	31.2%
Diagnosis—Lung Cancer	70.0	20.1%
Diagnosis—Ovarian Cancer	54.0	15.5%
Diagnosis—Other Malignancies	116.0	33.2%
Stage at Diagnosis—Stage IV	147.0	42.1%
Stage at Diagnosis—Stage III	103.0	29.5%
Stage at Diagnosis—Stage II	66.0	18.9%
Stage at Diagnosis—Stage I	33.0	9.5%

3. Resampling and Interval-Based Data Structuring

To optimize model performance, symptom data were grouped into intervals of 3, 4, 5, 6, or 7 days. Within each interval, symptom scores were averaged to capture overall symptom trends, rather than day-to-day fluctuations, while maintaining temporal relationships.

To ensure statistical robustness, only individuals with at least ($n \times 7$) days of continuous data were included in the analysis, where n represents the interval length. For example, for a 3-day interval, participants needed at least 21 days of data to be included in the model.

Individuals with insufficient records were excluded to ensure uniformity in training and testing datasets. Shorter intervals (e.g., 3 days) retained high temporal resolution, but increased data variability and longer intervals (e.g., 7 days) provided smoother trends but potentially masked short-term symptom escalations.

A binary classification variable was assigned for each interval: 1 (escalation detected) if the total symptom burden score increased beyond a predefined threshold and 0 (no escalation) if the symptom burden remained stable or decreased.

The predictive framework used data from past intervals (e.g., intervals 1–3) to forecast symptom escalation in the next interval (e.g., interval 4). This sliding-window approach ensured that the model learned from sequential patterns in symptom progression.

4. Deep Learning Model Architecture

Deep learning models were selected for their strong performance in modeling complex and temporal relationships in patient-reported outcome data. Long Short-Term Memory (LSTM) and Gated Recurrent Unit (GRU) are types of recurrent neural networks (RNNs) designed to capture sequential dependencies and long-term patterns across time-series data, making them well-suited for predicting symptom progression. Convolutional Neural Networks (CNNs), although originally developed for image analysis, have shown strong performance in extracting features from structured time-series data due to their ability to recognize localized patterns. These models were chosen to evaluate different learning mechanisms and identify the most effective approach for forecasting physical and mental symptom escalation during chemotherapy. The architectural details of each deep learning model are described in the following subsections.

4.1. Long Short-Term Memory (LSTM)

LSTM networks are designed to capture longitudinal dependencies within sequential data, making them well-suited for symptom prediction. The architecture included the following:

- A 50-unit LSTM layer to process temporal trends.
- A dropout layer (0.2 probability) to mitigate overfitting.
- A fully connected (dense) layer with sigmoid activation for binary classification.
- Binary cross-entropy loss function with the Adam optimizer for efficient learning.

4.2. Convolutional Neural Network (CNN)

CNNs were used to detect localized patterns in symptom data, recognizing critical escalation features across intervals. The model structure comprised the following:

- A 1D convolutional layer (64 filters, kernel size = 3) for feature extraction.
- Max-pooling and flattening layers to reduce data dimensionality.
- Dense layers with ReLU activation for feature refinement.
- A dropout layer for regularization.
- A sigmoid-activated output layer for binary classification.

4.3. Gated Recurrent Unit (GRU)

GRUs are an efficient alternative to LSTMs, designed to process sequential patterns with fewer computational requirements. The model included the following:

- A 50-unit GRU layer for learning temporal dependencies.
- Dropout regularization to prevent overfitting.
- A final sigmoid-activated layer for binary classification.

Each model was trained using 80% of the dataset, while 20% was reserved for evaluation. Performance was assessed using key classification metrics, including accuracy, precision, recall, F1 score, and area under the receiver operating characteristic curve (AUC).

An overview of the proposed symptom prediction framework is illustrated in Figure 1.

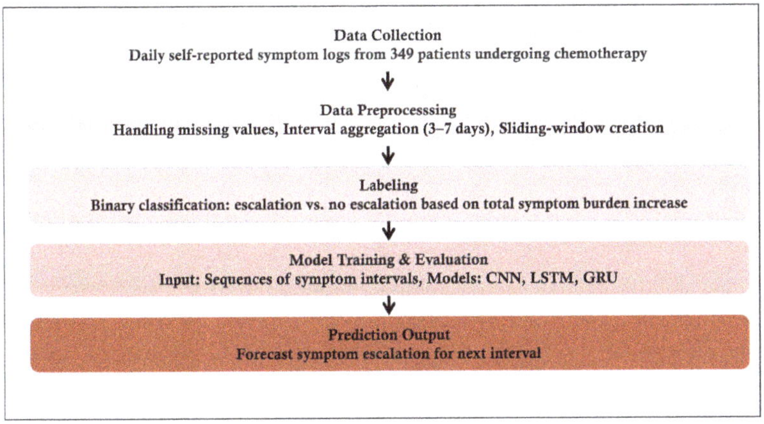

Figure 1. Workflow of the proposed deep learning-based framework for forecasting symptom escalation in chemotherapy patients.

5. Ethical Considerations

This study was conducted in compliance with ethical research standards and received Institutional Review Board (IRB) approval from the University of Utah (IRB protocol: IRB_00017472).

6. Results

The performance of deep learning models (CNN, LSTM, and GRU) was assessed for predicting physical and mental symptom escalation in chemotherapy patients. The dataset was analyzed using different interval lengths (3, 4, 5, 6, and 7 days), with model evaluation metrics including accuracy, precision, recall, F1 score, and AUC (area under the curve). A summary of the results across models and time intervals is provided in Tables 2–7.

Table 2. CNN performance for physical symptoms.

Interval	Accuracy	Precision	Recall	F1 Score	AUC
3	79.22%	83.74%	79.41%	81.51%	83.08%
4	77.02%	82.76%	79.18%	80.93%	81.89%
5	73.98%	81.47%	77.60%	79.49%	77.29%
6	76.59%	82.84%	82.35%	82.60%	80.20%
7	73.17%	83.50%	75.17%	79.12%	78.00%

For predicting physical symptom escalation, the 3-day interval consistently demonstrated the highest predictive accuracy across all models. The CNN, LSTM, and GRU models exhibited distinct strengths across the assessed metrics (Tables 2–4). Among them, GRU demonstrated the highest overall performance, achieving an accuracy of 80.05% and an F1 score of 82.50% at the 3-day interval, making it the most effective model for short-term symptom prediction.

Table 3. LSTM performance for physical symptoms.

Interval	Accuracy	Precision	Recall	F1 Score	AUC
3	79.22%	84.16%	78.81%	81.40%	83.76%
4	77.21%	83.04%	79.18%	81.06%	82.74%
5	74.55%	82.57%	77.10%	79.74%	78.45%
6	76.69%	82.58%	82.94%	82.76%	81.07%
7	74.59%	82.99%	78.50%	80.68%	78.70%

Table 4. GRU performance for physical symptoms.

Interval	Accuracy	Precision	Recall	F1 Score	AUC
3	80.05%	83.51%	81.53%	82.50%	83.77%
4	76.43%	83.26%	77.27%	80.15%	82.22%
5	73.33%	81.53%	76.22%	78.78%	77.45%
6	77.18%	83.68%	82.21%	82.94%	80.71%
7	74.35%	84.20%	76.40%	80.11%	78.48%

Table 5. CNN performance for mental symptoms.

Interval	Accuracy	Precision	Recall	F1 Score	AUC
3	77.36%	72.83%	60.64%	66.18%	77.26%
4	74.35%	71.68%	60.10%	65.38%	75.72%
5	70.65%	69.40%	61.45%	65.19%	72.98%
6	71.73%	69.52%	66.30%	67.87%	75.21%
7	70.33%	70.99%	63.00%	66.75%	72.96%

Table 6. LSTM performance for mental symptoms.

Interval	Accuracy	Precision	Recall	F1 Score	AUC
3	77.41%	71.49%	63.45%	67.23%	77.11%
4	74.28%	71.05%	61.07%	65.68%	75.76%
5	70.49%	69.68%	60.18%	64.59%	72.88%
6	71.73%	69.52%	66.30%	67.87%	75.03%
7	69.98%	69.84%	64.25%	66.93%	73.08%

Table 7. GRU performance for mental symptoms.

Interval	Accuracy	Precision	Recall	F1 Score	AUC
3	77.21%	71.65%	62.25%	66.62%	77.09%
4	74.28%	72.13%	58.97%	64.89%	75.62%
5	70.57%	69.11%	61.82%	65.26%	72.86%
6	71.53%	69.65%	65.20%	67.35%	75.01%
7	69.74%	69.46%	64.25%	66.75%	72.85%

For mental symptoms, Tables 5–7 present the performance metrics of each model across different interval lengths. Among the models, CNN exhibited a slight advantage in AUC, achieving 77.26%, whereas LSTM outperformed the others in recall (63.45%) and F1 score (67.23%) at the 3-day interval, indicating its effectiveness in capturing symptom escalation patterns over short-term periods.

All models demonstrated comparable effectiveness in predicting both physical and mental symptom escalation, with their highest performance metrics observed at the 3-day interval. As the interval length increased, a decline in predictive performance was evident across all models. While CNN, LSTM, and GRU exhibited slight variations in specific metrics, their overall performance remained relatively similar, suggesting that no single model consistently outperformed the others across all evaluation criteria.

7. Discussion

The findings of this study highlight the potential of deep learning models—particularly LSTM, CNN, and GRU—in predicting symptom escalation among chemotherapy patients. Model performance was strongest when using shorter intervals (n = 3 days). However, as the interval length increased, accuracy and recall declined across all models, though precision remained relatively stable. These results suggest that shorter intervals are more effective for tracking rapid symptom fluctuations, a common challenge in chemotherapy symptom management.

The comparative analysis of these models underscores their complementary strengths. While LSTMs and GRUs excel at learning sequential dependencies in symptom progression, CNNs enhance feature extraction, potentially improving prediction accuracy in structured patient-generated data. This multi-model approach can be adapted for various clinical applications, particularly in continuous symptom monitoring scenarios where early intervention is critical. Implementing these models in digital health systems could enable real-time symptom tracking and automated alerts for healthcare providers, facilitating proactive interventions for patients at high risk of symptom escalation. This aligns with the growing trend of integrating AI into oncological care, where early symptom management has been shown to improve clinical outcomes and patient satisfaction.

A key challenge in this study was the highly imbalanced dataset, with 84% of recorded symptom instances showing no escalation. To address this, symptom data were aggregated into multi-day intervals, reducing the dominance of zero scores and improving model training. However, the observed decline in predictive performance for longer intervals suggests that additional strategies are needed to manage class imbalance effectively. Future research should explore techniques such as oversampling, synthetic data generation, and advanced resampling strategies to further enhance the models' ability to detect symptom escalation across varying time frames.

Although our study included 349 participants, the dataset encompassed over 26,000 daily symptom entries, offering substantial longitudinal data for model training and evaluation. The application of temporal aggregation and sliding-window techniques enabled efficient use of this data by capturing dynamic symptom trends over time. However, we acknowledge that a larger and more demographically diverse participant pool could enhance the generalizability and robustness of the models.

This study focused on deep learning models due to their proven effectiveness in capturing temporal dependencies and complex nonlinear patterns in sequential health data. These architectures are particularly well-suited for modeling symptom progression over time, which is critical in the context of chemotherapy monitoring. While traditional machine learning models such as Random Forest and Support Vector Machines have shown utility in various clinical prediction tasks, they are often limited in their ability to handle time-series data without extensive feature engineering. Future work will include benchmarking against these classical models to provide a more comprehensive comparison and assess the added value of deep learning approaches in symptom prediction.

Our findings align closely with previous studies highlighting the potential of deep learning in predictive modeling of sequential patient-generated data [31–34,36]. Despite the promising results, several limitations should be considered. This study relied on self-reported symptom data, which may be subject to biases such as underreporting or inconsistencies in daily logging. Future research could integrate objective physiological markers (e.g., heart rate, activity levels) [37,38] and data from electronic health records (EHRs) [24,39] to supplement self-reported symptoms, enhancing prediction accuracy and robustness. Enrichment of self-reported symptoms by real-world data extracted from electronic health records (EHRs) can help improve the predictive model performance [40,41]. Clinical decision support for early identification of cancer symptom deterioration embedded into EHRs can potentially improve the quality of life of cancer patients undergoing chemotherapy [42,43]. Additionally, this study focused on chemotherapy patients, and further investigation is needed to assess the generalizability of these models across different cancer types and treatment regimens and broader patient populations [44].

8. Conclusions

This study demonstrates the effectiveness of deep learning models—CNN, LSTM, and GRU—in predicting symptom escalation in chemotherapy patients. By leveraging AI-driven symptom monitoring, healthcare providers can deliver more personalized, proactive care, potentially improving patient outcomes and quality of life. By integrating these models into digital health platforms or electronic health records, clinicians could receive real-time alerts, enabling timely interventions that may prevent complications, improve patient comfort, and support treatment adherence. Future work should focus on refining these models for extended time intervals, addressing data imbalance more effectively, and exploring their applicability across diverse clinical settings to maximize their impact on patient care.

Author Contributions: Methodology, J.F. and A.S.; Software, A.S.; Validation, J.F. and K.M.; Formal analysis, A.S.; Investigation, A.S.; Resources, J.F. and K.M.; Data curation, A.S., C.E. and K.M.; Writing—original draft, A.S.; Writing—review & editing, J.F.; Supervision, J.F. and K.M.; Project administration, A.S. and C.E.; Funding acquisition, J.F. and K.M. All authors have read and agreed to the published version of the manuscript.

Funding: The project was in part funded by the contract HT9425-24-1-0264-P00001 from the Congressionally Directed Medical Research Program (CDMRP).

Institutional Review Board Statement: This study was conducted in compliance with ethical research standards and received Institutional Review Board (IRB) approval from the University of Utah (IRB protocol: IRB_00017472, approval date 21 September 2019).

Informed Consent Statement: Informed consent was obtained from all subjects involved in the study.

Data Availability Statement: The data presented in this study are available on request from the corresponding author.

Conflicts of Interest: The authors declare no conflict of interest.

References

1. Lizán, L.; Pérez-Carbonell, L.; Comellas, M. Additional Value of Patient-Reported Symptom Monitoring in Cancer Care: A Systematic Review of the Literature. *Cancers* **2021**, *13*, 4615. [CrossRef] [PubMed]

2. Sanft, T.; Day, A.; Ansbaugh, S.; Armenian, S.; Baker, K.S.; Ballinger, T.; Demark-Wahnefried, W.; Dickinson, K.; Fairman, N.P.; Felciano, J.; et al. NCCN Guidelines® Insights: Survivorship, Version 1.2023. *J. Natl. Compr. Canc Netw.* **2023**, *21*, 792–803. [CrossRef] [PubMed]
3. Ream, E.; Hughes, A.E.; Cox, A.; Skarparis, K.; Richardson, A.; Pedersen, V.H.; Wiseman, T.; Forbes, A.; Bryant, A. Telephone interventions for symptom management in adults with cancer. *Cochrane Database Syst. Rev.* **2020**, *6*, CD007568. [CrossRef] [PubMed]
4. Kamdar, M.; Jethwani, K.; Centi, A.J.; Agboola, S.; Fischer, N.; Traeger, L.; Rinaldi, S.; Strand, J.; Ritchie, C.; Temel, J.S.; et al. A Digital Therapeutic Application (ePAL) to Manage Pain in Patients with Advanced Cancer: A Randomized Controlled Trial. *J. Pain Symptom Manag.* **2024**, *68*, 261–271. [CrossRef] [PubMed]
5. Agboola, S.; Kamdar, M.; Flanagan, C.; Searl, M.; Traeger, L.; Kvedar, J.; Jethwani, K. Pain management in cancer patients using a mobile app: Study design of a randomized controlled trial. *JMIR Res. Protoc.* **2014**, *3*, e76. [CrossRef] [PubMed] [PubMed Central]
6. Basch, E.; Schrag, D.; Henson, S.; Jansen, J.; Ginos, B.; Stover, A.M.; Carr, P.; Spears, P.A.; Jonsson, M.; Deal, A.M.; et al. Effect of Electronic Symptom Monitoring on Patient-Reported Outcomes Among Patients with Metastatic Cancer: A Randomized Clinical Trial. *JAMA* **2022**, *327*, 2413–2422. [CrossRef] [PubMed] [PubMed Central]
7. Daly, B.; Nicholas, K.; Flynn, J.; Silva, N.; Panageas, K.; Mao, J.J.; Gazit, L.; Gorenshteyn, D.; Sokolowski, S.; Newman, T.; et al. Analysis of a Remote Monitoring Program for Symptoms Among Adults with Cancer Receiving Antineoplastic Therapy. *JAMA Netw. Open* **2022**, *5*, e221078. [CrossRef]
8. Basch, E.; Leahy, A.B.; Dueck, A.C. Benefits of Digital Symptom Monitoring with Patient-Reported Outcomes During Adjuvant Cancer Treatment. *J. Clin. Oncol.* **2021**, *39*, 701–703. [CrossRef]
9. Patt, D.A.; Patel, A.M.; Bhardwaj, A.; Hudson, K.E.; Christman, A.; Amondikar, N.; Escudier, S.M.; Townsend, S.; Books, H.; Basch, E. Impact of Remote Symptom Monitoring with Electronic Patient-Reported Outcomes on Hospitalization, Survival, and Cost in Community Oncology Practice: The Texas Two-Step Study. *JCO Clin. Cancer Inform.* **2023**, *7*, e2300182. [CrossRef]
10. Liljeroos, M.; Arkkukangas, M. Implementation of Telemonitoring in Health Care: Facilitators and Barriers for Using eHealth for Older Adults with Chronic Conditions. *Risk Manag. Healthc. Policy* **2023**, *16*, 43–53. [CrossRef] [PubMed] [PubMed Central]
11. Aggelidis, X.; Kritikou, M.; Makris, M.; Miligkos, M.; Papapostolou, N.; Papadopoulos, N.G.; Xepapadaki, P. Tele-Monitoring Applications in Respiratory Allergy. *J. Clin. Med.* **2024**, *13*, 898. [CrossRef] [PubMed] [PubMed Central]
12. Ezeamii, V.C.; Okobi, O.E.; Wambai-Sani, H.; Perera, G.S.; Zaynieva, S.; Okonkwo, C.C.; Ohaiba, M.M.; William-Enemali, P.C.; Obodo, O.R.; Obiefuna, N.G. Revolutionizing Healthcare: How Telemedicine Is Improving Patient Outcomes and Expanding Access to Care. *Cureus* **2024**, *16*, e63881. [CrossRef] [PubMed] [PubMed Central]
13. Zini, E.M.; Lanzola, G.; Quaglini, S.; Bossi, P.; Licitra, L.; Resteghini, C. A pilot study of a smartphone-based monitoring in-tervention on head and neck cancer patients undergoing concurrent chemo-radiotherapy. *Int. J. Med. Inform.* **2019**, *129*, 404–412. [CrossRef] [PubMed]
14. Rusli, E.; Wujcik, D.; Galaznik, A. Remote Symptom Alerts and Patient-Reported Outcomes (PROS) in Real-World Breast Cancer Practice: Innovative Data to Derive Symptom Burden and Quality of Life. *Bioengineering* **2024**, *11*, 846. [CrossRef] [PubMed] [PubMed Central]
15. Fraterman, I.; Wollersheim, B.M.; Tibollo, V.; Glaser, S.L.C.; Medlock, S.; Cornet, R.; Gabetta, M.; Gisko, V.; Barkan, E.; di Flora, N.; et al. An eHealth App (CAPABLE) Providing Symptom Monitoring, Well-Being Interventions, and Educational Material for Patients with Melanoma Treated with Immune Checkpoint Inhibitors: Protocol for an Exploratory Intervention Trial. *JMIR Res. Protoc.* **2023**, *12*, e49252. [CrossRef] [PubMed] [PubMed Central]
16. Snyder, C.F.; Blackford, A.L.; Okuyama, T.; Akechi, T.; Yamashita, H.; Toyama, T.; Carducci, M.A.; Wu, A.W. Using the EORTC-QLQC30 in clinical practice for patient management: Identifying scores requiring a clinician's attention. *Qual. Life Res.* **2013**, *22*, 2685–2691. [CrossRef]
17. Jeon, S.; Given, C.W.; Sikorskii, A.; Given, B. The utility of screening in the design of trials for symptom management in cancer. *J. Pain. Symptom Manag.* **2009**, *38*, 606–614. [CrossRef]
18. Oldenmenger, W.H.; de Raaf, P.J.; de Klerk, C.; van der Rijt, C.C. Cut points on 0–10 numeric rating scales for symptoms included in the Edmonton Symptom Assessment Scale in cancer patients: A systematic review. *J. Pain. Symptom Manag.* **2013**, *45*, 1083–1093. [CrossRef]
19. Zhang, J.; Lv, X.N.; Wang, M.; Zhang, J.; Qi, F. Continuous nursing symptom management in cancer chemotherapy patients using deep learning. *Sci. Rep.* **2025**, *15*, 7990. [CrossRef]
20. Moraza, J.; Esteban-Aizpiri, C.; Aramburu, A.; García, P.; Sancho, F.; Resino, S.; Chasco, L.; Conde, F.J.; Gutiérrez, J.A.; Santano, D.; et al. Using machine learning to predict deterioration of symptoms in COPD patients within a telemonitoring program. *Sci. Rep.* **2025**, *15*, 7064. [CrossRef]
21. Wang, Y.; Van Dijk, L.; Mohamed, A.S.R.; Fuller, C.D.; Zhang, X.; Marai, G.E.; Canahuate, G. Predicting late symptoms of head and neck cancer treatment using LSTM and patient reported outcomes. In Proceedings of the 25th International Database Engineering

& Applications Symposium, Montreal, QC, Canada, 14–16 July 2021; Volume 2021, pp. 273–279. [CrossRef] [PubMed] [PubMed Central]
22. Wang, Y.; Van Dijk, L.; Mohamed, A.S.R.; Naser, M.; Fuller, C.D.; Zhang, X.; Marai, G.E.; Canahuate, G. Improving Prediction of Late Symptoms using LSTM and Patient-reported Outcomes for Head and Neck Cancer Patients. In Proceedings of the 2023 IEEE 11th International Conference on Healthcare Informatics (ICHI), Houston, TX, USA, 26–29 June 2023; Volume 2023, pp. 292–300. [CrossRef] [PubMed] [PubMed Central]
23. Badura, A.; Bienkowska, M.; Mysliwiec, A.; Pietka, E. Continuous Short-Term Pain Assessment in Temporomandibular Joint Therapy Using LSTM Models Supported by Heat-Induced Pain Data Patterns. *IEEE Trans. Neural Syst. Rehabil. Eng.* **2024**, *32*, 3565–3576. [CrossRef] [PubMed]
24. Lindvall, C.; Deng, C.Y.; Agaronnik, N.D.; Kwok, A.; Samineni, S.; Umeton, R.; Mackie-Jenkins, W.; Kehl, K.L.; Tulsky, J.A.; Enzinger, A.C. Deep Learning for Cancer Symptoms Monitoring on the Basis of Electronic Health Record Unstructured Clinical Notes. *JCO Clin. Cancer Inform.* **2022**, *6*, e2100136. [CrossRef] [PubMed] [PubMed Central]
25. Chae, S.; Street, W.N.; Ramaraju, N.; Gilbertson-White, S. Prediction of cancer symptom trajectory using longitudinal electronic health record data and long short-term memory neural network. *JCO Clin. Cancer Inform.* **2024**, *8*, e2300039. [CrossRef]
26. Zeinali, N.; Youn, N.; Albashayreh, A.; Fan, W.; Gilbertson White, S. Machine Learning Approaches to Predict Symptoms in People with Cancer: Systematic Review. *JMIR Cancer* **2024**, *10*, e52322. [CrossRef] [PubMed] [PubMed Central]
27. Papachristou, N.; Puschmann, D.; Barnaghi, P.; Cooper, B.; Hu, X.; Maguire, R.; Apostolidis, K.; Conley, Y.P.; Hammer, M.; Katsaragakis, S.; et al. Learning from data to predict future symptoms of oncology patients. *PLoS ONE* **2018**, *13*, e0208808. [CrossRef] [PubMed] [PubMed Central]
28. Pan, L.C.; Wu, X.R.; Lu, Y.; Zhang, H.Q.; Zhou, Y.L.; Liu, X.; Liu, S.L.; Yan, Q.Y. Artificial intelligence empowered digital health technologies in cancer survivorship care: A scoping review. *Asia Pac. J. Oncol. Nurs.* **2022**, *9*, 100127. [CrossRef] [PubMed] [PubMed Central]
29. Pinzon-Arenas, J.O.; Kong, Y.; Chon, K.H.; Posada-Quintero, H.F. Design and Evaluation of Deep Learning Models for Continuous Acute Pain Detection Based on Phasic Electrodermal Activity. *IEEE J. Biomed. Health Inform.* **2023**, *27*, 4250–4260. [CrossRef] [PubMed]
30. Metzger, M.H.; Gadji, A.; Haj Salah, N.; Kane, W.; Boue, F. Deep Learning Methods for Detecting Side Effects of Cancer Chemotherapies Reported in a Remote Monitoring Web Application. *Stud. Health Technol. Inform.* **2022**, *294*, 880–881. [CrossRef] [PubMed]
31. Verma, S.; Raj, S.; Kumar, S.; Raj, S.; Rautaray, S.S.; Pandey, M. Disease Predictive System Based on Symptom Analysis Using ML Algorithm. In *Smart Systems: Innovations in Computing*; Somani, A.K., Mundra, A., Gupta, R.K., Bhattacharya, S., Mazumdar, A.P., Eds.; SSIC 2023; Smart Innovation, Systems and Technologies; Springer: Singapore, 2024; Volume 392. [CrossRef]
32. Bhati, R.; Jones, J.; Durand, A. Interpret Your Care: Predicting the Evolution of Symptoms for Cancer Patients. *arXiv* **2023**, arXiv:2302.09659. [CrossRef]
33. Sannala, G.S.; Rohith, K.V.G.; Vyas, A.G.; Kavitha, C.R. Explainable Artificial Intelligence-Based Disease Prediction with Symptoms Using Machine Learning Models. In *IoT Based Control Networks and Intelligent Systems*; Joby, P.P., Alencar, M.S., Falkowski-Gilski, P., Eds.; ICICNIS 2023; Lecture Notes in Networks and Systems; Springer: Singapore, 2024; Volume 789. [CrossRef]
34. Floricel, C.; Nipu, N.; Biggs, M.; Wentzel, A.; Canahuate, G.; Van Dijk, L.; Mohamed, A.; Fuller, C.D.; Marai, G.E. THALIS: Human-Machine Analysis of Longitudinal Symptoms in Cancer Therapy. *arXiv* **2021**, arXiv:2108.02817. [CrossRef]
35. Mooney, K.H.; Beck, S.L.; Wong, B.; Dunson, W.; Wujcik, D.; Whisenant, M.; Donaldson, G. Automated home monitoring and management of patient-reported symptoms during chemotherapy: Results of the symptom care at home RCT. *Cancer Med.* **2017**, *6*, 537–546. [CrossRef] [PubMed]
36. Smiley, A.; Tsai, T.Y.; Zakashansky, E.; Gabriel, A.; Xhakli, T.; Cui, W.; Huo, X.; Havrylchuk, I.; Cui, H.; Finkelstein, J. Exercise Exertion Levels Prediction Based on Real-Time Wearable Physiological Signal Monitoring. *Stud. Health Technol. Inform.* **2023**, *305*, 172–175. [CrossRef] [PubMed]
37. D'Haese, P.F.; Finomore, V.; Lesnik, D.; Kornhauser, L.; Schaefer, T.; Konrad, P.E.; Hodder, S.; Marsh, C.; Rezai, A.R. Prediction of viral symptoms using wearable technology and artificial intelligence: A pilot study in healthcare workers. *PLoS ONE* **2021**, *16*, e0257997. [CrossRef] [PubMed] [PubMed Central]
38. Cay, G.; Sada, Y.H.; Dehghan Rouzi, M.; Uddin Atique, M.M.; Rodriguez, N.; Azarian, M.; Finco, M.G.; Yellapragada, S.; Najafi, B. Harnessing physical activity monitoring and digital biomarkers of frailty from pendant based wearables to predict chemotherapy resilience in veterans with cancer. *Sci. Rep.* **2024**, *14*, 2612. [CrossRef] [PubMed] [PubMed Central]
39. Bandyopadhyay, A.; Albashayreh, A.; Zeinali, N.; Fan, W.; Gilbertson-White, S. Using real-world electronic health record data to predict the development of 12 cancer-related symptoms in the context of multimorbidity. *JAMIA Open* **2024**, *7*, ooae082. [CrossRef] [PubMed] [PubMed Central]

40. Hickin, M.P.; Shariff, J.A.; Jennette, P.J.; Finkelstein, J.; Papapanou, P.N. Incidence and Determinants of Dental Implant Failure: A Review of Electronic Health Records in a U.S. Dental School. *J. Dent. Educ.* **2017**, *81*, 1233–1242. [CrossRef] [PubMed]
41. Finkelstein, J.; Zhang, F.; Levitin, S.A.; Cappelli, D. Using big data to promote precision oral health in the context of a learning healthcare system. *J. Public. Health Dent.* **2020**, *80* (Suppl. S1), S43–S58. [CrossRef] [PubMed] [PubMed Central]
42. Paranjpe, I.; Russak, A.J.; De Freitas, J.K.; Lala, A.; Miotto, R.; Vaid, A.; Johnson, K.W.; Danieletto, M.; Golden, E.; Meyer, D.; et al. Retrospective cohort study of clinical characteristics of 2199 hospitalised patients with COVID-19 in New York City. *BMJ Open* **2020**, *10*, e040736. [CrossRef] [PubMed] [PubMed Central]
43. Finkelstein, J.; Gabriel, A.; Schmer, S.; Truong, T.T.; Dunn, A. Identifying Facilitators and Barriers to Implementation of AI-Assisted Clinical Decision Support in an Electronic Health Record System. *J. Med. Syst.* **2024**, *48*, 89. [CrossRef] [PubMed] [PubMed Central]
44. Smiley, A.; Reategui-Rivera, C.M.; Villarreal-Zegarra, D.; Escobar-Agreda, S.; Finkelstein, J. Exploring Artificial Intelligence Biases in Predictive Models for Cancer Diagnosis. *Cancers* **2025**, *17*, 407. [CrossRef] [PubMed] [PubMed Central]

diagnostics

MDPI

Article

Advanced Assessment of Oxidative Stress and Inflammation in Military Personnel: Development of a Novel IIRPM Score Using Artificial Intelligence

Florina-Diana Mihai [1], Emil-Tiberius Trasca [2,3,*], Patricia-Mihaela Radulescu [4,*], Razvan Mercut [5,†], Elena-Irina Caluianu [2,3], Eleonora Daniela Ciupeanu-Calugaru [6,†], Dan Marian Calafeteanu [3,7], Georgiana-Andreea Marinescu [1], Suzana Danoiu [8] and Dumitru Radulescu [2,3,†]

[1] UMF Craiova Doctoral School, University of Medicine and Pharmacy Craiova, 200349 Craiova, Romania; staicu_diana2002@yahoo.com (F.-D.M.); marinescu_georgiana.andreea@yahoo.com (G.-A.M.)
[2] Department of Surgery, University of Medicine and Pharmacy Craiova, 200349 Craiova, Romania; irina.caluianu@umfcv.ro (E. I.C.); dr_radulescu_dumitru@yahoo.com (D.R.)
[3] The Military Emergency Clinical Hospital, 'Dr. Stefan Odobleja' Craiova, 200749 Craiova, Romania; danutcalafeteanu@yahoo.com
[4] Department of Pneumology, University of Medicine and Pharmacy Craiova, 200349 Craiova, Romania
[5] Department of Plastic and Reconstructive Surgery, University of Medicine and Pharmacy of Craiova, 200349 Craiova, Romania; mercut.razvan@umfcv.ro
[6] Department of Biology and Environmental Engineering, University of Craiova, 200585 Craiova, Romania; ciupeanudaniela@gmail.com
[7] Department of Ortopedics, University of Medicine and Pharmacy Craiova, 200349 Craiova, Romania
[8] Department of Pathophysiology, University of Medicine and Pharmacy of Craiova, 200349 Craiova, Romania; suzanadanoiu@yahoo.com
* Correspondence: etrasca@yahoo.com (E.-T.T.); patricia.radulescu@umfcv.ro (P.-M.R.)
† These authors contributed equally to this work.

Abstract: Background/Objectives: The health of military personnel in modern operational settings is critical for sustaining defense readiness. Extended exposure to extreme conditions can cause oxidative stress and systemic inflammation, potentially affecting performance. To address this problem, we developed an innovative diagnostic tool, the Post-Mission Integrated Risk Index (IIRPM), which integrates hematologic markers with key clinical variables. A novel aspect of the approach is the incorporation of ΔNLR, thus quantifying the change in the neutrophil-to-lymphocyte ratio measured before and after deployment, thereby providing a sensitive indicator of the inflammatory impact of operational stress. **Methods:** In this retrospective study, we analyzed comprehensive clinical and biological data from 443 military personnel over a ten-year period, with measurements taken before and after missions. We applied robust statistical techniques, including paired *t*-tests and Pearson correlation analyses, to assess variations in hematologic and metabolic parameters. Data segmentation was performed using Gaussian mixture models, and the predictive performance of the resulting model was validated with a multi-layer perceptron (MLP) neural network. **Results:** The analysis revealed significant post-mission increases in both the baseline NLR and ΔNLR, accompanied by notable shifts in metabolic markers. Data segmentation identified three distinct profiles: a reference profile characterized by stable immunologic parameters, an acute inflammatory response profile, and a proinflammatory metabolic profile marked by elevated cholesterol levels and higher mean age. Remarkably, the MLP model achieved 100% accuracy on the test set, with an average cross-validation accuracy of 97%. **Conclusions:** The IIRPM—which incorporates ΔNLR, age, mission duration, and cholesterol levels—offers a novel strategy to assess inflammatory risk among military personnel, thus facilitating personalized preventive interventions. Further validation in multicenter and longitudinal studies is anticipated to

 https://doi.org/10.3390/diagnostics15070832

consolidate the clinical utility of this tool, ultimately fostering a more adaptive approach in military medicine to address the complex challenges of modern operational theaters.

Keywords: oxidative stress; systemic inflammation; military personnel; integrative inflammatory risk post-mission index (IIRPM); ΔNLR (Delta NLR); neutrophil-to-lymphocyte ratio (NLR); artificial intelligence (AI); machine learning; risk stratification; military medicine

1. Introduction

In contemporary operational settings, the well-being of military personnel is paramount to maintaining an effective defense capability. Service members are frequently exposed to environments characterized by extreme physical demands, intense stress, and hostile conditions. Prolonged exposure to such adverse factors, including chronic sleep deprivation, excessive physical exertion, and significant psychological stress, can initiate oxidative stress and systemic inflammation. These processes, when sustained over time, have the potential to compromise both operational performance and rapid response capabilities. Consequently, continuous and comprehensive health monitoring is essential to prevent long-term physiological decline and maintain operational readiness [1,2].

Traditional assessment methodologies, which typically emphasize isolated measurement of individual biomarkers, often fail to capture the complex interplay between the immune response and oxidative stress. However, recent investigations have illuminated the value of integrated hematological indices, such as the neutrophil-to-lymphocyte ratio (NLR), platelet-to-lymphocyte ratio (PLR), and monocyte-to-lymphocyte ratio (MLR) as reliable indicators of systemic inflammation and oxidative stress. In particular, the NLR has emerged as a sensitive and specific marker of inflammation, closely associated with an overproduction of reactive oxygen species that can disrupt cell integrity by overwhelming endogenous antioxidant defenses [3–5]. Elevated NLR values are not only indicative of acute inflammatory responses but also signal an increased predisposition to chronic diseases, including cardiovascular disease [6–10]. Integrating these hematological markers with critical clinical parameters such as age, duration of mission, and cholesterol levels offers the promise of a comprehensive risk assessment, allowing personalized and preventive interventions.

Despite these advances, conventional biomarker assessments are often hampered by their fragmented and labor-intensive nature, which hinders rapid and holistic data interpretation. The absence of a standardized framework for data integration further complicates the comparability of results across studies and may lead to an underestimation of systemic risk factors. In this context, the incorporation of artificial intelligence (AI) methodologies emerges as a promising solution. Machine learning techniques—exemplified by Gaussian mixture models (GMM) and multi-layer perceptron (MLP) neural networks—are capable of processing large datasets concurrently, uncovering complex patterns, and building predictive models with exceptional precision [11,12]. By synergistically correlating hematological parameters with clinical and demographic information, these AI-driven approaches facilitate a more comprehensive assessment of inflammatory status and provide a robust framework for the ongoing monitoring of military health.

Consequently, the main objective of this study is to develop and validate the IIRPM Score, a composite metric designed to quantify post-mission inflammatory risk. This integrative score combines measures of NLR, PLR, and MLR with clinical variables such as age, duration of mission, and cholesterol levels to allow for precise risk stratification.

Using artificial intelligence capabilities, the approach seeks to minimize human error and detect early patterns of inflammatory response, thereby supporting the implementation of customized preventive strategies. The adoption of such an integrated model holds significant promise in improving operational performance and strengthening resilience against extreme stressors [1,13–16]. Furthermore, the convergence of molecular biology, precision medicine, and AI-driven IT solutions paves the way for the personalization of preventive and therapeutic strategies, informed by the unique profiles of individual military personnel and a refined understanding of adaptive mechanisms to operational stress.

2. Materials and Methods

2.1. Study Design

This retrospective investigation was carried out at the Military Hospital "Dr. Ștefan Odobleja" in Craiova over a decade-long period, from 1 October 2014 to 31 October 2024. The primary objective was to conduct an in-depth assessment of oxidative stress and inflammation in military personnel. To effectively capture the impact of operational environmental changes, the study focused exclusively on service members deployed on international missions. Clinical and biological data were collected systematically at both the time of deployment and after return.

Initially, 632 eligible military personnel were identified (Figure 1).

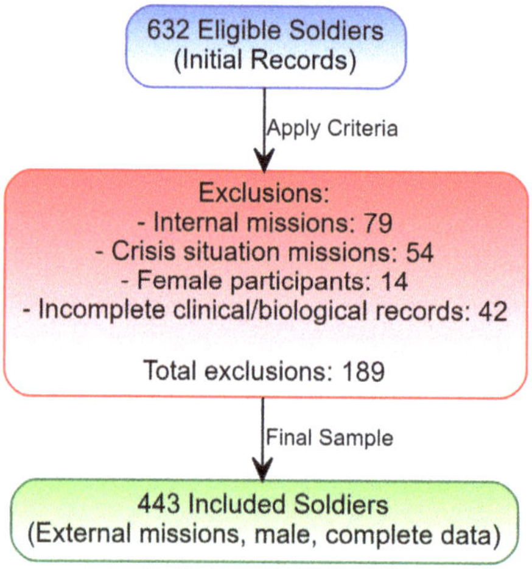

Figure 1. Study population selection flowchart for military personnel.

After applying stringent inclusion and exclusion criteria, the final sample was refined to 443 participants, ensuring sample homogeneity and the integrity of subsequent analyses.

2.2. Inclusion Criteria

The study considered only soldiers who had participated in international missions aimed at defending national territory within the framework of collective defense alliances (e.g., NATO), maintaining international peace and stability, or engaging in operations against international terrorism. To ensure the robustness and reliability of the analyses, only complete clinical and biological records were included—adhering to institutional protocols available in the electronic database of the Military Hospital "Dr. Ștefan Odobleja".

2.3. Exclusion Criteria

Service members who participated exclusively in domestic missions were excluded, as the study was specifically designed to evaluate the impact of a changing operational environment and its associated effects. Furthermore, individuals participating in missions under crisis conditions (such as emergency interventions or periods of international tension) or in active combat operations during wartime were not included, given that both biological and psychoemotional parameters are profoundly influenced in such contexts. Furthermore, the female subgroup was omitted from the analysis due to the very limited number of cases (14 women), which could potentially skew the statistical results. As a result, the final cohort comprised only male military personnel who had participated in overseas missions under comparable conditions and timeframes.

2.4. Data Collection

For each participant, clinical, biological, and demographic data were extracted from the electronic database of the Military Hospital "Dr. Ștefan Odobleja" in Craiova, with the objective of capturing changes from the point of deployment to the moment of return. The parameters selected for analysis included inflammatory markers, indicators of oxidative stress, and other biomarkers pertinent to a comprehensive evaluation of general health status. Rigorous validation procedures were implemented that involved independent verification and cross-correlation of data, and any records that were found to be inconsistent or incomplete were excluded from the study. This research protocol received approval from the Medical and Ethics Council of the Military Hospital "Dr. Ștefan Odobleja" in Craiova, in compliance with international regulations for medical research and the Declaration of Helsinki guidelines (approval number A/OR1-972/27 September 2023). Furthermore, ethical clearance was granted by the Ethics Committee of the University of Medicine and Pharmacy in Craiova (approval number 355/17 September 2024).

2.5. Statistical Analysis

Data processing was performed using SPSS (version 26.0, IBM Corporation, Armonk, NY, USA), Python (version 3.11) and specialized libraries (pandas, numpy, scikit-learn, imbalanced-learn, Matplotlib (version 3.7.3), and Seaborn (version 0.12.2)). Continuous variables that follow a normal distribution are presented as means $\pm$ standard deviations, whereas categorical variables are reported as percentages. Group comparisons were performed using the independent samples *t*-test, the Mann–Whitney U test for non-parametric data, and Fisher's Exact Test for categorical variables with low frequencies.

The methodological diagram (Figure 2) provides a clear overview of the study's workflow. Initially, data were collected both pre- and post-mission and then preprocessed through cleaning and normalization. Key features—including ΔNLR, age, mission duration, and cholesterol—were extracted from the dataset.

These features were used in two parallel AI-based analyses: first, a Gaussian mixture model was applied to segment the participants into distinct clusters, forming the basis for computing the Post-Mission Integrated Risk Score (IIRPM); second, the same features were fed into a multi-layer perceptron neural network to classify the profiles, with its performance evaluated via cross-validation. This dual approach—clustering with GMM and classification with MLP—ensures a robust assessment of inflammatory risk in military personnel.

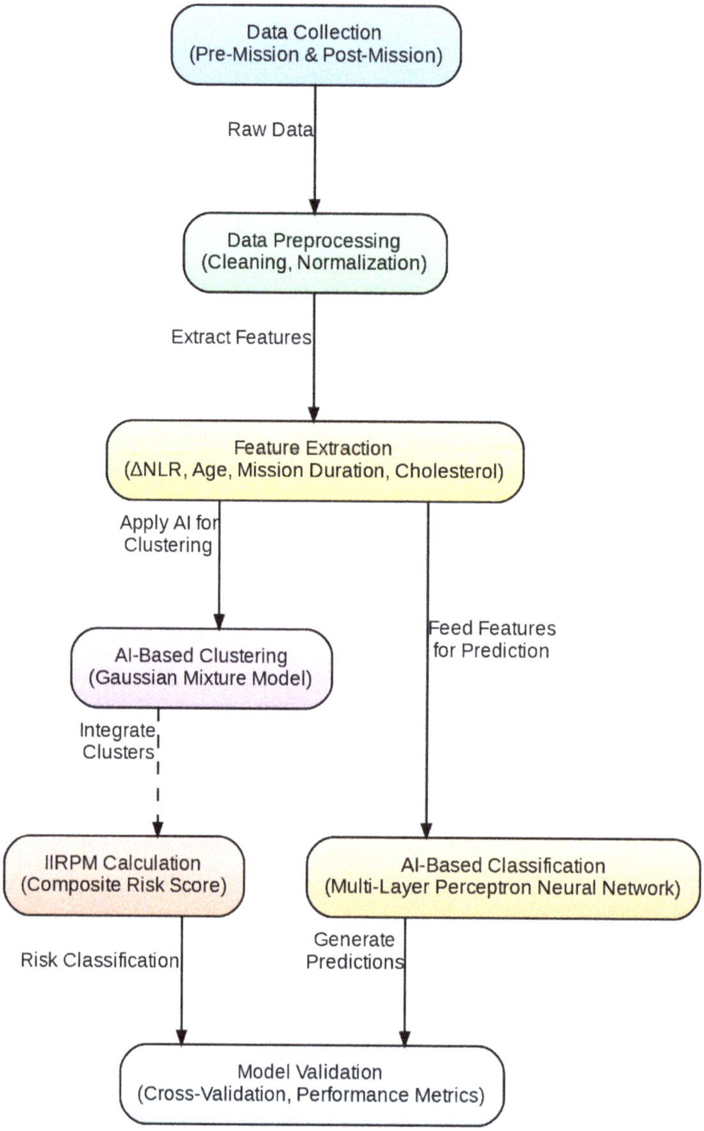

Figure 2. Overview of the research framework for post-mission risk assessment.

2.5.1. Data Preprocessing

Before advanced analysis, the dataset was meticulously cleaned and standardized. Continuous variables were normalized using the MinMaxScaler method to constrain them within a unit interval. Categorical variables were appropriately encoded using either one-hot or label encoding, depending on their nature. Incomplete records were excluded, and outlier values were rigorously evaluated and removed if they could not be justified on methodological or clinical grounds.

2.5.2. Data Augmentation and Balancing

To address the imbalance among different military profiles (identified later in the clustering analysis) and to prevent the model from being disproportionately influenced by underrepresented classes, an oversampling strategy using SMOTE (Synthetic Minority Over-Sampling Technique) was employed. This algorithm generated new synthetic instances based on existing characteristics, contributing to a more balanced training set and reducing the risk of overfitting to the majority classes.

This data augmentation method was integrated into a processing pipeline that encompassed both the preprocessing steps and the neural network training.

2.5.3. Neural Network Model

An MLP was developed to classify military personnel according to their inflammatory and oxidative stress profiles. The input variables used to train the MLP model were specifically the normalized values of mission duration and the post-mission neutrophil-to-lymphocyte ratio, as these features demonstrated the strongest discriminatory power in the clustering analysis (Figure 3).

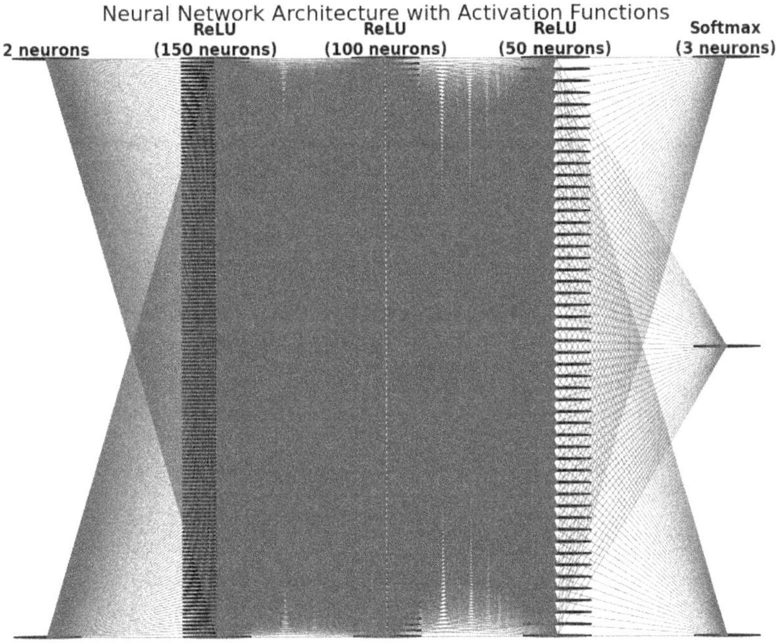

Figure 3. Neural network architecture for post-mission risk classification.

The neural network architecture consisted of an input layer with two neurons corresponding to these features, three hidden layers with 150, 100, and 50 neurons, respectively (all utilizing the ReLU activation function), and an output layer with three neurons corresponding to the identified clusters. A Softmax function was applied to the output to facilitate multiclass classification. Optimization was achieved using the Adam optimizer with an adaptive learning rate, complemented by regularization techniques, namely early stopping and L2 penalization, to ensure both the stability and robustness of the model.

2.5.4. Model Validation

Due to the relatively small size of the dataset (443 military personnel), we opted for 5-fold cross-validation rather than 10-fold CV, as this approach ensures that each fold contains approximately 88 samples, thereby providing more stable and reliable performance estimates compared to having only about 44 samples per fold. Key performance metrics included accuracy, precision, recall, F1-score, the Matthews correlation coefficient, and Cohen's Kappa. This rigorous validation framework was instrumental in detecting any signs of overfitting and verifying that the model was capturing meaningful associations between the variables related to inflammation and oxidative stress. Our examination of the confusion matrix and learning curves further illuminated the structure of misclassifications and the complexity inherent in the dataset.

2.5.5. Capturing Variable Interactions

The neural network was specifically engineered to uncover complex, nonlinear interactions among clinical and biochemical variables. This design allowed for the detection of synergistic effects, such as the amplification of inflammation under conditions of increased oxidative stress, as well as antagonistic interactions that might mitigate the impact of certain pro-inflammatory factors.

2.5.6. Advanced Clustering for Profile Identification

An initial analysis of all available variables revealed that mission duration and the post-mission neutrophil-to-lymphocyte ratio provided the strongest discrimination between participant profiles. Post-mission NLR was chosen because it directly reflects the intensity of the inflammatory response induced by prolonged operational stress, while mission duration was included as it directly affects the level of exposure to stressors, exhibiting clear differences across subgroups. Together, these two parameters enabled a robust and clinically relevant segmentation of the military personnel.

To delineate clinically homogeneous subgroups, the participants were segregated using a Gaussian mixture model (GMM) clustering algorithm. Both features were normalized using the MinMaxScaler to ensure comparability. The GMM was configured with three components (n_components = 3) to capture the natural heterogeneity within the data, with a random_state set to 42 for reproducibility and n_init equal to 10 to ensure robust initialization. The clustering solution was validated by computing the silhouette score, which confirmed that a three-cluster configuration provided a good separation of profiles. Furthermore, a dimensionality reduction through Principal Component Analysis (PCA) enabled a two-dimensional visualization of the clusters, thereby corroborating the internal consistency of the clustering results.

Furthermore, dimensionality reduction through Principal Component Analysis (PCA) enabled a two-dimensional visualization of the clusters, which corroborated the internal consistency of the clustering results.

2.5.7. Calculation of the Post-Mission Integrated Risk Index (IIRPM)

The Post-Mission Integrated Risk Index (IIRPM) was computed by summing the individual scores of four clinically relevant parameters: ΔNLR, age, mission duration, and post-mission cholesterol level. Each parameter was assigned a score ranging from 0 to 2 points based on clinically meaningful thresholds derived from the statistical analyses (see Section 3, Table 6). The total IIRPM score thus spans from 0 (minimal risk) to 8 (maximum risk), facilitating straightforward risk stratification.

3. Results

3.1. Descriptive Analysis of Hematological and Biochemical Parameters

Within the final cohort of 443 military personnel, comparative analyses of hematological and biochemical data obtained at deployment and upon return revealed statistically significant variations in several parameters (see Table 1).

Table 1. Hematological and biochemical parameters before and after deployment.

Biological Parameter	Mean ± SD (Pre-Mission)	Mean ± SD (Post-Mission)	*p*-Value (*t*-Test)
Basophils ($\times 10^3/\mu L$)	0.03 ± 0.02	0.03 ± 0.02	0.4311
Total Cholesterol (mg/dL)	194.69 ± 37.16	196.69 ± 38.25	0.4275
Creatinine (mg/dL)	0.92 ± 0.18	0.91 ± 0.15	0.8151
Eosinophils ($\times 10^3/\mu L$)	0.29 ± 2.18	0.19 ± 0.12	0.3613
Glucose (mg/dL)	96.51 ± 8.62	96.69 ± 8.12	0.7446
Neutrophils ($\times 10^3/\mu L$)	3.61 ± 1.11	4.29 ± 1.57	<0.0001 *
Hematocrit (%)	44.74 ± 3.94	44.20 ± 2.46	0.0136 *
Hemoglobin (g/dL)	15.33 ± 1.70	15.43 ± 0.95	0.2705
Lymphocytes ($\times 10^3/\mu L$)	2.51 ± 4.03	2.37 ± 0.62	0.4668
MCH (pg)	30.00 ± 2.49	30.19 ± 1.51	0.1824
MCHC (g/dL)	34.24 ± 2.76	34.92 ± 0.91	<0.0001 *
MCV (fL)	88.09 ± 8.24	86.47 ± 4.01	0.0002 *
Monocytes ($\times 10^3/\mu L$)	1.30 ± 14.72	0.66 ± 0.19	0.3637
MPV (fL)	10.82 ± 1.21	10.67 ± 0.92	0.0433 *
PCT (%)	0.28 ± 0.61	0.24 ± 0.05	0.2709
Platelets ($\times 10^3/\mu L$)	232.72 ± 55.13	231.59 ± 50.56	0.7495
RBC ($\times 10^6/\mu L$)	5.20 ± 2.10	5.12 ± 0.37	0.4241
RDW (%)	13.14 ± 3.59	13.05 ± 0.84	0.6034
AST (U/L)	24.69 ± 7.75	23.05 ± 8.63	0.0029 *
ALT (U/L)	29.28 ± 13.45	27.43 ± 13.65	0.0416 *
Triglycerides (mg/dL)	121.96 ± 63.27	150.15 ± 107.00	<0.0001 *
ESR (mm/hr)	8.02 ± 5.12	7.33 ± 5.01	0.0444 *
WBC ($\times 10^3/\mu L$)	6.74 ± 1.57	7.54 ± 1.96	<0.0001 *

* statistically significant ($p < 0.05$).

Paired *t*-tests were used to assess differences in mean values before and after missions. In particular, the neutrophil count increased significantly (from 3.61 ± 1.11 to 4.29 ± 1.57; $p < 0.0001$), suggesting an augmented immune response associated with operational stress. In parallel, a significant decrease in hematocrit was observed ($p = 0.0136$), potentially indicative of mild hemodilution. Furthermore, triglyceride levels showed a marked elevation (from 121.96 ± 63.27 mg/dL to 150.15 ± 107.00 mg/dL; $p < 0.0001$), which may reflect metabolic influences on the inflammatory response.

In terms of derived inflammatory indices, NLR increased significantly—from 1.62 ± 0.54 to 1.90 ± 0.80 ($p < 0.0001$)—signaling a more pronounced systemic immune activation. Similar trends were observed in other indices, such as the Systemic Inflammation Response Index (SIRI) and the Systemic Immune-Inflammation Index (SII), further supporting the presence of increased oxidative stress and an exaggerated inflammatory response (Table 2).

Table 2. Inflammatory markers before and after deployment.

Inflammatory Marker	Mean ± SD (Pre-Mission)	Mean ± SD (Post-Mission)	*p*-Value (*t*-Test)
NLR	1.62 ± 0.54	1.90 ± 0.80	<0.0001 *
PLR	105.14 ± 30.98	103.46 ± 32.80	0.4336
MLR	0.27 ± 0.18	0.29 ± 0.09	0.0853
SIRI	0.99 ± 0.54	1.28 ± 0.72	<0.0001 *
SII	377.79 ± 163.92	443.79 ± 234.42	<0.0001 *
IIC	1.86 ± 0.72	2.14 ± 0.94	<0.0001 *

* statistically significant ($p < 0.05$).

Marked increases in NLR and SIRI support the hypothesis of an amplified inflammatory response after deployment, while the cumulative inflammatory index (IIC) demonstrated a significant rise (from 1.86 ± 0.72 to 2.14 ± 0.94). However, the evaluation of individual parameters alone proved insufficient to precisely stratify military personnel by degree of impact. Consequently, a clustering approach was subsequently employed to identify distinct inflammatory and metabolic response patterns.

3.2. Selection of the Inflammatory Marker and Development of the NLR-Based Risk Score

To elucidate how operational conditions influence the inflammatory response, several hematological indices were analyzed, namely NLR, SIRI, SII, and IIC, with a primary focus on NLR measured before and after deployment. Pearson's correlation analysis revealed that while SII exhibited a very high correlation (r = 0.7094), its limited variability reduced its sensitivity to detect acute changes. In contrast, NLR showed a moderate correlation (r = 0.6299) with a highly significant difference between the pre- and post-deployment values ($p = 1.43 \times 10^{-50}$) (Table 3).

Table 3. Pearson correlation analysis for inflammatory markers.

Marker	Pearson Correlation (r)	*p*-Value
NLR_2—NLR_3	0.6299	$p < 0.0001$ (11.43×10^{-50})
$SIRI_2$—$SIRI_3$	0.4938	$p < 0.0001$ (9.87×10^{-29})
SII_2—SII_3	0.7094	$p < 0.0001$ (2.67×10^{-69})
IIC_2—IIC_3	0.5747	$p < 0.0001$ (1.79×10^{-40})

$_2$—pre-deployment; $_3$—post-deployment.

Based on these findings, a new variable—ΔNLR—was defined as the difference between post-deployment and pre-deployment NLR values (NLR_3—NLR_2). This derived parameter serves as an individualized indicator of change, allowing for a more nuanced classification of participants according to their response to operational stress. To further explore the interplay among ΔNLR, age, mission duration, and post-mission cholesterol levels, a pair plot was generated (Figure 4), which confirmed the presence of potentially complex interrelationships between these variables.

Subsequently, a regression model was constructed with post-deployment NLR ($NLR_{\_pred}$) as the dependent variable and ΔNLR, age, mission duration, and cholesterol measured upon return as predictors. The model formulation is as follows:

$$NLR_{pred} = \beta_0 + \beta_1 \times \Delta NLR + \beta_2 \times Age + \beta_3 \times Mission\ Duration + \beta_4 \times Post\text{-}Mission\ Cholesterol$$

The coefficients obtained (Table 4) indicated that each predictor contributed significantly to the variations observed in the NLR after deployment. Notably, ΔNLR was particularly effective in capturing acute inflammatory changes, while post-deployment cholesterol emerged as a significant predictor due to its correlation with elevated inflammatory risk.

The post-deployment data were then subjected to clustering analysis, which segregated the participants into three distinct groups: Cluster 0 ("Basal Profile"), Cluster 1 ("Acute Inflammatory Profile"), Cluster 2 ("Metabolic Proinflammatory Profile").

In Cluster 1, the post-deployment NLR reached its highest value (2.53 ± 1.31), with ΔNLR increasing by +0.70 and associated with elevated cholesterol levels (210.30 ± 40.8 mg/dL). In contrast, Cluster 2 exhibited a more moderate increase in NLR (+0.31), but this was accompanied by significantly higher cholesterol levels and a higher mean age (Table 5).

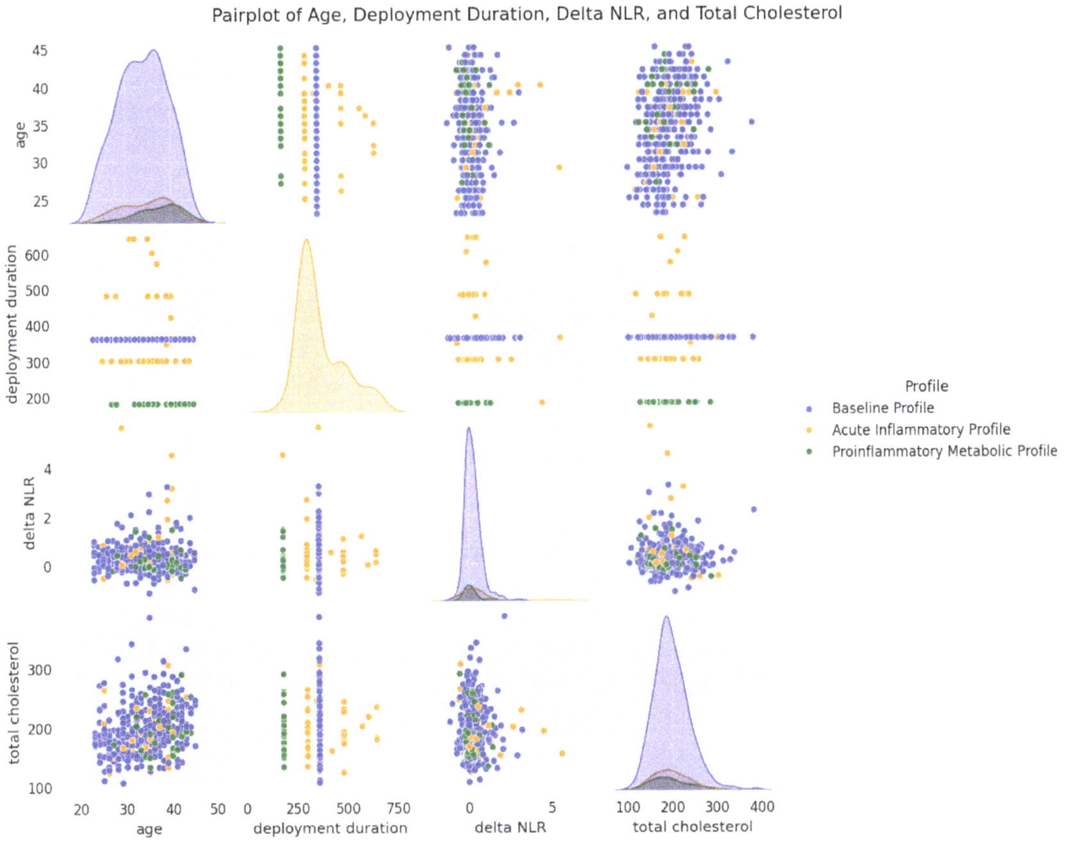

Figure 4. Distribution and intercorrelations among ΔNLR, age, mission duration, and post-mission cholesterol.

Table 4. Regression coefficients for the NLR-based model.

Variable	Coefficient (β)	Standard Error	*p*-Value
Intercept	−1.20	0.33	<0.001 *
ΔNLR	2.05	0.42	<0.001 *
Age (years)	0.07	0.03	0.005 *
Mission Duration (days)	0.0048	0.0018	0.017 *
Post-Mission Cholesterol (mg/dL)	0.011	0.003	0.004 *

* statistically significant ($p < 0.05$).

Table 5. Comparison of key biological parameters across clusters.

Parameter	Cluster 0 (*n* = 354)	Cluster 1 (*n* = 58)	Cluster 2 (*n* = 31)	*p*-Value
Age (years)	34.00 ± 5.4	34.60 ± 5.3	37.80 ± 4.5	0.0003
Mission Duration (days)	360.00 ± 0.7	369.80 ± 98.6	180.00 (fix)	<0.0001
NLR (post-deployment)	1.80 ± 0.57	2.53 ± 1.31	1.76 ± 1.12	<0.0001
ΔNLR	0.21 ± 0.44	0.70 ± 1.07	0.31 ± 0.90	<0.0001
Cholesterol (mg/dL)	196.50 ± 39.3	210.30 ± 40.8	225.60 ± 46.6	<0.0001
Triglycerides (mg/dL)	140.30 ± 86.5	158.20 ± 68.1	176.70 ± 78.5	<0.0001

Table 5. *Cont.*

Parameter	Cluster 0 (n = 354)	Cluster 1 (n = 58)	Cluster 2 (n = 31)	p-Value
Glucose (mg/dL)	96.80 ± 8.12	98.30 ± 8.62	100.50 ± 9.0	<0.0001
Creatinine (mg/dL)	0.91 ± 0.14	0.93 ± 0.11	0.95 ± 0.15	0.0080
Hematocrit (%)	44.20 ± 2.46	43.70 ± 2.50	44.00 ± 2.45	0.0020
Hemoglobin (g/dL)	15.40 ± 0.95	15.20 ± 1.00	15.30 ± 0.98	0.1250
Platelets ($10^3/\mu L$)	231.60 ± 50.56	228.10 ± 48.98	230.90 ± 51.20	0.0007
Leukocytes ($10^3/\mu L$)	7.54 ± 1.96	8.62 ± 2.00	7.12 ± 1.75	<0.0001

These results indicate that personnel in Cluster 1 show a more robust inflammatory response, while those in Cluster 2 tend to display a metabolic profile that predisposes them to inflammation.

To ensure comparability between different measurement units, all parameters were standardized using the Z-Score method. This standardization, illustrated in the radar chart (Figure 5), allowed for a fair comparison by placing all variables on a common scale, thus facilitating a clear visualization of the differences and variations among the identified profiles.

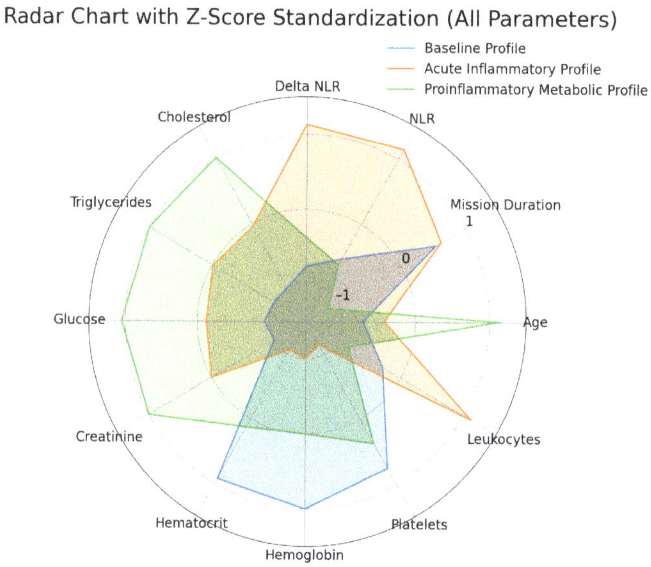

Figure 5. Radar chart of profiles with parameter standardization using Z-score.

Based on these conclusions, the Post-Mission Integrated Risk Index (IIRPM) was developed, with a composite score calculated by summing the individual scores of four clinically relevant parameters: ΔNLR, age, mission duration, and post-mission cholesterol level. Each parameter was assigned a score ranging from 0 to 2 points according to clearly defined intervals reflecting clinical relevance (Table 6).

Specifically, higher ΔNLR values indicate acute inflammatory responses, increased age and elevated cholesterol levels reflect greater cardiometabolic risk, and longer mission duration represents extended exposure to operational stressors. The sum of these individual scores yields a total IIRPM score ranging from 0 (minimal risk) to 8 (maximum risk), facilitating clear risk stratification (Table 7).

Table 6. Calculation of the Post-Mission Integrative Inflammatory Risk Index (IIRPM).

Parameter	Interval/Values	Assigned Score
ΔNLR (Delta NLR)	<0.2	0
	0.2–0.5	1
	≥0.5	2
Age (years)	<35	0
	35–40	1
	>40	2
Mission Duration (days)	<300	0
	300–360	1
	≥360	2
Post-Mission Cholesterol (mg/dL)	<190	0
	190–220	1
	>220	2

Table 7. Classification of inflammatory risk based on IIRPM Score.

Total Score	Risk Level	Interpretation
<2 points	Low	Minimal risk; no significant concerns.
3–4 points	Moderate	Present risk; warrants monitoring.
≥5 points	High	Elevated risk; requires enhanced monitoring and potential clinical intervention.

Elevated cholesterol levels were incorporated into the index based on their significantly different distribution between clusters and their association with NLR changes, suggesting a metabolic environment conducive to inflammation.

Through this integrative approach, a practical tool has been developed that can be readily implemented in military clinical practice. This instrument facilitates the rapid identification of personnel at high risk for acute inflammation and metabolic imbalances post-deployment, thereby supporting personalized preventive interventions and continuous health monitoring in the context of military operations.

3.3. Evaluation of Model Performance

The MLP neural network, designed to classify military personnel according to their post-mission inflammatory and metabolic profiles, was rigorously evaluated using several key performance metrics: accuracy, precision, recall, F1-score, the Matthews correlation coefficient (MCC), and Cohen's Kappa. Together, these metrics provide a robust assessment of the model's ability to detect physiological and biochemical alterations associated with operational stress.

3.4. Performance on the Test Set

When applied to the test dataset, the model achieved a perfect accuracy of 100%. The confusion matrix (Figure 6) clearly demonstrates that almost all instances were correctly classified, with only one misclassification, where a case belonging to Profile 1 was incorrectly identified as Profile 0.

Both precision and recall were 100%, and the F1 score was recorded at 1.00, highlighting the exceptional performance of the model. Furthermore, the MCC was calculated at 0.99, indicating an extremely strong correlation between the predictions of the model and the actual labels, while Cohen's Kappa also reached 0.99, reflecting an excellent level of agreement.

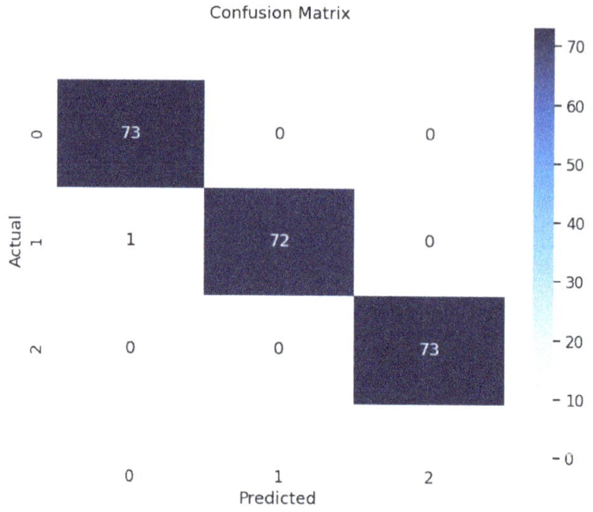

Figure 6. Confusion matrix of the neural network model.

3.5. Learning Curve and Training Stability

To assess the stability of the training and the overall efficiency of the learning process, the neural network learning curve was analyzed (Figure 7).

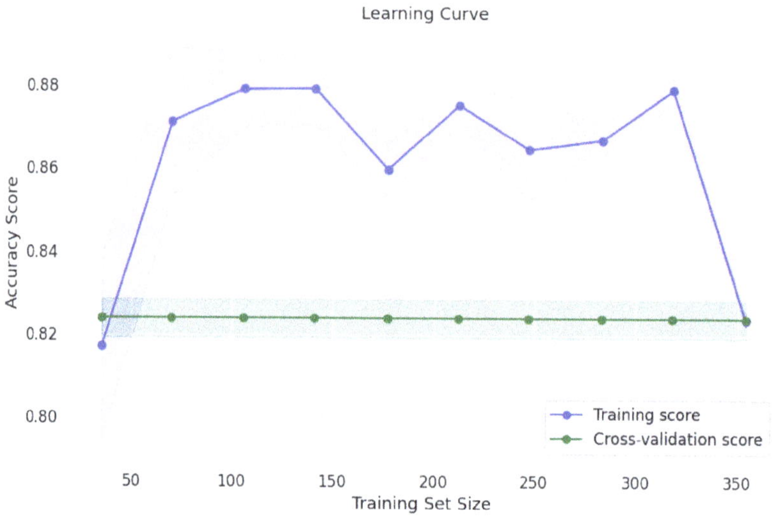

Figure 7. Learning curve of the neural network.

This curve provides insight into the progression of the model's performance over time, illustrating its ability to generalize to unseen data. The observed reduction in the training accuracy at the largest training set size (final data point) is due to averaging the performance across cross-validation folds, reflecting variations inherent to smaller training subsets within certain folds. At smaller subset sizes, the training performance metric may appear elevated due to easier memorization of fewer instances; however, as the dataset size approaches its maximum, the average training accuracy reflects the consistent generalization across all folds, stabilizing toward the true generalization performance. Thus, this observed fluctuation does not indicate decreased model learning capacity but rather highlights the model's behavior when averaging performance across varied subsets within the cross-validation procedure. In particular, the accuracy of the training experienced a rapid increase before stabilizing at approximately 88%. In parallel, the accuracy of the validation remained steady at around 82%, suggesting an optimal balance that minimizes the risks of both under- and over-fitting. The relatively narrow confidence band around the learning curve further supports the robustness and consistency of the model.

3.6. Model Validation via Cross-Validation

A 5-fold cross-validation approach was employed to further verify the model's generalizability. Across the folds, the accuracy of the model ranged from 93.26% to 100%, with an average accuracy of approximately 97% and a standard deviation of 2%. The weighted precision and recall were recorded at 98% and 97%, respectively, which confirms the robustness of the classification performance.

The MCC values in the folds varied between 0.828 and 1.000, yielding an average of 0.91 (standard deviation = 0.06). Similarly, Cohen's Kappa values ranged from 0.811 to 1.000, with an average of 0.91 (standard deviation = 0.07). These high values strongly indicate a robust correlation between predicted classifications and true labels and underscore a high level of agreement between the predictions of the model and the observed class distribution between the military personnel (Figure 8).

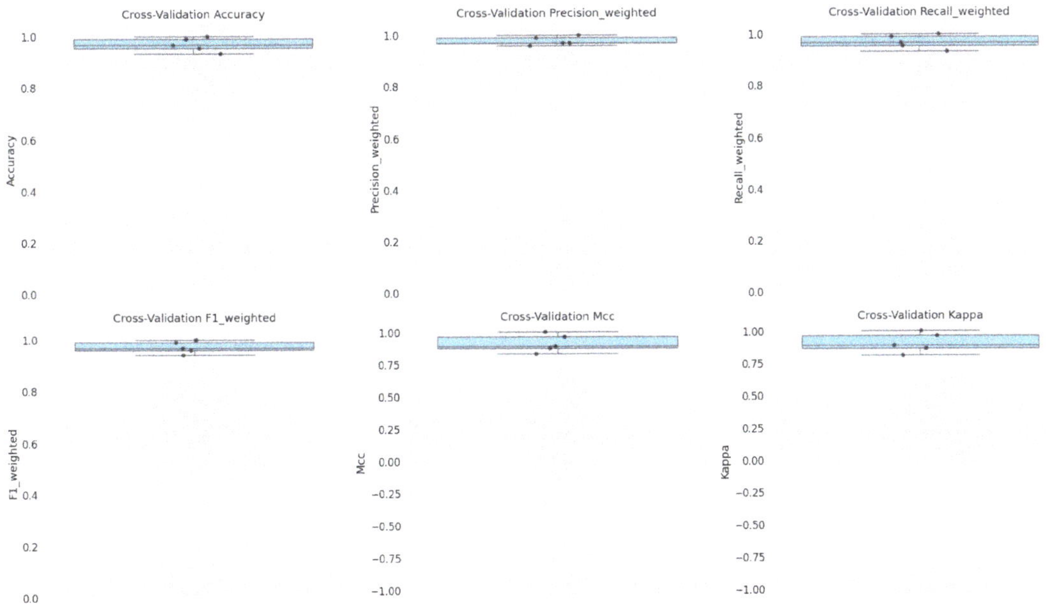

Figure 8. Cross-validation scores for accuracy, precision, recall, and F1-score.

More specifically, the MCC values for each fold were 0.964, 0.828, 1.000, 0.871, and 0.888, while the corresponding Cohen's Kappa values were 0.963, 0.811, 1.000, 0.862, and 0.888. These figures further confirm the strong predictive performance of the model and its ability to reliably capture the distribution of the inflammatory and metabolic changes observed after deployment (Figure 9).

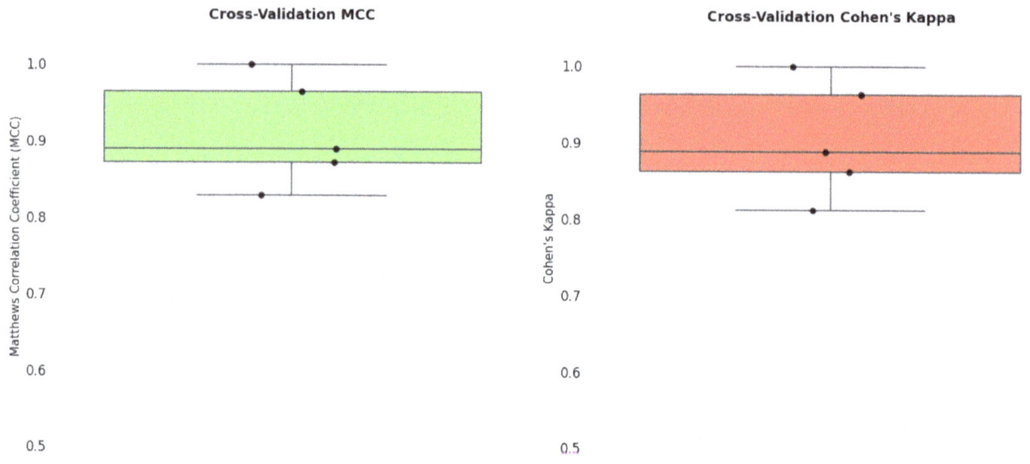

Figure 9. MCC and Cohen's Kappa across the 5 folds.

4. Discussion

This study was designed to advance the evaluation of oxidative stress and inflammation in military personnel returning from international missions by employing an integrative approach that combines rigorous statistical analysis with advanced artificial intelligence techniques. Based on data collected from 443 military subjects over a ten-year period, the findings offer a detailed account of how prolonged exposure to hostile operational conditions affects hematological and metabolic parameters. Furthermore, by segmenting the data into three distinct clusters and constructing a predictive model, the Post-Mission Integrated Risk Index (IIRPM) was derived, which integrates NLR and its change (ΔNLR) with key clinical factors such as age, post-mission cholesterol levels, and duration of the mission.

4.1. Cluster Segmentation and Biological Significance

Cluster analysis revealed three distinct response profiles that underscore the individual variability between military personnel. The first cluster, labeled the "Reference Profile" and comprising approximately 80% of the sample, is characterized by relative immunologic stability, with only a minimal increase in ΔNLR ($+0.21 \pm 0.44$). This observation is consistent with previous literature suggesting that, in the absence of acute inflammatory stress, the NLR remains close to baseline values [17]. In addition, earlier studies on military populations have shown that most individuals return to normal physiological parameters after a mission, without major inflammatory alterations [18].

In contrast, the "Acute Inflammatory Response" cluster (approximately 13.1% of participants) is marked by a significant increase in ΔNLR ($+0.70 \pm 1.07$), suggesting an intense inflammatory reaction and potentially increased oxidative stress. This response is frequently associated with sustained physical exertion and intense psychological stress—factors known to exacerbate systemic inflammation and increase the risk of cardiovascular events [19,20].

The third cluster, termed the "Metabolic Proinflammatory Profile" (7% of the sample), is characterized by a moderate ΔNLR increase ($+0.31 \pm 0.90$) combined with elevated cholesterol levels and a higher mean age. These findings imply an underlying predisposition to chronic inflammation and cardiometabolic risk, supporting the hypothesis that aging and dyslipidemia may synergistically sustain a proinflammatory state [21–23].

4.2. Relevance of ΔNLR and Its Correlation with the Cumulative Inflammatory Index

The differential analysis of NLR, captured by ΔNLR, emerged as a central parameter in quantifying the inflammatory response to operational stress. The significant increase in ΔNLR, particularly observed in the "Acute Inflammatory Response" cluster, highlights the marker's sensitivity to rapid changes induced by intense physical and psychological stress [24]. Furthermore, the positive correlation between ΔNLR and the Cumulative Inflammatory Index (IIC) indicates that dynamic monitoring of this marker may effectively predict the long-term impact of operational stress on an individual's inflammatory status [3,25]. Mechanistically, neutrophils activation results in increased production of reactive oxygen species (ROS), thereby intensifying oxidative stress, while the concomitant reduction in lymphocyte count contributes to immune imbalance [26–29].

4.3. Predictive Model and the Role of Artificial Intelligence

Beyond descriptive and cluster analyses, a predictive model was developed using an MLP neural network to classify inflammatory profiles based on ΔNLR, age, mission duration, and post-mission cholesterol levels. The model achieved 100% accuracy on the test set and an average of 97% accuracy in cross-validation, underscoring the robustness of AI in capturing complex, non-linear relationships among clinical and biological variables [5,30,31]. This machine learning approach offers a distinct advantage over traditional statistical methods by simultaneously processing large volumes of data and detecting subtle patterns that might otherwise be overlooked. When implemented in a digital application, this model can enable medical personnel to quickly compute the IIRPM score using standard clinical data, thus facilitating prompt and informed clinical decision-making.

4.4. Age, Mission Duration, and Cholesterol: Foundations of the IIRPM

The linear regression analysis confirmed the cumulative impact of ΔNLR, age, mission duration, and post-mission cholesterol on the inflammatory response. With advancing age, the process of "inflammaging"—characterized by a decline in antioxidant capacity and increased low-grade inflammation—can exacerbate the inflammatory response, particularly when compounded by dyslipidemia [32]. Elevated cholesterol levels, especially when associated with reduced HDL levels, further intensify oxidative stress and may lead to endothelial dysfunction, promoting atherosclerosis [33,34]. In addition, extended mission durations reflect prolonged exposure to adverse environmental conditions such as high temperatures, pollution, or sleep deprivation, all of which deplete antioxidant reserves and raise inflammatory markers [1,35,36]. Incorporating these variables into the IIRPM score provides a comprehensive assessment of post-mission inflammatory risk.

4.5. Clinical Implications and Operational Context

The IIRPM score represents a novel, practical tool for military medicine, enabling the rapid stratification of inflammatory and oxidative risks. In operational contexts where rapid response and resource allocation are critical, this score can identify individuals who require focused monitoring and personalized intervention. Personnel with elevated IIRPM scores can benefit from intensive recovery protocols, targeted nutritional interventions (e.g., cholesterol reduction and antioxidant supplementation), and psychological support to mitigate long-term cardiovascular and metabolic complications [21,22,37–41]. The integration of this AI-based evaluation into digital platforms offers the potential for real-time clinical decision-making, especially in resource-limited operational settings.

4.6. Influence of Environmental and Psychological Factors

In addition to biological and metabolic parameters, environmental and psychological factors play a crucial role in shaping the post-mission inflammatory response. Exposure to extreme conditions, such as pollution, radiation, or even microgravity during space missions, can catalyze oxidative stress [42–44]. Simultaneously, chronic psychological stress, anxiety, and existential fears can activate the hypothalamic–pituitary–adrenal axis, leading to increased glucocorticoid secretion that further amplifies inflammation and oxidative stress [29,40]. These findings underscore the importance of a multidisciplinary approach in assessing military health, integrating environmental and psychological factors into comprehensive preventive and intervention strategies.

4.7. Study Limitations

Despite its promising findings, this study has several limitations. First, the sample consisted exclusively of male military personnel, which may limit the generalizability of the results to the entire military population, including female service members. Second, the analysis focused on international missions conducted under relatively homogeneous operational conditions, excluding crisis situations or domestic deployments where stressors might be more variable or severe. Furthermore, the study did not include detailed psychoemotional assessments, such as measures of anxiety or post-traumatic stress, nor did it incorporate genetic or epigenetic markers that might influence the inflammatory response to operational stress. These limitations suggest important avenues for future research aimed at further refining and expanding the IIRPM model.

4.8. Implications and Future Perspectives

This study underscores the critical importance of an integrated evaluation of hematological, metabolic, and clinical parameters in quantifying post-mission inflammatory risk. Through cluster segmentation, differential analysis of ΔNLR, and the integration of variables such as age, mission duration, and cholesterol levels, an innovative risk score, the IIRPM, was developed, which can guide personalized preventive interventions in military medicine. The application of advanced AI techniques not only optimizes data analysis and minimizes interpretative errors but also opens up new possibilities for expanding this research. Future studies should consider incorporating additional variables, such as psychological and genetic factors, and validate the model in diverse populations. Furthermore, the development of digital applications based on this model could enable the rapid integration of the IIRPM score into military health monitoring systems, facilitating swift and effective management of inflammatory and metabolic risks.

5. Conclusions

The findings of this study underscore the complexity of the inflammatory and oxidative responses in military personnel returning from international missions, revealing the presence of at least three distinct profiles: a baseline profile marked by immunological stability, an acute inflammatory response profile, and a metabolic pro-inflammatory profile. In this context, ΔNLR emerged as an exceptionally sensitive marker, capable of rapidly detecting both immune alterations induced by operational stress and potential cardiometabolic risks.

The innovative approach, which integrates multiple parameters—including age, mission duration, and cholesterol levels—into a predictive model based on advanced artificial intelligence techniques, demonstrated outstanding classification performance. The robust results obtained through modern statistical segmentation and validation with an MLP neural network support the reliability and clinical utility of the IIRPM score as an effective tool for triaging and monitoring post-mission risk.

From a practical point of view, the IIRPM score can be implemented as a digital application within military health systems, thus facilitating the early identification of vulnerable personnel and guiding personalized preventive interventions aimed at reducing oxidative stress and managing inflammation. Consequently, the results of this study not only contribute significantly to our understanding of complex biological mechanisms but also open new avenues for research and clinical applications.

In general, effective health management among military personnel requires an integrated approach that combines careful monitoring of inflammatory biomarkers with comprehensive assessments of demographic, metabolic, psychological, and environmental factors. Further validation of the IIRPM score through multicenter, expansive, and longitudinal studies will consolidate the relevance of this innovative instrument and establish a new standard in military medicine, tailored to the multifaceted and often unpredictable challenges encountered in operational theaters.

Author Contributions: Conceptualization, D.R. and E.-T.T.; methodology, D.R. and P.-M.R.; software, R.M.; validation, D.R., E.-I.C. and E.-T.T.; formal analysis, D.R. and D.M.C.; investigation, D.R. and G.-A.M.; resources, S.D. and E.D.C.-C.; data curation, D.R. and P.-M.R.; writing—original draft preparation, D.R.; writing—review and editing, D.R. and F.-D.M.; visualization, R.M. and E.D.C.-C.; supervision, D.R. and E.-T.T.; project administration, D.R.; funding acquisition, P.-M.R. All authors have read and agreed to the published version of the manuscript.

Funding: The article processing charges were funded by the University of Medicine and Pharmacy of Craiova, Romania, 200349 Craiova, Romania.

Institutional Review Board Statement: This research protocol received approval from the Medical and Ethics Council of the Military Hospital "Dr. Ștefan Odobleja" in Craiova, in compliance with international regulations for medical research and the Declaration of Helsinki guidelines (approval number A/CR 1-972/27 September 2023). Furthermore, ethical clearance was granted by the Ethics Committee of the University of Medicine and Pharmacy in Craiova (approval number 335/17 September 2024).

Informed Consent Statement: Informed consent was obtained from all subjects involved in the study.

Data Availability Statement: The authors declare that the data of this research are available from the corresponding authors, upon reasonable request.

Conflicts of Interest: The authors declare no conflicts of interest.

References

1. Kargl, C.K.; Gage, C.R.; Forse, J.N.; Koltun, K.J.; Bird, M.B.; Lovalekar, M.; Martin, B.J.; Nindl, B.C. Inflammatory and Oxidant Responses to Arduous Military Training: Associations with Stress, Sleep, and Performance. *Med. Sci. Sports Exerc.* **2024**, *56*, 2315–2327. [CrossRef] [PubMed]
2. Sun, Y.; Rawish, E.; Nording, H.M.; Langer, H.F. Inflammation in Metabolic and Cardiovascular Disorders—Role of Oxidative Stress. *Life* **2021**, *11*, 672. [CrossRef] [PubMed]
3. Firment, J.; Hulin, I. Zahorec index or Neutrophil-to-lymphocyte ratio, valid biomarker of inflammation and immune response to infection, cancer and surgery. *Bratisl. Lek. Listy.* **2024**, *125*, 75–83. [CrossRef] [PubMed]
4. Wu, H.; Cao, T.; Ji, T.; Luo, Y.; Huang, J.; Ma, K. Predictive value of the neutrophil-to-lymphocyte ratio in the prognosis and risk of death for adult sepsis patients: A meta-analysis. *Front. Immunol.* **2024**, *15*, 1336456. [CrossRef] [PubMed]
5. Adamstein, N.H.; Ridker, P.M. The neutrophil-lymphocyte ratio: Considerations for clinical application. *Eur. Heart J.* **2021**, *42*, 2216–2217. [CrossRef] [PubMed]

6. Liao, Q.Q.; Mo, Y.J.; Zhu, K.W.; Gao, F.; Huang, B.; Chen, P.; Jing, F.T.; Jiang, X.; Xu, H.Z.; Tang, Y.F.; et al. Platelet-to-Lymphocyte Ratio (PLR), Neutrophil-to-Lymphocyte Ratio (NLR), Monocyte-to-Lymphocyte Ratio (MLR), and Eosinophil-to-Lymphocyte Ratio (ELR) as Biomarkers in Patients with Acute Exacerbation of Chronic Obstructive Pulmonary Disease (AECOPD). *Int. J. Chron. Obstruct. Pulmon. Dis.* **2024**, *19*, 501–518. [CrossRef] [PubMed]
7. Liu, H.; Zhan, F.; Wang, Y. Evaluation of monocyte-to-high-density lipoprotein cholesterol ratio and monocyte-to-lymphocyte ratio in ischemic stroke. *J. Int. Med. Res.* **2020**, *48*, 300060520933806. [CrossRef] [PubMed]
8. Pritzker, K.P.H. Blood-based biomarkers of chronic inflammation. *Expert. Rev. Mol. Diagn.* **2023**, *23*, 495–504. [CrossRef] [PubMed]
9. Hoffmeister, A.; Rothenbacher, D.; Kunze, M.; Brenner, H.; Koenig, W. Prognostic value of inflammatory markers alone and in combination with blood lipids in patients with stable coronary artery disease. *Eur. J. Intern. Med.* **2005**, *16*, 47–52. [CrossRef]
10. Morrisette-Thomas, V.; Cohen, A.A.; Fülöp, T.; Riesco, É.; Legault, V.; Li, Q.; Milot, E.; Dusseault-Bélanger, F.; Ferrucci, L. Inflamm-aging does not simply reflect increases in pro-inflammatory markers. *Mech. Ageing Dev.* **2014**, *139*, 49–57. [CrossRef] [PubMed]
11. Ulusoy, C.O.; Kurt, A.; Seyhanli, Z.; Hizli, B.; Bucak, M.; Agaoglu, R.T.; Oguz, Y.; Yucel, K.Y. Role of Inflammatory Markers and Doppler Parameters in Late-Onset Fetal Growth Restriction: A Machine-Learning Approach. *Am. J. Reprod. Immunol.* **2024**, *92*, e70004. [CrossRef] [PubMed]
12. Li, W.; Zeng, L.; Yuan, S.; Shang, Y.; Zhuang, W.; Chen, Z.; Lyu, J. Machine learning for the prediction of cognitive impairment in older adults. *Front. Neurosci.* **2023**, *17*, 1158141. [CrossRef] [PubMed]
13. Radulescu, D.; Mihai, F.D.; Trasca, M.E.; Caluianu, E.I.; Calafeteanu, C.D.M.; Radulescu, P.M.; Mercut, R.; Ciupeanu-Calugaru, E.D.; Marinescu, G.A.; Siloşi, C.A.; et al. Oxidative Stress in Military Missions-Impact and Management Strategies: A Narrative Analysis. *Life* **2024**, *14*, 567. [CrossRef] [PubMed]
14. Holliday, S.B.; DeSantis, A.; Germain, A.; Buysse, D.J.; Matthews, K.A.; Troxel, W.M. Deployment Length, Inflammatory Markers, and Ambulatory Blood Pressure in Military Couples. *Mil. Med.* **2017**, *182*, e1892–e1899. [CrossRef] [PubMed]
15. Almer, A.; Weber, A.; Haid, F.; Paletta, L.; Schneeberger, M.; Ladstätter, S.; Wallner, D.; Glanz, P.; Klöckl, P.; Eder, D.; et al. Real-time remote stress monitoring based on specific stress modelling considering load characteristics of different military forces. In *Cognitive Computing and Internet of Things*; Paletta, L., Ayaz, H., Asgher, U., Eds.; AHFE (2023) International Conference; AHFE Open Access; AHFE International: Orlando, FL, USA, 2023; Volume 73.
16. Beckner, M.E.; Main, L.; Tait, J.L.; Martin, B.J.; Conkright, W.R.; Nindl, B.C. Circulating biomarkers associated with performance and resilience during military operational stress. *Eur. J. Sport. Sci.* **2022**, *22*, 72–86. [CrossRef] [PubMed]
17. Daoub, M.; Mustafa, A. The Neutrophil Lymphocyte Ratio (NLR); recycled as Predictor of Angiographic Coronary Artery Disease Severity in stable Ischaemic Heart Disease. *J. Clin. Cardiol. Cardiovasc. Interv.* **2022**, *5*. [CrossRef]
18. Tait, J.L.; Bulmer, S.; Drain, J.R.; Main, L.C. Associations between inflammatory markers and well-being during 12 weeks of basic military training. *Eur. J. Appl. Physiol.* **2021**, *121*, 849–860. [CrossRef] [PubMed]
19. Bizuti, M.R.; Meneghel, D.; Schwede ED, C.; Jost, L.N. Physical Exercise As a Modulator of Oxidative Stress and Inflammation in Atherosclerotic Plaque. *J. Adv. Med. Med. Res.* **2020**, *32*, 36–44. [CrossRef]
20. Serra, R.; Ielapi, N.; Licastro, N.; Provenzano, M.; Andreucci, M.; Bracale, U.M.; Jiritano, F.; de Franciscis, S.; Mastroroberto, P.; Serraino, G.F. Neutrophil-to-lymphocyte Ratio and Platelet-to-lymphocyte Ratio as Biomarkers for Cardiovascular Surgery Procedures: A Literature Review. *Rev. Recent. Clin. Trials.* **2021**, *16*, 173–179. [CrossRef] [PubMed]
21. Aljuraiban, G.S.; Alharbi, F.J.; Aljohi, A.O.; Almeshari, A.Z.; Alsahli, A.S.; Alotaibi, B.S.; Abudawood, M.; Alfawaz, W.; Abulmeaty, M. Systemic immune-inflammation index and its relation to blood pressure and dyslipidemia in adults: A retrospective study. *Medicine* **2024**, *103*, e38810. [CrossRef] [PubMed]
22. Ridker, P.M.; Lei, L.; Louie, M.J.; Haddad, T.; Nicholls, S.J.; Lincoff, A.M.; Libby, P.; Nissen, S.E.; CLEAR Outcomes Investigators. Inflammation and Cholesterol as Predictors of Cardiovascular Events Among 13,970 Contemporary High-Risk Patients With Statin Intolerance. *Circulation* **2024**, *149*, 28–35. [CrossRef] [PubMed]
23. Church, M.C.; Workman, J.L.; Suganuma, T. Macrophages, Metabolites, and Nucleosomes: Chromatin at the Intersection between Aging and Inflammation. *Int. J. Mol. Sci.* **2021**, *22*, 10274. [CrossRef] [PubMed]
24. Bennett, N.; Lawrence-Wood, E.; McFarlane, A. Is inflammatory change associated with psychological risk and resilience in high-risk military personnel? *BMJ Mil. Health.* **2024**, *170*, 396–401. [CrossRef] [PubMed]
25. Radulescu, P.M.; Davitoiu, D.V.; Baleanu, V.D.; Padureanu, V.; Ramboiu, D.S.; Surlin, M.V.; Bratiloveanu, T.C.; Georgescu, E.F.; Streba, C.T.; Mercut, R.; et al. Has COVID-19 Modified the Weight of Known Systemic Inflammation Indexes and the New Ones (MCVL and IIC) in the Assessment as Predictive Factors of Complications and Mortality in Acute Pancreatitis? *Diagnostics* **2022**, *12*, 3118. [CrossRef] [PubMed]
26. Islam, M.R.; Habib, M.A.; Lia, F.A.; Noor Islam, L. Role of oxidase and antioxidant enzymes in neutrophils and blood circulation in patients with acute coronary syndrome. *J. Blood Biol. Disord.* **2023**, *8*, 020890351. [CrossRef]

27. Hu, X.T.; Chen, B.W.; Cao, Y.J.; Zhou, C.; Li, H.B.; Wang, D.H. Enhanced oxidative stress is associated with tissue neutrophilia and poor steroid response in chronic rhinosinusitis with nasal polyps. *World J. Otorhinolaryngol. Head. Neck Surg.* **2023**, *9*, 320–327. [CrossRef] [PubMed]
28. Zendelovska, D.; Petrushevska, M.; Atanasovska, E.; Spasovska, K.; Gjorgjievska, K.; Pavlovska, K.; Grozdanovski, K. COVID-19 disease induced alteration of oxidative stress and clinical laboratory parameters in moderate and severe patients. *Eur. Rev. Med. Pharmacol. Sci.* **2022**, *26*, 5611–5617. [PubMed]
29. Somani, A.; Singh, A.K.; Gupta, B.; Nagarkoti, S.; Dalal, P.K.; Dikshit, M. Oxidative and Nitrosative Stress in Major Depressive Disorder: A Case Control Study. *Brain Sci.* **2022**, *12*, 144. [CrossRef] [PubMed]
30. Mercuţ, R.; Ciurea, M.E.; Traşcă, E.T.; Ionescu, M.; Mercuţ, M.F.; Rădulescu, P.M.; Călăraşu, C.; Streba, L.; Ionescu, A.G.; Rădulescu, D. Applying Neural Networks to Analyse Inflammatory, Sociodemographic, and Psychological Factors in Non-Melanoma Skin Cancer and Colon Cancer: A Statistical and Artificial Intelligence Approach. *Diagnostics* **2024**, *14*, 2759. [CrossRef] [PubMed]
31. Buican, I.L.; Gheorman, V.; Udriştoiu, I.; Olteanu, M.; Rădulescu, D.; Calafeteanu, D.M.; Nemeş, A.F.; Călăraşu, C.; Rădulescu, P.M.; Streba, C.T. Interactions between Cognitive, Affective, and Respiratory Profiles in Chronic Respiratory Disorders: A Cluster Analysis Approach. *Diagnostics* **2024**, *14*, 1153. [CrossRef] [PubMed]
32. Moshtagh, M.; Moodi, M.; Moezi, S.A.; Sharifi, F.; Khazdair, M.R. Inflammatory and Oxidative Stress Biomarkers in the Elderly, the Birjand Longitudinal Aging Study. *Biomed. Res. Int.* **2023**, *2023*, 4683542. [CrossRef]
33. Babcock, M.C.; DuBose, L.E.; Witten, T.L.; Stauffer, B.L.; Hildreth, K.L.; Schwartz, R.S.; Kohrt, W.M.; Moreau, K.L. Oxidative Stress and Inflammation Are Associated With Age-Related Endothelial Dysfunction in Men With Low Testosterone. *J. Clin. Endocrinol. Metab.* **2022**, *107*, e500–e514. [CrossRef] [PubMed]
34. Ye, H.; Liu, Q.; Wang, Y.; Zhen, X.; Yan, N. The Effect of Cholesterol Efflux on Endothelial Dysfunction Caused by Oxidative Stress. *Int. J. Mol. Sci.* **2023**, *24*, 5939. [CrossRef] [PubMed]
35. Bachmann, M.C.; Bellalta, S.; Basoalto, R.; Gómez-Valenzuela, F.; Jalil, Y.; Lépez, M.; Matamoros, A.; von Bernhardi, R. The Challenge by Multiple Environmental and Biological Factors Induce Inflammation in Aging: Their Role in the Promotion of Chronic Disease. *Front. Immunol.* **2020**, *11*, 570083. [CrossRef] [PubMed]
36. Guan, J. The interplay between aging and inflammation and its role in chronic disease development. *Theor. Nat. Sci.* **2024**, *48*, 45–54. [CrossRef]
37. Sekhar, R.; Taffet, G.; Kumar, P. Glynac supplementation in older adults protects from meal driven oxidative stress and inflammation: Results of a rct. *Innov. Aging* **2022**, *6* (Suppl. S1), 814–815. [CrossRef]
38. Prata, C.; Angeloni, C.; Maraldi, T. Strategies to Counteract Oxidative Stress and Inflammation in Chronic-Degenerative Diseases 2.0. *Int. J. Mol. Sci.* **2024**, *25*, 5026. [CrossRef] [PubMed]
39. Blagov, A.V.; Summerhill, V.I.; Sukhorukov, V.N.; Zhigmitova, E.B.; Postnov, A.Y.; Orekhov, A.N. Potential use of antioxidants for the treatment of chronic inflammatory diseases. *Front. Pharmacol.* **2024**, *15*, 1378335. [CrossRef] [PubMed]
40. Şahin, F.; Koşar, A.F.; Aslan, A.F.; Yiğitbaş, B.; Uslu, B. Serum biomarkers in patients with stable and acute exacerbation of chronic obstructive pulmonary disease: A comparative study. *J. Med. Biochem.* **2019**, *38*, 503. [CrossRef] [PubMed]
41. Sipahi, H.; Mat, A.F.; Ozhan, Y.; Aydin, A. The Interrelation between Oxidative Stress, Depression and Inflammation through the Kynurenine Pathway. *Curr. Top. Med. Chem.* **2023**, *23*, 415–425. [CrossRef] [PubMed]
42. Lee, K.; Kim, J. Abstract LB144: The short-term associations of air pollutants with inflammation and oxidative stress markers in the Korean population. *Cancer Res.* **2024**, *84*, LB144. [CrossRef]
43. Cahoon, D.S.; Rabin, B.M.; Fisher, D.R.; Shukitt-Hale, B. Effects of HZE-Particle Exposure Location and Energy on Brain Inflammation and Oxidative Stress in Rats. *Radiat. Res.* **2023**, *200*, 431–443. [CrossRef] [PubMed]
44. Olaniyan, M.F.; Muhibi, M.A.; Olaniyan, T.B. Oxidative Stress and Inflammatory Response Interplay. *J. Prev. Diagn. Treat. Strateg. Med.* **2023**, *2*, 94–100. [CrossRef]

diagnostics

MDPI

Review

Artificial Intelligence for the Diagnosis and Management of Patellofemoral Instability: A Comprehensive Review

Michele Mercurio [1,2], Federica Denami [1,*], Andrea Vescio [1], Filippo Familiari [1,2], Umile Giuseppe Longo [3,4], Olimpio Galasso [5], Giorgio Gasparini [1,2] on behalf of the Italian Orthopaedic Research Society (IORS) and David H. Dejour [6]

[1] Department of Orthopaedic and Trauma Surgery, Magna Graecia University, "Renato Dulbecco" University Hospital, 88100 Catanzaro, Italy; michele.mercurio@unicz.it (M.M.); andreavescio88@gmail.com (A.V.); filippofamiliari@unicz.it (F.F.); gasparini@unicz.it (G.G.)
[2] Research Center on Musculoskeletal Health, MusculoSkeletal Health@UMG, Magna Graecia University, 88100 Catanzaro, Italy
[3] Fondazione Policlinico Universitario Campus Bio-Medico, 00128 Roma, Italy; g.longo@policlinicocampus.it
[4] Research Unit of Orthopaedic and Trauma Surgery, Department of Medicine and Surgery, Università Campus Bio-Medico di Roma, 00128 Rome, Italy
[5] Department of Medicine, Surgery and Dentistry, University of Salerno, 84081 Salerno, Italy; ogalasso@unisa.it
[6] Lyon Ortho Clinic, Clínica de la Sauvegarde, 69009 Lyon, France; dr.dejour@lyon-ortho-clinic.com
* Correspondence: federica.denami@studenti.unicz.it; Tel.: +39-0961-3647002

Abstract

Patellofemoral instability (PFI) is a multifactorial orthopedic condition affecting predominantly young and active individuals. Accurate diagnosis and personalized treatment planning remain challenging due to the complex interplay of anatomical and biomechanical factors. Recently, artificial intelligence (AI), particularly machine learning (ML) and deep learning (DL), has gained attention for its role in musculoskeletal imaging and orthopedics care. This review explores the current and potential applications of AI in diagnosis and management of PFI. A total of 11 relevant articles were identified and included in the review. Articles originated from six countries, with China having the most contributions ($n = 4$), followed by Finland ($n = 3$), and Korea, Japan, USA and Portugal with 1 each. In the results section, findings are grouped into three themes: (A) Diagnosis, (B) Outcomes and Complications and (C) Challenges, Limitations and Future Directions. The review also discussed advancements in automated image analysis, predictive modeling and outcome prediction. Overall, AI has the potential to improve consistency, efficiency, and personalization of care in patients with PFI, although still requiring technological developments for implementation in daily practice. Existing studies are limited by small datasets, methodological heterogeneity, and lack of external validation. Future research should focus on multicenter data integration, explainable AI frameworks, and clinical validation to enable translation into routine orthopedic practice.

Keywords: artificial intelligence; deep learning; machine learning; patellofemoral instability; Rx; MRI; CT

1. Introduction

Patellofemoral instability (PFI) is a common orthopedic condition characterized by the abnormal movement of the patella outside the femoral trochlea, ranging from partial subluxation to full dislocation. This condition primarily affects adolescents and young active adults aged 10 to 16 years old [1,2], particularly females, and represents a significant cause of anterior knee pain, functional limitation, and recurrent joint complaints. The clinical spectrum ranges from a single episode of acute patellar dislocation to chronic instability with recurrent dislocations, often associated with a profound impact on sport participation and quality of life [3–5].

The pathophysiology of PFI is multifactorial, involving a complex interplay between static and dynamic stabilizers of the patellofemoral joint. Key anatomical risk factors include trochlear dysplasia, patella alta, increased tibial tuberosity-trochlear groove (TT–TG) distance, coronal plane malalignment, and rotational abnormalities of the femur or tibia [6–8]. It can also be associated with generalized ligamentous laxity and other co-morbidities including connective tissue disorders (i.e., Marfan's syndrome, Ehlers-Danlos syndrome) and genetic diseases (i.e., nail syndrome, small patella syndrome) which also have multisystem manifestations [9–11]. Accurate diagnosis and classification of PFI are essential for guiding treatment selection and optimizing outcomes, which may include conservative rehabilitation, medial patellofemoral ligament (MPFL) reconstruction, tibial tubercle osteotomy, lateral release, and trochleoplasty [12,13]. If not treated properly, it can lead to the that is also known as interobserver variability. In recent years, artificial intelligence (AI) and deep learning (DL) applications have emerged as promising tools for enhancing objectivity, consistency, and efficiency in musculoskeletal imaging; these techniques have shown promise in automating image-based measurements, identifying pathological features, and predicting outcomes based on complex data integration [14–17]. While these technologies offer the potential to enhance diagnostic accuracy and personalize treatment strategies, their integration into clinical practice remains limited and requires further validation.

While previous reviews have highlighted AI applications across various orthopedic areas—such as anterior cruciate ligament (ACL) injuries [18–20], surgical planning [21], knee arthroplasty [22,23], and assessment of degenerative joint diseases [24,25]—these have largely focused on tasks like ligament tear detection, surgical guidancedevelopment of an osteoarthritic (OA) condition [26–29]. The algorithm needs to be characterized by objective, reliable, and measurable data. As stated by the Lyon school [30], the knowledge of patient's medical and conducting a clinical examination are essential components but not sufficient; the ultimate determination relies on a thorough evaluation of both X-ray images and slices imaging. A clinical exam, including assessment of lower limb alignment, quadriceps trophism, apprehension sign and J sign, is essential for the suspected diagnosis. Radiographic examinations confirm suspected diagnosis and assess for concomitant injuries. In particular, signs such patellar height, patellar tilt and trochlear dysplasia should be evaluated with X-rays, and femoral anteversion, tibial rotation and TT-TG distance should be evaluated with computer tomography scans (CT). Otherwise, the whole description of patellofemoral abnormalities could be evaluated with magnetic resonance imaging (MRI) which is also a better option for evaluating loose bodies, assessing MPFL and localization of injury, and also plays a crucial role in the early detection and comprehensive evaluation of complications [31–34]. Overall, no single imaging parameter is sufficient for diagnosis and there may also be a clinical-radiological mismatch. In addition, current imaging techniques usually provide static information [35], which may not capture the dynamic nature of PFI. Among other limitations, knee position, flexion, and rotation during scanning can affect measurements; also, different radiologists may report different findings or measurements, a condition, implant design, and predicting postoperative outcomes. In these contexts, explainable AI frameworks have been integrated to varying degrees, with clinical validation ranging from retrospective performance assessment to limited prospective implementation. In contrast, the patellofemoral joint presents unique diagnostic and biomechanical challenges, and AI applications specifically addressing PFI have not yet been systematically reviewed.

The aim of this review is to provide a synthesis of the available evidence on AI applications specific to PFI, thus providing insights into its current role and future potential in improving patient care. To the best of our knowledge, this is the first study to comprehensively explore the applications of AI in the diagnosis and management of PFI.

2. Materials and Methods

A literature review was conducted and reported in accordance with the Preferred Reporting Items for Systematic Reviews and Meta-Analyses statement (PRISMA) [36] guidelines (Figure 1). A comprehensive search of PubMed, MedLine, Scopus, and Cochrane Central was performed in June 2025. The search strategy, to retrieve relevant articles, included the following terms: "deep learning", "artificial intelligence", "machine learning", "patellofemoral instability" "MRI", "CT", "Radiography", "diagnosis", and "treatment".

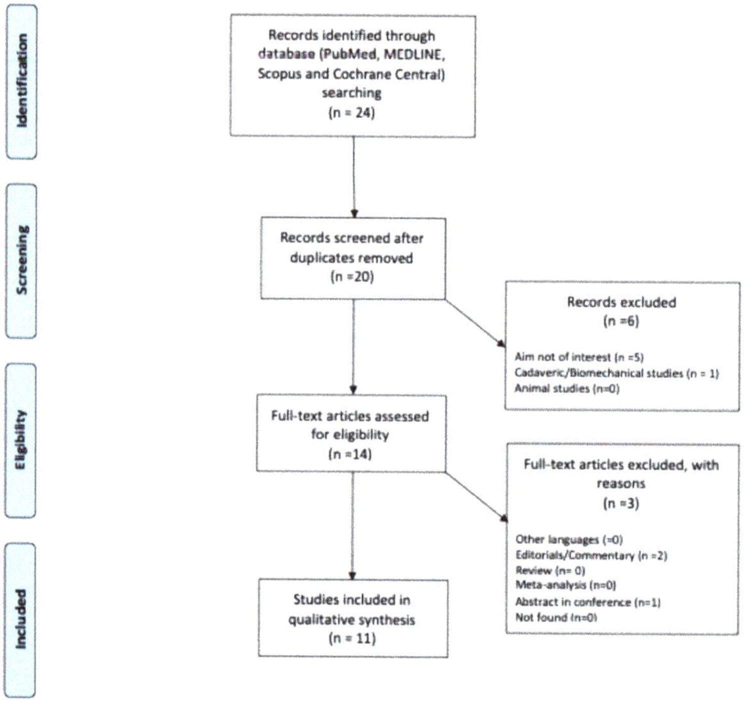

Figure 1. Flowchart PRISMA.

Studies were included if they met the following criteria: (1) original research articles, observational studies, or clinical trials; (2) focused on AI applications for PFI; (3) published in English; (4) reported quantitative or qualitative outcomes relevant to diagnosis, management, or prediction of PFI. Exclusion criteria comprised reviews, editorials, conference abstracts without full text, and preclinical studies not involving human participants. Studies including fewer than five patients were excluded to ensure meaningful analysis. Only articles published in the last five years were considered. Two reviewers (F.D. and A.V.) independently screened records and abstracts to identify articles for inclusion, contacting a third senior author (M.M.) in cases of disagreement. The reference list of each included article, as well as the available gray literature at our institution, were screened for potential additional articles. Other reviews, editorials, letters to the editor, and expert opinions were also considered but not included. Emphasis was placed on studies applying AI to diagnosis, imaging, outcome prediction, or treatment planning for PFI. The include articles are summarized in Table 1.

Table 1. Included studies, (A) Diagnosis, (B) Outcomes and complications and (C) Future Directions and Challenges, Machine learning (ML), Artificial intelligence (AI), Convolutional neural network (CNN), Support Vector Machines (SVM), Visual geometry group 16 (VGG-16), Insall-Salvati index (ISI), Caton-Deschamps index (CDI), modified, Caton-Deschamps index (MCDI), Keerati index (KI), Patellofemoral osteoarthritis (PFOA), International knee documentation committee (IKDC), Femoral trochlear dysplasia (FTD), Kujala score (KS), Sulcus angle (SA), Trochlear facet asymmetry (TFA), Trochlear groove depth (TGD), Lateral trochlear inclination (LTI), Modified Insall-Salvati index (MISI), Caton Deschamps index (CDI), Patell trochlear index (PTI), Western Ontario and McMaster Universities osteoarthritis index (WOMAC), Congruence angle (CA), Lateral patellar tilt (LPT), Inter class correlation (ICC), Area under the curve (AUC), Receiver Operating Characteristic (ROC), and positive and negative predictive values (PPV and NPV, respectively).

N	Authors (Year) Country	Journal	AI	Sample	Aim	Result	Limits
1	Ye et al. (2020) China [37]	Eur. Radiol.	CNN (VGG-16)	1018 left knee radiographs	Determine the patellar height using lateral knee radiographs.	ISI, CDI, and KI (ICC = 0.91–0.95,) MCDI (left knee ICC = 0.65). The performance of the algorithm met or exceeded that of manual determination of ISI, CDI, and KI by radiologists.	Training size and category; lack of standard and ancillary information.
2	Bayramoglu et al. (2021) Finland [38]	Osteo. Cart.	CNN	2803 patients (19% PFOA at X-rays)	Detect PFOA from lateral view plain radiographs.	ROC AUC (0.958).	Multicenter Osteoarthritis study data alone; limited X-rays view; model explanations.
3	Bayramoglu et al. (2022) Finland [39]	Int. J. Med. Inf	CNN	5507 knees (953 PFOA)	Predict PFOA based on texture patches analysis of lateral knee radiographs.	Age, sex, BMI, WOMAC score, tibiofemoral KL grade to predict PFOA AUC (0.817).	Lack of external data.
4	Tuya et al. (2023) China [40]	Eur. Radiol.	U-Net	1431 consecutive Laurin views	Calculated radiographic parameters using the Laurin view.	SA, CA, LPT (ICC = 0.85–0.97).	Small sample size; lack of a gold standard and the inherent variation in manual measurement.
5	Xu et al. (2023) China [41]	WJCC	CNN	464 MRI 1.5 T Knee (202 FTD)	Detect FTD from knee MRI scans.	Sensitivity, Specificity, PPV and NPV of the AI model (0.74–0.96).	Single axial 1.5T MRI image.
6	Barbosa et al. (2024) Portugal [42]	Eur. Radiol.	U-Net	763 knee MRI slices (95 patients)	Index measurements in knee MRI slices (axial and sagittal).	LTI, TGD, ISI, CDI and PTI (ICC > 0.9), and SA, TFA and MISI (ICC > 0.75).	Less robust models, landmarks positioning.
7	Kwak et al. (2025) Korea [43]	KSSTA	ML	108 Patients (54 dislocated patella) (1.5–3.0 MRI)	Early diagnosis and personalized treatment planning in young patients.	KS AUC (0.87), Wiberg index AUC (0.85), IS method AUC (0.84); patellar tilt AUC (0.81) and total AUC (0.934).	Retrospective design; lack of CT and WLLRx, only logistic regression.
8	Bayramoglu et al. (2024) Finland [44]	Methods Inf. Med	CNN (VGG-16)	1832 subjects, (3276 knees)	Predict the radiographic progression of PFOA over a 7 year period using lateral knee radiographs.	AUC (0.856).	Single population trained model; No PFOA potential predictors progression consideration.
9	Nagawa et al. (2024) Japan [45]	Sci. Rep.	ML-based prediction model (SVM)	49 patients (19 PFI)	Predictive model for patellofemoral instability based on MRI.	Accuracy (0.909 ± 0.015); AUC (0.939 ± 0.009).	Small sample size; only the distal femur evaluation.
10	Sieberer et al. (2025) USA [46]	Knee	AI algorithm	60 patients (30 dislocated patella)	AI-derived measurements patellar tilt segmenting 3D CT scans.	Predicted ICC (0.86–0.90).	lack of gold standard; CT supine position.
11	Zhan et al. (2024) China [47]	Arthroscopy	ML	218 patients	Develop a ML model to predict clinical outcomes after MPFLR.	Score Accuracies Lysholm (0.884); IKDC (0.859); Kujala (0.969) Tegner (0.756).	Retrospective nature; selected knee surgery; no external validation; small sample size; short follow-up.

A quality assessment of the methodology was carried out independently by three authors (FD, AV, and MM) using the modified Newcastle–Ottawa Quality Assessment Scale [48] (Table 2). Substantial interobserver agreement (Cohen kappa coefficients ranging between 0.59 and 0.74) was achieved. According to the overall score, the quality was categorized as "low" (0–3), "medium" (4–6), and "high" (7–9). The criteria included: 1, representativeness of the exposed cohort; 2, selection of the unexposed cohort; 3, ascertainment of exposure; 4, the proof that the outcome of interest was not observed at the start; 5, the comparability of cohorts based on structure or analysis; 6, the evaluation of the outcome; 7, a follow-up period long enough to capture the findings; 8, the adequacy of the follow-up of the cohorts. Each study received a score with a maximum of one or two points for each numbered criterion within the categories, in accordance with the modified Newcastle–Ottawa scale rules.

Table 2. Quality assessment of included studies according to the Modified Newcastle–Ottawa scale.

	Criteria								Total	Quality
	1	2	3	4	5	6	7	8		
Ye et al. (2020) [37]	1	1	1	1	1	1	1	1	8	High
Bayramoglu et al. (2021) [38]	1	1	1	1	1	1	1	1	8	High
Bayramoglu et al. (2022) [39]	1	1	1	1	1	1	1	1	8	High
Tuya et al. (2023) [40]	1	1	1	1	1	1	1	1	8	High
Xu et al. (2023) [41]	1	0	0	1	1	1	1	0	5	Medium
Barbosa et al. (2024) [42]	1	1	1	1	1	1	1	1	8	High
Kwak et al. (2025) [43]	1	1	1	1	1	1	1	1	8	High
Bayramoglu et al. (2024) [44]	1	1	1	1	1	1	1	1	8	High
Nagawa et al. (2024) [45]	1	1	1	1	1	1	1	1	8	High
Sieberer et al. (2025) [46]	1	1	1	1	1	1	1	1	8	High
Zhan et al. (2024) [47]	1	1	1	1	1	1	1	1	8	High

3. Results and Discussion

A total of 24 articles were identified through the initial search, resulting in 11 studies [37–47] that were included in the review (Figure 1). The selected articles originated from six countries, with China contributing the largest number (n = 4), followed by Finland (n = 3), and Korea, Japan, USA and Portugal with 1 each.

In the results section, findings are grouped into three thematic domains: (A) Diagnosis, (B) Outcomes and Complications, and (C) Challenges, Limitations and Future Directions.

Across the included studies, a variety of AI algorithms were applied for diagnostic and predictive purposes. DL architectures, mainly convolutional neural networks (CNNs) and hybrid DL models, were the most used and demonstrated high accuracy in automating radiographic measurements and identifying key morphological parameters associated with PFI. Traditional machine learning algorithms, including support vector machines (SVMs) were employed to predict instability risk factors and postoperative outcomes. Specifically, only two studies [37,44] reported the use of specific architecture type: in particular, VGG-16. Furthermore, three studies [38,39,41] referred broadly to the use of CNN, while two studies [40,42] specified the use of a U-Net architecture; however, these works did not provide further information on the specific model configuration or implementation details. Some authors, to mitigate constraints posed by constrained dataset sizes, used domain adaptation methodologies and approaches such as data augmentation [49]. Notably, only a subset of studies reported the full neural architecture used (e.g., VGG-16, U-Net). Several studies referred broadly to "deep learning" without specifying layer structure, training settings, or validation workflows, which limits reproducibility and comparability across models. This heterogeneity highlights the need for standardized reporting and multicenter model validation before clinical translation.

Although most models demonstrated excellent internal performance, their implementation in clinical workflows remains limited. None of the included studies reported full integration into radiology systems or clinical decision-support software; AI was primarily used as a research tool to assist image quantification or outcome prediction rather than as a real-time diagnostic aid.

A schematic representation of the AI workflow for the diagnosis and management of PFI is provided in Figure 2. The diagram summarizes the data sources, feature extraction process, modeling approaches, and clinical applications discussed in this review.

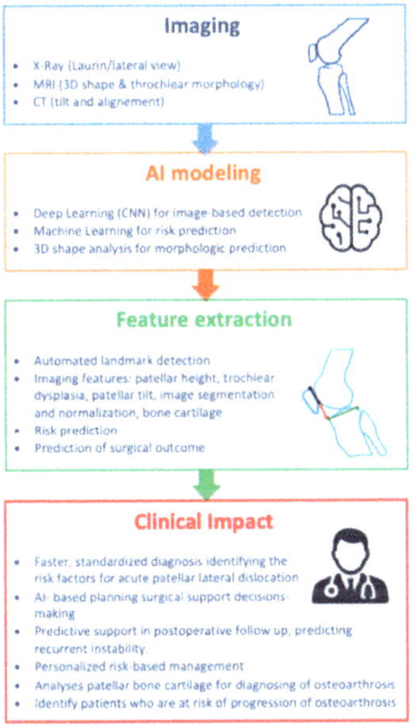

Figure 2. Graphical abstract summarizing AI applications in the diagnosis and prediction of patellofemoral instability (PFI). Workflow illustrating the process from imaging data acquisition through feature extraction and selection, followed by AI model application, leading to clinical decision support. The figure highlights how selected imaging features contribute to improved diagnostic consistency and treatment planning in orthopedic practice.

3.1. Diagnosis

Recent advances have underscored the value of machine learning (ML) algorithms combined with optimization strategies for identifying key risk factors for PFI in pediatric and adolescent populations.

In order to mitigate operator-dependent bias inherent in the manual interpretation of radiographic images, recent studies have increasingly adopted AI algorithms to automate the quantification of critical radiological parameters, including patellar tilt and patellar height. Notably, the diagnostic performance of CNN-based model was comparable in accuracy to that of radiology specialists in the assessment of the Insall-Salvati Index (ISI), Caton-Deschamps Index (CDI), modified Caton-Deschamps Index (MCDI), and Keerati Index (KI) [26]. Ye et al. developed a CNN system for automatic patellar height, that consists of a landmark detection network (VGG16) and mathematical formulas to determine the patellar height using lateral knee radiographs [37]. Compared with the reference standard (manual measurement), the algorithm showed high accuracy in predicting the ISI, CDI, and KI (ICC = 0.91–0.95), but not the MCDI. Similarly, Tuya et al. [40] employed a deep learning method using U-Net to identify the landmarks of the patellofemoral joint (PFJ) by analyzing the Laurin. Subsequently, various parameters were determined, such as the sulcus angle (SA), congruence angle (CA), patellofemoral ratio (PFR), and lateral patellar tilt (LPT). Model performance was evaluated via the percentage of correct keypoints (PCK), intraclass correlation coefficient (ICC), mean absolute difference (MAD), root mean square (RMS) and 95% limits of agreement (LoA). Comparing the results with the mean of three radiologists, the U-Net show good performance; high ICC values (0.85–0.97), showing strong agreement with expert radiologists. The model-maintained accuracy even in cases with patellar instability or osteoarthritis. Compared to Ye et al., the U-net for segmenting landmarks using PCK at the 2 mm threshold showed larger results.

Although radiographic examinations are simple and cost-effective, their utility is limited by the lack of standardized radiographic evaluation criteria, the absence of normative reference values, and the need for proper imaging technique and views acquisition. For these reasons, other authors [41–43,45] have been committed to uniform the PFI assessment with MRI, demonstrating that it will be the future standard. In a 2024 study [43], researchers developed a predictive ML model using a dataset of 1.5–3.0 T MRI derived morphological measurements, including the Koshino-Sugimoto (KS) index, Wiberg classification, and TT-TG distance. One hundred and eight patients divided into two cohorts, lateral patellar dislocation (54 subjects) and control (54 subjects) groups were included in the study. The ML approach employed supervised learning techniques, training the algorithm on labeled data to distinguish between stable and unstable patellofemoral joints. Genetic algorithm-based optimization was integrated to select the most relevant features and fine-tune the model parameters, enhancing prediction accuracy and reducing overfitting. The final model demonstrated excellent diagnostic performance, with an area under the curve (AUC) of 0.934, reflecting high sensitivity and specificity in detecting patients at risk of PFI. The KS index was the main risk factor (AUC: 0.87) and, in combination with the Wiberg index (AUC: 0.85), showed the strongest association with lateral patellar dislocation. More extended trial, including the patellar height measurement, was performed by Barbosa et al. [42]. The authors suggested utilizing a deep learning algorithm (U-Net) to automatically identify the positions of landmarks and calculate index measurements in knee MRI images (both axial and sagittal). Findings indicated that the suggested approach is dependable for automatically quantifying the primary PFI indices mentioned in existing research (ISI, CDI, as well as SA, trochlear facet asymmetry (TFA), trochlear groove depth (TGD) and lateral trochlear inclination (LTI)). This method, when compared to the measurements taken by an expert musculoskeletal radiologist, significantly aids radiologists by decreasing the time required and lessening the complexity of the task involved. in terms of SA, it is the only parameter that obtained a higher intraclass correlation coefficient (ICC = 0.85–0.97 vs. ICC > 0.75) by using the U-Net-based deep learning approach develop by Tuya et al. The radiographic Laurin view offers a more detailed perspective of the trochlea, and these differences in imaging techniques might have played a role in the results that were noted. [42]. Additional femoral trochlear dysplasia (FTD) evidence was reported by Xu et al. [41], that developed a DL model to automatically detect FTD from knee MRI scans (axial image-1.5 T). Using a dataset of 464 knee MRI cases (202 with FTD and 252 normal), the authors trained a CNN with heatmap regression to identify key anatomical landmarks. The AI model's diagnostic accuracy was 88%, with sensitivity, specificity, positive predictive value and negative predictive value ranging from 74% to 96%, outperforming junior and intermediate clinicians and matching the performance of senior experts. AI model significantly reduced diagnostic time (0.14 ± 0.11 s vs. 102.97 ± 21.26 s) compared to less experienced physicians. Furthermore, it was discovered that assessing the angle of the lateral trochlea and the depth of the trochlear groove yielded more reliable results than evaluating the ratio of the medial to lateral facets, when considering both the consistency within groups and the accuracy of disease diagnosis. In fact, MRI offers a superior view of the femoral trochlea's structure in comparison to X-rays. On the other hand, the authors simplified the exam involving a single MRI level. As highlighted, no further information is available on multi-levels imaging or superior resolution exams. As a result, when utilizing MRI for diagnosing FTD, the choice of parameters tends to focus on assessing the angle of the lateral trochlea and the depth of the trochlear groove.

Recently, Nagawa et al. [45] integrated 3D statistical shape analysis (SSA) based on MRI with ML techniques to develop a predictive model for patellofemoral instability. According to the 3D trochlea reconstruction, the authors extracted principal components describing morphological variations that distinguish unstable knees from normal ones. Using a linear support vector machine (SVM) classifier, the model achieved an accuracy exceeding 90%, demonstrating the potential of this method to effectively discriminate anatomical features associated with the condition. The pointwise distance map revealed that the height of the trochlea in the PFI models, when compared to the normal models, was noted at the central part of the proximal trochlea floor. This approach represents a promising step toward more objective and automated diagnostic tools, with potential applications in personalized surgical planning.

Sieberer et al. developed and reported the results of a selection 2D slice methodology for calculating patellar tilt. AI was employed to analyze 3D CT scans in order to obtain patellar tilt from significant surface reference points. The findings were benchmarked against the conventional approach and the manual positioning of reference points conducted by one of the researchers involved in the study, revealing a high level of concordance between the various methods [46].

Despite promising results, heterogeneity across studies limits direct comparison of model performance.

Variations in imaging modalities (radiography, CT, MRI), preprocessing methods, and validation strategies create inconsistencies in outcome metrics. Sample sizes were generally small and single-center, often lacking external validation. Moreover, while DL models achieved superior segmentation and measurement accuracy, they remain limited by poor interpretability, whereas ML approaches, though more explainable, depend heavily on handcrafted features and smaller datasets. These discrepancies underscore the need for standardized imaging protocols, harmonized datasets, and transparent performance reporting.

3.2. Outcomes and Complications

While evidence regarding the application of AI in post-operative care remains limited, emerging data in the literature are promising. Recent studies have demonstrated the potential of machine learning models to predict clinical outcomes following MPFL reconstruction.

Zhan et al. developed ML algorithms that reliably forecast patient recovery and risk of complications, supporting more personalized surgical planning and postoperative management. Authors built 42 predictive models addressing seven clinical outcomes, achieving up to 97% accuracy in predicting return to pre-injury sports activity. Significantly, a low preoperative Tegner score, a reduced interval before surgery, and no severe trochlear dysplasia are key indicators for resuming preinjury sports. In contrast, the lack of severe trochlear dysplasia along with patellar alta were important factors predicting the return to pivoting sports [50]. Additionally, advanced age, being female, and a low preoperative Lysholm score strongly indicate the likelihood of experiencing recurrent instability. These predictive tools contribute to optimizing treatment strategies by integrating diverse clinical and demographic data, highlighting the growing role of AI in managing PFI [47]. A notable limitation of the available evidence is the short-term follow-up period. This is particularly relevant given the growing interest in the development of patellofemoral osteoarthritis (PFOA) as a long-term outcome following treatment for PFI, which has increasingly attracted the attention of researchers. The integration of AI-based tools, in particular DL, into outcome analysis may reasonably enhance immediate surgical results and help mitigate the risk of chronic complications, such as PFOA, through early detection and the implementation of individualized follow-up strategies.

In 2021, a study introduced a completely automated technique (CNN) for identifying PFOA in lateral view plain radiographs, based on the Multicenter Osteoarthritis Study (MOST), which is a significant multicenter dataset, employing deep learning. The developed model underwent assessment in a subject-wise stratified cross-validation framework to evaluate its reliability. The final model demonstrated a strong discriminative capacity (AUC 0.958) [38].

By analyzing large datasets that integrate imaging, kinematic, and clinical follow-up data, DL algorithms can identify early predictors of degenerative changes in the patellofemoral joint. Bayramoglu et al. [44] proposed a deep CNN (VGG-16) capable of predicting the radiographic progression of PFOA over a 7 year period using lateral knee radiographs. For purposes of comparison, a machine learning model (LightGBM—Gradient Boosting Machine, Microsoft, Redmond, Washington, USA) was developed using clinical factors such as age, gender, body mass index (BMI), the overall score from the Western Ontario and McMaster Universities Arthritis Index (WOMAC), and the tibiofemoral Kellgren and Lawrence (KL) grading. Notably, the integrated model achieved the best performance (AUC = 0.865), demonstrating its effectiveness in distinguishing patients at risk for developing PFOA and not. These findings highlight the potential of hybrid AI models in supporting early risk stratification and personalized follow-up in patients treated for PFI. In addition to predicting disease progression, Bayramoglu [39] also investigated the use of both LightGBM classifiers and deep CNN methods to predict PFOA based on texture patches analysis of lateral knee radiographs. Specifically, they compared models trained on image-based texture patches from the patellar region with those using conventional clinical data and participant characteristics. Notably, the model relying solely on texture features extracted from the superior and inferior region of interest (ROI) of the patella significantly outperformed the clinical-based model (AUC = 0.884 vs. 0.817). These results underscore the potential of patellar texture analysis as a valuable imaging biomarker for early and accurate osteoarthritis diagnosis.

3.3. *Challenges, Limitations and Future Directions*

Although not strictly categorized as AI, the work of Van Haver et al. [51] employed statistical shape modeling (SSM) to objectively characterize and classify trochlear dysplasia based on 3D CT data. By capturing shape variation through principal component analysis, the model achieved high sensitivity (85%) and specificity (95%) in distinguishing dysplastic from normal femur. This early computational approach laid important groundwork for the later development of AI-driven tools aimed at automatic morphological assessment and classification.

One of the most promising areas for future development in the evaluation of PFI lies in the integration of dynamic imaging, such dynamic measurement of PFJ alignment using weight-bearing MRI [52] or dynamic axial CT [53], and AI [54,55]. However, this is promising mostly for research because the availability of the machine is limited. Considering conventional radiological techniques limits, which provide static images of an inherently dynamic condition, there is a clear need for diagnostic approaches capable of analyzing joint behavior during movement. Emerging technologies such as cine-MRI and 4D-CT allow visualization of patellar tracking throughout flexion-extension but remain limited by technical challenges, costs, and accessibility [56]. In this context, the application of DL algorithms could enhance the analysis of these data by automating the recognition of dynamic maltracking patterns and improving the reproducibility of assessments. AI could also contribute to the development of integrated predictive models that combine morphological and functional information to support early diagnosis and personalized treatment planning. DL capable of processing sequential and temporal data (e.g., recurrent neural networks, time-series convolutional models, or transformer-based approaches) have the potential to analyze patellar tracking, alignment changes, and soft tissue interactions during movement [57,58]. By quantifying these dynamic parameters, AI could provide a more physiologically accurate assessment of instability, guide personalized rehabilitation or surgical planning, and predict postoperative outcomes. However, such applications remain in early conceptual stages and require standardized acquisition protocols, large dynamic datasets, and close collaboration between engineers and clinicians for successful translation into practice. Future research should therefore focus on the development and clinical validation of these tools to translate the theoretical potential of AI-assisted dynamic analysis into practical orthopedic applications.

Despite the growing interest and promising results regarding the use of AI in PFI, several limitations characterize the current literature [59]. First, the current body of literature remains limited, with most studies focusing on isolated applications such as automated imaging measurements or outcome prediction in small, retrospective cohorts. Large-scale, prospective studies with standardized datasets are lacking, limiting the generalizability and clinical translation of existing AI models.

Second, the heterogeneity in imaging protocols, anatomical landmarks, and diagnostic criteria across studies can hinder reproducibility and external validation of AI tools. Many models are developed using single-institution data, which may not reflect the variability encountered in broader clinical practice. On the other hand, no specific standard protocols are present regarding the number of radiographic images or patients for AI training, validation, and assessment. Standard radiographs differ in projections, patient positioning, and acquisition parameters, resulting in variable measurements of patellar height, tilt, and alignment. Similarly, MRI and CT protocols vary in slice thickness, acquisition planes, and sequences. This aspect highlights the need for a shared and standardized pathway as recently proposed with an MRI protocol for patellar height and trochlear classification [34]. Task of governmental institutions and supranational orthopedic societies should collaborate to provide guidelines for the standardization and acceptability of AI tools [35].

Another limitation should be that standard CT and MRI scans are typically acquired with the patient in a supine position, ignoring the extensor apparatus [60,61]. As a result, there is no available data on how, for example, these methods evaluate patellar tilt under weightbearing (WB) conditions, where the patella's position may significantly differ [62]. Furthermore, definitions of anatomical landmarks and diagnostic criteria are not standardized across studies, limiting reproducibility and external validation of AI models. Recent advances in imaging techniques, such as the use of weight-bearing cone-beam CT (CBCT) with 3D spatial measurements, have demonstrated improved assessment of patellofemoral alignment under functional conditions [63]. These methods offer precise quantification of patellar tilt and shift along multiple axes, providing valuable diagnostic insights beyond traditional supine imaging. However, such analyses currently rely on manual landmark identification and geometric calculations, which can be time-consuming and operator-dependent. In this context, AI—Particularly DL—holds significant promise. Future applications may include the development of automated 3D segmentation and alignment analysis tools trained on CBCT datasets, allowing for faster and more reproducible assessment [64]. Moreover, AI-based predictive models could integrate dynamic 3D parameters with patient-specific clinical and anatomical data to enhance surgical planning and stratify the risk of recurrent dislocation.

Third, while DL models often demonstrate high accuracy, they frequently operate as "black boxes," providing limited interpretability for clinicians. This lack of transparency can raise concerns about reliability and clinical trust, particularly in high-stakes decision-making such as surgical planning. To address this, interpretable AI approaches—such as saliency maps, attention mechanisms, and feature importance analysis—can be applied to highlight which anatomical features, measurements, or imaging landmarks drive model predictions. In our review, the studies selected focus on models that allow visualization of key patellofemoral parameters, ensuring that AI outputs provide clinically meaningful and transparent information to support surgical planning.

Fourth, there are important ethical and legal considerations surrounding the use of AI in clinical practice, including data privacy, informed consent for model use, and the potential for algorithmic bias—especially when training datasets are not representative of diverse patient populations [14,65].

Finally, the integration of AI into clinical workflows remains challenging [66]. There is a need for user-friendly interfaces, education of healthcare professionals, and robust validation through randomized clinical trials to confirm that AI-assisted tools improve diagnostic accuracy, surgical outcomes, and long-term patient care in PFI. Clinical barriers encompass limited workflow integration, lack of real-time application, and clinician skepticism due to limited interpretability of DL models. Regulatory and ethical challenges involve patient data privacy, algorithm accountability, and compliance with healthcare regulations [67–69]. To overcome these obstacles, future efforts should focus on developing multicenter annotated datasets, implementing explainable AI frameworks, standardizing imaging and labeling protocols, and designing AI tools that seamlessly integrate into existing clinical decision-making workflows. Addressing these factors is crucial to translate the theoretical promise of AI into routine orthopedic practice

Despite promising developments, several challenges remain in adopting AI for PFI. Future effort should prioritize multicenter collaborations to generate high-quality annotated datasets, integration of AI tools into PACS and surgical planning software [70], and clinical trials to evaluate the impact of AI on patient outcomes [71]. Interdisciplinary cooperation between clinicians, engineers, and data scientists will be essential to realize the full potential of AI in this domain.

Furthermore, ML models could be trained to distinguish between patients likely to maintain favorable outcomes and those at higher risk for complications, thereby facilitating tailored rehabilitation protocols or closer radiographic monitoring. Additional developments may also include AI-assisted dynamic simulations to model joint stress evolution post-surgery and predict long-term cartilage wear.

4. Conclusions

Artificial intelligence represents a promising strategy to enhance the diagnosis, classification, and management of patellofemoral instability. In this study, the comparative analyses performed between the evaluated AI models and standard radiological parameters demonstrated that the integration of automated feature extraction and predictive algorithms can improve both the consistency and reproducibility of PFI assessment. These comparisons were essential for achieving the research goals, as they quantified the added value of the proposed approach relative to conventional methods and highlighted which algorithmic components most strongly contributed to performance improvements. Current studies demonstrate potential to enhance consistency, efficiency, and personalization of care; despite these encouraging findings, clinical implementation remains limited by small, single-center datasets, heterogeneous imaging protocols, and a lack of external validation.

Future research should therefore prioritize the creation of large, multicenter datasets, the development of interpretable and transparent AI algorithms, and integration of AI tools into clinical workflows. Collaborative efforts between clinicians, data scientists, and engineers will be essential to translate these technologies from research to practice. By overcoming these barriers, AI has the potential to meaningfully support evidence-based, personalized care for patients with patellofemoral instability.

Author Contributions: Conceptualization, M.M., F.D. and D.H.D.; methodology, M.M., F.D. and A.V.; data curation, M.M., F.D. and A.V.; writing—original draft preparation, M.M., F.D. and D.H.D.; writing—review and editing, M.M., F.D., A.V., F.F., U.G.L., O.G., G.G. and D.H.D.; supervision, M.M., F.D., A.V., F.F., O.G., G.G. and D.H.D.; project administration, M.M. and F.D. All authors have read and agreed to the published version of the manuscript.

Funding: This research received no external funding.

Institutional Review Board Statement: Not applicable.

Informed Consent Statement: Not applicable.

Data Availability Statement: The data presented in this study are available on reasonable request from the corresponding author.

Acknowledgments: Michele Mercurio and Giorgio Gasparini are members of the Executive Board of the Italian Orthopaedic Research Society (IORS).

Conflicts of Interest: The authors declare no conflicts of interest.

References

1. Mercurio, M.; Corona, K.; Galasso, O.; Cerciello, S.; Morris, B.J.; Guerra, G.; Gasparini, G. Soccer Players Show the Highest Seasonal Groin Pain Prevalence and the Longest Time Loss from Sport among 500 Athletes from Major Team Sports. *Knee Surg. Sports Traumatol. Arthrosc.* **2022**, *30*, 2149–2157. [CrossRef] [PubMed]
2. Wolfe, S.; Varacallo, M.; Thomas, J.D.; Carroll, J.J.; Kahwaji, C.I. *Patellar Instability*; StatPearls: Tampa, FL, USA, 2018.
3. Dejour, D.H.; Mesnard, G.; Giovannetti de Sanctis, E. Updated Treatment Guidelines for Patellar Instability: "Un Menu à La Carte". *J. Exp. Orthop.* **2021**, *8*, 109. [CrossRef] [PubMed]
4. Blønd, L.; Askenberger, M.; Stephen, J.; Akmeşe, R.; Balcarek, P.; El Attal, R.; Chouliaras, V.; Ferrua, P.; Monart, J.M.; Pagen-stert, G.; et al. Management of First-Time Patellar Dislocation: The ESSKA 2024 Formal Consensus—Part 1. *Knee Surg. Sports Traumatol. Arthrosc.* **2025**, *33*, 1925–1932. [CrossRef]
5. Barbosa, R.M.; Da Silva, M.V.; Macedo, C.S.; Santos, C.P. Imaging Evaluation of Patellofemoral Joint Instability: A Review. *Knee Surg. Relat. Res.* **2023**, *35*, 7. [CrossRef]
6. Schoettle, P.B.; Zanetti, M.; Seifert, B.; Pfirrmann, C.W.; Fucentese, S.F.; Romero, J. The Tibial Tuberosity–Trochlear Groove Distance; a Comparative Study between CT and MRI Scanning. *Knee* **2006**, *13*, 26–31. [CrossRef]
7. Dai, Z.-Z.; Sha, L.; Zhang, Z.-M.; Liang, Z.-P.; Li, H.; Li, H. Comparing the Tibial Tuberosity–Trochlear Groove Distance between CT and MRI in Skeletally Immature Patients with and without Patellar Instability. *Orthop. J. Sports Med.* **2021**, *9*, 2325967120973665. [CrossRef]
8. Chen, J.; Wu, C.; Ye, Z.; Zhao, J.; Xie, G. Tibial Tuberosity-Trochlear Groove Distance and Its Components in Patients with and without Episodic Patellar Dislocation: A Study of 781 Knees. *J. Bone Jt. Surg.* **2022**, *104*, 504–511. [CrossRef]
9. Al-Dadah, O.; Hing, C. Patellofemoral Instability. *Knee* **2022**, *37*, A1–A2. [CrossRef]
10. Park, S.J.; Won, S.H.; Park, M.S.; Sung, K.H. Normative Values of Tibial Tubercle–Trochlear Groove Distance and Tibial Tubercle–Posterior Cruciate Ligament Distance in Children. *Am. J. Sports Med.* **2023**, *51*, 1785–1791. [CrossRef]
11. Camp, C.L.; Heidenreich, M.J.; Dahm, D.L.; Stuart, M.J.; Levy, B.A.; Krych, A.J. Individualizing the Tibial Tubercle–Trochlear Groove Distance: Patellar Instability Ratios That Predict Recurrent Instability. *Am. J. Sports Med.* **2016**, *44*, 393–399. [CrossRef]
12. Pineda, T.; Dejour, D.H. [Artículo Traducido] Menú a La Carta Para Inestabilidad Patelar Recurrente. *Rev. Esp. Cir. Ortop. Traumatol.* **2025**, *69*, T544–T550.

13. Pauyo, T.; Park, J.P.; Bozzo, I.; Bernstein, M. Patellofemoral Instability Part I: Evaluation and Nonsurgical Treatment. *JAAOS-J. Am. Acad. Orthop. Surg.* **2022**, *30*, e1431–e1442. [CrossRef] [PubMed]
14. Mercurio, M.; Denami, F.; Melissaridou, D.; Corona, K.; Cerciello, S.; Laganà, D.; Gasparini, G.; Minici, R. Deep Learning Models to Detect Anterior Cruciate Ligament Injury on MRI: A Comprehensive Review. *Diagnostics* **2025**, *15*, 776. [CrossRef] [PubMed]
15. Alsoof, D.; McDonald, C.L.; Kuris, E.O.; Daniels, A.H. Machine Learning for the Orthopaedic Surgeon: Uses and Limitations. *J. Bone Jt. Surg.* **2022**, *104*, 1586–1594. [CrossRef]
16. Familiari, F.; Galasso, O.; Massazza, F.; Mercurio, M.; Fox, H.; Srikumaran, U.; Gasparini, G. Artificial Intelligence in the Management of Rotator Cuff Tears. *Int. J. Environ. Res. Public Health* **2022**, *19*, 16779. [CrossRef]
17. Vescio, A.; Testa, G.; Sapienza, M.; Familiari, F.; Mercurio, M.; Gasparini, G.; de Salvatore, S.; Donati, F.; Canavese, F.; Pavone, V. Artificial Intelligence in Pediatric Orthopedics: A Comprehensive Review. *Medicina* **2025**, *61*, 954. [CrossRef]
18. Andriollo, L.; Picchi, A.; Sangaletti, R.; Perticarini, L.; Rossi, S.M.P.; Logroscino, G.; Benazzo, F. The Role of Artificial Intelligence in Anterior Cruciate Ligament Injuries: Current Concepts and Future Perspectives. *Healthcare* **2024**, *12*, 300. [CrossRef]
19. Wolfgart, J.M.; Hofmann, U.K.; Praster, M.; Danalache, M.; Migliorini, F.; Feierabend, M. Machine Learning to Recognise ACL Tears: A Systematic Review. *Appl. Sci.* **2025**, *15*, 4636. [CrossRef]
20. Alaiti, R.K.; Vallio, C.S.; da Silva, A.G.M.; Gobbi, R.G.; Pécora, J.R.; Helito, C.P. Predicting ACL Reconstruction Failure with Machine Learning: Development of Machine Learning Prediction Models. *Orthop. J. Sports Med.* **2025**, *13*, 23259671251324519. [CrossRef]
21. Elkohail, A.; Soffar, A.; Khalifa, A.M.; Omar, I.; Mosaad, M.; Abdulaziz, M.; Elsaket, A.; Panhwer, H.S.; Abdelglil, M.; Teama, M.; et al. AI-Enhanced Surgical Decision-Making in Orthopedics: From Preoperative Planning to Intraoperative Guidance and Real-Time Adaptation. *Cureus* **2025**, *17*, 92762. [CrossRef]
22. Rodriguez, H.C.; Rust, B.D.; Roche, M.W.; Gupta, A. Artificial Intelligence and Machine Learning in Knee Arthroplasty. *Knee* **2025**, *54*, 28–49. [CrossRef]
23. Lan, Q.; Li, S.; Zhang, J.; Guo, H.; Yan, L.; Tang, F. Reliable Prediction of Implant Size and Axial Alignment in AI-Based 3D Preoperative Planning for Total Knee Arthroplasty. *Sci. Rep.* **2024**, *14*, 16971. [CrossRef]
24. Kumar, R.; Sporn, K.; Borole, A.; Khanna, A.; Gowda, C.; Paladugu, P.; Ngo, A.; Jagadeesan, R.; Zaman, N.; Tavakkoli, A. Biomarker-Guided Imaging and AI-Augmented Diagnosis of Degenerative Joint Disease. *Diagnostics* **2025**, *15*, 1418. [CrossRef]
25. Choi, E.; Shin, S.; Lee, K.; An, T.; Lee, R.K.; Kim, S.; Son, Y.; Kim, S.T. Artificial Intelligence-Enhanced Diagnosis of Degenera-tive Joint Disease Using Temporomandibular Joint Panoramic Radiography and Joint Noise Data. *Sci. Rep.* **2025**, *15*, 1823.
26. Familiari, F.; Madonna, V.; Mercurio, M.; Cinque, M.E.; Gasparini, G.; Galasso, O.; Moatshe, G. Outcomes and Complications of Inlay versus Onlay Patellofemoral Arthroplasty: A Systematic Review. *Knee* **2023**, *41*, 124–136. [CrossRef] [PubMed]
27. Sava, M.-P.; Neopoulos, G.; Leica, A.; Hirschmann, M.T. Patellofemoral Arthroplasty with Onlay Prosthesis Leads to Higher Rates of Osteoarthritis Progression than Inlay Design Implants: A Systematic Review. *Knee Surg. Sports Traumatol. Arthrosc.* **2023**, *31*, 3927–3940. [CrossRef] [PubMed]
28. Vella-Baldacchino, M.; Chughtai, D.; Kow, J.; Carr, C.; Coyle, A.; Farrow-Foster, A.; Russell, J.; Liddle, A.D. Outcomes of Pa-tellofemoral Joint Arthroplasty: A Systematic Review of Revision Timelines and Complication Rates. *J. Orthop. Surg.* **2025**, *20*, 289. [CrossRef]
29. Erquicia, J.I.; Jiménez, D.M.; Riverola, A.P.; Cavalieri, E.; Gasol, B.; Camprubí, E.; Bonet, J.G.; Blanquet, J.L. Standard Versus Dysplastic Inlay Implant for Patellofemoral Arthroplasty: Surgical Technique and Decision-Making. *Arthrosc. Tech.* **2024**, *13*, 102962. [CrossRef]
30. Dejour, D.H.; Mazy, D.; Pineda, T.; Cance, N.; Dan, M.J.; de Sanctis, E.G. Patellar Instability: Current Approach. *EFORT Open Rev.* **2025**, *10*, 378–387. [CrossRef]
31. Gupta, H.; Batta, N.; Kataria, H.; Batra, V.; Upadhyay, A.; Jain, V.; Mishra, P.; Goel, N. A Comparison of the Reliability of the Patellar Tendon-Trochlear Groove (PTTG) Distance and the Tibial Tuberosity-Trochlear Groove (TTTG) Distance Measured on MRI. *Malays. Orthop. J.* **2020**, *14*, 34.
32. Familiari, F.; Tollefson, L.V.; Izzo, A.; Mercurio, M.; LaPrade, R.F.; Di Vico, G. A High-Grade Lachman's Exam Predicts a Ramp Tear of the Medial Meniscus in Patients with Anterior Cruciate Ligament Tear: A Prospective Clinical and Radiological Evaluation. *J. Clin. Med.* **2024**, *13*, 683. [CrossRef] [PubMed]
33. Giovannetti de Sanctis, E.; Toanen, C.; Guarino, A.; Pineda, T.; Deroche, E.; Resurg; Dejour, D.H. The Role of the Most Cranial Trochlear Orientation in Patellar Maltracking to Better Characterise Trochlear Morphology. *Knee Surg. Sports Traumatol. Arthrosc.* **2024**, *32*, 2909–2918. [CrossRef] [PubMed]
34. Dejour, D.H.; de Sanctis, E.G.; Müller, J.H.; Deroche, E.; Pineda, T.; Guarino, A.; Toanen, C.; Group, P.I.; Amarossi, A.; Baujard, A.; et al. Adapting the Dejour Classification of Trochlear Dysplasia from Qualitative Radiograph-and CT-Based Assessments to Quantitative MRI-Based Measurements. *Knee Surg. Sports Traumatol. Arthrosc.* **2025**, *33*, 2833–2846. [CrossRef] [PubMed]

35. Minici, R.; Mercurio, M.; Iannò, B.; Galasso, O.; Gasparini, G.; Laganà, D. Advantages of the Use of Axial Traction Magnetic Resonance Imaging (MRI) of the Shoulder in Patients with Suspected Rota-Tor Cuff Tears: An Exploratory Pilot Study. *Healthcare* **2023**, *11*, 724. [CrossRef]
36. Moher, D.; Liberati, A.; Tetzlaff, J.; Altman, D.G.; The PRISMA Group. Preferred Reporting Items for Systematic Reviews and Meta-Analyses: The PRISMA Statement. *Ann. Intern. Med.* **2009**, *151*, 264–269. [CrossRef]
37. Ye, Q.; Shen, Q.; Yang, W.; Huang, S.; Jiang, Z.; He, L.; Gong, X. Development of Automatic Measurement for Patellar Height Based on Deep Learning and Knee Radiographs. *Eur. Radiol.* **2020**, *30*, 4974–4984. [CrossRef]
38. Bayramoglu, N.; Nieminen, M.T.; Saarakkala, S. Automated Detection of Patellofemoral Osteoarthritis from Knee Lateral View Radiographs Using Deep Learning: Data from the Multicenter Osteoarthritis Study (MOST). *Osteoarthr. Cartil.* **2021**, *29*, 1432–1447. [CrossRef]
39. Bayramoglu, N.; Nieminen, M.T.; Saarakkala, S. Machine Learning Based Texture Analysis of Patella from X-Rays for Detecting Patellofemoral Osteoarthritis. *Int. J. Med. Inf.* **2022**, *157*, 104627. [CrossRef]
40. Tuya, E.; Nai, R.; Liu, X.; Wang, C.; Liu, J.; Li, S.; Huang, J.; Yu, J.; Zhang, Y.; Liu, W.; et al. Automatic Measurement of the Patellofemoral Joint Parameters in the Laurin View: A Deep Learning–Based Approach. *Eur. Radiol.* **2023**, *33*, 566–577.
41. Xu, S.-M.; Dong, D.; Li, W.; Bai, T.; Zhu, M.-Z.; Gu, G.-S. Deep Learning-Assisted Diagnosis of Femoral Trochlear Dysplasia Based on Magnetic Resonance Imaging Measurements. *World J. Clin. Cases* **2023**, *11*, 1477. [CrossRef]
42. Barbosa, R.M.; Serrador, L.; da Silva, M.V.; Macedo, C.S.; Santos, C.P. Knee Landmarks Detection via Deep Learning for Automatic Imaging Evaluation of Trochlear Dysplasia and Patellar Height. *Eur. Radiol.* **2024**, *34*, 5736–5747. [CrossRef] [PubMed]
43. Kwak, Y.H.; Ko, Y.J.; Kwon, H.; Koh, Y.-G.; Aldosari, A.M.; Nam, J.-H.; Kang, K.-T. Application of a Machine Learning and Optimization Method to Predict Patellofemoral Instability Risk Factors in Children and Adolescents. *Knee Surg. Sports Traumatol. Arthrosc.* **2025**, *33*, 487–499. [CrossRef] [PubMed]
44. Bayramoglu, N.; Englund, M.; Haugen, I.K.; Ishijima, M.; Saarakkala, S. Deep Learning for Predicting Progression of Patellofemoral Osteoarthritis Based on Lateral Knee Radiographs, Demographic Data, and Symptomatic Assessments. *Methods Inf. Med.* **2024**, *63*, 001–010. [CrossRef] [PubMed]
45. Nagawa, K.; Inoue, K.; Hara, Y.; Shimizu, H.; Tsuchihashi, S.; Matsuura, K.; Kozawa, E.; Sugita, N.; Niitsu, M. Three-Dimensional Magnetic Resonance Imaging-Based Statistical Shape Analysis and Machine Learning-Based Prediction of Patellofemoral Instability. *Sci. Rep.* **2024**, *14*, 11390. [CrossRef]
46. Sieberer, J.; Rancu, A.; Park, N.; Desroches, S.; Manafzadeh, A.R.; Tommasini, S.; Wiznia, D.H.; Fulkerson, J. Patellar Tilt Calculation Utilizing Artificial Intelligence on CT Knee Imaging. *Knee* **2025**, *54*, 217–221. [CrossRef]
47. Zhan, H.; Kang, X.; Zhang, X.; Zhang, Y.; Wang, Y.; Yang, J.; Zhang, K.; Han, J.; Feng, Z.; Zhang, L.; et al. Machine-Learning Models Reliably Predict Clinical Outcomes in Medial Patellofemoral Ligament Reconstruction. *Arthrosc. J. Arthrosc. Relat. Surg.* **2024**, *41*, 1896–1908.e2. [CrossRef]
48. Available online: https://www.Ohri.ca/Programs/Clinical_epidemiology/Oxford.Asp (accessed on 1 September 2025).
49. Shorten, C.; Khoshgoftaar, T.M.; Furht, B. Text Data Augmentation for Deep Learning. *J. Big Data* **2021**, *8*, 101. [CrossRef]
50. Mercurio, M.; Cerciello, S.; Corona, K.; Guerra, G.; Simonetta, R.; Familiari, F.; Galasso, O.; Gasparini, G. Factors Associated with a Successful Return to Performance After Anterior Cruciate Ligament Reconstruction: A Multiparametric Evaluation in Soccer Players. *Orthop. J. Sports Med.* **2024**, *12*, 23259671241275663. [CrossRef]
51. Van Haver, A.; Mahieu, P.; Claessens, T.; Li, H.; Pattyn, C.; Verdonk, P.; Audenaert, E. A Statistical Shape Model of Trochlear Dysplasia of the Knee. *Knee* **2014**, *21*, 518–523. [CrossRef]
52. Mariani, S.; La Marra, A.; Arrigoni, F.; Necozione, S.; Splendiani, A.; Di Cesare, E.; Barile, A.; Masciocchi, C. Dynamic Measurement of Patello-Femoral Joint Alignment Using Weight-Bearing Magnetic Resonance Imaging (WB-MRI). *Eur. J. Radiol.* **2015**, *84*, 2571–2578. [CrossRef]
53. Pınar, H.; Akseki, D.; Karaoğlan, O.; Genç, İ. Kinematic and Dynamic Axial Computed Tomography of the Patello-Femoral Joint in Patients with Anterior Knee Pain. *Knee Surg. Sports Traumatol. Arthrosc.* **1994**, *2*, 170–173. [CrossRef] [PubMed]
54. Yoon, Y.E.; Kim, S.; Chang, H.-J. Artificial Intelligence and Echocardiography. *J. Cardiovasc. Imaging* **2021**, *29*, 193. [CrossRef] [PubMed]
55. Sermesant, M.; Delingette, H.; Cochet, H.; Jaïs, P.; Ayache, N. Applications of Artificial Intelligence in Cardiovascular Imaging. *Nat. Rev. Cardiol.* **2021**, *18*, 600–609. [CrossRef] [PubMed]
56. Chen, Y.; Liu, X.; Sheng, B.; Yuan, M.; Lv, F.; Lv, F.; Yu, F.; Li, J. Abnormal Sagittal Patellar Tilt during Active Knee Flexion and Extension on 4DCT Might Be Associated with Patellofemoral Pain. *BMC Musculoskelet. Disord.* **2025**, *26*, 132. [CrossRef]
57. Hwang, I.; Saravanan, K.; Coralli, C.V.; Tu, S.J.; Mellon, S.J. DG-PPU: Dynamical Graphs Based Post-Processing of Point Clouds Extracted from Knee Ultrasounds. In Proceedings of the 2025 IEEE 22nd International Symposium on Biomedical Imaging (ISBI), London, UK, 14–17 April 2025; IEEE: New York, NY, USA, 2025; pp. 1–5.

58. Buchanan, R.; Tu, S.J.; Camurri, M.; Mellon, S.J.; Fallon, M. 3d Freehand Ultrasound Using Visual Inertial and Deep Inertial Odometry for Measuring Patellar Tracking. In Proceedings of the 2024 IEEE International Symposium on Medical Measurements and Applications (MeMeA), Eindhoven, The Netherlands, 26–28 June 2024; IEEE: New York, NY, USA, 2024; pp. 1–6.
59. Amirian, S.; Carlson, L.A.; Gong, M.F.; Lohse, I.; Weiss, K.R.; Plate, J.F.; Tafti, A.P. Explainable AI in Orthopedics: Challenges, Opportunities, and Prospects. In Proceedings of the 2023 Congress in Computer Science, Computer Engineering, & Applied Computing (CSCE), Las Vegas, NV, USA, 24–27 July 2023; IEEE: New York, NY, USA, 2023; pp. 1374–1380.
60. Bruno, F.; Barile, A.; Arrigoni, F.; Laporta, A.; Russo, A.; Carotti, M.; Splendiani, A.; Di Cesare, E.; Masciocchi, C. Weight-Bearing MRI of the Knee: A Review of Advantages and Limits. *Acta Bio Med. Atenei Parm.* **2018**, *89*, 78.
61. Hansen, P.; Harving, M.; Øhlenschlæger, T.; Brinch, S.; Lavard, P.; Krogsgaard, M.; Boesen, M. Comparison between Conventional MRI and Weight-Bearing Positional MRI Reveals Important Differences in Radiological Measurements of the Patellofemoral Joint. *Skelet. Radiol.* **2023**, *52*, 1525–1534. [CrossRef]
62. Tennant, S.; Williams, A.; Vedi, V.; Kinmont, C.; Gedroyc, W.; Hunt, D. Patello-Femoral Tracking in the Weight-Bearing Knee: A Study of Asymptomatic Volunteers Utilising Dynamic Magnetic Resonance Imaging: A Preliminary Report. *Knee Surg. Sports Traumatol. Arthrosc.* **2001**, *9*, 155–162. [CrossRef]
63. Chen, Y.; Yu, F.; Rong, F.; Lv, F.; Lv, F.; Li, J. Analysis of Spatial Patellofemoral Alignment Using Novel Three-Dimensional Measurements Based on Weight-Bearing Cone-Beam CT. *Insights Imaging* **2025**, *16*, 1. [CrossRef]
64. Tiribilli, E.; Bocchi, L. Deep Learning-Based Workflow for Bone Segmentation and 3D Modeling in Cone-Beam CT Orthopedic Imaging. *Appl. Sci.* **2024**, *14*, 7557. [CrossRef]
65. Radanliev, P.; Santos, O.; Brandon-Jones, A.; Joinson, A. Ethics and Responsible AI Deployment. *Front. Artif. Intell.* **2024**, *7*, 1377011. [CrossRef]
66. Koski, E.; Murphy, J. AI in Healthcare. In *Nurses and Midwives in the Digital Age*; IOS Press: Amsterdam, The Netherlands, 2021; pp. 295–299.
67. Korb, R.; Peter, E. *Integration of Artificial Intelligence into Clinical Workflows: Barriers and Best Practices*; ResearchGate: Berlin, Germany, 2025.
68. Mennella, C.; Maniscalco, U.; De Pietro, G.; Esposito, M. Ethical and Regulatory Challenges of AI Technologies in Healthcare: A Narrative Review. *Heliyon* **2024**, *10*, e26297. [CrossRef]
69. Nizamullah, F.; Fahad, M.; Abbasi, N.; Qayyum, M.U.; Zeb, S. Ethical and Legal Challenges in AI-Driven Healthcare: Patient Privacy, Data Security, Legal Framework, and Compliance. *Int. J. Innov. Res. Sci. Eng. Technol.* **2024**, *13*, 15216–15223.
70. Purnomo, G.; Yeo, S.-J.; Liow, M.H.L. Artificial Intelligence in Arthroplasty. *Arthroplasty* **2021**, *3*, 37. [CrossRef]
71. Misir, A.; Yuce, A. AI in Orthopedic Research: A Comprehensive Review. *J. Orthop. Res.* **2025**, *43*, 1508–1527. [CrossRef]

diagnostics

MDPI

Review

Artificial Intelligence-Powered Chronic Obstructive Pulmonary Disease Detection Techniques—A Review

Abdul Rahaman Wahab Sait [1,2,*] and Mujeeb Ahmed Shaikh [2,3]

1 Department of Archives and Communication, Center of Documentation and Administrative Communication, King Faisal University, P.O. Box 400, Hofuf 31982, Saudi Arabia
2 King Salman Center for Disability Research, Riyadh 11614, Saudi Arabia
3 Department of Basic Medical Science, College of Medicine, AlMaarefa University, Diriyah 13713, Saudi Arabia; smujeeb@um.edu.sa
* Correspondence: asait@kfu.edu.sa

Abstract

Chronic obstructive pulmonary disease (COPD) is a progressive respiratory condition, contributing significantly to global morbidity and mortality. Traditional diagnostic tools are effective in diagnosing COPD. However, these tools demand specialized equipment and expertise. Advances in artificial intelligence (AI) provide a platform for enhancing COPD diagnosis by leveraging diverse data modalities. The existing reviews primarily focus on single modalities and lack information on interpretability and explainability. Thus, this review intends to synthesize the AI-powered frameworks for COPD identification, focusing on data modalities, methodological innovation, evaluation strategies, and reporting limitations and potential biases. By adhering to Preferred Reporting Items for Systematic Reviews and Meta-Analyses (PRISMA) guidelines, a systematic search was conducted across multiple repositories. From an initial pool of 1978 records, 22 studies were included in this review. The included studies demonstrated exceptional performance in specific settings. Most studies were retrospective and limited in diversity, lacking generalizability and external or prospective validation. This review presents a roadmap for advancing AI-assisted COPD detection. By highlighting the strengths and limitations of existing studies, it supports the development of future research. Future studies can utilize the findings to build models using prospective, multicenter, and multi-ethnic validations, ensuring generalizability and fairness.

Keywords: chronic obstructive pulmonary disease; artificial intelligence; lung disease; medical imaging; computed tomography; chest radiography; spirogram; computed tomography

1. Introduction

Chronic obstructive pulmonary disease (COPD) poses significant risks to public health across the globe, ranking among the leading causes of morbidity and mortality [1–3]. Due to the complex nature of early symptoms and the underutilization of spirometry, the condition is frequently unrecognized [4,5]. The widespread adoption of spirometry is limited by several factors, including the limited availability of equipment, the need for competent technicians, and patient effort constraints, which can result in delayed diagnosis and loss of opportunities for timely intervention [6–8]. Although imaging modalities, including chest radiography (CXR) and computed tomography (CT), symptom questionnaires, and electronic health records (EHRs) are used extensively in clinical workflows, these modalities are insufficient to serve as standalone diagnostic tools for COPD diagnosis [9–11]. Early diagnosis of COPD is crucial for improving patient outcomes. However, it remains a persistent challenge in routine practice due to the shortcomings of traditional diagnostic approaches [12–15].

Recent advances in artificial intelligence (AI) offer novel prospects for COPD screening [16–18]. By using massive amounts of complicated clinical data, AI can identify subtle disease signatures [19]. At the imaging level, deep learning algorithms can identify anatomical abnormalities associated with COPD, such as emphysema and airway remodeling [20]. Analyzing respiratory sound recordings with convolutional neural networks (CNNs) enables the automatic classification of airflow obstruction [21–23]. EHR data, including structured factors (demographics, smoking history, comorbidities, and laboratory tests) and unstructured clinical narratives evaluated through natural language processing, can be utilized for phenotyping and risk prediction [24]. Recently, wearable and physiological signals, including capnography, photoplethysmography, and nocturnal oximetry, have been investigated as potential low-cost alternatives for COPD identification [25]. The wide range of modalities highlights the significance of AI systems in enhancing conventional diagnostic processes [26–28]. The performance of the AI applications relies on the quality and type of features extracted from these diverse modalities [29]. AI's clinical decision support capability makes it crucial for identifying COPD [30]. The integration of probability scores, predicted lung function indicators, and customized risk profiles enables AI models to generate meaningful outcomes, supporting clinicians in making effective decisions [31–34]. It enhances triage decisions, accelerates treatment, and reduces underdiagnoses in primary care [35]. AI models can benefit from multimodal fusion, analyzing imaging, physiological, acoustic, and electronic health record data to better understand disease heterogeneity. In addition, AI applications have the potential to correlate imaging-derived features to exacerbation risk and mortality, highlighting their relevance in long-term therapy [35]. These advancements emphasize AI as a key breakthrough for redesigning COPD screening, staging, and monitoring.

In the context of AI-based COPD screening, several review studies have been conducted. However, these studies have significant shortcomings, which limit their applicability in guiding research and clinical translation. The majority of the reviews have a limited modality focus, focusing solely on imaging-based approaches (CT or CXR) or limiting their application in AI-powered COPD screening approaches [36–40]. Furthermore, these studies are unable to incorporate diverse data sources, such as respiratory sounds, electronic health records (EHR), and wearable physiological signals [41,42]. The existing studies emphasize algorithmic performance indicators rather than rigorously evaluating the model's effectiveness. The need for external validation on separate cohorts to determine a study's practical usefulness is overlooked in existing reviews. Furthermore, implementation, fairness, and explainability are underemphasized in the existing studies. A limited number of studies explore algorithmic bias, subgroup performance differences, or deployment equity across demographic or geographic groups. Likewise, the integration of workflows, cost-effectiveness, and real-world viability is underexplored. The existing reviews lack in reporting methodological standards, knowledge gaps, or significant advancements, such as multimodal fusion, semi-supervised learning, and uncertainty quantification. These factors motivate us to conduct this review.

This study intends to investigate the potential of AI applications for COPD identification using imaging, spirometry, respiratory sounds, EHR, and physiological inputs. Unlike existing studies, it assesses methodological rigor, validation quality, and deployment readiness, bridging the gap between technological advancement and clinical application. It provides researchers, clinicians, and policymakers with a consolidated evidence base, presenting a set of actionable recommendations for advancing AI in the identification of COPD.

The remaining part of this study is organized as follows: Section 2 presents the review protocol, including the databases, searching strategy, and eligibility criteria. It explains the screening process based on the PRISMA guidelines, including the extraction of study characteristics, AI approaches, datasets, validation strategies, outcomes, and the assessment of risk of bias. Section 3 highlights the findings of this review. It discusses the role of methodological innovations, dataset diversities, and generalization, contextualizing the study findings with current clinical practice and research gaps. Finally, Section 4 provides key insights, underscoring the potential of AI in identifying COPD. It outlines the study's contribution and provides recommendations for future research.

2. Materials and Methods

The purpose of this study is to synthesize existing research on the use of AI for detecting COPD. In accordance with the updated Preferred Reporting Items for Systematic Reviews and Meta-Analyses (PRISMA) guidelines [43–45], we extracted and reviewed the studies associated with AI-driven COPD identification. Although biomedical reviews are prospectively registered in PROSPERO, this study was not registered due to the consideration of computational methodology and AI-based COPD identification. The evolving nature of AI research necessitates flexibility in methods and scope, which is not compatible with fixed registration protocols. To mitigate the absence of PROSPERO registration and to preserve methodological credibility, we implemented a predefined governance and amendment plan. The review's parameters, including objectives, search strategy, eligibility criteria, and primary outcomes, were predetermined and remain constant throughout the process. We identified potential areas for amendments, such as expanding inclusion to preprints and updating search terms to capture emerging AI architectures. Subsequently, we documented the rationale, the exact modification, and its effect on the synthesis. For instance, each adjustment in search vocabulary required a full re-run of the database search and independent dual screening of all new entries. An amendment log was used to document decisions, and the results highlighted the downstream influence of study inclusion and interpretation. Using these strategies, we maintained the core principles of PROSPERO, handling the protocol deviations in a systematic manner to strengthen the trustworthiness of the review process.

2.1. Research Questions

This study is designed in order to address the following research questions:

Research question (RQ) 1: What AI techniques and data modalities have been introduced to the identification of COPD?

RQ2: What evaluation strategies and performance metrics are employed to determine the model's performance?

RQ3: What limitations, biases, and challenges are reported in the existing literature?

2.2. Data Sources and Search Strategy

A comprehensive literature search was conducted across multiple biological and technical databases, including PubMed/MEDLINE, Embase, IEEE Xplore, Scopus, and Web of Science. Additionally, arXiv and medRxiv were searched in order to find preprints and upcoming research highlighting the rapid evolution of AI. To capture the increasing importance of deep learning and advanced machine learning in healthcare, this review included studies published between January 2010 and April 2025. Boolean operators, keywords, and controlled vocabulary terms were combined to capture variation in terminology. While the

COPD concept was expressed through terms such as "chronic obstructive pulmonary disease," "COPD," "chronic bronchitis," and "emphysema," AI concepts were captured with terms such as "artificial intelligence," "machine learning," "deep learning," "neural networks," "support vector machines," "transformers," "ensemble methods," "convolutional neural networks," and "computer-aided diagnosis." These were further combined with terms related to diagnostic activity, such as "identification," "classification," "screening," "prediction," and "detection."

2.3. Study Selection

Table 1 outlines the eligibility criteria for extracting the studies from the databases. The inclusion and exclusion criteria were designed to ensure methodological rigor, clinical relevance, and comparability across the selected studies.

Table 1. Inclusion and exclusion criteria.

Inclusion	Exclusion
Original research articles and preprints with methodological detail.	Narrative reviews, systematic reviews, and conference abstracts that lack sufficient data.
Studies based on human-derived datasets.	Animal studies and simulated data without clinical relevance.
AI-based COPD detection, classification, or diagnosis.	Statistical models without algorithmic learning.
Studies reporting quantitative performance metrics.	Studies without measurable performance outcomes.
Studies published in the English language between 2010 and 2025.	Non-English publications.

2.4. Data Extraction

We used customized syntax according to the database. A reference management system was used to import citations and remove duplicates. Two distinct steps were involved in the selection process. The first step was to evaluate the titles and abstracts in order to exclude irrelevant studies. In the second step, methodological relevance and performance indicators of eligible articles were examined. We retained studies related to AI-based COPD screening that report quantitative performance indicators, including accuracy, sensitivity, specificity, and area under the receiver operating characteristic curve (ROC). Two reviewers conducted independent screening, and disagreements were resolved through consensus.

To ensure consistency across studies, a structured data extraction form was used. Using this form, we extracted variables, including bibliographic information, the country of origin, the data modality (CT, CXR, spirometry, respiratory sounds, and EHR), the size of the dataset, the AI methodology (CNNs, transformers, ensemble methods), preprocessing steps, validation strategies, reported performance metrics, and interpretability approaches (SHAP, Grad-CAM, and feature importance). Additionally, clinical integration, ethical considerations, and data restrictions were recorded.

2.5. Risk of Bias and Quality Assessment

We aimed for methodological rigor and openness in assessing the quality of included studies through the application of QUADAS-2 and PROBAST. QUADAS-2 assesses diagnostic accuracy research, whereas PROBAST was utilized to evaluate prediction model studies. The quality of the dataset, the potential for overfitting, the appropriateness of validation procedures, and the precision of outcome definitions were considered during these assessments, enabling a uniform evaluation of methodological rigor across a diverse collection of studies.

Reviewers calibrated a subset of studies prior to formal assessment to maintain uniformity in signaling question and applicability domain interpretations. To avoid subjective bias, two reviewers independently evaluated each study using tools and addressed conflicts through consensus discussions throughout the primary review process. In order to formally monitor inter-rater reliability, Cohen's kappa (κ) was determined for each tool at different stages of the evaluation. The level of agreement across reviewers was confirmed by the substantial agreement ($\kappa > 0.80$). After reaching a consensus through structured consensus discussions, any disagreements were acknowledged and documented. We used QUADAS-2 and PROBAST in a systematic and repeatable approach by integrating dual independent assessment, computation of inter-rater agreement metrics, and consensus resolution.

Through systematic evaluation of the included studies, we addressed potential publication biases. By including peer-reviewed literature and preprints from repositories, publication biases were mitigated. The inclusion of preprints supports this study in capturing cutting-edge methodological developments and reducing the risk of time-lag bias. The reported performance indicators were examined for clustering around exceptionally high values, indicating potential issues such as selective reporting, overfitting, or lack of transparency in validation procedures. We reported algorithmic biases, limiting the AI applications in delivering equitable performance across diverse patient populations.

2.6. Data Synthesis and Ethical Considerations

We followed a structured narrative synthesis due to the heterogeneity of study designs, AI architectures, dataset sources, and reported outcomes. The included studies were classified based on data modality, reflecting the primary source of information used by AI applications. Under each modality, individual studies were compared on multiple dimensions, including dataset characteristics, methodology, validation strategy, and performance metrics, providing a nuanced understanding of the current landscape of AI-based COPD identification. Moreover, ethical considerations were documented, addressing issues of patient privacy, data protection regulations, and the implications of the studies' findings for clinical deployment.

Using a PRISMA flow diagram, the study selection processes were documented and visualized, presenting the number of records retrieved from each database, the removal of duplicates, the number of studies excluded during title and abstract screening, the number of studies assessed for full-text eligibility, and the final set of included studies. The explicit reporting of these processes strengthens the reproducibility of this review, synthesizing current evidence and establishing a framework for future studies.

3. Results and Discussions

Figure 1 summarizes the review process, ensuring the inclusion of high-quality studies associated with AI-powered COPD identification. A total of 1978 records were identified across multiple databases, reflecting the impact of research studies in medical imaging, machine learning, and computational health sciences. The final set of 22 studies is synthesized in this review, underscoring the rigorous selection process, guaranteeing transparency and reproducibility. The included studies cover various approaches to COPD identification utilizing CT scans, CXR, spirometry, lung sounds, and multimodal data, highlighting the significance of AI in COPD detection. In line with the research objectives, this section is structured around four RQs, outlining the implications, limitations, potential biases, and future research directions of the included studies.

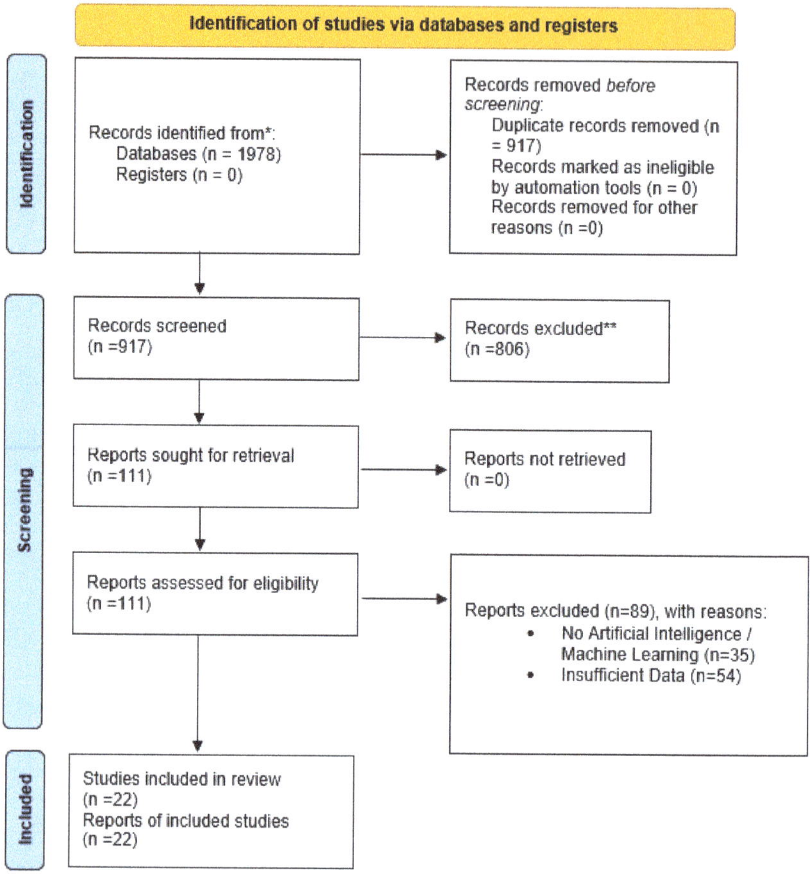

Figure 1. PRISMA-based study selection process. * denotes the primary source and ** denotes the excluded records.

3.1. RQ1: What AI Techniques Have Been Introduced to the Identification of COPD?

The synthesis of this review demonstrates the use of diverse data modalities for identifying COPD using distinct methodological innovations based on AI techniques tailored to each modality. The heterogeneity of COPD conditions necessitates adaptive analytical approaches that integrate structural, functional, and symptomatic data. Unlike traditional clinical approaches, AI applications exploit diverse data sources to uncover latent patterns associated with COPD. AI techniques, including conventional machine learning algorithms such as support vector machines (SVMs) and decision trees, as well as more advanced deep learning architectures like convolutional neural networks (CNNs), residual networks, attention-based multiple instance learning (MIL), and self-supervised learning, have been applied to the identification of COPD. RQ1 highlights the diverse range of AI methods for detecting COPD using diverse data modalities. Each modality has its own set of strengths and limitations. CT offers structural accuracy, chest radiography provides scalability, spirometry offers functional insights, and lung sounds/EHR approaches emphasize accessibility and systemic integration. These methods provide the groundwork for evaluating AI's ability to handle the multidimensionality of COPD.

3.1.1. CT-Based COPD Identification

The CT modality has been widely used for the identification of COPD due to its capacity to detect emphysema, the thickness of the airway wall, and other structural abnormalities. Figure 2 reveals the sample COPD and normal CT images derived from the Lung Image Database Consortium and Image Database Resource Initiative (LIDC-IDRI) repository [46]. It highlights the extraction of latent structural and functional signatures of COPD from CT images, translating the outcomes into clinically actionable insights. Additionally, it illustrates the structural differences between a normal lung and a lung affected by COPD. The CT features, including emphysema quantification, airway wall thickness, lumen diameter, and measures of air-trapping on inspiratory–expiratory scans, support AI models in differentiating emphysema-predominant and airway-predominant phenotypes.

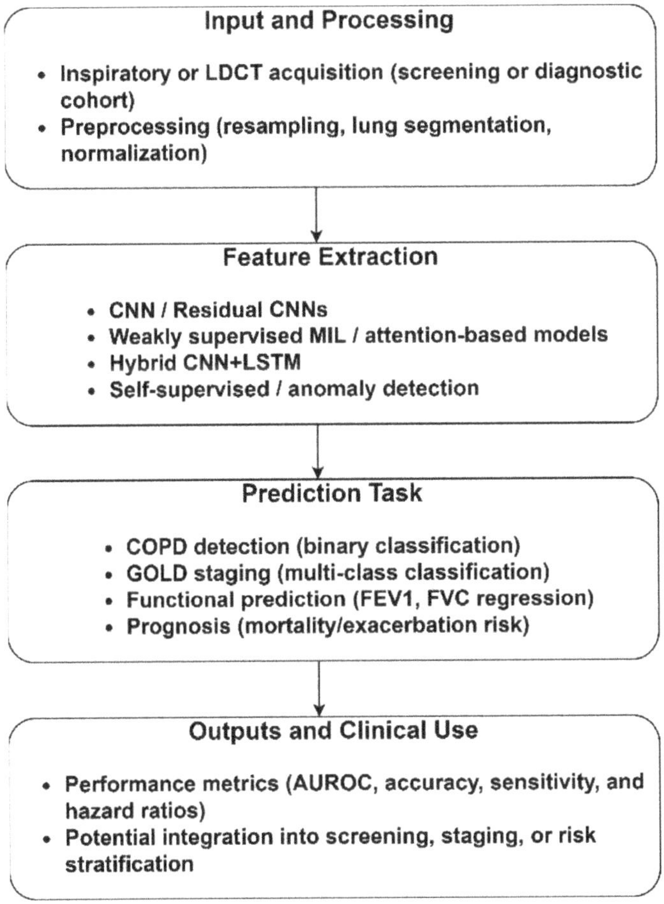

Figure 2. COPD identification using CT images.

Figure 2 summarizes the generalized methodological pipeline for COPD identification using low-dose CT (LDCT) scans. Pre-processing steps, including resampling, lung segmentation, and intensity normalization, are crucial for reducing scanner variability and standardizing inputs for downstream algorithms. The feature extraction enables the models to identify subtle COPD patterns. Based on the study's objectives, the prediction tasks are classified into binary and multi-class classification, regression, and prognosis.

Finally, outputs and clinical use are reported using ROC, sensitivity, specificity, accuracy, and hazard ratios. The sample CT images are presented in the Supplementary Material, Figure S1: (a) Normal and (b) COPD CT Images.

Table 2 presents the characteristics of the included studies, including the dataset details, AI approach, validation design, quantitative performance, and limitations. The individual studies highlight the potential of supervised [47,48], weakly supervised [49–52], and self-supervised [53,54] approaches. The comparative synthesis reveals critical differences in their generalizability. Traditional supervised models [47,48] achieve exceptional outcomes on well-annotated datasets. However, these models show reduced transferability across populations. In contrast, weakly supervised approaches [49–52] report improved adaptability to partially labeled data, rendering them suitable for real-world deployment. Self-supervised learning strategies [53,54] extend generalizability through robust feature representations that transfer across ethnic and demographic subgroups. Overall, supervised CNN architectures excel in single-center settings, whereas weakly and self-supervised approaches offer resilience to label noise and cross-population diversity, providing a clinically realistic path toward broader implementation.

3.1.2. CXR-Based COPD Identification

The CXR images are widely applied and cost-effective imaging modalities in the evaluation of respiratory diseases. These images are less sensitive compared to the LDCT scans. However, they provide valuable insights into COPD markers. The included studies extract radiographic patterns related to airway obstruction and emphysema. The findings demonstrated that AI-powered CXR analysis can stratify disease severity and predict prognosis, offering a powerful, scalable, and clinically practical approach to early disease detection and risk stratification.

Figure 3 outlines the CXR-based COPD identification pipeline. In the input and preprocessing steps, resizing, normalization, lung segmentation, and artifact reduction were performed to standardize image quality. Feature extraction used diverse deep learning techniques to extract COPD features. Using these features with classification approaches, COPD and non-COPD CXR images were classified. Additionally, disease staging, spirometric index estimation, and prognostic estimates of mortality or exacerbation risk were achieved through the included studies. The model's performance was evaluated using metrics, including AUROC, accuracy, sensitivity, specificity, calibration, and hazard ratios, rendering the CXR-based COPD identification model a practical tool for large-scale COPD screening and monitoring. The sample CXR images are presented in the Supplementary Material, Figure S2: (a) COPD and (b) Normal CXR Images.

Table 2. Findings of CT-based COPD identification approaches.

Study	Dataset Number of Participants (n)	AI Approach	Validation Design	Quantitative Performance	Limitations
Tang et al. [47]	Training Dataset: $n = 2589$ (Male: 1440 and Female: $n = 1149$) Location: Canada External Dataset: $n = 2195$ (Male: 1318 and Female: 877) Location: ECLIPSE (Multinational)	Fine-tuned Residual CNNs architecture	Three-fold cross-validation (CV) on PanCan; external test on ECLIPSE with no model change.	CV-AUC 0.889 ± 0.017; external AUC 0.886 ± 0.017; positive predictive value (PPV) 0.847 ± 0.056, negative predictive value (NPV) 0.755 ± 0.097	Screening bias, retrospective, and limited generalization
González et al. [48]	$n = 7983$ COPDGene (US, multicenter smokers) + $n = 1672$ ECLIPSE (multinational smokers)	2D CNN using four canonical CT views for COPD detection, Global Initiative for Chronic Obstructive Lung Disease (GOLD) staging, and prognosis.	Internal test in COPDGene; external test in ECLIPSE; logistic/Cox models for events & mortality.	AUC = ~0.85 for COPD Accuracy = 74.95%	Smoker-only cohorts and cross-study CT protocol differences.
Sun et al. [49]	Multicenter China CT cohort: $n = 1393$ from four large public hospitals; labels from spirometry; external validation on NLST subset (~620 cases).	Weakly supervised CT DL (multiple-instance/patch-bag paradigm) for COPD detection + GOLD staging.	Internal split in the Chinese cohort; external check on National Lung Screening Trial (NLST).	GOLD grading accuracy ≈ 76.4% with weighted $\kappa \approx 0.619$	Retrospective and site-specific protocols.
Xue et al. [50]	$n = 800$ for training and testing. $n = 260$ for the external validation	Two-Stage-Attention MIL (TSA-MIL) using slice/patch bags; compares against conventional MIL and CNN baselines.	Cross-validation; external test set included.	Internal accuracy ≈ 92%, AUC ≈ 0.95; external AUC ≈ 0.87	Potential label noise from weak supervision, single-country data, and limited reporting on scanner harmonization.
Park et al. [51]	$n = 16{,}148$ with mean age of 55 ± 10 (standard deviation)	Volumetric CT deep learning and regression/classification techniques to predict PFTs (FEV_1, FVC, FEV_1/FVC) and flag abnormality.	Train/validation/test splits, internal validation, and threshold-based screening analyses.	Reported sensitivities were 61.6%, 46.9%, and 36.1% for different abnormality thresholds.	Single-country screening population and limited generalization.
Humphries et al. [52]	COPDGene test cohort $n = 7143$; external ECLIPSE $n = 1962$; US/multinational smokers with baseline inspiratory CT and outcomes.	CNNs + LSTM to automate emphysema grading on CT.	Internal testing (COPDGene) + external testing (ECLIPSE).	Weighted κ (DL vs. visual) 0.60; mortality hazard ratios vs. "no emphysema": 1.5, 1.7, 2.9, 5.3, 9.7	Smoker-enriched cohorts and demand substantial computational resources.
Almeida et al. [53]	COPDGene: train/val/test $n = 3144$/ $n = 786$/$n = 1310$; external COSYCONET $n = 446$ (Germany).	SSL representation + anomaly-detection on 3D CT patches to quantify COPD severity as "anomaly score."	Internal test (COPDGene) and external test (COSYCONET); compared to supervised DL baselines; linked anomaly score to PFTs, SGRQ, emphysema, and air-trapping.	AUC = 84.3 ± 0.3 (COPDGene) and AUC = 76.3 ± 0.6 (COSYCONET) for COPD versus low-risk; the anomaly score is significantly associated with lung function, symptoms, and exacerbations ($p < 0.001$).	Scanner/protocol variability and anomaly approach improve generalization. However, interpretability and thresholds for clinical use are in an emerging stage.
Almeida et al. [54]	COPDGene: train/val/test $n = 3144$/$n = 786$/$n = 1310$	SSL versus Supervised CNN for COPD Detection: Uncertainty Estimation and Fairness Analysis.	Cross-ethnic internal/external style evaluation.	SSL showed significantly higher AUC than supervised across ethnic groups ($p < 0.001$; article emphasizes generalization rather than a single pooled AUC).	US-centric cohorts, limited emphasis on generalization and fairness metrics.

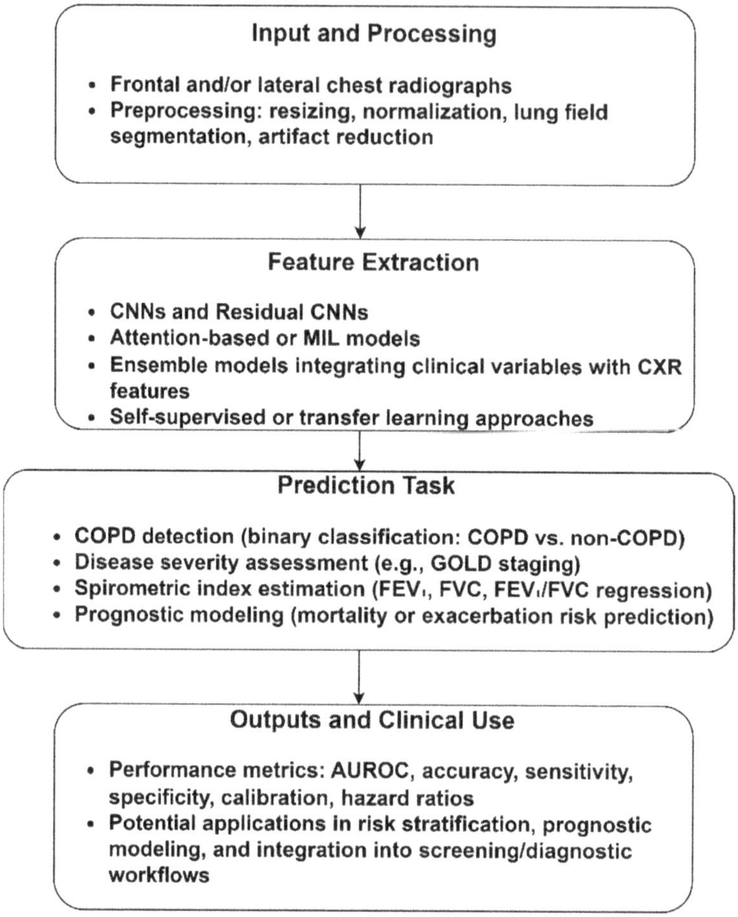

Figure 3. COPD identification using CXR images.

Table 3 highlights the contributions of the included studies based on CXR images, which advance COPD detection and prognosis through the use of AI techniques. The review findings demonstrate the significance of supervised and ensemble learning strategies for CXR-based COPD identification. Early supervised models [55] achieve reliable detection of airflow obstruction. However, the reliance on a single-center dataset introduces institutional bias that restricts its generalizability to diverse healthcare settings. Ueda et al. [56] addressed this limitation by conducting multi-institutional studies. They used regression-based estimation of spirometric indices. However, the variations in image quality may affect the model's generalization ability. Prognostic models [57,58] expanded the application of CXR-based COPD identification into survival prediction and risk stratification. These models were validated in homogeneous ethnic populations, limiting confidence in broader applicability. The advanced ensemble and multimodal approach [59] outperforms the traditional supervised models through its ensemble learning functionality. These comparisons report the inherent limitations of supervised CNN architectures.

Table 3. Findings of CXR-based COPD identification approaches.

Study	Dataset Number of Participants (n)	AI Approach	Validation Design	Quantitative Performance	Limitations
Nam et al. [55]	4225 patients Training ($n = 3475$), validation ($n = 435$), and test ($n = 315$)	DL survival model (DLSP_CXR and integrated DLSP_integ). Outcomes via time-to-event modeling.	Development + validation cohorts; time-dependent AUC analyses vs. established indices.	The time-dependent AUC of the DL model showed no difference compared to BODE (0.87 vs. 0.80; $p = 0.34$), ADO (0.86 vs. 0.89; $p = 0.51$), SGRQ (0.86 vs. 0.70; $p = 0.09$), and was higher than CAT (0.93 vs. 0.55; $p < 0.001$); good calibration.	Prognostic (not diagnostic), Korean cohorts, and treatment decisions require prospective testing.
Ueda et al. [56]	Multi-institution Japan; 81,902 patients with 141,734 CXR-spirometry pairs from five hospitals and external tests at two independent institutions (n = 2137 CXRs; $n = 5290$).	DL model to estimate FVC and FEV1 from a single CXR (regression).	Training/validation/testing on three sites, external testing on two sites.	FVC r = 0.91/0.90, ICC = 0.91/0.89, MAE = 0.31 L/0.31 L; FEV1 r = 0.91/0.91, ICC = 0.90/0.90, MAE = 0.28 L/0.25 L.	Retrospective, Japan-only cohorts, and estimate lung function (not a COPD label).
Schroeder et al. [57]	Single-institution (USA); 6749 two-view CXRs (2012–2017) from 4436 subjects with near-concurrent PFTs ($\leq$180 days).	ResNet-18 (frontal + lateral) trained on PFT labels to predict airflow obstruction. Compared with an NLP model of radiology reports.	Training/validation/testing subject splits.	AUC 0.814 for obstructive lung disease (FEV1/FVC < 0.70); for severe COPD (FEV1 < 0.5), AUC 0.837; both > NLP (0.704 and 0.770; $p < 0.001$).	Single-center, retrospective, and limited generalizability.
Doroodgar Jorshery et al. [58]	Ever-smokers ($n = 12{,}550$) (mean age 62·4 ± 6·8 years, 48.9% male, 12.4% rate of 6-year COPD) and never-smokers ($n = 15{,}298$) (mean age 63.0 ± 8.1 years, 42.8% male, 3.8% rate of 6-year COPD), collected at Massachusetts General Brigham (MGB) hospital, Boston, USA.	Uses pre-trained CXR-Lung-Risk CNN to stratify risk for incident COPD from a single baseline CXR.	External retrospective validation; time-to-event analyses for incident COPD.	Reports risk stratification for 6-year incident COPD; (focuses on HRs/C-indices rather than diagnostic AUC)	Retrospective design and single-site primary cohort.
Zou et al. [59]	Multicenter China; 1055 participants (COPD $n = 535$, controls $n = 520$) with frontal CXR + clinical data; internal test $n = 284$; external test $n = 105$.	Ensemble DL combining CXR features + clinical parameters for COPD screening and GOLD staging.	Internal split + external test from another site.	COPD detection AUC: internal 0.969 (fusion), external 0.934; CXR-only 0.946; clinical-only 0.963. Staging AUC: 0.894 (3-class) and 0.852 (5-class).	Retrospective; modest external cohort; exclusion of many comorbid lung diseases may overstate real-world performance.

3.1.3. Spirometry/Spirogram-Based COPD Identification

Figure 4 illustrates the significance of spirometry and flow-volume curves in diagnosing and classifying COPD, highlighting the transformation of raw spirograms into clinically meaningful outputs. The preprocessing steps, including normalization, quality filtering, and augmentation, addressed the variability in device calibration. Using MLP, CNNs, and SSL, the included studies enable the exploitation of suboptimal curves. Prediction tasks uncover novel genetic associations, linking respiratory functions to COPD susceptibility loci. Through diagnostic, prognostic, and genetic dimensions, AI-based spirometry holds promise for earlier detection and risk stratification.

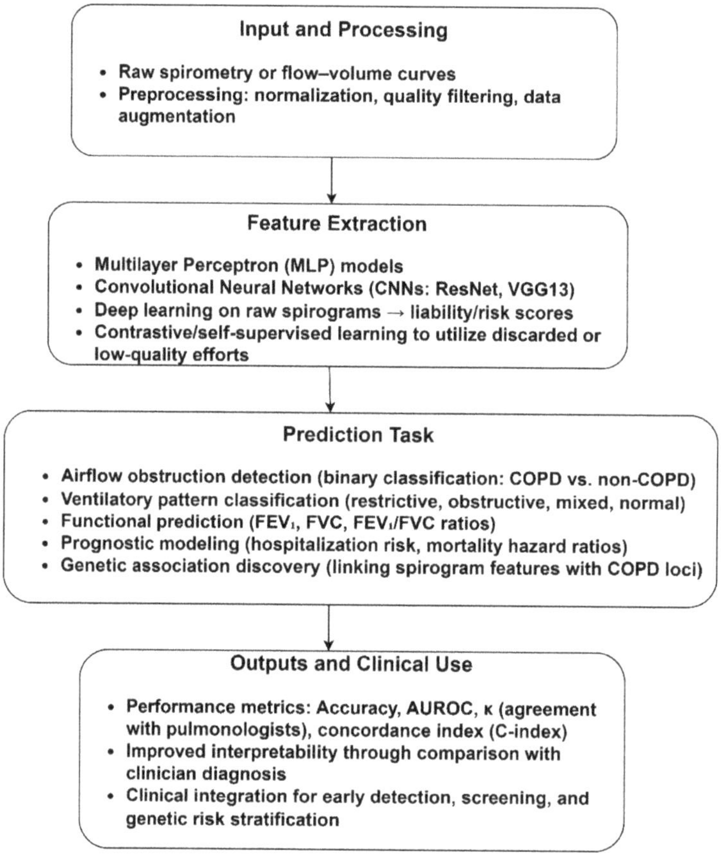

Figure 4. COPD identification using spirogram.

Table 4 outlines the significant contributions of the studies based on spirometry and spirogram analysis. Spirometry-based COPD identification approaches highlight the differences between supervised learning and advanced self-supervised strategies. Supervised models [60,61] demonstrate their diagnostic potential by outperforming clinicians in controlled settings. However, the models' performance relies on data quality and device calibration. Self-supervised and contrastive learning [62,63] address these shortcomings through the extraction of latent features from raw or suboptimal spirograms, improving generalizability across diverse populations. Compared to supervised CNN architectures, self-supervised approaches show exceptional robustness across heterogeneous datasets, rendering them suitable for clinical deployment.

Table 4. Findings of Spirometry-based COPD identification approaches.

Study	Dataset Number of Participants (n)	AI Approach	Validation Design	Quantitative Performance	Limitations
Mac et al. [60]	~1400 patients, Toronto General Hospital, Canada; single-center cohort with spirometry + plethysmography	Multilayer perceptron (MLP) deep learning vs. pulmonologists	Internal validation with cross-validation; performance compared against clinicians and PFT "gold standard"	Outperformed pulmonologists in classification; comparable to complete PFT diagnostic acumen (exact accuracy not specified, $\kappa > 0.7$ reported)	Single-center, relatively small sample, limited external validation, restricted to Canadian patients, and may not capture device/institutional variability
Wang et al. [61]	18,909 subjects, First Affiliated Hospital of Guangzhou Medical University, China; large hospital-based PFT dataset	CNN-based models (ResNet, VGG13) on flow–volume curves	Split into training, validation, and test sets; compared DL vs. pulmonologists and primary care physicians	VGG13 accuracy 95.6%; pulmonologists 76.9% ($\kappa = 0.46$); primary care physicians 56.2%	Single-institution dataset, Chinese-only population, retrospective, limited interpretability, imbalance across ventilatory patterns
Cosentino et al. [62]	~350,000 participants, UK Biobank, United Kingdom; raw spirograms (ages 40–69, general population)	Deep learning on raw spirograms → COPD liability score	Training/validation/test splits within UK Biobank; evaluated against traditional phenotypes and genetic associations.	AUROC ~0.82 for COPD; AUROC ~0.89 for COPD hospitalization; HR ~1.22 for mortality prediction; identified 67 novel loci.	Labels are noisy due to their reliance on EHR/ICD codes, a UK-only cohort (limited generalizability), no bronchodilator data, and limited ethnic diversity.
Hill et al. [63]	~350,000 participants, UK Biobank, United Kingdom; included QC-passed and suboptimal spirograms.	Contrastive learning (Spiro-CLF) using all efforts, incl. discarded curves.	Train-test split within the UK Biobank and held-out test set.	AUROC of 0.981 for obstruction; C-index 0.654 for mortality (vs. ~0.59 best effort only).	UK-only cohort (limited generalizability), limited ethnic diversity, and retrospective.

3.1.4. Other Modalities

Figure 5 illustrates the importance of lung sounds, EHR, and multimodal imaging in detecting and managing COPD. Using lung sound analysis, features, such as spectral, cepstral, and time–frequency, can be used to identify lung abnormalities, offering a low-cost, non-invasive screening for primary care or resource-limited settings. EHR-based approaches that combine structured data and unstructured clinical notes have demonstrated substantial predictive value for COPD case finding and risk stratification. Unlike an unimodal pipeline, a multimodal model shows the application of CT-derived features with blood transcriptomic profiles, enabling the discovery of clinically relevant subtypes associated with COPD and non-COPD. It highlights underlying biological pathways, advancing precision medicine.

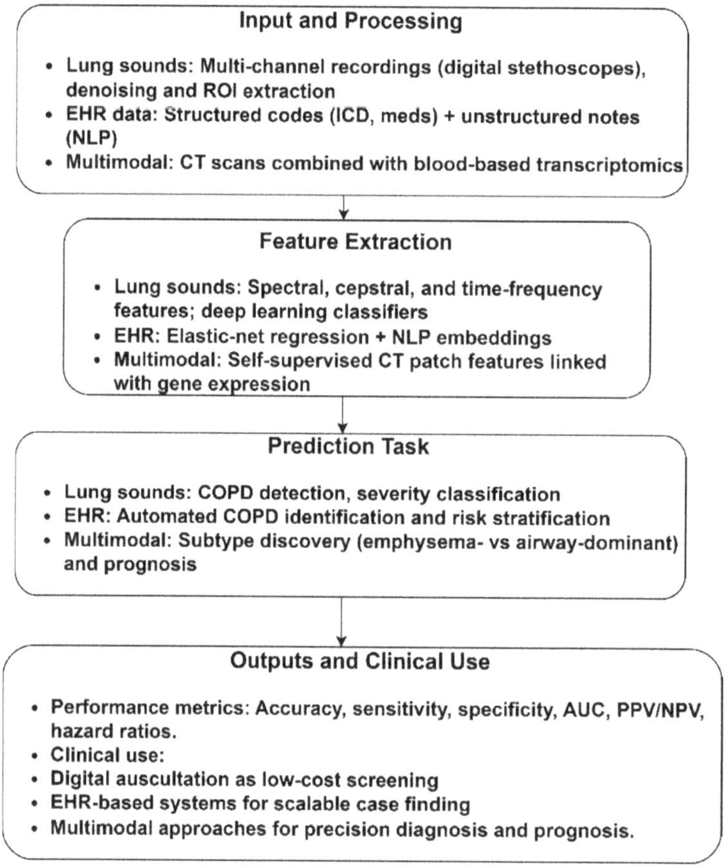

Figure 5. COPD identification using other modalities.

Table 5 summarizes the role of diverse data modalities, including lung sounds, EHR, and multi-omics data, in detecting COPD. The included studies reveal the performance of traditional supervised learning and emerging self-supervised representation learning strategies. Lung sound-based COPD diagnosis and screening strategies [64–66] employed supervised models, relying on fused acoustic features. While they report impressive accuracies, the reliance on a single source on public datasets may lead to overfitting and limited generalization. The lack of external validation undermines their translational potential. Additionally, the supervised feature–classifier pipelines tend to learn dataset-specific patterns rather than robust disease signatures. Similarly, Chu et al. [42] demonstrated the performance of a supervised elastic-net logistic regression approach. However, the model's sensitivity reflects the shortcomings of the supervised model, missing critical COPD features in clinical settings. Chen et al. [67] showed the potential of self-supervised learning through a context-aware representation learning strategy that extracts multimodal image expression with transcriptomic data. Unlike supervised learning, the self-supervised model unveils biologically meaningful subtypes. The cross-validation and independent replication in COPDGene underscore its robustness, uncovering latent disease structure.

3.2. *RQ2: What Evaluation Strategies and Performance Metrics Are Employed to Determine the Model's Performance?*

The evaluation of AI-driven COPD identification represents a pivotal determinant of its clinical credibility. Although the focus is on algorithmic innovation, the applicability of the included studies relies on the robustness and appropriateness of their evaluations. A wide variety of validation procedures and performance measurements were reported throughout the studies, covering regression and classification. The integration of various methods shows how assessment procedures have progressed while highlighting the gaps that hinder clinical readiness.

The use of internal validation was consistent across modalities. A significant number of studies have employed random train–validation–test splits or k-fold cross-validation in order to quantify the model's performance on unseen data. This method was widely used in CXR and spirometry-based studies due to the relatively smaller datasets and the need to make optimal use of the data. In the attention-based CT model, Xue et al. [50] applied cross-validation to minimize the sampling variance and optimize the amount of knowledge gained from a small number of cohorts. Tang et al. [47] validated the pre-trained model, reporting stable AUROC values of ~0.89. Similarly, Schroeder et al. [57] and Zou et al. [59] applied the AUROC metric to evaluate the chest radiography-based COPD detection approaches. Sun et al. [49] and Almeida et al. [53,54] employed multicenter and multi-ethnic cohorts, highlighting the importance of evaluation strategies incorporating fairness and inclusivity. Park et al. [51] reported the mean absolute error and concordance correlation coefficients in order to evaluate CT-based prediction. Ueda et al. [56] extended this framework by including intra-class correlation coefficients and Pearson correlations. Gonzalez predicted mortality using hazard ratios.

Due to their dual role in diagnosis and prognosis, CT studies typically emphasized AUROC and hazard ratios. CXR studies employed regression measures to estimate spirometric indices. Spirometry-based models prioritize sensitivity and specificity. Due to the limited size of the datasets, lung-sound models have maintained high levels of accuracy and AUROC. However, these studies lack external validation. In order to highlight their incorporation of structured and unstructured clinical data, EHR-based and multimodal models focused on specificity, PPV, and incremental AUROC. A significant improvement over relying on AUROC is the incorporation of prognostic indicators, multicenter diversity, and external validation. The majority of the included studies were in the preparation stage rather than being ready for clinical deployment due to the inconsistent use of calibration, fairness testing, and clinical utility metrics. Limited validation in homogeneous groups increases the likelihood that models may underperform in diverse clinical contexts. High AUROC scores without calibration or decision-curve analysis may lead to inflated confidence and obscure practical limitations. Overall, the findings highlight the lack of standardized assessment frameworks.

Table 5. Findings of other modalties-based COPD identification approaches.

Study	Dataset Number of Participants (n)	AI Approach	Validation Design	Quantitative Performance	Limitations
Altan et al. [64]	41 patients underwent 12-channel auscultations (posterior/anterior chest points) in Turkey.	Feature engineering through 3D second-order difference plots (chaos plots); quantization; Deep Extreme Learning Machine.	Retrospective single-dataset development; internal evaluation only (no independent external site).	Overall accuracy 94.31%, weighted sensitivity 94.28%, weighted specificity 98.76%, AUC 0.9659 for five-class COPD severity.	Small, single-source dataset, no external validation, and explicit external testing not reported.
Naqvi & Choudhry [65]	The International Conference on Biomedical and Health Informatics (ICBHI) dataset comprises 920 recordings and 126 subjects in total. The study subset utilized 703 recordings for the COPD, pneumonia/healthy classes, making it a multi-site public dataset.	Region of Interest (ROI) extraction + denoising, fusion of time/cepstral/spectral features; backward elimination feature selection; classifiers compared.	Internal cross-validation and hold-out evaluation on ICBHI; no self-collected or clinical external cohort	Best model Accuracy 99.70%, TPR > 99%, FNR < 1% on selected fused features	Limited patient metadata, public mixed-source recordings, potential label/device noise, and no external clinical validation.
Yu et al. [66]	12-channel lung-sound recordings from 42 COPD patients (age 38–68; 34 men/8 women). Data recorded by pulmonologists with Littmann 3200.	Hand-engineered Hilbert–Huang Transform (EEMD) time–frequency–energy features → ReliefF channel/feature selection → SVM classifier (compared to Bayes, decision tree, DBN). Uses 4 channels (L1–L4) after selection.	Retrospective model development on the public dataset; experiments compare multi-class tasks (mild vs. moderate + severe; moderate vs. severe). Internal resampling; no external cohort.	For mild vs. moderate + severe: Accuracy 89.13%, Sensitivity 87.72%, Specificity 91.01%. For moderate vs. severe: Accuracy 94.26%, Sensitivity 97.32%, Specificity 89.93%.	Small sample, single public dataset, and no external validation.
Chu et al. [42]	Mass General Brigham (MGB) Biobank (Boston, MA)—3420 screen-positive candidates, gold-standard chart-review labels by pulmonologists; train/test gold standards n = 182/100 (77/46 COPD cases). External validation: Marshfield Clinic (Wisconsin) independent EHR/biobank sample.	Elastic-net logistic models using structured EHR (ICD, meds, etc.) + NLP features (SAFE) from notes; compared models with/without spirometry features.	Internal testing on MGB gold-standard test set; independent external validation at Marshfield with identical screening/filtering and blinded chart review.	Internal MGB: PPV 91.7%, Sensitivity 71.7%, Specificity 94.4%. External (Marshfield): FPV 93.5%, Sensitivity 61.4%, Specificity 90%.	Trained in biobank/EHR populations; sensitivity drops without spirometry; portability shown across two U.S. systems; However, international generalizability is not investigated.
Chen et al. [67]	1223 participants with inspiratory/expiratory CT + blood RNA-seq (50% female; 82% NHW, 18% African American; mean age 67). Train/test split 923/300; additional independent replication on 1527 COPDGene participants with CT but without RNA-seq. The Siemens B31F kernel is included for analysis.	CT patch features via context-aware self-supervised representation learning (CSRL) → MLP to learn image-expression axes (IEAs) linking CT structure and blood transcriptome; associations tested with clinical traits and Cox survival models; pathway enrichment.	Nested 5-fold CV within training; held-out test set; independent replication in non-RNA-seq COPDGene subset; focuses on associations and prognosis rather than binary classification.	Identified emphysema-predominant, airway-predominant strongly correlated with CT emphysema/airway measures and lung function; significant associations with outcomes via Cox models and enriched biological pathways (adjusted $p < 0.001$).	Single vendor/kernel (Siemens b31f) constraint; U.S. smoker cohort; not a straightforward "COPD vs. non-COPD" classifier; generalizability beyond COPDGene not demonstrated.

3.3. RQ3: What Limitations, Biases, and Challenges Are Reported in the Existing Literature?

The AI-based COPD literature exhibits methodological and practical limitations, including dataset and spectrum bias, acquisition and label heterogeneity, retrospective design, class imbalance, and limited fairness and interpretability.

CT-based COPD screening relies on cohorts enriched with smokers, such as COPDGene, ECLIPSE, or lung cancer screening programs. These datasets strengthen the detection of emphysema and airway abnormalities, restricting the models' applicability to non-smokers and underdiagnosed populations. CXR studies were based on specific countries or health systems, leading to a spectrum bias that limits their generalizability. The reliance on the UK Biobank dataset limits the applicability of the spirogram-based models. The lung sound datasets were small and device-specific. Similarly, EHR-driven approaches depend on the specific coding and documentation practices, presenting challenges in deploying these models in heterogeneous settings.

The heterogeneity in acquisition and labeling has the potential to generate domain shift and complicates benchmarking. A wide variety of scanner manufacturers and reconstruction kernels are considered in CT databases, which contain the inspiratory and expiratory phases. In the absence of harmonization, models can mistakenly learn scanner artifacts rather than disease signatures. The reliability of the CXR-based models may be compromised by differences in projection, equipment (portable vs. stationary), and patient position. In contrast to lung-sound recordings, which vary in terms of microphone quality, channel number, and background noise, spirometry is highly dependent on the patient's efforts and the calibration of the specific equipment. EHR-based studies face challenges, including uneven categorization, various note styles, and missing information. In addition, there is an inconsistency in reference labeling. The fixed-ratio criteria exaggerate the prevalence in older persons, the GOLD staging suffers from moderate repeatability, and the code-based phenotyping approach causes misclassification. Spirometry is not foolproof due to time discrepancies between image or sound capture and lung function measurement, reducing comparability across studies.

Study design limitations undermine the trustworthiness of the studies' findings. The majority of the studies were based on a retrospective dataset. A few CT and CXR models used independent external cohorts, while many utilized internal splits with cross-validation. There was a lack of prospective assessment across the modalities. Dependence on retrospective processes leads to data leakage, especially when multiple images from the same patient are included in both training and test sets, or when hyperparameters are accidentally tuned on test data. Another widespread challenge is class imbalance. Most studies reported overall accuracy or AUROC, leading to poor sensitivity or specificity in minority subgroups. There was a lack of reporting of precision–recall measures, F1-scores, calibration plots, and decision-curve studies, leading to misinterpretation of the model's performance. The incorporation of saliency maps or attention overlays into some CT and CXR models has been identified. However, these representations tend to be unstable and have not been thoroughly evaluated against radiological markers. In the spirogram and lung-sound-based studies, the physiological or acoustic correlates of model predictions were rarely clarified. As a result, clinicians may face challenges in making informed decisions based on the findings of these models. EHR approaches rely on documentation artifacts rather than disease biology, reducing their interpretability and explainability.

Across the studies, another critical gap is the limited use of robust external validation. For instance, CT and CXR-based models were trained and validated on hospital-specific datasets. These models may encounter challenges in handling diversity in scanner protocols, demographic distributions, and disease prevalence. Models trained on COPDGene and ECLIPSE datasets demonstrate improved robustness across populations and acquisition settings. The UK Biobank dataset facilitates the training and discovery of genetic associations using spirometry-based models for COPD identification. However, the ethnic homogeneity restricts the model's applicability to non-European populations. EHR-based models-based on two U.S. healthcare datasets, indicate the importance of cross-institutional validation. However, the differences in practice-specific coding may impact the model's performance. These findings underscore the need for large, multi-institutional datasets with demographic and geographic diversity.

The included studies lack a comprehensive assessment of the subgroup. Despite reporting aggregate accuracy or AUROC, limited studies have assessed performance across age, sex, ethnicity, or geography, which are crucial to generalizability and fairness. As a result of this exclusion, there is a possibility of overlooking systemic biases that might impair equitable clinical deployment. For instance, the spirometry model using the UK Biobank dataset [61,63] benefitted from a large sample size and high-quality measurement. However, the data were derived from a predominantly White British cohort. Ethnic homogeneity poses uncertainties regarding applicability to non-Europeans with different lung function norms, smoking behaviors, and COPD prevalence. In the absence of rigorous subgroup validation, these models have the potential to incorrectly categorize underrepresented groups. The majority of CT and CXR models were trained on older male smokers, restricting their applicability to women, younger individuals, and never-smokers with distinct disease trajectories. Due to datasets derived from single institutions or local health systems, lung-sound and EHR-based techniques confront similar challenges. Variations in clinical practice, diagnostic labeling, and environmental exposures may result in the inability of predictors learnt in these settings to transfer consistently across other geographic or cultural contexts.

The significance of subgroup analysis is shown by concrete examples from other domains of AI-based medical diagnosis. The use of comparable subgroup reporting in COPD research would reveal hidden biases and facilitate the implementation of remedial procedures. Methodological improvements are needed to address subgroup performance. The strategies, including targeted data augmentation for underrepresented groups, fairness-aware loss functions during training, or transfer learning, can be used to improve COPD-identification models' performance across regions and cohorts. Interpretability tools, such as SHAP values and attention overlays, can reveal subgroup-specific feature dependencies, such as the distribution of emphysema across ethnic groups.

3.4. Future Directions

AI-driven COPD diagnosis and categorization have demonstrated significant potential across imaging, physiological, acoustic, and EHR modalities. Future research should adhere to a staged roadmap that prioritizes short-term feasibility, mid-term consolidation, and long-term innovation in order to transform the methodological advancements into therapeutically beneficial and clinically trusted tools.

In the short term, reducing spectrum bias and strengthening external validation are the key priorities. Assessing AI models in a real-world environment requires prospective, multicenter studies. To promote fairness and worldwide applicability, these initiatives should target underrepresented populations, including women, younger individuals, never-smokers, and low- and middle-income patients. Additionally, it is essential to implement standardized reporting frameworks, such as TRIPOD-AI, PROBAST-AI, and CONSORT-AI, to foster transparency, comparability, and reproducibility.

The mid-term research should emphasize multimodal integration and interpretability. We identified a potential combination of modalities for developing multimodality-based COPD diagnosis and screening. The complementary value of structural and functional information is shown by CXR-derived features combined with spirometry or clinical data, outperforming imaging-only models in staging and prognostic tasks. The integration of genomic or transcriptome data with CT-based models has shown promise for extending precision medicine beyond diagnosis by revealing molecular pathways and identifying subtypes of COPD. Combining EHR-driven models with spirometry can improve prediction accuracy, addressing coding variability. Although the lung-sound classifiers deliver reasonable performance with limited computational costs, they remain underexplored in multimodal contexts. By combining structural and functional modalities and clinical phenotypes with molecular profiles, an effective COPD identification model can be developed. Future research should evaluate integrative approaches in multicenter, demographically diverse cohorts and explicitly correlate AI-derived features with pathophysiological markers, such as airway wall thickening, emphysema subtypes, and acoustic wheeze signatures, to enhance the interpretability of COPD identification models.

Long-term research should focus on addressing fairness, sustainability, and clinical application. Sustainable computing approaches and energy-efficient architectures should be standard procedures in future work to mitigate the environmental impacts of training AI models on a broader scale. In order to guarantee an equitable and clinically reliable deployment, it is recommended that future research on COPD artificial intelligence include comprehensive subgroup studies (based on age, gender, ethnicity, and geographic location) and combine them with interpretability frameworks. AI-derived outputs, such as risk score, PFT values, or imaging-derived severity indices, can support current diagnostic workflows through quantitative decision support. Using this integration, personalized treatment planning and earlier diagnosis can be streamlined. However, the barriers, including a lengthy regulatory approval process, ethical challenges, and limited infrastructure, should be addressed in order to facilitate the seamless adoption. With extensive external validation, multimodal, interpretable models, and fairness-aware, sustainable healthcare systems, promising research may be transformed into reliable, equitable, and globally deployable AI solutions for COPD diagnosis and treatment.

3.5. The Review's Limitations and Potential Biases

The limitations of this study should be addressed to contextualize its findings. Publication bias may exist despite a comprehensive multi-database search strategy. High-performance measures or unique approaches are likely to be published, whereas negative or underperforming data may be unpublished, leading to overestimation of AI model efficacy. The review was limited to English-language publications that may introduce language bias. This may have excluded potentially relevant studies from other languages, primarily from regions with high COPD prevalence. AI architectures, data acquisition protocols, labeling standards, and outcome measures varied across the included studies, limiting the feasibility of a quantitative meta-analysis. While narrative synthesis provides a qualitative overview, it reduces the comparability of the performance of the included studies. The inclusion of preprints ensured coverage of the recent developments in COPD screening and diagnosis. However, these studies typically lack the rigor of peer review. These studies may change their findings upon further analysis or methodological refinements, introducing uncertainty to the evidence base. Furthermore, the possibility of time-lag bias exists in any review that delves into an emerging field of study, presenting a current snapshot rather than a final and comprehensive account of AI applications in COPD detection due to the exclusion of recently published or ongoing studies.

4. Conclusions

This review synthesized 22 studies covering CT, CXR, spirometry, lung sounds, and EHR-based approaches, enabling the detection and prognosis of COPD. CT-based studies demonstrated discriminative ability, underscoring their prognostic potential. CXR-based studies have shown promising outcomes, supporting population-level screening and providing a reliable estimate of spirometric indices. Spirometry-driven approaches achieved exceptional accuracy in detecting airflow obstruction. Emerging modalities, including lung sounds, EHR, and multimodal data, illustrated the capability of AI in harnessing non-imaging data to identify COPD-associated risks. However, the majority of these studies were retrospective, which reduced their representativeness and global applicability. Methodological limitations, such as inconsistent external validation and insufficient subgroup analysis to assess fairness across the population, hinder clinical trust and adoption. This review acknowledges its limitations. The dependence on the English-language studies may have excluded relevant non-English studies. The heterogeneity in methodological approaches and performance metrics prevents a formal meta-analysis. The findings of this review set a pathway for future research. Prospective validation and multicenter datasets are required to guarantee fairness and generalizability. Incorporating multimodal data can capture the multifaceted dimensions of COPD, improving risk prediction.

Supplementary Materials: The following supporting information can be downloaded at: https://www.mdpi.com/article/10.3390/diagnostics15202562/s1, Figure S1: (a) Normal and (b) COPD CT Images; Figure S2: (a) COPD and (b) Normal CXR Images.

Funding: The authors extend their appreciation to the King Salman Center for Disability Research for funding this work through Research Group No. KSRG-2024-353.

Institutional Review Board Statement: Not applicable.

Informed Consent Statement: Not applicable.

Data Availability Statement: Not applicable.

Conflicts of Interest: The authors declare no conflict of interest.

References

1. Adeloye, D.; Song, P.; Zhu, Y.; Campbell, H.; Sheikh, A.; Rudan, I. Global, regional, and national prevalence of, and risk factors for, chronic obstructive pulmonary disease (COPD) in 2019: A systematic review and modelling analysis. *Lancet Respir. Med.* **2022**, *10*, 447–458. [CrossRef]
2. Safiri, S.; Carson-Chahhoud, K.; Noori, M.; Nejadghaderi, S.A.; Sullman, M.J.M.; Heris, J.A.; Ansarin, K.; Mansournia, M.A.; Collins, G.S.; Kolahi, A.-A.; et al. Burden of chronic obstructive pulmonary disease and its attributable risk factors in 204 countries and territories, 1990-2019: Results from the Global Burden of Disease Study 2019. *BMJ* **2022**, *378*, e069679. [CrossRef]
3. Wang, Y.; Han, R.; Ding, X.; Feng, W.; Gao, R.; Ma, A. Chronic obstructive pulmonary disease across three decades: Trends, inequalities, and projections from the Global Burden of Disease Study 2021. *Front. Med.* **2025**, *12*, 1564878. [CrossRef]
4. Li, Y.; Tang, X.; Zhang, R.; Lei, Y.; Wang, D.; Wang, Z.; Li, W. Research progress in early states of chronic obstructive pulmonary disease: A narrative review on PRISm, pre-COPD, young COPD and mild COPD. *Expert Rev. Respir. Med.* **2025**, *19*, 1063–1079. [CrossRef]
5. Faner, R.; Cho, M.H.; Koppelman, G.H.; Melén, E.; Verleden, S.E.; Dharmage, S.C.; Meiners, S.; Agusti, A. Towards early detection and disease interception of COPD across the lifespan. *Eur. Respir. Rev.* **2025**, *34*, 240243. [CrossRef]
6. Long, H.; Li, S.; Chen, Y. Digital health in chronic obstructive pulmonary disease. *Chronic Dis. Transl. Med.* **2023**, *9*, 90–103. [CrossRef]
7. d'Elia, A.; Jordan, R.E.; Jordan, R.; Cheng, K.K.; Chi, C.; Correia-de-Sousa, J.; Dickens, A.P.; Dickens, A.; Enocson, A.; Farley, A.; et al. COPD burden and healthcare management across four middle-income countries within the Breathe Well research programme: A descriptive study. *Glob. Health Res.* **2024**, *18*, 1–7. [CrossRef]
8. Roberts, N.J.; Smith, S.F.; Partridge, M.R. Why is spirometry underused in the diagnosis of the breathless patient: A qualitative study. *BMC Pulm. Med.* **2011**, *11*, 37. [CrossRef]
9. Farha, F.; Abass, S.; Khan, S.; Ali, J.; Parveen, B.; Ahmad, S.; Parveen, R. Transforming pulmonary health care: The role of artificial intelligence in diagnosis and treatment. *Expert Rev. Respir. Med.* **2025**, *19*, 575–595. [CrossRef]
10. Kumar, Y.; Koul, A.; Singla, R.; Ijaz, M.F. Artificial intelligence in disease diagnosis: A systematic literature review, synthesizing framework and future research agenda. *J. Ambient. Intell. Humaniz. Comput.* **2023**, *14*, 8459–8486. [CrossRef]

11. Gupta, J.; Mehrotra, M.; Aggarwal, A.; Gashroo, O.B. Meta-Learning Frameworks in Lung Disease Detection: A survey. *Arch. Comput. Methods Eng.* **2025**, *1*, 1–31. [CrossRef]
12. Robertson, N.M.; Centner, C.S.; Siddharthan, T. Integrating artificial intelligence in the diagnosis of COPD globally: A way forward. *Chronic Obstr. Pulm. Dis. J. COPD Found.* **2023**, *11*, 114–120. [CrossRef]
13. Kaplan, A.; Cao, H.; FitzGerald, J.M.; Iannotti, N.; Yang, E.; Kocks, J.W.H.; Kostikas, K.; Price, D.; Reddel, H.K.; Tsiligianni, I.; et al. Artificial intelligence/machine learning in respiratory medicine and potential role in asthma and COPD diagnosis. *J. Allergy Clin. Immunol. Pract.* **2021**, *9*, 2255–2261. [CrossRef]
14. Calzetta, L.; Pistocchini, E.; Chetta, A.; Rogliani, P.; Cazzola, M. Experimental drugs in clinical trials for COPD: Artificial intelligence via machine learning approach to predict the successful advance from early-stage development to approval. *Expert Opin. Investig. Drugs* **2023**, *32*, 525–536. [CrossRef]
15. Lin, C.-H.; Cheng, S.-L.; Chen, C.-Z.; Chen, C.-H.; Lin, S.-H.; Wang, H.-C. Current progress of COPD early detection: Key points and novel strategies. *Int. J. Chronic Obstr. Pulm. Dis.* **2023**, *18*, 1511–1524. [CrossRef]
16. Díaz, A.A.; Nardelli, P.; Wang, W.; Estépar, R.S.J.; Yen, A.; Kligerman, S.; Maselli, D.J.; Dolliver, W.R.; Tsao, A.; Orejas, J.L.; et al. Artificial intelligence–based CT assessment of bronchiectasis: The COPDGene Study. *Radiology* **2023**, *307*, e221109. [CrossRef]
17. Ajitha, E.; Abishekkumaran, S.; Deva, J. Enhancing diagnostic accuracy in lung disease: A ViT approach. In Proceedings of the 2024 International Conference on Advances in Data Engineering and Intelligent Computing Systems (ADICS) 2024, Chennai, India, 18–19 April 2024; pp. 1–6.
18. Sabir, M.W.; Farhan, M.; Almalki, N.S.; Alnfiai, M.M.; Sampedro, G.A. FibroVit—Vision transformer-based framework for detection and classification of pulmonary fibrosis from chest CT images. *Front. Med.* **2023**, *10*, 1282200. [CrossRef]
19. Kabir, F.; Akter, N.; Hasan, K.; Ahmed, T.; Akter, M. Predicting Chronic Obstructive Pulmonary Disease Using ML and DL Approaches and Feature Fusion of X-Ray Image and Patient History. *Int. J. Adv. Comput. Sci. Appl.* **2024**, *15*, 149–158. [CrossRef]
20. Hadhoud, Y.; Mekhaznia, T.; Bennour, A.; Amroune, M.; Kurdi, N.A.; Aborujilah, A.H.; Al-Sarem, M. From binary to multi-class classification: A two-step hybrid cnn-vit model for chest disease classification based on x-ray images. *Diagnostics* **2024**, *14*, 2754. [CrossRef]
21. Rabby, A.S.; Chaudhary, M.F.; Saha, P.; Sthanam, V.; Nakhmani, A.; Zhang, C.; Barr, R.G.; Bon, J.; Cooper, C.B.; Curtis, J.L.; et al. Light Convolutional Neural Network to Detect Chronic Obstructive Pulmonary Disease (COPDxNet): A Multicenter Model Development and External Validation Study. *medRxiv* **2025**. [CrossRef]
22. Nakrani, H.; Shahra, E.Q.; Basurra, S.; Mohammad, R.; Vakaj, E.; Jabbar, W.A. Advanced Diagnosis of Cardiac and Respiratory Diseases from Chest X-Ray Imagery Using Deep Learning Ensembles. *J. Sens. Actuator Netw.* **2025**, *14*, 44. [CrossRef]
23. Mezina, A.; Burget, R. Detection of post-COVID-19-related pulmonary diseases in X-ray images using Vision Transformer-based neural network. *Biomed. Signal Process. Control* **2024**, *87*, 105380. [CrossRef]
24. Saha, P.K.; Nadeem, S.A.; Comellas, A.P. A survey on artificial intelligence in pulmonary imaging. *WIREs Data Min. Knowl. Discov.* **2023**, *13*, e1510. [CrossRef]
25. Abdullah; Fatima, Z.; Abdullah, J.; Rodríguez, J.L.O.; Sidorov, G. A Multimodal AI Framework for Automated Multiclass Lung Disease Diagnosis from Respiratory Sounds with Simulated Biomarker Fusion and Personalized Medication Recommendation. *Int. J. Mol. Sci.* **2025**, *26*, 7135. [CrossRef]
26. Yadav, S.; Rizvi, S.A.M.; Agarwal, P. Advancing pulmonary infection diagnosis: A comprehensive review of deep learning approaches in radiological data analysis. *Arch. Comput. Methods Eng.* **2025**, *32*, 3759–3786. [CrossRef]
27. Liu, X.; Pan, F.; Song, H.; Cao, S.; Li, C.; Li, T. MDFormer: Transformer-Based Multimodal Fusion for Robust Chest Disease Diagnosis. *Electronics* **2025**, *14*, 1926. [CrossRef]
28. Caliman Sturdza, O.A.; Filip, F.; Terteliu Baitan, M.; Dimian, M. Deep Learning Network Selection and Optimized Information Fusion for Enhanced COVID-19 Detection: A Literature Review. *Diagnostics* **2025**, *15*, 1830. [CrossRef]
29. Abhishek, S.; Ananthapadmanabhan, A.J.; Anjali, T.; Reyma, S.; Perathur, A.; Bentov, R.B. Multimodal Integration of an Enhanced Novel Pulmonary Auscultation Real-Time Diagnostic System. *IEEE Multimed.* **2024**, *31*, 18–43. [CrossRef]
30. Damaševičius, R.; Jagatheesaperumal, S.K.; Kandala, R.N.V.P.S.; Hussain, S.; Alizadehsani, R.; Gorriz, J.M. Deep learning for personalized health monitoring and prediction: A review. *Comput. Intell.* **2024**, *40*, e12682. [CrossRef]
31. Akhter, Y.; Singh, R.; Vatsa, M. AI-based radiodiagnosis using chest X-rays: A review. *Front. Big Data* **2023**, *6*, 1120989. [CrossRef]
32. Aburass, S.; Dorgham, O.; Al Shaqsi, J.; Abu Rumman, M.; Al-Kadi, O. Vision Transformers in Medical Imaging: A Comprehensive Review of Advancements and Applications Across Multiple Diseases. *J. Imaging Inform. Med.* **2025**, *12*, 1–17. [CrossRef]
33. Jha, T.; Suhail, S.; Northcote, J.; Moreira, A.G. Artificial Intelligence in Bronchopulmonary Dysplasia: A Review of the Literature. *Information* **2025**, *16*, 262. [CrossRef]
34. Chaudhari, D.; Kamboj, P. Harnessing Machine Learning and Deep Learning for Non-Communicable Disease Diagnosis: An In-Depth analysis. *Arch. Comput. Methods Eng.* **2025**, *7*, 1–45. [CrossRef]

35. Fischer, A.M.; Varga-Szemes, A.; Martin, S.S.; Sperl, J.I.; Sahbaee, P.; Neumann, D.M.; Gawlitza, J.; Henzler, T.; Johnson, C.M.B.; Nance, J.W.; et al. Artificial intelligence-based fully automated per lobe segmentation and emphysema-quantification based on chest computed tomography compared with global initiative for chronic obstructive lung disease severity of smokers. *J. Thorac. Imaging* **2020**, *35*, S28–S34. [CrossRef]
36. Ebrahimian, S.; Digumarthy, S.R.; Bizzo, B.; Primak, A.; Zimmermann, M.; Tarbiah, M.M.; Kalra, M.K.; Dreyer, K.J. Artificial intelligence has similar performance to subjective assessment of emphysema severity on chest CT. *Acad. Radiol.* **2022**, *29*, 1189–1195. [CrossRef]
37. Yevle, D.V.; Mann, P.S.; Kumar, D. AI Based Diagnosis of Chronic Obstructive Pulmonary Disease: Acomparative Review. *Arch. Comput. Methods Eng.* **2025**, *4*, 1–38. [CrossRef]
38. Feng, Y.; Wang, Y.; Zeng, C.; Mao, H. Artificial intelligence and machine learning in chronic airway diseases: Focus on asthma and chronic obstructive pulmonary disease. *Int. J. Med. Sci.* **2021**, *18*, 2871–2889. [CrossRef] [PubMed]
39. Exarchos, K.P.; Aggelopoulou, A.; Oikonomou, A.; Biniskou, T.; Beli, V.; Antoniadou, E.; Kostikas, K. Review of artificial intelligence techniques in chronic obstructive lung disease. *IEEE J. Biomed. Health Inform.* **2021**, *26*, 2331–2338. [CrossRef] [PubMed]
40. Bian, H.; Zhu, S.; Zhang, Y.; Fei, Q.; Peng, X.; Jin, Z.; Zhou, T.; Zhao, H. Artificial Intelligence in Chronic Obstructive Pulmonary Disease: Research Status, Trends, and Future Directions—A Bibliometric Analysis from 2009 to 2023. *Int. J. Chronic Obstr. Pulm. Dis.* **2024**, *19*, 1849–1864.
41. Xu, Y.; Long, Z.A.; Setyohadi, D.B. A comprehensive review on the application of artificial intelligence in Chronic Obstructive Pulmonary Disease (COPD) management. In Proceedings of the 2024 18th International Conference on Ubiquitous Information Management and Communication (IMCOM), Kuala Lumpur, Malaysia, 3–5 January 2024; pp. 1–8.
42. Chu, S.H.; Wan, E.S.; Cho, M.H.; Goryachev, S.; Gainer, V.; Linneman, J.; Scotty, E.J.; Hebbring, S.J.; Murphy, S.; Lasky-Su, J.; et al. An independently validated, portable algorithm for the rapid identification of COPD patients using electronic health records. *Sci. Rep.* **2021**, *11*, 19959. [CrossRef] [PubMed]
43. Rauf, A.; Muhammad, N.; Mahmood, H.; Aftab, M. Healthcare service quality: A systematic review based on PRISMA guidelines. *Int. J. Qual. Reliab. Manag.* **2025**, *42*, 837–850. [CrossRef]
44. Veroniki, A.A.; Hutton, B.; Stevens, A.; McKenzie, J.E.; Page, M.J.; Moher, D.; McGowan, J.; Straus, S.E.; Li, T.; Munn, Z.; et al. Update to the PRISMA guidelines for network meta-analyses and scoping reviews and development of guidelines for rapid reviews: A scoping review protocol. *JBI Evid. Synth.* **2025**, *23*, 517–526. [CrossRef] [PubMed]
45. Aggarwal, R.; Sounderajah, V.; Martin, G.; Ting, D.S.W.; Karthikesalingam, A.; King, D.; Ashrafian, H.; Darzi, A. Diagnostic accuracy of deep learning in medical imaging: A systematic review and meta-analysis. *npj Digit. Med.* **2021**, *4*, 65. [CrossRef] [PubMed]
46. LIDC-IDRI Dataset. Available online: https://www.cancerimagingarchive.net/collection/lidc-idri/ (accessed on 9 September 2025).
47. Tang, L.Y.W.; Coxson, H.O.; Lam, S.; Leipsic, J.; Tam, R.C.; Sin, D.D. Towards large-scale case-finding: Training and validation of residual networks for detection of chronic obstructive pulmonary disease using low-dose CT. *Lancet Digit. Health* **2020**, *2*, e259–e267. [CrossRef]
48. González, G.; Ash, S.Y.; Vegas-Sánchez-Ferrero, G.; Onieva, J.O.; Rahaghi, F.N.; Ross, J.C.; Díaz, A.; Estépar, R.S.J.; Washko, G.R.; Copdgene, F.T. Disease staging and prognosis in smokers using deep learning in chest computed tomography. *Am. J. Respir. Crit. Care Med.* **2018**, *197*, 193–203. [CrossRef]
49. Sun, J.; Liao, X.; Yan, Y.; Zhang, X.; Sun, J.; Tan, W.; Liu, B.; Wu, J.; Guo, Q.; Gao, S.; et al. Detection and staging of chronic obstructive pulmonary disease using a computed tomography–based weakly supervised deep learning approach. *Eur. Radiol.* **2022**, *32*, 5319–5329. [CrossRef]
50. Xue, M.; Jia, S.; Chen, L.; Huang, H.; Yu, L.; Zhu, W. CT-based COPD identification using multiple instance learning with two-stage attention. *Comput. Methods Programs Biomed.* **2023**, *230*, 107356. [CrossRef]
51. Park, H.; Yun, J.; Lee, S.M.; Hwang, H.J.; Seo, J.B.; Jung, Y.J.; Hwang, J.; Lee, S.H.; Lee, S.W.; Kim, N. Deep learning–based approach to predict pulmonary function at chest CT. *Radiology* **2023**, *307*, e221488. [CrossRef]
52. Humphries, S.M.; Notary, A.M.; Centeno, J.P.; Strand, M.J.; Crapo, J.D.; Silverman, E.K.; Lynch, D.A.; For the Genetic Epidemiology of COPD (COPDGene) Investigators. Deep learning enables automatic classification of emphysema pattern at CT. *Radiology* **2020**, *294*, 434–444. [CrossRef]
53. Almeida, S.D.; Norajitra, T.; Lüth, C.T.; Wald, T.; Weru, V.; Nolden, M.; Jäger, P.F.; von Stackelberg, O.; Heußel, C.P.; Weinheimer, O.; et al. Prediction of disease severity in COPD: A deep learning approach for anomaly-based quantitative assessment of chest CT. *Eur. Radiol.* **2024**, *34*, 4379–4392. [CrossRef]
54. Almeida, S.D.; Norajitra, T.; Lüth, C.T.; Wald, T.; Weru, V.; Nolden, M.; Jäger, P.F.; von Stackelberg, O.; Heußel, C.P.; Weinheimer, O.; et al. How do deep-learning models generalize across populations? Cross-ethnicity generalization of COPD detection. *Insights Into Imaging* **2024**, *15*, 198. [CrossRef]
55. Nam, J.G.; Kang, H.-R.; Lee, S.M.; Kim, H.; Rhee, C.; Goo, J.M.; Oh, Y.-M.; Lee, C.-H.; Park, C.M. Deep learning prediction of survival in patients with chronic obstructive pulmonary disease using chest radiographs. *Radiology* **2022**, *305*, 199–208. [CrossRef]

56. Ueda, D.; Matsumoto, T.; Yamamoto, A.; Walston, S.L.; Mitsuyama, Y.; Takita, H.; Asai, K.; Watanabe, T.; Abo, K.; Kimura, T.; et al. A deep learning-based model to estimate pulmonary function from chest x-rays: Multi-institutional model development and validation study in Japan. *Lancet Digit. Health* **2024**, *6*, e580–e588. [CrossRef]
57. Schroeder, J.D.; Bigolin Lanfredi, R.; Li, T.; Chan, J.; Vachet, C.; Paine, R., III; Srikumar, V.; Tasdizen, T. Prediction of obstructive lung disease from chest radiographs via deep learning trained on pulmonary function data. *Int. J. Chronic Obstr. Pulm. Dis.* **2020**, *5*, 3455–3466. [CrossRef]
58. Doroodgar Jorshery, S.; Chandra, J.; Walia, A.S.; Stumiolo, A.; Corey, K.; Zekavat, S.M.; Zinzuwadia, A.N.; Patel, K.; Short, S.; Mega, J.L.; et al. Leveraging Deep Learning of Chest Radiograph Images to Identify Individuals at High Risk for Chronic Obstructive Pulmonary Disease. *medRxiv* **2024**. [CrossRef]
59. Zou, X.; Ren, Y.; Yang, H.; Zou, M.; Meng, P.; Zhang, L.; Gong, M.; Ding, W.; Han, L.; Zhang, T. Screening and staging of chronic obstructive pulmonary disease with deep learning based on chest X-ray images and clinical parameters. *BMC Pulm. Med.* **2024**, *24*, 153. [CrossRef]
60. Mac, A.; Xu, T.; Wu, J.K.Y.; Belousova, N.; Kitazawa, H.; Vozoris, N.; Rozenberg, D.; Ryan, C.M.; Valaee, S.; Chow, C.-W. Deep learning using multilayer perception improves the diagnostic acumen of spirometry: A single-centre Canadian study. *BMJ Open Respir. Res.* **2022**, *9*, e001396. [CrossRef] [PubMed]
61. Wang, Y.; Li, Q.; Chen, W.; Jian, W.; Liang, J.; Gao, Y.; Zhong, N.; Zheng, J. Deep Learning-based analytic models based on flow-volume curves for identifying ventilatory patterns. *Front. Physiol.* **2022**, *13*, 824000. [CrossRef]
62. Cosentino, J.; Behsaz, B.; Alipanahi, B.; McCaw, Z.R.; Hill, D.; Schwantes-An, T.-H.; Lai, D.; Carroll, A.; Hobbs, B.D.; Cho, M.H.; et al. Inference of chronic obstructive pulmonary disease with deep learning on raw spirograms identifies new genetic loci and improves risk models. *Nat. Genet.* **2023**, *55*, 787–795. [CrossRef] [PubMed]
63. Hill, D.; Torop, M.; Masoomi, A.; Castaldi, P.; Dy, J.; Cho, M.; Hobbs, B. Deep Learning Utilizing Discarded Spirometry Data to Improve Lung Function and Mortality Prediction in the UK Biobank. In Proceedings of the A95. the Idea Generator: Novel Risk Factors and Fresh Approaches to Disease Characterization 2022, San Francisco, CA, USA, 13–18 May 2022; p. A2145.
64. Altan, G.; Kutlu, Y.; Gökçen, A. Chronic obstructive pulmonary disease severity analysis using deep learning on multi-channel lung sounds. *Turk. J. Electr. Eng. Comput. Sci.* **2020**, *28*, 2979–2996. [CrossRef]
65. Naqvi, S.Z.H.; Choudhry, M.A. An automated system for classification of chronic obstructive pulmonary disease and pneumonia patients using lung sound analysis. *Sensors* **2020**, *20*, 6512. [CrossRef] [PubMed]
66. Yu, H.; Zhao, J.; Liu, D.; Chen, Z.; Sun, J.; Zhao, X. Multi-channel lung sounds intelligent diagnosis of chronic obstructive pulmonary disease. *BMC Pulm. Med.* **2021**, *21*, 321. [CrossRef] [PubMed]
67. Chen, J.; Xu, Z.; Sun, L.; Yu, K.; Hersh, C.P.; Boueiz, A.; Hokanson, J.E.; Sciurba, F.C.; Silverman, E.K.; Castaldi, P.J.; et al. Deep learning integration of chest computed tomography imaging and gene expression identifies novel aspects of copd. *Chronic Obstr. Pulm. Dis. J. COPD Found.* **2023**, *10*, 355–368. [CrossRef] [PubMed]

diagnostics

MDPI

Review

Transforming Breast Imaging: A Narrative Review of Systematic Evidence on Artificial Intelligence in Mammographic Practice

Andrea Lastrucci [1], Nicola Iosca [1], Yannick Wandael [1], Angelo Barra [1], Renzo Ricci [1], Jacopo Nori Cucchiari [2], Nevio Forini [3], Graziano Lepri [4] and Daniele Giansanti [5,*]

[1] Department of Allied Health Professions, Azienda Ospedaliero-Universitaria Careggi, 50134 Florence, Italy; ioscan@aou-careggi.toscana.it (N.I.); wandaely@aou-careggi.toscana.it (Y.W.); barraa@aou-careggi.toscana.it (A.B.); riccire@aou-careggi.toscana.it (R.R.)
[2] Breast Imaging Unit, Department of Radiology, Azienda Ospedaliero-Universitaria Careggi, 50134 Florence, Italy; norij@aou-careggi.toscana.it
[3] Dipartimento di Medicina e Chirurgia, Università degli Studi di Perugia, Piazzale Settimio Gambuli, 1, 06129 Perugia, Italy; nevio.forini@unipg.it
[4] Unità Sanitaria Locale Umbria 1, Via Guerriero Guerra 21, 06127 Perugia, Italy; graziano.lepri@uslumbria1.it
[5] Centre TISP, Istituto Superiore di Sanità, 00161 Rome, Italy
* Correspondence: daniele.giansanti@iss.it

Abstract

Background: Breast cancer is still the most common type of cancer worldwide. Advances and the global use of artificial intelligence (AI) have opened up new opportunities to improve diagnostic accuracy and optimize breast cancer screening. This review summarizes the findings from systematic reviews to assess the current situation of AI integration in mammography. **Methods**: A total of 28 systematic reviews were included and analyzed using a standardized narrative checklist to assess the impact of AI on mammography imaging. Bibliometric analysis and thematic synthesis were used to assess trends, evaluate the performance of AI in different modalities and identify challenges and opportunities for clinical implementation. **Results and Discussion**: AI technologies show an overall performance comparable to radiologists in terms of sensitivity and specificity, especially when integrated with human interpretation to detect breast cancer in mammography. However, most studies are retrospective, which raises concerns about their generalizability to real-world clinical settings. Key limitations include potential dataset bias—often stemming from the over-representation of specific imaging equipment or clinical environments—limited ethnic and demographic diversity, the lack of model explainability that hinders clinical trust, and an unclear or evolving legal and regulatory framework that complicates integration into standard practice. **Conclusions**: AI has the potential to transform mammography screening, but its integration into the real world requires prospective validation, ethical safeguards and robust regulatory oversight. Coordinated international efforts are essential to ensure that AI is used safely, fairly and effectively in breast cancer diagnostics.

Keywords: mammography; artificial intelligence; breast cancer

1. Introduction

1.1. Breast Cancer Epidemiology and Clinical Features

Breast cancer is the most frequently diagnosed cancer worldwide. In 2020, 2.3 million new cases were reported globally, accounting for 1 in every 8 cancers diagnosed and making it the most common cancer overall, according to data from the International Agency for

Research on Cancer (IARC) [1]. That same year, breast cancer caused approximately 685,000 deaths, making it the leading cause of cancer death among women and the fifth leading cause of cancer mortality overall [1].

Although the disease predominantly affects women, male breast cancer occurs in about 1% of cases [2]. Incidence rates are highest in high-income countries—such as Australia, Western Europe, and North America—but are increasing in many low- and middle-income countries (LMICs), where demographic transitions and lifestyle changes are shifting cancer patterns [1,3].

From a clinical perspective, breast cancer is biologically and histologically heterogeneous, arising most frequently in ductal or lobular epithelium, and is categorized into molecular subtypes based on hormone receptor and HER2 status [4]. These subtypes are key in determining prognosis and guiding personalized treatment approaches.

Despite significant advances in early detection and therapeutic strategies—especially in high-resource settings—breast cancer remains a major global health challenge, with substantial disparities in access to care and survival outcomes [1,3,5].

1.2. Evolution of Mammographic Imaging

The origins of mammographic imaging can be traced back to the early 20th century. In 1913, German surgeon Albert Salomon was the first to systematically study breast tissue using X-rays, comparing radiographic findings with histological samples from over 3000 mastectomies. His pioneering work laid the foundation for the use of X-ray imaging in breast cancer diagnosis [6].

However, it was not until the 1950s and 1960s that mammography began to emerge as a distinct clinical tool. The development of dedicated mammography units, lower-dose radiation techniques, and improved film-screen combinations marked a major shift from general radiography to breast-specific imaging. The introduction of xeromammography in the 1960s, although later abandoned, represented an early effort to enhance image clarity and lesion detection [7].

By the 1970s and 1980s, mammography had become more widely adopted in clinical settings, particularly after studies began to demonstrate its efficacy in early cancer detection. Landmark trials such as the Health Insurance Plan (HIP) study in New York showed that routine mammographic screening could significantly reduce breast cancer mortality among women aged 50 and older [8].

The transition to digital mammography in the late 1990s and early 2000s represented a major technological leap. Unlike analog systems, Full-Field Digital Mammography (FFDM) offered enhanced contrast resolution, image storage flexibility, and the potential for advanced image processing and telemedicine applications [9]. These benefits were validated in large comparative trials, including the Digital Mammographic Imaging Screening Trial (DMIST), which demonstrated the superior sensitivity of digital mammography in women under 50 and those with dense breasts [9].

More recently, the advent of digital breast tomosynthesis (DBT)—also known as 3D mammography—has further refined diagnostic accuracy. By acquiring multiple low-dose images at different angles, DBT reconstructs a pseudo-3D representation of the breast, improving lesion visibility and reducing recall rates [10].

Today, mammographic imaging is a cornerstone of breast cancer screening and diagnosis. Its evolution reflects a continuous pursuit of greater sensitivity and specificity, driven by technological innovation and a deeper understanding of breast cancer biology.

1.3. Artificial Intelligence Integration in Mammography

This long-standing trajectory has laid the groundwork for the integration of artificial intelligence (AI) into mammographic workflows—a development aimed at optimizing interpretation, reducing diagnostic variability, and addressing the growing demand for radiological services.

The integration of artificial intelligence (AI) into mammographic imaging represents a promising frontier aimed at enhancing breast cancer detection and diagnosis. Initial explorations of AI in mammography began several decades ago, inspired by the potential of computer-aided detection (CAD) systems developed in the late 20th century [11].

Early CAD systems were designed to assist radiologists by highlighting suspicious areas in mammograms, thus acting as a "second reader." Despite improving sensitivity in some cases, these first-generation tools often suffered from high false-positive rates, limiting their widespread adoption [12].

With advances in machine learning and, more recently, deep learning techniques, AI applications in mammography have experienced significant renewed interest. These advanced models are capable of analyzing complex imaging patterns beyond human visual perception, offering the potential to improve diagnostic accuracy, reduce inter- and intra-observer variability, and streamline radiologists' workflow. Consequently, AI has shown promise not only as a second reader but also as a tool for prioritizing cases and assisting in risk stratification [13].

However, the gradual integration of AI tools into clinical mammography has raised important questions and discussions within the medical community. These concern the need for rigorous clinical validation, the transparency of AI decision-making processes, and their seamless integration into existing diagnostic pathways to ensure safety, reliability, and acceptance by practitioners [14].

1.4. Current Challenges and Opportunities in AI-Driven Breast Cancer Screening

The COVID-19 pandemic has significantly disrupted routine breast cancer screening programs worldwide, leading to delayed diagnoses and increased challenges for healthcare systems [15]. In response to these challenges, there has been a rapid acceleration in the adoption and development of artificial intelligence (AI) applications in mammography. AI-driven tools have been explored to support remote screening workflows, prioritize high-risk cases, and manage increased workloads, thereby helping to mitigate the impact of service disruptions [16,17]. This surge in interest highlights AI's potential role not only in improving diagnostic accuracy but also in enhancing the resilience and efficiency of breast cancer screening programs during healthcare crises.

Recent advances in artificial intelligence (AI) have introduced powerful techniques such as machine learning (ML), artificial neural networks (ANNs), and deep learning (DL), which are revolutionizing many fields including medicine [18]. These AI methods enable automated decision-making by learning from complex and large datasets, simulating aspects of human cognition through interconnected processing layers. In the medical domain, these approaches have demonstrated promising potential to enhance diagnostic speed, accuracy, and efficiency across various applications [18], with potential also in breast cancer screening. Specifically, AI tools can support mammographic image analysis by improving lesion detection and classification, facilitating earlier diagnosis and personalized patient care. Nevertheless, the integration of AI into clinical workflows still faces important challenges. Key among these is the need for the explainability and transparency of AI systems, which are essential to build clinician trust, address ethical concerns, and comply with regulatory standards [19]. Overcoming these barriers is crucial for the widespread adoption of AI-assisted mammography and for fully realizing AI's potential to improve breast cancer detection outcomes.

Simultaneously, the evolution of breast cancer imaging encompasses a wide range of conventional and emerging modalities, with AI positioned as a transformative component in this landscape [20].

These developments highlight both exciting opportunities and complex obstacles, underscoring the critical need for the comprehensive synthesis and evaluation of existing evidence to guide safe and effective AI implementation in mammography.

1.5. Framing the Research: Key Questions and Aims of the Narrative Review

The rapid advancement of artificial intelligence (AI) technologies has opened new horizons in mammographic breast cancer screening, yet a comprehensive understanding of their impact remains essential. Several broad and fundamental questions arise in this evolving field:

First, what is the current state of AI applications in mammography across clinical, technical, and research domains?

Second, how does the integration of AI influence diagnostic accuracy, workflow efficiency, and healthcare delivery in breast imaging?

Third, what are the main barriers and facilitators affecting the adoption and implementation of AI technologies in breast cancer screening programs? And finally, what ethical, legal, and social implications emerge from the use of AI in this context?

Addressing these questions is critical to guide future research, optimize clinical applications, and support informed policy decisions for the safe and responsible integration of AI into breast cancer detection and management.

Aim

The purpose of this study is to conduct a narrative review to comprehensively explore the role of artificial intelligence (AI) in mammographic breast cancer screening. This review aims to aggregate and synthesize findings from existing systematic reviews in order to provide a consolidated and high-level understanding of how AI is currently applied within mammography. By identifying and analyzing key themes and trends emerging from these reviews, this study seeks to highlight significant advancements such as improvements in diagnostic accuracy, workflow efficiency, and clinical outcomes and examine the challenges related to implementation, standardization, and ethical considerations.

Specific aims:

- Trend analysis: Map recent trends in the scientific literature on AI in mammography, highlighting growth areas, publication volume, and thematic shifts using bibliometric insights.
- Themes and categorization: Identify and organize the main themes emerging from existing systematic reviews, focusing on AI applications that enhance breast cancer detection and diagnostic processes in mammography.
- Opportunities and challenges: Analyze the opportunities and challenges reported in the literature, including benefits related to diagnostic performance and clinical workflow, alongside barriers encountered in real-world adoption and integration.

2. Materials and Methods

This work was conducted as a narrative review, aiming to collect and synthesize existing systematic reviews and meta-analyses on the use of artificial intelligence (AI) in mammography, with a specific focus on practical applications in breast cancer screening. This review followed the ANDJ narrative checklist.

A targeted literature search was performed on PubMed, Scopus and the Web of Science using a composite query designed to identify relevant reviews. The search string is reported in Box 1.

Box 1. Used search keys.

("artificial intelligence" OR "machine learning" OR "deep learning" OR "convolutional neural networks," "transformers," or "radiomics") AND ("mammography" OR "breast cancer screening")

The search retrieved articles without date restrictions, although most of the studies included were published within the last ten years.

During the selection process, we prioritized reviews that investigated the actual implementation and clinical application of AI methods in mammography—such as diagnostic support, lesion detection, triage strategies, and risk stratification. Reviews with only general, theoretical, or purely mathematical overviews of AI, without reference to mammographic practice, were excluded.

Each study was evaluated through a structured quality checklist based on prior methodological guidance. For each included review, six key parameters were assessed:

- N1: Clarity of the study's rationale.
- N2: The appropriateness of the design.
- N3: The transparency of the described methods.
- N4: Clarity in presenting results.
- N5: Coherence between results and conclusions.
- N6: The disclosure of conflicts of interest.

Parameters N1 to N5 were graded on a 5-point scale (1 = very poor, 5 = excellent), while N6 was assessed binary: "Yes" if conflicts of interest were clearly disclosed or "No" if not.

Only studies meeting the following criteria were included in the final synthesis:

- A "Yes" rating for N6 (conflict of interest disclosure).
- A score of 3 or higher on each of the five graded parameters (N1–N5).

The selected reviews were then analyzed through a focused investigation with particular care, for example, on the following:

- The types of AI algorithms applied (e.g., CNNs, ensemble learning),
- The clinical tasks and workflow integration,
- The datasets and validation strategies used,
- The reported strengths, weaknesses, and evidence gaps.

This process enabled a comprehensive overview of the current state of AI applications in mammography, highlighting both converging evidence and areas requiring further investigation.

Each study was independently evaluated by two reviewers (AL and DG). In cases of disagreement, a third reviewer (either GL or NF) acted as adjudicator to reach consensus.

The anonymized assessment, seen in Table S1, listing the included studies is reported in the Supplementary Materials.

Potential sources of bias were considered at multiple stages of the review process. Selection bias was minimized by applying predefined eligibility criteria and performing independent dual screening. Assessment bias was reduced through the structured checklist and the adjudication process in cases of reviewer disagreement.

A total of 28 studies were included in the study as they matched the focus of this review [21–48].

3. Results

3.1. Trend Analysis

To better understand the growth trajectory and maturity of artificial intelligence (AI) research applied to mammography, we conducted a comparative trend analysis across several adjacent clinical fields. The aim of this analysis is twofold: first, to characterize the specific evolution of AI-focused mammography literature over time, and second, to contextualize this growth by comparing it with broader trends in AI research in radiology, oncology, and breast cancer at large.

This comparison is important to establish whether mammography AI research is following a unique path or whether it mirrors more general patterns seen in medical AI literature. By identifying shared or divergent trends, we gain insight into how mammography sits within the wider AI–healthcare landscape—whether as a lagging, leading, or aligned subfield.

To do so, we employed four targeted literature searches (Search Keys 1–4, shown in Box S1 in the Supplementary Materials), which represent increasing levels of generalization:

- Search Key 1 focuses on mammography and AI (our core interest).
- Keys 2, 3, and 4 expand the scope to radiology, oncology, and breast cancer, respectively, still retaining AI as a central theme.

Using Search Key 1 from Box S1, on the core focus of this review on artificial intelligence (AI) applied to mammography, we identified a total of 1748 studies published between 1989 and 2024 on PubMed. Among these, 221 were reviews or systematic reviews, indicating a mature body of synthesized evidence in this niche area.

Publication trends show a clear acceleration over the past decade, with 1312 studies (about 75%) published in the last 10 years and a substantial 1042 studies (60%) in just the last 5 years. Notably, this means that nearly 80% of the last decade's output was concentrated in the most recent half—a strong indicator of recent intensified research activity.

Several factors likely contribute to this surge. Technologically, advances in deep learning architectures, the increasing availability of large annotated mammographic datasets, and improvements in computational resources have made AI applications in mammography more feasible and effective. Systemically, many health systems worldwide have prioritized digital transformation initiatives, fostering the development and deployment of AI tools for diagnostic imaging.

Importantly, the COVID-19 pandemic appears to have acted as a catalyst accelerating this growth. During the pandemic, radiology departments faced critical workforce shortages, backlog pressures, and triage complexities, all of which heightened interest in AI-driven solutions to maintain diagnostic throughput and resilience. Moreover, the pandemic's push towards digital health and remote care created a conducive environment for AI innovation and evaluation, particularly in imaging fields.

To contextualize these findings, we compared this focused trend with broader AI research in related clinical domains using other key search strings from Box S1:

- For Key 2 (*"artificial intelligence" AND "radiology"*), a vast total of 32,854 publications since 1960 were found, with an overwhelming 87.9% (28,864) published in the last 10 years and 74.0% (24,317) in the last 5 years. The most recent 5 years alone represent about 84.3% of the publications produced in the preceding 5-year period (from 10 to 5 years ago), demonstrating a pronounced clustering of research activity.
- For Key 3 (*"artificial intelligence" AND "oncology"*), there have been 43,252 publications since 1961, with 81.7% (35,337) from the last decade and 65.7% (28,423) from the last 5 years. The most recent 5 years account for approximately 80.5% of the output of the prior 5-year interval, reflecting a similarly strong acceleration.

- For Key 4 (*"artificial intelligence" AND "breast cancer"*), a more focused yet significant dataset of 7292 publications since 1986 was identified, with 83.3% (6077) from the last 10 years and 66.8% (4872) from the last 5 years. The most recent 5 years make up about 80.2% of the preceding 5-year output, highlighting a consistent pattern of concentrated growth in AI research specific to breast cancer.

Overall, these comparisons reveal a strikingly consistent pattern: across the domains of radiology, oncology, breast cancer, and mammography-focused AI research, roughly 80% to 84% of the research output in the last five years corresponds to the research produced in the preceding five-year period. In other words, about four-fifths of the publications from the last decade were generated in just the most recent half of that time span.

This convergence around the 80% mark highlights a strong clustering of research activity in the most recent years, reflecting a common, rapid acceleration of AI-driven studies across these related but distinct fields.

Mammography-focused research (Key 1), despite being smaller in total volume, aligns clearly with this pattern, illustrating its role as an emerging but integral component within the broader AI and cancer imaging research ecosystem.

This shared trajectory underscores how advances in computational power, machine learning methods, and the availability of large-scale annotated datasets, combined with systemic incentives such as digital health policies and clinical needs, are collectively fueling this surge.

Additionally, the COVID-19 pandemic likely acted as a catalyst across all domains, increasing the urgency of and resource allocation to AI research aimed at improving diagnostic capacity, workflow resilience, and remote care options during a period of unprecedented healthcare strain.

In summary, these aligned trends demonstrate that AI research in mammography is not isolated but part of a broader, interlinked expansion of AI applications in medical imaging and oncology—all experiencing a similarly steep growth curve driven by technological innovation and healthcare challenges.

3.2. The Integration of AI in Mammography: The Focus on Emerging Themes and Technological Innovations

A total of 28 articles were included in this study as they matched the focus of this narrative review [21–48]. An analysis of the studies was conducted with a particular focus on the integration of AI technology in mammography, which is summarized in Table 1. A brief supplementary summary of the systematic reviews included can be found below.

The study by Abu Abeelh and Abuabeileh [21] reports that AI in screening mammography has the potential to improve diagnostic accuracy, reduce false-positive results and reduce radiologists' workload. Although generally comparable or even superior to traditional methods, challenges such as false-positive results and variability in subgroup performance require further research.

The study by Yoon et al. [22] found that standalone AI in screening digital mammography performs comparably or better than radiologists, particularly in reader studies and digital breast tomosynthesis. AI showed higher sensitivity but lower specificity, highlighting both its potential and current limitations.

The review by Zeng et al. [23] is focused on the frequency and characteristics of AI errors in reading screening mammography and it reported that AI errors primarily involve false positives and false negatives, with their frequency varying by algorithm threshold and version. Other error types like localization and technical errors are under-reported, limiting the full understanding of AI limitations.

The review by Freeman et al. [24] found that most AI systems were less accurate than radiologists in large, retrospective studies, and none outperformed double reading. While smaller studies showed promise, there is insufficient evidence to support AI replacing radiologists in breast cancer screening without further prospective evaluation.

The study by Laws et al. [25] highlights significant gaps in mammography datasets used for AI development, including limited global representation, poor documentation, and a lack of demographic transparency. Only a small fraction of datasets are publicly accessible, and most lack diversity data critical for equitable AI advancement.

The study by Branco et al. [26] found that AI algorithms in mammography screening generally perform comparably to radiologists and improve diagnostic accuracy when used alongside them. AI can support radiologists, especially less experienced ones, by enhancing lesion detection and overall evaluation accuracy.

In the review by Schopf et al. [27], it is reported that AI models using only mammography images predict future breast cancer risk more accurately than traditional clinical risk tools, with median area under the receiver operating characteristic curve (AUC) of 0.72 versus 0.61. Adding clinical data to AI models provided minimal to no additional predictive benefit.

The systematic review by Avanzo et al. [28] examined the application of AI in medical imaging, with a section dedicated to mammography. The review highlights that AI technologies support breast cancer detection and characterization by enhancing diagnostic accuracy, reducing false negatives, and facilitating precision medicine. Advanced methods such as deep convolutional neural networks (CNNs), clustering algorithms, and classifiers significantly improve lesion detection across various imaging modalities, including digital mammography, contrast-enhanced spectral mammography (CESM), and tomosynthesis.

The systematic review by Rentiya et al. [29] highlights the evolving role of AI in breast cancer detection and treatment, emphasizing its potential to improve diagnostic accuracy and efficiency beyond traditional methods like computer-aided detection. While AI integration shows promise, the review underscores the importance of addressing challenges related to data quality, validation, ethics, and regulation to fully realize its benefits in clinical practice.

The review by Batchu et al. [30] summarizes evidence on AI's utility in mammography, highlighting its potential to reduce false positives, increase sensitivity (up to 91%), and assist in both diagnosis and risk prediction. Despite heterogeneity across studies and the need for more prospective research, AI shows promise in reducing radiologist workload and improving diagnostic performance.

The study by Xavier et al. [31] demonstrates that deep learning (DL)-based triage can significantly reduce radiologist workload—by over 68%—while maintaining high sensitivity (93.1%) in detecting breast cancer, supporting its potential as an effective tool in screening workflows. However, high heterogeneity across studies and systems highlights the need for standardized implementation frameworks and more prospective validation.

The systematic review and meta-analysis by Hickman et al. [32] found that standalone machine learning algorithms in screening mammography can match or exceed human reader performance (AUC 0.89 vs. 0.85), with the potential for significant workflow optimization through triage. However, the results are largely retrospective and limited in scope, emphasizing the urgent need for prospective validation in real-world conditions to confirm these promising results.

The study by Liu et al. [33] confirms the high diagnostic accuracy of ML methods in mammography, especially convolutional neural networks (CNNs), which outperformed other models with a pooled AUC of 0.974, a sensitivity of 96.1% and a specificity of 95.0%. These results emphasize the great potential of CNNs in breast cancer screening workflows, although prospective, real-world studies are needed to validate their clinical impact.

The review by Anderson et al. [34] emphasizes that while AI algorithms for mammography screening show a modest improvement in diagnostic accuracy, especially when combined with radiologists, the current evidence is limited by retrospective designs and methodological weaknesses. Few studies have used robust real-world results, emphasizing the urgent need for high-quality, prospective external validation to establish the true clinical benefits of AI.

The study by Bhalla et al. [35] analyzes DL studies for breast cancer detection at mammography, focusing on reproducibility and best practice. Most studies showed a high risk of bias due to unrepresentative patient selection. Only four studies met appropriate quality standards, using models such as ResNet and RetinaNet, with the best AUC values of 0.93–0.95. Combining AI with radiologist assessments improved accuracy and specificity. However, none of the studies provided meaningful explanations beyond lesion localization or assessed AI–radiologist interaction in real clinical settings.

The review by Goh et al. [36] highlights a critical gap in the current DL literature on mammography: despite promising diagnostic performance (e.g., AUCs up to 0.955 with combined AI-radiologist readings), most studies lack reproducibility and explainability. An overwhelming 96% were flagged for a high risk of bias, largely due to non-representative datasets. Few studies train robust, transparent models, and none assess real-world AI–radiologist interaction or offered interpretable insights beyond localization.

The study by Gurmessa and Jimma [37] examines explainable AI (XAI) methods for breast cancer diagnosis using mammography and ultrasound images. Most studies highlighted issues with datasets as a key research gap. The relationship between accuracy and explainability remains unclear, and real-world assessments of XAI reliability are lacking. Overall, the review emphasizes the need for further research to improve explainability, dataset quality, and confidence in XAI systems for clinical use.

The review by Hussain et al. [38] examines how DL and AI are used to predict breast cancer risk by analyzing imaging, genetic, and clinical data. Traditional models rely mostly on demographics and history, but AI offers more personalized predictions. AI techniques like natural language processing can improve risk assessment and support better screening and management. The review provides a clear overview of current progress and future possibilities in AI-based breast cancer risk prediction.

The review by Oh et al. [39] analyzed radiomics—a technique used for extracting detailed data from medical images—to differentiate benign from malignant breast lesions. Results from MRI, mammography, and ultrasound showed high accuracy, with sensitivities around 79–92% and specificities around 81–85%. Radiomics shows promise as a non-invasive diagnostic aid for breast cancer, but biopsy remains the definitive standard due to current technological and study limitations.

The study by Hussain et al. [40] examines the applications of DL, radiomics, and radio genomics in digital breast tomosynthesis (DBT), an advanced 3D mammography technique rapidly replacing traditional 2D mammography. The study highlights how these AI-driven approaches enhance breast cancer detection and patient stratification by linking imaging features with genetic information. The review provides insights into the current landscape and future directions of DL, radiomics, and radio genomics in DBT imaging for early breast cancer diagnosis.

The review by Madani et al. [41] examines how DL improves breast cancer detection using different imaging methods, including mammography. Early detection is vital but current manual screening is slow, expensive, and error-prone. AI, especially DL, offers automated, more accurate analysis to support radiologists. The paper discusses the pros and cons of various imaging techniques, summarizes recent AI research, and highlights key datasets for training models.

The review by Gardezi [42] examines the use of ML and DL for breast cancer diagnosis using mammography data. Traditional methods are limited, while DL shows significant improvements despite challenges such as data scarcity and high computational costs, which are partially addressed by data augmentation and higher computational power. The detection of masses in dense breast tissue is more challenging compared to calcifications.

The study by Yassin et al. [43] reviews the current state of CAD systems for breast cancer using different imaging modalities. The review focuses on ML-based classifiers and image types used in CAD systems and highlights advances and areas for future research to improve the objectivity and efficiency of breast cancer detection and diagnosis.

The review by Singh and Singh [44] examines the use of breast thermography for the early detection of breast cancer. Recent advancements in artificial neural networks and ML have improved diagnostic accuracy by improving image analysis steps such as segmentation and classification. Despite some challenges, such as false positives, the integration of numerical simulations and newer ML methods promises more reliable real-time breast cancer screening in the future.

The study by Sorin et al. [45] focuses on DL applications in contrast-enhanced mammography (CEM), a newer imaging modality that improves breast cancer diagnosis. The DL models focused on lesion classification, detection and segmentation and achieved a wide range of accuracy (AUC 0.53 to 0.99). Attention-based models showed high accuracy (~88–89%), and combining DL with radiomics or radiological input further improved performance. Most studies, while promising, are retrospective and emphasize the need for prospective clinical validation to confirm DL's real-world effectiveness in CEM.

The relevance of AI-enhanced mammography is further reinforced by a recent systematic review and meta-analysis by Ciurescu et al. [46], who evaluate the diagnostic and prognostic value of AI-assisted mammography in conjunction with the Systemic Immune–Inflammation Index (SII). Their work explores the synergy between imaging biomarkers and systemic markers, indicating new horizons for integrated AI-driven assessment in breast cancer.

While not focused exclusively on mammography, the systematic review by Rostami et al. [47] discusses AI's role in identifying cancers of unknown primary, reinforcing the cross-cutting impact of AI in oncologic imaging and diagnostics. Their findings highlight how radiomics and AI-guided workflows contribute to narrowing diagnostic uncertainty in highly complex cases.

Finally, Bennett et al. [48] present an updated systematic review on breast cancer screening, emphasizing not only the evolving evidence base but also the implications for national screening guidelines. Although AI is not the central focus, the review acknowledges the increasing relevance of technology-assisted strategies in improving early detection, reinforcing the system-level integration of AI into preventive health efforts.

Table 1 presents the common themes that emerged from the included studies concerning the application of AI in mammographic practice.

Table 1. Common themes identified across included systematic reviews.

Common Theme	Summary	Key References
Reader cancer detection comparison	Most systematic reviews explore AI systems that show comparable sensitivity and specificity to radiologists in mammography and suggest they are an advanced technique for cancer detection.	[21,22,24,29,31,32,34–36,40–46,48]
Radiologist workload reduction	AI can triage low-risk mammograms, thereby reducing the number of images requiring human interpretation without compromising sensitivity.	[21,30,31]
Error types	AI errors are typically quantified in terms of false positives and negatives, which vary based on positivity thresholds, algorithm version, and study quality.	[23]
Ethical implication	Many studies explore the ethical implication, challenges and frameworks on the use of AI software in clinical practice.	[29,36,37]
Methodological limitations	Many studies are retrospective, with concerns about bias, limited generalizability, and the inconsistent reporting of accuracy metrics, highlighting the necessity of performing more rigorous prospective studies.	[24,29,32–34,45,47]
Combined AI and radiologist performance	The integration of AI with radiologist interpretation frequently results in improved diagnostic accuracy compared to using radiologists alone.	[26,34,35]
Prospective and future applications	AI technology shows promise for future risk-based screening, early detection, and personalized screening strategies based on imaging features.	[27,29,37,38,44]
Performance on advanced imaging technique	AI has been applied to modalities such as DBT and CEM, showing promising yet preliminary results.	[22,38,40,45]

AI: artificial intelligence; CEM: contrast-enhanced mammography; DBT: digital breast tomosynthesis.

Table 2 goes deep into technological implementations and details on AI applications. Numerous studies have explored and confirmed the potential of artificial intelligence (AI) to improve the early diagnosis of breast cancer through mammography. AI is primarily applied to assist the reading of radiographic images, reduce the workload of radiologists, improve diagnostic sensitivity and specificity, and reduce false positives that cause unnecessary recalls and anxiety in patients [21,22,30].

Diagnostic Performance and Types of Algorithms

AI developed for mammography typically employs machine learning (ML) and deep learning (DL) models, with the widespread use of convolutional neural networks (CNNs) for automated image analysis [33,42]. CNNs demonstrate superior performance compared to other techniques such as artificial neural networks (ANNs) or support vector machines (SVMs), reaching sensitivity over 95% and AUC (area under the ROC curve) values close to 0.97 [33].

Most studies evaluate AI algorithms either as standalone systems or in combination with clinical assessment by radiologists [22,26,34]. Meta-analytic results indicate that standalone algorithms can match or surpass radiologists' sensitivity, though often with slightly lower specificity, while the human–machine combination tends to improve overall accuracy [22,34].

Reduction in False Positives and Workload

A key feature of AI is its ability to significantly reduce false positives, with reductions reported up to 69% [30]. This has a strong clinical impact as it lowers unnecessary recalls, improving the cost-effectiveness of screening. Additionally, deep learning-based systems have been studied as triage tools capable of excluding low-risk cases, reducing the radiologist's workload by up to 68% without compromising sensitivity, which remains above 90% [31].

Datasets and Generalizability

A critical issue highlighted is the quality and representativeness of datasets used to train and validate AI models. Many datasets are private, with poor or absent demographic descriptions, limiting the generalizability and fairness of AI across diverse populations [25]. Moreover, variability in algorithm performance based on population and clinical setting underscores the need for external and multicenter validations, which remain infrequent [26,34].

Errors and Technical Challenges

AI is not free from errors, with frequent false positives and false negatives depending on decision thresholds and algorithm versions [23]. Some reviews also report a lack of transparency and difficulty in explainability of AI decisions, which is an important limitation for clinical adoption and operator trust [35,37].

Clinical Integration and Governance

The literature emphasizes the complexity of integrating AI into mammographic screening workflows due to factors such as technological interoperability, staff training, regulation, and ethical and legal issues [27,36]. Governance frameworks based on evidence standards, continuous monitoring, and strategies to build trust are necessary for safe and sustainable AI adoption [36].

Multidisciplinary Applications and Future Perspectives

Beyond mammography, AI is also applied to complementary imaging modalities such as digital breast tomosynthesis, magnetic resonance imaging, and ultrasound, often integrating radiomics and radio genomics techniques for more accurate diagnosis and personalized risk stratification [38–40]. The combined use of clinical, genomic, and imaging data through deep learning models promises to transform breast cancer management, from early diagnosis to prognosis and treatment.

Table 2. Insights on the use of AI and on technological integration.

Ref.	Brief Description	AI Applications and Technical Details
[21]	Systematic review on AI in screening mammography focusing on diagnostic accuracy, reductions in false positives, and radiologist support. Analyzes 13 studies on AI performance in breast cancer detection.	AI algorithms assist in mammography readings, sometimes outperforming double radiologist readings. Techniques improve specificity, reduce unnecessary recalls, and lower workload. Challenges include false positives and variation in performance across demographics.
[22]	Meta-analysis assessing standalone AI performance in digital mammography and digital breast tomosynthesis (DBT) screening. Includes 16 studies with over 1 million exams.	Standalone AI evaluated via reader and cohort studies. AI shows higher AUC than radiologists in digital mammography and DBT. AI demonstrates higher sensitivity but lower specificity compared to radiologists. Uses QUADAS-2 for study quality assessment.

Table 2. *Cont.*

Ref.	Brief Description	AI Applications and Technical Details
[23]	Systematic review focusing on error types and frequencies in AI mammography readings, analyzing false-positive and false-negative rates across 7 retrospective studies.	Errors analyzed include false positives and false negatives varying by AI threshold and algorithm version. Meta-analysis of pooled error rates conducted. Sparse reporting of other AI error types such as location or technical errors.
[24]	Systematic review of AI test accuracy in breast cancer screening programs including 12 studies (131,822 women). Examines AI alone or combined with radiologists.	Most AI systems less accurate than single radiologists and far less than double readings. Some small studies show promise in lab settings. AI used for triage screens out low-risk women but can miss some cancers. No prospective clinical studies found. QUADAS-2 tool used for quality assessment.
[25]	Review of mammography datasets used in AI development, focusing on dataset diversity, inclusivity, traceability, and accessibility.	Identifies 254 datasets with most privately held; poor demographic reporting (race/ethnicity, sex/gender). Highlights global representation gaps and documentation transparency issues, impacting AI model generalizability and fairness.
[26]	Systematic review of external validation studies for AI algorithms in mammography breast cancer screening (30 studies, 2014–2024).	AI algorithms demonstrate comparable AUC and sensitivity to radiologists alone. Combining AI with radiologists improves accuracy statistically. Studies include diverse populations and validation datasets. Emphasizes need for external validation.
[27]	Systematic review on integration of AI in breast cancer screening workflows, focusing on clinical implementation challenges and real-world performance.	Discusses AI deployment in clinical settings, highlighting variability in algorithm performance, integration with radiologists, regulatory considerations, and workflow optimization. Emphasizes importance of prospective studies and continuous monitoring of AI tools.
[28]	Systematic review of AI applied to medical imaging research in Italy (2015–2020). Main imaging modalities: MRI (44%), CT (12%), radiography/mammography (11%). Focuses on neurological diseases (29%) and cancer diagnosis (25%). AI tasks: classification (57%), segmentation (16%). Methods: 65% machine learning, 35% deep learning. Rapid growth in AI research observed.	AI used primarily for image classification and segmentation across multiple imaging modalities. Machine learning and deep learning models analyzed. Emphasis on building common frameworks, data sharing, and collaborations.
[29]	Review of AI advancements in breast cancer detection and treatment, highlighting shift from CAD to AI-based methods. Discusses challenges like data quality, regulation, ethics, and validation. Promising potential to improve early diagnosis and patient outcomes.	AI applications in automated interpretation of mammograms and tomosynthesis. Deep learning methods improve accuracy and efficiency in detection. Challenges include algorithm validation and clinical integration.
[30]	Systematic review of AI in mammography focusing on diagnosis and prediction of breast malignancies. Reports reduction in false positives (up to 69%) and increased sensitivity (84–91%). AI models can independently classify suspicious findings comparable to radiologists.	Machine learning models applied to reduce radiologist workload, improve diagnosis accuracy, and predict breast cancer risk. Calls for larger prospective studies to confirm clinical utility.

Table 2. *Cont.*

Ref.	Brief Description	AI Applications and Technical Details
[31]	Meta-analysis on deep learning (DL) software for triaging breast cancer screening mammograms. Shows 68.3% reduction in radiologist workload with 93.1% sensitivity. Highlights complexity of AI implementation but promising healthcare optimization.	DL algorithms used for triage of mammograms to exclude low-risk cases, maintaining high sensitivity. Meta-analysis of commercially available DL software with performance metrics reported.
[32]	Systematic review and meta-analysis of standalone machine learning (ML) algorithms for screening mammography workflow. ML algorithms achieve or exceed human reader performance with pooled sensitivity of 75.4%, specificity of 90.6%, AUC of 0.89.	Standalone ML models for mammogram detection and triage, evaluated independently from human readers. Evidence based on retrospective studies; external prospective validation needed.
[33]	Meta-analysis of ML methods (CNN, ANN, SVM) in mammography diagnosis for breast cancer screening. CNN showed highest sensitivity (96.1%), specificity (95.0%) and AUC (0.974). Emphasizes need for prospective studies.	Evaluation of different ML methods for breast cancer diagnosis on mammography images. CNNs demonstrate superior performance compared to ANN and SVM.
[34]	Systematic review of independent external validation studies of AI algorithms for screening mammography. Some AI algorithms improve accuracy over radiologists alone; combined AI and radiologist interpretation shows further improvement.	External validation of commercial AI tools for mammography cancer detection. Studies include retrospective reader and simulation designs. AI improves diagnostic accuracy, especially when combined with radiologists.
[35]	Systematic review evaluating reproducibility and explainability of deep learning in mammography for breast cancer detection. Found high risk of bias in most studies; only few of adequate quality. Common architectures include ResNet and RetinaNet. Highest AUC reported was ~0.945. Combined AI and radiologist readings improve performance. Lack of explainability and real-world interaction studies noted.	Analysis of deep learning models' reproducibility and clinical validity. Emphasis on need for explainable AI and real-world validation. Ensemble models and patch classifiers common. Highest diagnostic performance when AI assists radiologists.
[36]	Systematic review identifying challenges in AI implementation for breast cancer screening. Key issues: reproducibility, evidentiary standards, tech integration, trust, ethics, legal and societal concerns. Uses CFIR framework to propose governance strategies.	Mainly AI in mammography (19 studies) and ultrasound (1 study). Highlights needs for robust evidence, trust-building, addressing ethical/legal aspects, and structured governance. CFIR helps map challenges to solutions for clinical adoption.
[37]	Review of explainable AI (XAI) methods applied to breast cancer diagnosis via mammography and ultrasound. Investigates evaluation methods, ethical challenges, and trust in XAI systems.	Analyzes 14 studies on XAI for breast cancer imaging. Finds limited evaluation of user trust and confidence. Dataset quality and related issues highlighted as key research gaps. Calls for systematic evaluation of XAI trustworthiness in clinical settings.
[38]	Systematic review on machine learning and deep learning for breast cancer risk prediction using imaging, radiomics, genomics, and clinical data. Discusses current approaches and future potential.	Covers 20 studies using DL models for personalized risk prediction integrating multi-modal data. Explores NLP applications on imaging and non-imaging features to improve clinical decision-making. Provides overview for researchers on AI risk assessment techniques.

Table 2. *Cont.*

Ref.	Brief Description	AI Applications and Technical Details
[39]	Systematic review and meta-analysis on radiomics to differentiate benign and malignant breast lesions. Assesses diagnostic accuracy across imaging modalities including MRI, mammography, ultrasound, and CT.	Includes 31 studies with 8773 patients. Radiomics showed high sensitivity and specificity across MRI, mammography, and ultrasound, with CT data limited. Supports radiomics as promising adjunct or alternative diagnostic tool, while biopsy remains gold standard.
[40]	Comprehensive review of deep learning, radiomics, and radiogenomics applications in digital breast tomosynthesis (DBT). Focus on DBT's potential for enhanced early breast cancer detection.	Thirty studies reviewed on DL, radiomics, and radiogenomics applied to DBT, synthetic mammography, and full-field digital mammography. Emphasizes interdisciplinary approaches and new model development for clinical deployment of AI in DBT imaging.
[41]	Systematic review of deep learning in breast cancer detection using multiple imaging modalities. Discusses limitations of current manual analysis and benefits of AI-assisted interpretation.	Reviews latest AI and DL models across mammograms, ultrasound, MRI, and histopathology images. Reports on datasets and algorithm development supporting early detection and improved diagnostic accuracy. Highlights AI's role in reducing false positives and improving efficiency.
[42]	Systematic review of ML and DL for breast cancer detection using mammographic data. Highlights evolution from traditional ML to deep learning improving CAD systems.	Deep learning methods (CNNs, deep feature learning) enhance diagnostic accuracy in breast cancer CAD; issues include data scarcity and computational cost, mitigated by data augmentation and improved DL architectures.
[43]	Systematic review of machine learning CAD systems for breast cancer using various imaging modalities.	Analysis of ML classifiers and image modalities for breast cancer detection; discussion on improving CAD systems objectivity and efficiency.
[44]	Review on infrared breast thermography for early breast cancer detection, covering image acquisition, segmentation, feature extraction, and classification.	Use of artificial neural networks to improve thermographic image classification; numerical simulation to reduce false positives; ML techniques for real-time applications recommended.
[45]	Systematic review on deep learning applications in contrast-enhanced mammography (CEM).	CNN models dominate; used for lesion classification, detection, segmentation; attention mechanisms improve accuracy; integration with radiomics and radiologist assessments enhances diagnostic performance; mostly retrospective studies, need for prospective validation.
[46]	Meta-analysis of AI-assisted mammography and prognostic role of Systemic Immune–Inflammation Index (SII) in breast cancer.	AI shows high diagnostic accuracy (AUC up to 0.93), reduces radiologist workload and improves detection in dense breasts. SII is prognostic biomarker linked to survival. Challenges include cut-off variability and need for prospective studies.
[47]	Systematic review on imaging modalities for cancer of unknown primary (CUP).	Use of CT, MRI, FDG-PET/CT, emerging whole-body MRI, FAPI-PET/CT, AI and radiomics to improve detection and characterization of primary tumors; evolving imaging tech increases diagnostic precision.
[48]	Systematic review update on breast cancer screening informing Canadian guidelines. Although not focused solely on mammography, this study offers important updated evidence on breast cancer screening, helping to contextualize AI's role within current screening guidelines.	Machine learning employed to prioritize screening literature; synthesis of RCT and observational data on screening benefits and harms; ML used in research prioritization.

3.3. Opportunities and Challenges for Applying Artificial Intelligence in Mammography

The incorporation of AI in mammography is transforming breast cancer screening and diagnosis. Whereas AI has huge potential for enhanced diagnostic accuracy, streamlined processes, and personalized care, its clinical deployment is qualified by issues related to data representativeness, regulations, and credibility.

One of its most promising advantages is improved diagnostic performance. Some studies demonstrate that deep learning models, namely convolutional neural networks (CNNs), are comparable to, if not better than, experienced radiologists. For example, Liu et al. reported that CNN-based models achieve an AUC value of 0.974, outperforming conventional ML algorithms such as support vector machines and artificial neural networks (ANNs) [33]. Similarly, Yoon et al. found that independent AI models performed better than radiologists on DBT alone, achieving a higher AUC (0.90 vs. 0.79), although specificity was slightly lower [22]. These results reflect the promise of AI to improve the early detection of cancer, a key factor in patient outcomes.

AI may also reduce radiologists' workload, a major problem in high-volume screening programs. Several systematic reviews reported that the use of AI-assisted triage systems can reliably rule out 68% of low-risk mammograms, with diagnostic sensitivity exceeding 90% [31,32]. Improving workflow in this way not only reduces the burden on medical staff but also increases efficiency and potentially reduces report turnaround time.

Personalized risk prediction is another new possibility. Standard models typically use clinical and demographic information—such as breast density, family history and age—to predict a woman's risk of breast cancer later in life. However, AI models based directly on mammography images offer better predictive ability [27,28].

In addition, AI can support a radiologist's assessment if it is used as a complement, not a substitute. Castelo Branco et al. and Anderson et al. concluded in their systematic reviews that performance regularly improved when human interpretation and AI were used together and that improvements in AUC ranged from 0.02 to 0.13 [26,34].

In addition, AI is regularly applied to other advanced imaging modalities. Sorin et al. show that CNN-based algorithms have already achieved AUCs of 0.99 or higher when retrospectively analyzing CEM [45]. The future of AI-assisted mammography beyond routine 2D mammography seems clear, especially for more complex imaging conditions such as DBT and CE mammography.

Despite these encouraging developments, significant challenges remain. The biggest obstacle is the lack of validation and generalization beyond training and test data. As highlighted by Freeman et al. and Anderson et al., most studies to date are retrospective and based on highly curated data that are not rich in natural diversity and complexity [24,34]. In the absence of large prospective studies, it is difficult to assess performance in routine clinical practice, where data heterogeneity and variability in surgery cannot be avoided.

The representativeness of the dataset is another related and equally important problem. Laws et al. explain that only 12% of the datasets used for training AI are related to ethnicity or ethnicity and the data are mainly from high-income areas such as Europe, North America and East Asia [25]. Such non-diversification may lead to biases in the AI training algorithms, which could then perform worse in unrepresented populations.

Ethical, legal and regulatory issues also limit the use of AI. The review by Goh et al. has identified several main problems, including inadequate frameworks, uncertainties regarding liability for errors in algorithms and the protection of patient data privacy [36]. In addition, there is the difficulty of establishing universal standards for the safety and performance of AI models. In most countries, regulatory standards for the use of medical image AI are either underdeveloped or unevenly enforced. Finally, the heterogeneity of technologies contributes to the overall complexity of the field. As documented by Batchu et al. and Madani et al. the use of different AI architectures, imaging modalities, and validation methods hampers direct comparison across studies and prevents meaningful synthesis of results [30,41].

Overall, AI holds great potential for mammographic imaging, from improved diagnostic accuracy to personalized screening protocols and reduced clinician burden. However, realizing these benefits comes with significant hurdles in terms of data diversity, explainability, approvability and clinical validation. The potential integration of AI into breast screening soon will depend on interdisciplinary collaboration between clinicians, data scientists, regulators and ethicists. Only through multilateral collaboration can AI be transitioned from an experimental promise to routine clinical practice in a safe, fair and trustworthy manner.

Figure 1 presents a graphical summary of the key challenges and opportunities previously described regarding the application of AI technology in mammography imaging.

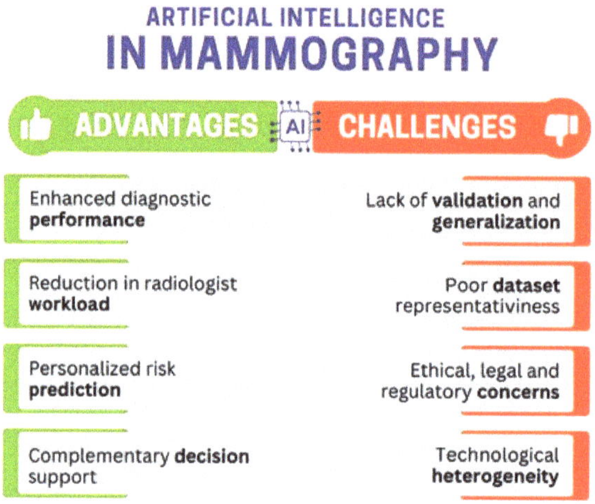

Figure 1. Graphical summary of key opportunities and challenges in applying AI to mammography imaging.

4. Discussion

4.1. Current Trends and Evidence Synthesis on AI Applications in Mammography

In recent years, the application of artificial intelligence (AI) in mammography has attracted growing attention from researchers, clinicians, and healthcare stakeholders alike. This surge reflects the promise of AI to enhance breast cancer detection, improve diagnostic accuracy, and alleviate the workload on radiologists. The field has experienced a rapid expansion in scientific publications, fueled by technological advancements, the availability of large, annotated imaging datasets, and increased computational capabilities.

A search for studies combining the terms "mammography" and "artificial intelligence" reveals an impressive growth in publications over the last three decades, with over 75% of the research produced in just the past ten years and 60% in the last five years alone. This trend mirrors the broader momentum in AI applications within radiology and oncology, where similar exponential growth patterns are observed.

Several factors have contributed to this accelerated development. Advances in deep learning algorithms and imaging technology, alongside global digital health initiatives, have paved the way for innovative AI tools in breast cancer screening. The COVID-19 pandemic further acted as a catalyst, compelling healthcare systems worldwide to adopt digital solutions for maintaining diagnostic services amid workforce challenges and social distancing requirements.

To provide a comprehensive synthesis of the rapidly growing but fragmented literature, a narrative review was conducted. This review aimed to integrate existing systematic reviews and meta-analyses on AI applications in mammography, thereby overcoming the heterogeneity and methodological variability of individual studies. By analyzing 28 systematic reviews, the narrative review offers a higher-level perspective that consolidates diverse data sources and highlights both consensus and gaps in current knowledge.

The added value of this narrative review lies in several key aspects: first, its capacity to assess the robustness of evidence across varied populations, AI models, and clinical settings, thus offering guidance for future research priorities and clinical implementation strategies; second, its identification of methodological strengths and limitations that inform best practices for AI validation; third, its comprehensive evaluation of AI's impact on radiologist workload and diagnostic performance; and finally, its critical examination of challenges related to algorithm explainability, data bias, and regulatory frameworks

This multi-dimensional analysis is crucial for translating AI innovations into safe, effective, and equitable clinical tools.

Key findings from the synthesized systematic reviews and meta-analyses confirm that AI holds significant potential to improve diagnostic sensitivity, reduce radiologists' workload, and optimize clinical workflows. For instance, Abu Abeelh and Abuabeileh [21] and Yoon et al. [22] report that AI systems can match or even outperform radiologists in breast cancer screening, though limitations remain concerning false positives and false negatives. Zeng et al. [23] further emphasize that AI errors are mostly related to false-positive and false-negative rates, which are influenced by threshold settings and different algorithm versions.

Nevertheless, multiple reviews underscore the pressing need for further prospective and standardized studies to validate AI's clinical effectiveness in real-world settings. Freeman et al. [24] and Anderson et al. [34] caution against considering AI as a substitute for radiologists without robust prospective validation, highlighting that most existing evidence derives from retrospective studies with notable methodological limitations. Similarly, Hickman et al. [32] advocate for prospective clinical trials to confirm the promising results generated by machine learning algorithms.

Another important finding pertains to workload reduction for radiologists. Studies such as Batchu et al. [30] and Xavier et al. [31] demonstrate that AI systems—especially those based on deep learning—can effectively triage low-risk mammograms, significantly decreasing the volume of images requiring manual review without compromising diagnostic sensitivity.

A recurrent theme in the literature is the synergistic combination of AI and human radiologists. Many studies indicate that integrating AI outputs with clinical evaluation improves diagnostic performance compared to either AI or radiologists alone [35,36]. However, Goh et al. [36] and Gurmessa and Jimma [37] point out challenges related to the explainability and reproducibility of AI models, which are crucial for clinical acceptance and patient safety. The lack of transparency and biases due to non-representative datasets remain significant hurdles [35,36].

Data quality and representativeness are also critical concerns. Laws et al. [25] highlight significant gaps in available datasets, especially regarding global representativeness and demographic transparency, which are essential for developing equitable and generalizable AI models.

Advances have also been observed in AI applications to advanced mammographic modalities such as digital breast tomosynthesis and contrast-enhanced mammography. In these contexts, the integration of deep learning, radiomics, and radiogenomics has shown promise in enhancing diagnostic accuracy and risk stratification [28,40,45].

From an ethical and regulatory standpoint, Rentiya et al. [29] and Hussain et al. [38] emphasize the need for continued attention to validation processes, privacy concerns, bias mitigation, and governance frameworks to ensure safe and responsible AI deployment in clinical practice.

4.2. Advances in Breast Cancer Research and Mammographic Technologies: The Role of AI

The field of breast cancer research has experienced significant expansion in recent years, driven by rising incidence rates globally and a growing emphasis on early detection, personalized therapies, and improved patient outcomes. Market analyses indicate that the global breast cancer therapeutics sector was valued at approximately USD 29.85 billion in 2023 and is projected to reach around USD 60.78 billion by 2033, growing at a compound annual growth rate (CAGR) of 7.37% from 2024 to 2033 [49].

Concurrently, advancements in mammographic technologies, particularly digital breast tomosynthesis (DBT), are reshaping breast cancer diagnostics. DBT offers improved cancer detection rates and reduced false positives compared to traditional 2D mammography, leading to increased adoption globally. The global mammography market, encompassing imaging hardware, AI-driven software, and related diagnostic services, was valued at over USD 2.93 billion in 2023 and is expected to expand at a CAGR of approximately 8.68% through 2031 [50,51].

Moreover, the integration of artificial intelligence (AI) tools into mammography is accelerating, supporting enhanced image interpretation, risk assessment, and workflow efficiency in clinical settings. The global AI in medical imaging market was valued at USD 1.29 billion in 2023 and is projected to grow by 22.4% to reach USD 1.65 billion in 2024 [52]. Specifically, AI in the mammography sector is forecasted to increase from USD 509.58 million in 2024 to USD 844.52 million by 2034, growing at a CAGR of 3.3% from 2025 to 2034 [53]. This rapid growth is driven by ongoing improvements in deep learning algorithms, expanding annotated imaging datasets, and greater regulatory approvals for AI-assisted diagnostic tools.

These interrelated sectors—breast cancer therapeutics, mammography technologies, and AI integration—are poised for continued expansion as research advances, regulatory approvals progress, and clinical adoption widens. Together, they highlight a rapidly evolving ecosystem focused on improving early detection, diagnostic accuracy, workflow optimization, and ultimately, patient survival and quality of life [49–53].

4.3. Towards Routine Integration: Coordinated Efforts for AI in Mammography

Recent advancements in mammographic technologies combined with the integration of artificial intelligence (AI) are revolutionizing breast cancer diagnostics. However, despite promising developments, several critical challenges must be overcome before AI can be reliably and routinely implemented in clinical practice. Among these challenges, ensuring the quality, representativeness, and diversity of imaging datasets is fundamental to avoid biases and to guarantee algorithmic robustness across different populations and imaging conditions.

Furthermore, AI systems must offer explainability to clinicians to build trust and facilitate transparent diagnostic decisions. Prospective validation in real-world clinical environments remains essential to confirm the clinical utility and safety of these tools. Regulatory frameworks governing AI applications in healthcare are still in a state of flux, requiring clearer guidance to streamline approval and adoption processes while safeguarding patient safety.

Beyond these technical and regulatory concerns, additional factors critically influence the integration of AI in mammography. The impact of AI on radiologist training and continuing education must be carefully considered, as reliance on automated systems could affect the development and maintenance of human diagnostic skills. Moreover, medico-legal responsibilities surrounding AI-assisted diagnoses are complex and need clear definitions to allocate liability appropriately.

Finally, the patient–clinician relationship may evolve with AI involvement. It is imperative to understand how AI influences communication, patient trust, and shared decision-making, ensuring that technology complements rather than compromises the human aspects of care.

Addressing these multifaceted challenges through interdisciplinary research and policy development is vital to harness AI's full potential in breast cancer screening and diagnosis, ensuring equitable, safe, and effective care.

In the United States, the FDA has released a Draft Guidance on Artificial Intelligence-Enabled Device Software Functions, proposing a Total Product Lifecycle (TPLC) regulatory approach which is directly applicable to imaging-based AI systems, including those used in mammography [54]—aspects crucial to ensure the fairness and robustness of AI tools across diverse populations, addressing concerns about dataset bias and algorithmic transparency. Furthermore, in collaboration with Health Canada and the UK's MHRA, the FDA introduced the concept of Predetermined Change Control Plans, designed to manage real-world updates to approved AI tools, including those used in breast imaging workflows [55]—highlighting the need for continuous oversight and adaptive regulation in a rapidly evolving AI landscape, which also raises questions about ongoing medico-legal responsibilities. Professional societies such as the American College of Radiology (ACR) have emphasized that AI in mammography should serve as a decision-support tool—augmenting rather than replacing radiologists—particularly in the role of a second reader [56]—reinforcing the importance of maintaining human oversight and considering the impact of AI on radiologist training and clinical workflows.

In the European Union, the Artificial Intelligence Act—effective from August 2024—classifies AI used in mammography as a high-risk medical application. This mandates strict safeguards, including transparent data handling, human oversight, and ongoing post-deployment monitoring [57,58]—measures that directly address ethical standards and patient safety, while also underscoring challenges in integrating AI without disrupting patient–clinician relationships. Supporting these policies, the European Society of Breast Imaging (EUSOBI) has published guidance specific to the safe and effective adoption of AI in breast imaging. Their initiatives—such as the 2025 symposium "Mammography & Beyond: Special Focus on AI"— represent guidance in evolution and reiterreiterate the importance of integrating AI within evidence-based mammography practices [57]—promoting multidisciplinary collaboration to balance technological innovation with clinical realities.

Across North America and Europe, radiology organizations including the ACR, the Canadian Association of Radiologists (CAR), and the EUSOBI are setting standards for AI implementation in mammography. Their guidelines focus on ensuring image quality, enhancing interpretive accuracy, and improving workflow efficiency. Collaborative projects, such as the ACR's partnership with Densitas, are already contributing to AI-driven quality assurance protocols in mammographic positioning and acquisition [59]—demonstrating practical steps to improve diagnostic performance, yet also requiring consideration of how such tools affect professional roles and responsibilities.

Importantly, the sustained transition from experimental AI tools to routine clinical mammography requires harmonized multistakeholder efforts. Regulatory agencies must maintain flexible yet rigorous approval pathways; scientific societies should generate shared, evidence-based protocols for AI in breast imaging; and large-scale infrastructures such as the UK NHS AI Lab and the European Health Data Space must continue to invest in diverse, multicenter validation initiatives. Notable efforts include the NHS's prospective evaluation of AI tools in large-scale mammography programs, as well as pilot studies at Imperial College London and Leeds Teaching Hospitals, which test AI integration in symptomatic and screening settings [60]—highlighting the importance of prospective clinical validation and large-scale data to support safe and effective AI adoption.

In parallel, it is essential to address less frequently discussed but equally critical challenges such as the impact of AI on radiologist training pathways, the evolving medico-legal responsibilities surrounding AI-assisted diagnoses, and the shifting dynamics in patient–clinician communication and trust.

Altogether, these coordinated developments reflect a growing consensus: fully realizing the clinical promise of AI-enhanced mammography depends on aligned standards, regulatory maturity, and scientifically guided implementation—ensuring that technological progress ultimately translates into better early detection, diagnosis, and outcomes for patients.

4.4. From Promise to Practice: Advancing AI in Mammography Through Trials, Innovation, and Translation

In light of emerging recommendations from systematic reviews—which represent the foundational evidence base of this narrative review—and recent clinical guidelines, it is strategically essential to broaden the scope of analysis by integrating cutting-edge research outputs, especially those arising from prospective clinical trials, randomized controlled trials (RCTs), and the latest studies disseminated through IEEE and ACM conferences and preprint repositories.

The studies included in this analysis were rigorously selected following the search strategy and keyword criteria outlined in Section 2. This approach ensured the inclusion of the most relevant and recent evidence contributing novel insights to the field. Specifically, the selection encompassed systematic reviews and meta-analyses that synthesize current knowledge, alongside prospective clinical trials and RCTs that provide high-level evidence on the clinical efficacy and safety of AI applications in mammography. Additionally, technical papers from IEEE and ACM venues were incorporated to capture recent algorithmic innovations, system design, and implementation challenges that are often not yet reflected in the clinical literature.

This comprehensive integration is crucial for several reasons. First, systematic reviews and clinical guidelines primarily synthesize existing evidence to offer a consolidated understanding of the current state of knowledge, but they often lag behind the most recent technological and methodological innovations due to the inherent delays in publication and guideline updates. Incorporating fresh empirical data from high-quality clinical trials—particularly RCTs—provides robust, prospective, and contextually relevant evidence that can confirm, nuance, or challenge previous conclusions derived from retrospective or more controlled study designs.

Second, studies published in technical forums such as the IEEE and ACM often present novel algorithmic developments, optimization techniques, and real-world implementation insights that are not yet fully captured in traditional systematic reviews. These contributions provide valuable perspectives on practical challenges, including model generalizability across heterogeneous populations and imaging settings, workflow integration, explainability, and human–AI interaction—elements that are critical for successful clinical adoption but frequently under-reported in guideline documents.

Third, preprint platforms accelerate the dissemination of pioneering research, introducing novel approaches and hypotheses that push the boundaries of AI in mammography.

Although these studies require cautious interpretation due to the absence of formal peer review, their early availability promotes timely scientific dialog and can inspire rapid advancements and collaborative validation efforts.

By synergistically combining evidence from systematic reviews, guidelines, prospective trials, technical conference papers, and preprints, this narrative discussion gains a multidimensional perspective. Such a comprehensive approach not only strengthens the robustness of the conclusions but also aligns with the complex, interdisciplinary nature of AI integration in breast cancer screening. It underscores the importance of addressing technical performance alongside clinical, organizational, ethical, and regulatory dimensions, ultimately facilitating the translation of AI innovations into safe, effective, and equitable diagnostic tools.

Bridging Evidence and Practice: What Clinical Trials Reveal About AI in Mammography

While recent guidelines and systematic reviews have thoroughly outlined the technical, ethical, and regulatory barriers to clinical implementation of AI in mammography, prospective clinical trials and RCTs add essential layers of evidence that either reinforce or nuance these concerns [61–73]. First, real-world trials offer a unique opportunity to evaluate AI systems on heterogeneous populations, under non-curated conditions, and with clinical endpoints that go beyond model accuracy. Unlike retrospective studies, which often rely on idealized datasets, these trials can expose the fragility of models when applied across different imaging devices, clinical workflows, and patient demographics.

The MASAI trial [61,69], one of the most robust RCTs to date, exemplifies this transition by demonstrating non-inferiority of AI-supported screening compared to standard double reading. Importantly, the AI-assisted arm maintained sensitivity while significantly reducing reader workload, suggesting a promising avenue to alleviate radiologist shortages without compromising diagnostic accuracy. This type of prospective, population-based evaluation is a crucial milestone toward clinical translation, particularly in settings where human resource constraints threaten the scalability of breast screening programs.

Notably, some RCTs confirm the problem of generalizability, revealing performance drops when AI is tested outside its original training domain—thereby substantiating concerns raised in systematic reviews about dataset representativeness and algorithmic bias [24,25]. For example, while studies like Dembrower et al. [68] and Salim et al. [65] confirmed the high concordance of AI predictions with radiologist assessments in Swedish and Nordic cohorts, similar results are not guaranteed in more diverse or resource-constrained settings. Here, the role of trials is not merely to reproduce findings but to stress-test them under real-world variability.

Moreover, hybrid AI–radiologist workflows, although sometimes associated with improved accuracy, have been found to increase recall rates and workload, potentially leading to overdiagnosis—subtleties that are often overlooked in traditional benchmarking studies. This highlights the importance of outcome measures that extend beyond sensitivity and specificity, incorporating downstream clinical and organizational impacts.

Clinical trials also bring to light pragmatic insights on explainability and usability. While many systematic reviews emphasize the "black box" nature of deep learning, empirical data reveal that explainability tools (e.g., heatmaps or saliency maps) are frequently underutilized or misunderstood by clinicians, limiting their real-world effectiveness. Similarly, integrating AI into existing workflows entails logistical and cognitive burdens not always captured by technical assessments. The multireader study by Rangarajan et al. [64] underscores this by evaluating how AI tools function in educational contexts, offering insights into human–machine interaction beyond diagnostic metrics.

From a regulatory standpoint, trials help inform nuanced risk–benefit analyses and reveal the lack of context-specific evaluation frameworks. Even high-performing AI systems may falter in adoption due to documentation gaps, misalignment with health IT infrastructures, or lack of interoperability standards. In this sense, trials can act as a bridge between laboratory performance and regulatory readiness, identifying implementation bottlenecks early.

Emerging directions such as radiomics-based personalization [67,70] and AI-driven risk stratification [65] show promise in tailoring screening protocols. Yet, these approaches remain at the feasibility stage, and longitudinal outcome data are still scarce. Moreover, the methodological heterogeneity across trials—ranging from prospective paired-reader designs to retrospective validations—makes it difficult to synthesize findings in a standardized way. This calls for harmonized reporting standards and multicenter collaborations to enable meaningful meta-analyses.

Overall, prospective trials and RCTs not only validate or contest prior findings from systematic reviews and guidelines but also shift the conversation toward operational, behavioral, and implementation-related challenges. Bridging the gap between AI potential and clinical trustworthiness requires interdisciplinary collaboration, robust prospective evidence, and attention to the social and organizational dimensions of care.

Based on the current evidence, we recommend several key priorities to accelerate the safe and equitable integration of AI into mammography screening. First, expanding prospective multicenter trials across diverse healthcare systems and patient populations is essential to improve the generalizability of AI models and reduce potential biases. It is also important to incorporate outcome measures that go beyond simple accuracy metrics, including recall rates, workflow efficiency, clinician trust, and patient experience, to fully capture AI's impact in clinical practice.

The standardization of explainability tools and comprehensive clinician training must be prioritized to ensure that healthcare professionals can reliably interpret and trust AI outputs during diagnostic workflows. Furthermore, regulatory alignment should be strengthened by designing clinical trials that proactively address documentation requirements and interoperability standards, facilitating smoother adoption and oversight. Finally, fostering interdisciplinary partnerships among AI developers, clinicians, patients, and policy-makers is critical to ensure that technological innovations are closely aligned with real-world clinical needs and ethical considerations.

Ultimately, clinical trials must evolve from being post hoc validations to becoming proactive instruments of AI co-design, contextualization, and continuous learning in mammographic care.

Next-Gen AI for Mammography: Multimodal Learning and Optimization Strategies

To complement existing systematic reviews and clinical guidelines, recent articles from the ACM Digital Library provide cutting-edge algorithmic innovations and optimization strategies that address practical challenges in mammography AI, offering fresh empirical evidence and highlighting diverse methodological approaches.

Recent advancements in AI-driven mammography diagnosis demonstrate significant progress in addressing the complex challenges of early breast cancer detection, with recent studies exploring multi-granularity, optimization-based, and YOLO-based approaches [74–76], which exemplify different strategies for improving AI-based mammography diagnosis.

Wei and Fan [74] propose a multi-granularity, knowledge-guided multimodal pretraining approach (MM-CLIP) specifically tailored to breast cancer diagnosis. Their method stands out by effectively focusing on the small, complex lesion areas that distinguish mammogram analysis from conventional natural image recognition. By capturing diverse lesion morphologies and accounting for anatomical variability, this approach enhances diagnostic accuracy beyond prior CLIP-based models, marking a promising direction for multimodal AI integration in clinical mammography.

Complementing this, Doma et al. [75] leverage Weighted Particle Swarm Optimization (WPSO) to optimize the extraction of texture features from segmented mammogram images. This approach specifically targets microcalcifications—a critical early sign of breast cancer—enabling more precise classification into normal, benign, or malignant categories. Their AI framework reduces manual diagnostic overhead and supports the rapid detection of cancerous regions in hospital-derived mammogram datasets, highlighting the value of evolutionary optimization techniques in improving diagnostic efficiency and accuracy.

Further advancing the field, using a YOLOv5-based CAD framework, breast masses were detected and classified across multiple datasets, including CBIS-DDSM, VinDr-Mammo, and INBreast, as shown by Aydemir et al. [76]. The approach employed transfer learning and data augmentation to enhance accuracy and generalizability. Fivefold cross-validation yielded mAP around 0.84, with precision up to 0.855 and recall up to 0.787. Testing on MIAS and private clinical datasets confirmed the model's potential to support radiologists in reliable and efficient breast cancer diagnosis [76]. Overall, these studies highlight several critical themes for the application of artificial intelligence in mammography. First, there is a clear need to focus on fine-grained, lesion-level information through multimodal and multi-granularity models to capture the complexity inherent in mammographic images. Additionally, optimization algorithms such as WPSO and Coati play a crucial role in enhancing feature extraction and selection, which directly impacts diagnostic accuracy. Another key advantage comes from hybrid architectures that combine localization, feature extraction, and robust classification to effectively manage the variability and complexity of mammographic data.

Looking ahead, future research and clinical deployment should prioritize further multimodal integration, combining imaging data with clinical and genetic information to develop more contextualized and precise diagnostic models. The prospective validation of these optimized AI models in diverse, real-world clinical settings is essential to ensure their generalizability and operational feasibility. Emphasis must also be placed on interpretability and clinician usability, making sure that AI outputs are actionable and trusted within clinical workflows. Lastly, the development of standardized benchmarking frameworks that incorporate lesion complexity and heterogeneity will be necessary to rigorously compare emerging AI methods and foster progress in the field.

By addressing these challenges, the field can accelerate the transition from promising algorithms to clinically reliable tools that improve breast cancer diagnosis and patient care.

From Lab to Clinic: Usability and Integration Lessons from IEEE Research

A glance at IEEE conference papers offers valuable additions to the knowledge base established by systematic reviews and clinical guidelines by emphasizing technological innovation and practical AI applications in mammography. While systematic reviews and guidelines primarily synthesize and standardize existing evidence to guide clinical practice, IEEE research frequently explores novel methodological approaches and addresses challenges in real-world deployment.

For instance, Islam et al. [77] demonstrate a significant advancement in breast cancer detection accuracy by applying a deep learning approach to the recently released RSNA Screening Mammography dataset. Their study goes beyond prior work by focusing in detail on image preprocessing techniques and the critical factor of breast density, which is often overlooked. By investigating these aspects, they reveal practical ways to enhance AI model performance, achieving a high classification accuracy of 97.6% using a tailored 15-layer CNN. This granular attention to imaging nuances offers a valuable complement to the broader recommendations found in guidelines.

Yang et al. [78] contribute by developing MABEL, an AI-powered mammographic lesion diagnostic system that is specifically designed to integrate seamlessly into clinical workflows. Their system not only reduces radiologists' workload but also accelerates diagnosis through an intuitive doctor-oriented annotation tool and web interface. Furthermore, MABEL's compatibility with hospital Picture Archiving and Communication Systems (PACSs) reflects a mature stage of translational research, emphasizing the importance of usability, scalability, and real-world application—factors that systematic reviews and clinical guidelines typically do not address in depth.

Similarly, Rath et al. [79] provide a comprehensive empirical comparison of multiple AI algorithms and preprocessing strategies for mammogram analysis. By assessing various classification models including SVMs, KNNs, Random Forest, Decision Trees, CNNs, and RCNs, they identify the strengths and limitations of each approach in practical scenarios. Their exploration of image segmentation and feature extraction methods further enriches the understanding of how preprocessing influences diagnostic accuracy. This type of comparative research informs clinicians and developers about optimal AI solutions for implementation, supplementing the evidence summaries provided by systematic reviews.

Together, these IEEE studies exemplify how conference research can push the field forward by introducing innovative methodologies, addressing practical clinical integration challenges, and providing empirical data to guide AI deployment decisions. This approach offers a dynamic perspective on advancing AI-assisted breast cancer diagnosis beyond the scope of traditional evidence synthesis.

The Frontier of Innovation: Emerging Trends in Preprints on AI for Mammography

While peer-reviewed publications remain the cornerstone for establishing reliable evidence and clinical guidelines, recent preprints available on open repositories like arXiv are increasingly shaping the forefront of AI research in mammography. These preprints serve as a valuable window into the very latest innovations and exploratory methodologies, often addressing topics and challenges not yet fully covered in the formal literature. However, it is crucial to interpret their findings with appropriate caution since these studies have not yet undergone thorough peer review or clinical validation, processes essential for confirming reproducibility, robustness, and safety in real-world applications.

The preprints highlighted here reveal several critical and very hot themes currently driving the field forward. For instance, the study by [80] introduces advanced deep learning architectures that aim to significantly improve the precision of lesion detection and characterization. These models incorporate novel feature extraction layers designed to better capture subtle imaging patterns indicative of malignancy. In parallel, ref. [81] explores the integration of clinical metadata—such as patient history and genetic markers—with imaging data, aiming to build more contextualized and personalized diagnostic AI models. This multimodal approach acknowledges the complexity of breast cancer diagnosis beyond image pixels alone.

Additionally, ref. [82] focuses on enhancing the interpretability of AI decisions through innovative attention mechanisms and explainability tools. Given that clinical adoption strongly depends on trust and transparency, such advances are critical to bridging the gap between black-box AI systems and radiologists' workflow. Finally, ref. [83] addresses the challenge of scalability by proposing efficient training strategies that allow AI models to be trained on large, heterogeneous mammography datasets, ensuring broader applicability across diverse populations and imaging devices.

Together, these preprints highlight exciting, forward-looking directions for AI in mammography, ranging from methodological innovation to practical deployment considerations. Nonetheless, to translate these promising research advances into safe and effective clinical tools, it is essential that future work rigorously validate these models through peer review, prospective clinical trials, and real-world implementation studies.

Therefore, we recommend that the AI research community maintain a balanced approach: continue to foster innovation by sharing and discussing preprint findings openly while prioritizing robust validation and interdisciplinary collaboration with clinicians. This pathway will help ensure that novel AI technologies are not only cutting-edge but also trustworthy, equitable, and ultimately beneficial for patient care.

4.5. Limitations

This narrative review synthesizes peer-reviewed systematic reviews and meta-analyses on artificial intelligence (AI) applications in mammography using a structured yet flexible and transparent methodology. Rather than adhering strictly to the format of a fully systematic review, we adopted a narrative review approach to better accommodate the rapidly evolving and highly diverse nature of this field, where AI techniques, clinical applications, and study designs vary widely.

This narrative approach enabled us to capture emerging trends and novel applications of AI that might be overlooked by more rigid frameworks, providing a timely and interpretative synthesis of the current state of the art. While this method does not follow exhaustive search protocols or formal risk-of-bias assessments typical of systematic reviews, we ensured methodological rigor by applying a standardized quality checklist to guide study selection and appraisal, maintaining internal consistency and reliability in the included evidence.

Our literature search focused on major biomedical databases including PubMed, Scopus, and the Web of Science, providing comprehensive coverage of systematic reviews and meta-analyses. To complement this core evidence base, we also incorporated findings and recommendations from clinical practice guidelines, randomized controlled trials (RCTs), and other prospective clinical studies. Additionally, databases such as the IEEE Xplore and ACM Digital Library, as well as preprint servers, were consulted to include the most recent and technologically oriented research outputs. This complementary approach enriched our synthesis by integrating high-level evidence and expert consensus alongside emerging clinical data.

Only English-language publications were included to maintain feasibility, which may have excluded some valuable regional or non-English research. Although access to scientific outputs from radiological and oncological societies in original languages would add further depth, the challenges related to comprehensive retrieval and translation exceed the scope of this broad narrative review and suggest an avenue for future focused studies.

In summary, this review provides a comprehensive and balanced overview of AI's role in mammography screening, highlighting its promising potential supported by a growing and varied evidence base. The integration of systematic reviews, clinical guidelines, RCTs, and other clinical studies forms a robust foundation to inform future research directions, clinical implementation strategies, and policy-making. This collective evidence supports cautious optimism toward AI adoption while emphasizing the need for further high-quality, prospective, multicenter trials to confirm effectiveness and safety in diverse clinical settings.

5. A Final Thought: Beyond the Hype—Unlocking the True Clinical Potential of AI in Mammography Through Multidimensional Evidence

Based on the comprehensive findings of the systematic review and complemented by clinical guidelines, randomized controlled trials (RCTs), prospective studies, emerging methodological innovations, and real-world implementation research, the future of artificial intelligence applied to mammography requires a multidimensional approach that goes well beyond mere technical validation, encompassing clinical, organizational, ethical, and regulatory aspects. The following strategic priorities can be outlined.

Expansion of multicenter prospective clinical trials

To improve the generalizability and robustness of AI models, it is essential to conduct studies on heterogeneous populations in real-world conditions that reflect the diversity of devices, clinical environments, and demographic groups. Only large-scale randomized controlled trials (RCTs) can confirm AI's efficacy and safety compared to established practices, reducing sampling bias and overcoming the limitations of retrospective analyses. *These trials should also address medico-legal responsibilities and accountability in diagnostic decision-making, ensuring clarity on the role of radiologists and AI tools within clinical workflows.*

Adoption of broader clinical and organizational metrics

Traditional diagnostic accuracy measures (sensitivity and specificity) should be integrated with indicators of clinical and organizational impact, such as recall rates, overdiagnosis, radiologist workload, clinician confidence, and patient experience. These endpoints allow the evaluation of AI's real effects on care pathways, avoiding unwanted consequences such as overload or increased false positives. *Importantly, patient-centered outcomes and changes in the patient–clinician relationship must be assessed to preserve trust and shared decision-making.*

Standardization and training on explainability

Explainability tools (e.g., heatmaps) must be standardized and incorporated into dedicated clinical training programs so healthcare professionals can correctly interpret and effectively use them in decision-making, reducing the perception of a "black box" and improving trust in AI. *Enhancing interpretability directly supports radiologist training and mitigates concerns over reliance on opaque algorithms.*

Integration with healthcare systems and interoperability

Clinical trials should include assessments of integration requirements with existing IT infrastructures such as PACSs and electronic health records, as well as adherence to regulatory standards. The lack of interoperability and complete documentation remains a crucial barrier to large-scale clinical adoption. *Moreover, potential disruptions to workflow, increased cognitive load, and risks of clinician burnout must be carefully managed.*

Development and validation of multimodal and personalized models

The future of AI in mammography will move from image-only models to multimodal systems that integrate clinical, genetic, and radiomic data for more precise and personalized diagnosis and risk stratification. These models require rigorous prospective validation and large longitudinal studies to confirm effectiveness and sustainability. *Ethical considerations, including data privacy, informed consent, and equitable access, become increasingly critical as these models incorporate sensitive patient information.*

Algorithmic optimization with evolutionary and hybrid methods

The adoption of advanced optimization techniques (e.g., Particle Swarm Optimization, Coati Optimization) and hybrid architectures (e.g., YOLOv7 + UNet) could represent an important direction to improve feature extraction, lesion localization, and classification, increasing accuracy and clinical reliability. *However, greater algorithmic complexity heightens the need for explainability and regulatory scrutiny.*

Research on hybrid workflows and human–machine interaction

New studies should explore how workflows integrating AI and radiologists affect not only diagnostic outcomes but also clinical organization and recall decisions. Understanding cognitive and organizational dynamics is essential to avoid overload and ensure effective and sustainable AI use. *This includes clarifying roles and responsibilities and understanding impacts on patient communication and shared decision-making.*

Interdisciplinary collaboration and stakeholder engagement

The development, validation, and implementation of AI in mammography require close collaboration among developers, clinicians, patients, regulators, and policymakers. This co-design approach fosters technological solutions that address real clinical needs, are ethically sustainable, and facilitate adoption in diverse healthcare settings. *The early engagement of patients and clinicians helps build trust and align expectations.*

Adoption of standardized reporting and benchmarking frameworks

To enable objective comparisons and shared progress, common standards are needed for reporting clinical trial results and performance studies, accounting for lesion complexity, data heterogeneity, and population variability. *Transparent reporting supports regulatory oversight and addresses reproducibility concerns.*

From post hoc validations to trials as tools for co-design and continuous learning

Clinical trials must evolve from simple validation tools to dynamic platforms for the co-design, adaptation, and continuous monitoring of AI performance, promoting constant model updates based on real-world data and clinical feedback. *This dynamic approach is crucial for managing algorithm updates and maintaining compliance with evolving ethical and legal frameworks.*

Overall, the transition from the "promised AI" to "clinical practice" in mammography requires a holistic and integrated approach that combines robust prospective evidence from systematic reviews, clinical guidelines, RCTs, and real-world studies with algorithmic innovation, usability focus, and strong interdisciplinary collaboration. *Addressing training needs, medico-legal challenges, organizational changes, and patient–clinician dynamics is essential to develop AI diagnostic tools that are reliable, safe, sustainable, and truly beneficial for patients.*

6. Conclusions

This narrative review is grounded in a comprehensive analysis of 28 systematic reviews and meta-analyses that evaluate the role of artificial intelligence (AI) in mammography. These high-level evidence syntheses collectively highlight a promising potential for AI technologies to improve diagnostic accuracy, sensitivity, and specificity in breast cancer screening compared to conventional methods. The integration of AI-assisted tools demonstrates encouraging advancements in lesion detection, reductions in false positives, and improved workflow efficiency. Complementing these syntheses, this review also examined available randomized controlled trials (RCTs) and other clinical studies investigating AI applications in mammographic screening. Although these prospective studies provide initial empirical support for AI's clinical utility, they remain limited in number, sample size, and methodological rigor. Many clinical investigations suffer from short follow-up durations, inconsistent outcome measures, and varying definitions of performance metrics, which restrict the generalizability of their findings. Moreover, a significant challenge identified across the evidence base is the heterogeneity of study designs, AI algorithms, datasets, and population characteristics. Retrospective data predominates the field, often lacking standardized protocols and blinded assessments, which can introduce bias and limit reproducibility. The variability in AI model training and validation strategies further complicates direct comparisons and the aggregation of results. Given these limitations, the current body of evidence, while promising, is insufficient to support broad implementation of AI systems in routine mammographic screening. There is a pressing need for rigorously designed, large-scale, multicenter prospective trials that adopt harmonized methodologies and standardized outcome reporting. Such studies are essential to accurately assess AI's clinical impact, safety, and cost-effectiveness across diverse healthcare settings. In addition to clinical validation, future research should also address ethical considerations, data privacy, and the practical challenges of integrating AI tools within existing diagnostic workflows. Transparency in AI decision-making processes and user training will be critical to foster clinician trust and optimize patient outcomes. In summary, this narrative review underscores AI's potential to transform breast cancer screening but advocates for a cautious and evidence-driven approach. Prioritizing high-quality prospective research and comprehensive evaluation frameworks will enable the responsible adoption of AI technologies, ensuring they deliver genuine clinical benefit while minimizing risks and disparities.

Supplementary Materials: The following supporting information can be downloaded at https://www.mdpi.com/article/10.3390/diagnostics15172197/s1, Table S1. Outcome of the assessment. Box S1. Used search keys in Section 3.1.

Funding: This research received no external funding. The APC was funded by Daniele Giansanti.

Institutional Review Board Statement: Not applicable.

Informed Consent Statement: Not applicable.

Data Availability Statement: Not applicable.

Conflicts of Interest: The authors declare no conflict of interest.

References

1. Available online: https://gco.iarc.who.int/media/globocan/factsheets/cancers/20-breast-fact-sheet.pdf (accessed on 12 July 2025).
2. Available online: https://www.who.int/news-room/fact-sheets/detail/breast-cancer (accessed on 12 July 2025).
3. Arnold, M.; Morgan, E.; Rumgay, H.; Mafra, A.; Singh, D.; Laversanne, M.; Vignat, J.; Gralow, J.R.; Cardoso, F.; Siesling, S.; et al. Current and future burden of breast cancer: Global statistics for 2020 and 2040. *Breast* **2022**, *66*, 15–23. [CrossRef] [PubMed] [PubMed Central]
4. Yersal, O.; Barutca, S. Biological subtypes of breast cancer: Prognostic and therapeutic implications. *World J. Clin. Oncol.* **2014**, *5*, 412–424. [CrossRef] [PubMed] [PubMed Central]
5. Ginsburg, O.; Yip, C.H.; Brooks, A.; Cabanes, A.; Caleffi, M.; Dunstan Yataco, J.A.; Gyawali, B.; McCormack, V.; McLaughlin de Anderson, M.; Mehrotra, R.; et al. Breast cancer early detection: A phased approach to implementation. *Cancer* **2020**, *126* (Suppl. 10), 2379–2393. [CrossRef] [PubMed] [PubMed Central]
6. Nicosia, L.; Gnocchi, G.; Gorini, I.; Venturini, M.; Fontana, F.; Pesapane, F.; Abiuso, I.; Bozzini, A.C.; Pizzamiglio, M.; Latronico, A.; et al. History of Mammography: Analysis of Breast Imaging Diagnostic Achievements over the Last Century. *Healthcare* **2023**, *11*, 1596. [CrossRef] [PubMed]
7. Gold, R.H. The evolution of mammography. *Radiol. Clin. N. Am.* **1992**, *30*, 1–19. [CrossRef] [PubMed]
8. Available online: https://cdas.cancer.gov/hipb/ (accessed on 12 July 2025).
9. Joe, B.N.; Sickles, E.A. The evolution of breast imaging: Past to present. *Radiology* **2014**, *273* (Suppl. 2), S23–S44. [CrossRef] [PubMed]
10. Available online: https://www.radiologyinfo.org/en/info/tomosynthesis (accessed on 12 July 2025).
11. Doi, K. Computer-aided diagnosis in medical imaging: Historical review, current status and future potential. *Comput. Med. Imaging Graph.* **2007**, *31*, 198–211. [CrossRef] [PubMed] [PubMed Central]
12. Freer, T.W.; Ulissey, M.J. Screening mammography with computer-aided detection: Prospective study of 12,860 patients in a community breast center. *Radiology* **2001**, *220*, 781–786. [CrossRef] [PubMed]
13. McKinney, S.M.; Sieniek, M.; Godbole, V.; Godwin, J.; Antropova, N.; Ashrafian, H.; Back, T.; Chesus, M.; Corrado, G.S.; Darzi, A.; et al. International evaluation of an AI system for breast cancer screening. *Nature* **2020**, *577*, 89–94. [CrossRef]
14. Lehman, C.D.; Wellman, R.D.; Buist, D.S.; Kerlikowske, K.; Tosteson, A.N.; Miglioretti, D.L.; Breast Cancer Surveillance Consortium. Diagnostic Accuracy of Digital Screening Mammography with and Without Computer-Aided Detection. *JAMA Intern. Med.* **2015**, *175*, 1828–1837. [CrossRef] [PubMed] [PubMed Central]
15. Printz, C. Cancer organizations, institutions mobilize together during the COVID-19 pandemic: When confronted with myriad patient and provider challenges, the international cancer community launched multiple collaborations. *Cancer* **2021**, *127*, 825–826. [CrossRef] [PubMed] [PubMed Central]
16. Dang, L.A.; Chazard, E.; Poncelet, E.; Serb, T.; Rusu, A.; Pauwels, X.; Parsy, C.; Poclet, T.; Cauliez, H.; Engelaere, C.; et al. Impact of artificial intelligence in breast cancer screening with mammography. *Breast Cancer* **2022**, *29*, 967–977. [CrossRef] [PubMed] [PubMed Central]
17. Richman, I.; Tessier-Sherman, B.; Galusha, D.; Oladele, C.R.; Wang, K. Breast cancer screening during the COVID-19 pandemic: Moving from disparities to health equity. *J. Natl. Cancer Inst.* **2023**, *115*, 139–145. [CrossRef] [PubMed] [PubMed Central]

18. Kufel, J.; Bargieł-Łączek, K.; Kocot, S.; Koźlik, M.; Bartnikowska, W.; Janik, M.; Czogalik, Ł.; Dudek, P.; Magiera, M.; Lis, A.; et al. What Is Machine Learning, Artificial Neural Networks and Deep Learning?—Examples of Practical Applications in Medicine. *Diagnostics* **2023**, *13*, 2582. [CrossRef] [PubMed]
19. Shifa, N.; Saleh, M.; Akbari, Y.; Al Maadeed, S. A review of explainable AI techniques and their evaluation in mammography for breast cancer screening. *Clin. Imaging* **2025**, *123*, 110492. [CrossRef] [PubMed]
20. Cerdas, M.G.; Farhat, J.; Elshafie, S.I.; Mariyam, F.; James, L.; Qureshi, A.K.; Potru, M.; Paliwei, P.; Joshi, M.R.; Abraham, G.; et al. Exploring the Evolution of Breast Cancer Imaging: A Review of Conventional and Emerging Modalities. *Cureus* **2025**, *17*, e82762. [CrossRef] [PubMed] [PubMed Central]
21. Abu Abeelh, E.; Abuabeileh, Z. Screening Mammography and Artificial Intelligence: A Comprehensive Systematic Review. *Cureus* **2025**, *17*, e79353. [CrossRef] [PubMed] [PubMed Central]
22. Yoon, J.H.; Strand, F.; Baltzer, P.A.T.; Conant, E.F.; Gilbert, F.J.; Lehman, C.D.; Morris, E.A.; Mullen, L.A.; Nishikawa, R.M.; Sharma, N.; et al. Standalone AI for Breast Cancer Detection at Screening Digital Mammography and Digital Breast Tomosynthesis: A Systematic Review and Meta-Analysis. *Radiology* **2023**, *307*, e222639. [CrossRef] [PubMed] [PubMed Central]
23. Zeng, A.; Houssami, N.; Noguchi, N.; Nickel, B.; Marinovich, M.L. Frequency and characteristics of errors by artificial intelligence (AI) in reading screening mammography: A systematic review. *Breast Cancer Res. Treat.* **2024**, *207*, 1–13. [CrossRef] [PubMed] [PubMed Central]
24. Freeman, K.; Geppert, J.; Stinton, C.; Todkill, D.; Johnson, S.; Clarke, A.; Taylor-Phillips, S. Use of artificial intelligence for image analysis in breast cancer screening programmes: Systematic review of test accuracy. *BMJ* **2021**, *374*, n1872. [CrossRef] [PubMed] [PubMed Central]
25. Laws, E.; Palmer, J.; Alderman, J.; Sharma, O.; Ngai, V.; Salisbury, T.; Hussain, G.; Ahmed, S.; Sachdeva, G.; Vadera, S.; et al. Diversity, inclusivity and traceability of mammography datasets used in development of Artificial Intelligence technologies: A systematic review. *Clin. Imaging* **2025**, *118*, 110369. [CrossRef] [PubMed]
26. Branco, P.E.S.C.; Franco, A.H.S.; de Oliveira, A.P.; Carneiro, I.M.C.; de Carvalho, L.M.C.; de Souza, J.I.N.; Leandro, D.R.; Cândido, E.B. Artificial intelligence in mammography: A systematic review of the external validation. *Rev. Bras. Ginecol. Obstet.* **2024**, *46*, e-rbgo71. [CrossRef] [PubMed] [PubMed Central]
27. Schopf, C.M.; Ramwala, O.A.; Lowry, K.P.; Hofvind, S.; Marinovich, M.L.; Houssami, N.; Elmore, J.G.; Dontchos, B.N.; Lee, J.M.; Lee, C.I. Artificial Intelligence-Driven Mammography-Based Future Breast Cancer Risk Prediction: A Systematic Review. *J. Am. Coll. Radiol.* **2024**, *21*, 319–328. [CrossRef] [PubMed] [PubMed Central]
28. Avanzo, M.; Porzio, M.; Lorenzon, L.; Milan, L.; Sghedoni, R.; Russo, G.; Massafra, R.; Fanizzi, A.; Barucci, A.; Ardu, V.; et al. Artificial intelligence applications in medical imaging: A review of the medical physics research in Italy. *Phys. Med.* **2021**, *83*, 221–241. [CrossRef] [PubMed]
29. Rentiya, Z.S.; Mandal, S.; Inban, P.; Vempalli, H.; Dabbara, R.; Ali, S.; Kaur, K.; Adegbite, A.; Intsiful, T.A.; Jayan, M.; et al. Revolutionizing Breast Cancer Detection With Artificial Intelligence (AI) in Radiology and Radiation Oncology: A Systematic Review. *Cureus* **2024**, *16*, e57619. [CrossRef] [PubMed] [PubMed Central]
30. Batchu, S.; Liu, F.; Amireh, A.; Waller, J.; Umair, M. A Review of Applications of Machine Learning in Mammography and Future Challenges. *Oncology* **2021**, *99*, 483–490. [CrossRef] [PubMed]
31. Xavier, D.; Miyawaki, I.; Campello Jorge, C.A.; Freitas Silva, G.B.; Lloyd, M.; Moraes, F.; Patel, B.; Batalini, F. Artificial intelligence for triaging of breast cancer screening mammograms and workload reduction: A meta-analysis of a deep learning software. *J. Med. Screen.* **2024**, *31*, 157–165. [CrossRef] [PubMed]
32. Hickman, S.E.; Woitek, R.; Le, E.P.V.; Im, Y.R.; Mouritsen Luxhøj, C.; Aviles-Rivero, A.I.; Baxter, G.C.; MacKay, J.W.; Gilbert, F.J. Machine Learning for Workflow Applications in Screening Mammography: Systematic Review and Meta-Analysis. *Radiology* **2022**, *302*, 88–104. [CrossRef] [PubMed] [PubMed Central]
33. Liu, J.; Lei, J.; Ou, Y.; Zhao, Y.; Tuo, X.; Zhang, B.; Shen, M. Mammography diagnosis of breast cancer screening through machine learning: A systematic review and meta-analysis. *Clin. Exp. Med.* **2023**, *23*, 2341–2356. [CrossRef] [PubMed]
34. Anderson, A.W.; Marinovich, M.L.; Houssami, N.; Lowry, K.P.; Elmore, J.G.; Buist, D.S.M.; Hofvind, S.; Lee, C.I. Independent External Validation of Artificial Intelligence Algorithms for Automated Interpretation of Screening Mammography: A Systematic Review. *J. Am. Coll. Radiol.* **2022**, *19 Pt A*, 259–273. [CrossRef] [PubMed] [PubMed Central]
35. Bhalla, D.; Rangarajan, K.; Chandra, T.; Banerjee, S.; Arora, C. Reproducibility and Explainability of Deep Learning in Mammography: A Systematic Review of Literature. *Indian. J. Radiol. Imaging* **2023**, *34*, 469–487. [CrossRef] [PubMed] [PubMed Central]
36. Goh, S.; Goh, R.S.J.; Chong, B.; Ng, Q.X.; Koh, G.C.H.; Ngiam, K.Y.; Hartman, M. Challenges in Implementing Artificial Intelligence in Breast Cancer Screening Programs: Systematic Review and Framework for Safe Adoption. *J. Med. Internet Res.* **2025**, *27*, e62941. [CrossRef] [PubMed] [PubMed Central]
37. Gurmessa, D.K.; Jimma, W. Explainable machine learning for breast cancer diagnosis from mammography and ultrasound images: A systematic review. *BMJ Health Care Inform.* **2024**, *31*, e100954. [CrossRef] [PubMed] [PubMed Central]

38. Hussain, S.; Ali, M.; Naseem, U.; Nezhadmoghadam, F.; Jatoi, M.A.; Gulliver, T.A.; Tamez-Peña, J.G. Breast cancer risk prediction using machine learning: A systematic review. *Front. Oncol.* **2024**, *14*, 1343627. [CrossRef] [PubMed] [PubMed Central]
39. Oh, K.E.; Vasandani, N.; Anwar, A. Radiomics to Differentiate Malignant and Benign Breast Lesions: A Systematic Review and Diagnostic Test Accuracy Meta-Analysis. *Cureus* **2023**, *15*, e49015. [CrossRef] [PubMed] [PubMed Central]
40. Hussain, S.; Lafarga-Osuna, Y.; Ali, M.; Naseem, U.; Ahmed, M.; Tamez-Peña, J.G. Deep learning, radiomics and radiogenomics applications in the digital breast tomosynthesis: A systematic review. *BMC Bioinform.* **2023**, *24*, 401. [CrossRef] [PubMed] [PubMed Central]
41. Madani, M.; Behzadi, M.M.; Nabavi, S. The Role of Deep Learning in Advancing Breast Cancer Detection Using Different Imaging Modalities: A Systematic Review. *Cancers* **2022**, *14*, 5334. [CrossRef] [PubMed] [PubMed Central]
42. Gardezi, S.J.S.; Elazab, A.; Lei, B.; Wang, T. Breast Cancer Detection and Diagnosis Using Mammographic Data: Systematic Review. *J. Med. Internet Res.* **2019**, *21*, e14464. [CrossRef] [PubMed] [PubMed Central]
43. Yassin, N.I.R.; Omran, S.; El Houby, E.M.F.; Allam, H. Machine learning techniques for breast cancer computer aided diagnosis using different image modalities: A systematic review. *Comput. Methods Programs Biomed.* **2018**, *156*, 25–45. [CrossRef] [PubMed]
44. Singh, D.; Singh, A.K. Role of image thermography in early breast cancer detection- Past, present and future. *Comput. Methods Programs Biomed.* **2020**, *183*, 105074. [CrossRef] [PubMed]
45. Sorin, V.; Sklair-Levy, M.; Glicksberg, B.S.; Konen, E.; Nadkarni, G.N.; Klang, E. Deep Learning for Contrast Enhanced Mammography—A Systematic Review. *Acad. Radiol.* **2025**, *32*, 2497–2508. [CrossRef] [PubMed]
46. Ciurescu, S.; Ciupici-Cladovan, M.; Buciu, V.B.; Ilaș, D.G.; Cîtu, C.; Sas, I. Systematic Review and Meta-Analysis of AI-Assisted Mammography and the Systemic Immune-Inflammation Index in Breast Cancer: Diagnostic and Prognostic Perspectives. *Medicina* **2025**, *61*, 1170. [CrossRef] [PubMed] [PubMed Central]
47. Rostami, S.; Stutterheim, H.W.; Maxouri, O.; Willemse, J.R.J.; Rodríguez Sánchez, D.I.; Schats, W.; van Golen, L.W.; Vollebergh, M.A.; Cheung, Z.; Vogel, W.V.; et al. Imaging of Cancer of Unknown Primary: A systematic literature review of the past, present, and future. *Br. J. Radiol.* **2025**, *98*, 1209–1226. [CrossRef] [PubMed]
48. Bennett, A.; Shaver, N.; Vyas, N.; Almoli, F.; Pap, R.; Douglas, A.; Kibret, T.; Skidmore, B.; Yaffe, M.; Wilkinson, A.; et al. Screening for breast cancer: A systematic review update to inform the Canadian Task Force on Preventive Health Care guideline. *Syst. Rev.* **2024**, *13*, 304. [CrossRef] [PubMed] [PubMed Central]
49. Available online: https://www.novaoneadvisor.com/report/breast-cancer-therapeutics-market (accessed on 12 July 2025).
50. Available online: https://www.marketsandata.com/industry-reports/mammography-market (accessed on 12 July 2025).
51. Available online: https://www.marketsandmarkets.com/Market-Reports/diagnostic-imaging-market-411.html (accessed on 12 July 2025).
52. Available online: https://www.marketsandmarkets.com/Market-Reports/ai-in-medical-imaging-market-21977207.html (accessed on 12 July 2025).
53. Available online: https://www.towardshealthcare.com/insights/ai-in-breast-imaging-market-size (accessed on 12 July 2025).
54. Available online: https://www.fda.gov/media/184856/download (accessed on 12 July 2025).
55. Available online: https://www.fda.gov/regulatory-information/search-fda-guidance-documents/marketing-submission-recommendations-predetermined-change-control-plan-artificial-intelligence (accessed on 12 July 2025).
56. Available online: https://www.acr.org/Clinical-Resources/Publications-and-Research/ACR-Bulletin/Bolstering-Breast-Cancer-Detection (accessed on 12 July 2025).
57. Available online: https://digital-strategy.ec.europa.eu/en/policies/regulatory-framework-ai (accessed on 12 July 2025).
58. Available online: https://www.eusobi.org/content-eusobi/uploads/EUSOBI-Mammography-beyond-2025_Preliminary-Programme.pdf (accessed on 12 July 2025).
59. Available online: https://densitashealth.com/news/densitas-acr-learning-network-strategic-collaboration-to-improve-mammography-positioning/ (accessed on 12 July 2025).
60. Available online: https://www.lunit.io/en/company/news/lunit-and-leeds-teaching-hospitals-nhs-trust-to-launch-worlds-first-prospective-ai-study-in-symptomatic-breast-clinic-setting (accessed on 12 July 2025).
61. Hernström, V.; Josefsson, V.; Sartor, H.; Schmidt, D.; Larsson, A.M.; Hofvind, S.; Andersson, I.; Rosso, A.; Hagberg, O.; Lång, K. Screening performance and characteristics of breast cancer detected in the Mammography Screening with Artificial Intelligence trial (MASAI): A randomised, controlled, parallel-group, non-inferiority, single-blinded, screening accuracy study. *Lancet Digit. Health* **2025**, *7*, e175–e183. [CrossRef] [PubMed]
62. Friedewald, S.M.; Sieniek, M.; Jansen, S.; Mahvar, F.; Kohlberger, T.; Schacht, D.; Bhole, S.; Gupta, D.; Prabhakara, S.; McKinney, S.M.; et al. Triaging mammography with artificial intelligence: An implementation study. *Breast Cancer Res. Treat.* **2025**, *211*, 1–10. [CrossRef] [PubMed] [PubMed Central]
63. Eisemann, N.; Bunk, S.; Mukama, T.; Baltus, H.; Elsner, S.A.; Gomille, T.; Hecht, G.; Heywang-Köbrunner, S.; Rathmann, R.; Siegmann-Luz, K.; et al. Nationwide real-world implementation of AI for cancer detection in population-based mammography screening. *Nat. Med.* **2025**, *31*, 917–924. [CrossRef] [PubMed] [PubMed Central]

64. Rangarajan, K.; Manivannan, V.V.; Singh, H.; Gupta, A.; Maheshwari, H.; Gogoi, R.; Gogoi, D.; Das, R.J.; Hari, S.; Vyas, S.; et al. Simulation training in mammography with AI-generated images: A multireader study. *Eur. Radiol.* **2025**, *35*, 562–571. [CrossRef] [PubMed]
65. Salim, M.; Liu, Y.; Sorkhei, M.; Ntoula, D.; Foukakis, T.; Fredriksson, I.; Wang, Y.; Eklund, M.; Azizpour, H.; Smith, K.; et al. AI-based selection of individuals for supplemental MRI in population-based breast cancer screening: The randomized ScreenTrustMRI trial. *Nat. Med.* **2024**, *30*, 2623–2630. [CrossRef] [PubMed] [PubMed Central]
66. McGuinness, J.E.; Anderson, G.L.; Mutasa, S.; Hershman, D.L.; Terry, M.B.; Tehranifar, P.; Lew, D.L.; Yee, M.; Brown, E.A.; Kairouz, S.S.; et al. Effects of vitamin D supplementation on a deep learning-based mammographic evaluation in SWOG S0812. *JNCI Cancer Spectr.* **2024**, *8*, pkae042. [CrossRef] [PubMed] [PubMed Central]
67. Chen, Y.; Jiang, H.; Li, J.; Zhang, J.; Wu, P.; Dai, Z. A Mammography-Based Radiomic Nomogram for Predicting Malignancy in Breast Suspicious Microcalcifications. *Acad. Radiol.* **2024**, *31*, 492–502. [CrossRef] [PubMed]
68. Dembrower, K.; Crippa, A.; Colón, E.; Eklund, M.; Strand, F. ScreenTrustCAD Trial Consortium. Artificial intelligence for breast cancer detection in screening mammography in Sweden: A prospective, population-based, paired-reader, non-inferiority study. *Lancet Digit. Health* **2023**, *5*, e703–e711; Erratum in *Lancet Digit. Health* **2023**, *5*, e646. https://doi.org/10.1016/S2589-7500(23)00181-4. [CrossRef] [PubMed]
69. Lång, K.; Josefsson, V.; Larsson, A.M.; Larsson, S.; Högberg, C.; Sartor, H.; Hofvind, S.; Andersson, I.; Rosso, A. Artificial intelligence-supported screen reading versus standard double reading in the Mammography Screening with Artificial Intelligence trial (MASAI): A clinical safety analysis of a randomised, controlled, non-inferiority, single-blinded, screening accuracy study. *Lancet Oncol.* **2023**, *24*, 936–944. [CrossRef] [PubMed]
70. Zhou, C.; Xie, H.; Zhu, F.; Yan, W.; Yu, R.; Wang, Y. Improving the malignancy prediction of breast cancer based on the integration of radiomics features from dual-view mammography and clinical parameters. *Clin. Exp. Med.* **2023**, *23*, 2357–2368. [CrossRef] [PubMed]
71. Sechopoulos, I.; Abbey, C.K.; van der Waal, D.; Geertse, T.; Tetteroo, E.; Pijnappel, R.M.; Broeders, M.J.M. Evaluation of reader performance during interpretation of breast cancer screening: The Recall and detection Of breast Cancer in Screening (ROCS) trial study design. *Eur. Radiol.* **2022**, *32*, 7463–7469. [CrossRef] [PubMed] [PubMed Central]
72. Ma, M.; Liu, R.; Wen, C.; Xu, W.; Xu, Z.; Wang, S.; Wu, J.; Pan, D.; Zheng, B.; Qin, G.; et al. Predicting the molecular subtype of breast cancer and identifying interpretable imaging features using machine learning algorithms. *Eur. Radiol.* **2022**, *32*, 1652–1662. [CrossRef] [PubMed]
73. Liu, H.; Chen, Y.; Zhang, Y.; Wang, L.; Luo, R.; Wu, H.; Wu, C.; Zhang, H.; Tan, W.; Yin, H.; et al. A deep learning model integrating mammography and clinical factors facilitates the malignancy prediction of BI-RADS 4 microcalcifications in breast cancer screening. *Eur. Radiol.* **2021**, *31*, 5902–5912. [CrossRef] [PubMed]
74. Wei, H.; Fan, H. MM-CLIP: Multi-granularity Mammography CLIP for Breast Cancer Diagnosis. In Proceedings of the 2025 9th International Conference on Digital Signal Processing (ICDSP '25), Chengdu, China, 21–23 February 2025; pp. 92–99. [CrossRef]
75. Doma, M.K.; Padmanandam, K.; Tambvekar, S.; Kumar, K.K.; Abdualgalil, B.; Thakur, R.N. Artificial Intelligence-Based Breast Cancer Detection Using WPSO. *Int. J. Oper. Res. Inf. Syst.* **2022**, *13*, 1–16. [CrossRef]
76. Aydemir, B.K.K.; Telatar, Z.; Güney, S.; Dengiz, B. Detecting and Classifying Breast Masses via YOLO-Based Deep Learning. *Neural Comput. Appl.* **2025**, *37*, 11555–11582. [CrossRef]
77. Islam, M.S.; Yasmin, S.; Chowdhury, T.A.; Sayem, A.; Mim, K. AI-Assisted Breast Cancer Diagnosis: Deep Learning on RSNA Mammogram Images for Improved Classification. In Proceedings of the 2023 26th International Conference on Computer and Information Technology (ICCIT), Cox's Bazar, Bangladesh, 13–15 December 2023. [CrossRef]
78. Yang, Z.; Cao, Z.; Zhang, Y.; Chang, P.; Wu, S.; Huang, L. MABEL: An AI-Powered Mammographic Breast Lesion Diagnostic System. In Proceedings of the 2020 IEEE International Conference on E-Health Networking, Application & Services (HEALTHCOM), Shenzhen, China, 1–2 March 2021. [CrossRef]
79. Rath, S.; Giri, K.; Dash, S.R.; Barra, P.; Abdullah, A.A. Application of Artificial Intelligence using Mammograms to Identify Breast Cancer. In Proceedings of the 2024 6th International Conference on Computational Intelligence and Networks (CINE), Bhubaneswar, India, 19–21 December 2024. [CrossRef]
80. Available online: https://arxiv.org/abs/2506.08677 (accessed on 12 July 2025).
81. Available online: https://arxiv.org/abs/2506.03177 (accessed on 12 July 2025).
82. Available online: https://arxiv.org/abs/2503.13309 (accessed on 12 July 2025).
83. Available online: https://www.arxiv.org/abs/2505.03018 (accessed on 12 July 2025).

diagnostics

MDPI

Review

Artificial Intelligence in Assessing Reproductive Aging: Role of Mitochondria, Oxidative Stress, and Telomere Biology

Efthalia Moustakli [1], Themos Grigoriadis [2,†], Sofoklis Stavros [3,*,†], Anastasios Potiris [3], Athanasios Zikopoulos [3], Angeliki Gerede [4], Ioannis Tsimpoukis [3], Charikleia Papageorgiou [3], Konstantinos Louis [3] and Ekaterini Domali [2]

[1] Laboratory of Medical Genetics, Faculty of Medicine, School of Health Sciences, University of Ioannina, 45110 Ioannina, Greece; ef.moustakli@uoi.gr
[2] First Department of Obstetrics and Gynecology, Alexandra Hospital, Medical School, National and Kapodistrian University of Athens, 11528 Athens, Greece; kdomali@yahoo.fr (E.D.)
[3] Third Department of Obstetrics and Gynecology, University General Hospital "ATTIKON", Medical School, National and Kapodistrian University of Athens, 12462 Athens, Greece; apotiris@med.uoa.gr (A.P.); thanzik92@gmail.com (A.Z.); giannistsimpoukis94@gmail.com (I.T.); charikleiapap@yahoo.gr (C.P.); kostaslouisss@gmail.com (K.L.)
[4] Department of Obstetrics and Gynecology, Democritus University of Thrace, 69100 Campus, Greece; agerede@otenet.gr
* Correspondence: sfstavrou@med.uoa.gr; Tel.: +30-(210)5832237
† These authors contributed equally to this work.

Abstract

Fertility potential ever more diminishes due to the complex, multifactorial, and still not entirely clarified process of reproductive aging in women and men. Gamete quality and reproductive lifespan are compromised by biologic factors like mitochondrial dysfunction, increased oxidative stress (OS), and incremental telomere shortening. Clinically confirmed biomarkers, including follicle-stimulating hormone (FSH) and anti-Müllerian hormone (AMH), are used to estimate ovarian reserve and reproductive status, but these markers have limited predictive validity and an incomplete representation of the complexity of reproductive age. Recent advances in artificial intelligence (AI) have the capacity to address the integration and interpretation of disparate and complex sets of data, like imaging, molecular, and clinical, for consideration. AI methodologies that improve the accuracy of reproductive outcome predictions and permit the construction of personalized treatment programs are machine learning (ML) and deep learning. To promote fertility evaluations, here, as part of its critical discussion, the roles of mitochondria, OS, and telomere biology as latter-day biomarkers of reproductive aging are presented. We also address the current status of AI applications in reproductive medicine, promises for the future, and applications involving embryo selection, multi-omics set integration, and estimation of reproductive age. Finally, to ensure that AI technology is used ethically and responsibly for reproductive care, model explainability, heterogeneity of data, and other ethical issues remain as residual concerns.

Keywords: artificial intelligence (AI); reproductive aging; oxidative stress; mitochondria; telomere biology; machine learning; reproductive medicine

1. Introduction

Reproductive aging of females and males is an intricate, multifactorial process that has significant effects on fertility, outcomes of pregnancy, and health of the offspring [1,2]. It is described in females as decreased quantity and quality of oocytes resulting in diminished

 https://doi.org/10.3390/diagnostics15162075

ovarian reserve (DOR), high aneuploidy rates, and decreased reproductive capability. It is described in males as alterations in the quality of the sperm, including oxidative injury, DNA fragmentation, and alterations of telomere length [3]. The epidemiological tendency of postponed birth has widened the medical relevance of reproductive aging, placing great priority on precise diagnosis techniques for the estimation of reproductive lifespan as well as tailoring treatment regimens.

Conventional markers, including antral follicle count (AFC), FSH, and AMH exhibit limited predictive accuracy for reproductive outcomes, although they provide valuable insights into ovarian reserve [4,5]. Conversely, conventional semen analysis in males primarily assesses morphology and motility, often overlooking the underlying cellular and molecular alterations associated with reproductive aging. The quality of gametes and embryos is largely determined by three interrelated biological processes, mitochondrial dysfunction, oxidative stress (OS), and telomere biology. Recent research in reproductive biology has identified these processes as key contributors to reproductive decline and poorer reproductive outcomes. Telomere shortening functions as a cellular aging clock that restricts reproductive longevity, OS degrades DNA, proteins, and lipids necessary for gamete function, and mitochondrial impairment lowers ATP synthesis and increases reactive oxygen species (ROS) generation. Compared to traditional clinical indicators, these events collectively offer a more thorough biological basis for reproductive aging [6]. Despite the promise for these indicators to improve the assessment of reproductive aging, their integration into clinical practice is limited by the complexity and diversity of the information they provide [7,8].

AI, particularly ML and deep learning techniques, offers effective and efficient remedies to these challenges. Such technologies can process and integrate molecular profiles, clinical measures, imaging variables, and other varied information to develop forecasting systems that are more precise and robust than conventional statistical approaches [9]. Applications of AI in reproductive medicine are expanding quickly, ranging from sperm quality analysis to ovarian reserve prediction and IVF embryo selection. However, there is still little research on how artificial intelligence might be used to analyze and correlate biomarkers of reproductive aging, such as mitochondrial competence, OS measurements, and telomere dynamics [10].

We discuss the current knowledge of telomere biology, mitochondria, and OS as important indicators of reproductive aging. Subsequently, the application of AI in reproductive medicine is explored, with an emphasis on how these technologies may revolutionize the diagnosis and management of reproductive aging. The challenges of algorithm interpretability, data heterogeneity, and ethical issues in the use of AI-driven solutions are finally covered.

2. Mitochondrial Dysfunction in Reproductive Aging

2.1. The Central Role of Mitochondria in Reproductive Aging

Cells generate energy through oxidative phosphorylation (OXPHOS), which is controlled by vital organelles called mitochondria. Gamete mitochondrial activity is particularly crucial given the high energy demands of oocyte maturation, fertilization, and early embryonic development [11,12]. Oocyte mitochondria provide adenosine triphosphate (ATP) and regulate calcium homeostasis, apoptosis, and redox balance, which are critical for maintaining developmental competence and genetic stability. Sperm mitochondrial activity maintains motility and the integrity of the paternal DNA [13]. Even within the same individual throughout time, it is crucial to understand that every gamete cohort—whether from males or females—represents a distinct metabolic and functional profile. Due to this variability, a significant therapeutic window exists during which couples still producing gametes can benefit from treatments that enhance OXPHOS, improve mitochondrial function, and reduce OS. The function, quality, and viability of gametes in the context of reproductive age may be enhanced by focusing on these pathways, which could increase fertility potential and enhance the results of ART.

Reduced fertility is a result of reproductive aging-related decreases in mitochondrial quantity and quality. The accumulation of mitochondrial DNA (mtDNA) mutations, a decrease in mitochondrial membrane potential, and reduced ATP production are hallmarks of aging oocytes. These changes impair meiotic spindle formation, increasing aneuploidy rates and decreasing embryo quality. In a similar vein, elderly sperm with mitochondrial malfunction exhibit decreased motility and greater DNA breakage [14,15].

There are several methods for directly measuring mitochondrial activity in gametes. Transmission electron microscopy (TEM) to examine morphology, ATP assays for energy production, and JC-1 or TMRE labeling to determine mitochondrial membrane potential are frequently used to analyze mitochondrial activity in sperm. ATP quantification, ROS imaging to identify OS, and TEM or confocal imaging to analyze structure and distribution are used to evaluate oocyte mitochondrial function [16]. ATP measurements and oxygen consumption rate (respirometry) are utilized to assess mitochondrial function in granulosa and cumulus cells. These assessments provide essential insights into gamete quality, fertilization potential, and early embryo developmental competence [17].

Gamete-Specific Impacts of Mitochondrial Dysfunction

The mitochondria in the midpiece are crucial for spermatozoa to produce the ATP required for motility and capacitation. The mitochondrial membrane potential (MMP) is decreased by aging-related mitochondrial dysfunction, though, and this results in impaired motility, a reduced acrosome reaction, and increased DNA fragmentation because of the overproduction of ROS. In sperm, abnormal mitochondrial morphology and compromised mtDNA integrity have been linked to poor embryo development and decreased fertilization ability.

Granulosa and cumulus cells' mitochondria are essential for oocyte maturation, antioxidant defense, and steroidogenesis in ovarian follicles. Functional follicular mitochondria reduce the oocyte's developmental capacity by affecting its metabolic and redox environment. Mitochondrial DNA alterations in follicular cells have been linked to decreased ovarian reserve, whereas decreased ATP generation in cumulus cells can disrupt nutrition and signal exchange with the contained oocyte.

The energy requirements of oocytes, which have the most mitochondria in the body, peak during meiotic spindle construction and fertilization. A decrease in oocyte mitochondrial quality with age raises the probability of aneuploidy, impairs spindle formation, and lowers ATP availability. Furthermore, the development of the embryo is further jeopardized by the accumulation of mtDNA mutations and structural damage.

2.2. Mitochondrial Biomarkers of Reproductive Aging

An assortment of mitochondrial features has been determined to include potential indicators for assessing reproductive age. Among these, the mitochondrial DNA copy number (mtDNA-CN) has garnered significant attention [18]. Studies have indicated a relationship between mtDNA-CN in oocytes and embryos and both developmental competence and implantation capability. Reports of alterations in mtDNA-CN levels in the granulosa cells and follicular fluid of older women have raised the possibility that it could serve as a surrogate indication of oocyte quality [19].

Another possible biomarker for mitochondrial function is the mitochondrial membrane potential, or MMP. Higher apoptotic susceptibility and decreased energy production are indicated by reduced MMP in aged gametes [20]. Although JC-1 staining and other fluorometric assays have been used to measure MMP, its clinical applicability is currently primarily in the experimental stage [21].

The production of ROS is a third crucial mitochondrial characteristic. An increased ROS is mostly caused by dysfunctional mitochondria, which exacerbate OS and cause DNA damage, lipid peroxidation, and protein oxidation in gametes [22]. ROS levels in seminal plasma and follicular fluid have been frequently associated with poor reproductive outcomes, including decreased fertilization rates and embryo quality [23].

Finally, a direct measure of mitochondrial energy generation is the concentration of ATP. Aging oocytes with lower ATP levels experience challenges with cytoskeletal dynamics and meiotic spindle assembly, leading to chromosomal defects and unsuccessful fertilization. Measuring the ATP content of oocytes and embryos can provide insights into their developmental potential, even though it is technically challenging [24,25]. Table 1 summarizes the key mitochondrial biomarkers implicated in reproductive aging, including their biological roles, assessment methods, clinical relevance, and current limitations. However, these conventional methods are inherently invasive and destructive, rendering the assessed gametes unusable for ART. Recent developments in AI-driven image processing, spectroscopy, and metabolic profiling present the potential for non-invasive, point-of-care, and real-time gamete assessment. For instance, deep learning algorithms and high-resolution, label-free imaging modalities can evaluate subcellular characteristics without endangering gamete viability, potentially allowing integration into ART workflows for prompt clinical decision-making.

Table 1. Key mitochondrial biomarkers implicated in reproductive aging, including their biological roles, assessment methods, clinical relevance, and current limitations.

Biomarker	Biological Role	Assessment Method	Clinical Relevance	Limitations
mtDNA-CN [26]	Indicator of mitochondrial biogenesis	Quantitative (qPCR), digital PCR	Lower copy number is associated with reduced oocyte developmental competence and poorer embryo implantation potential	Requires invasive sampling of oocytes/embryos; inter-assay variability due to extraction and quantification differences
MMP [27]	Reflects mitochondrial functionality	JC-1, TMRE, Rhodamine dyes	High MMP correlates with better fertilization and blastocyst formation rates	Fluorescent dyes may yield inconsistent results between labs; signal intensity affected by staining time and temperature
ROS [28]	Byproduct of mitochondrial dysfunction	Chemiluminescence, fluorometric assays	Elevated ROS is linked to oxidative damage, impaired fertilization, and reduced embryo quality	Levels fluctuate rapidly in response to handling, oxygen exposure, and culture conditions; requires rapid measurement post-collection
ATP Content [29]	Direct measure of energy production	Bioluminescence assays	Adequate ATP is essential for spindle assembly, chromosome segregation, and normal fertilization	Requires destruction of the gamete/embryo for measurement; susceptible to degradation during sample processing

2.3. Current Challenges in Clinical Translation

Several limitations prevent mitochondrial biomarkers from becoming commonplace in the clinic, although they have good potential. One of the most significant restrictions is that there is no standard assay for the quantitative measurement of aspects like MMP and mtDNA-CN. Variation between the sensitivity of tests, treatment of samples, as well as the interpretation of results, can all cause inconsistent results between studies [30].

Another obstacle is obtaining the invasive embryo or oocyte samples required for direct analysis of the mitochondria. While less invasive, the validity of surrogate samples such as cumulus cells and follicular fluid as predictors of oocyte mitochondrial health remains under study [31]. Age, obesity, smoking, environmental contaminants, metabolic illnesses, and other confounding factors that may independently impact mitochondrial function make it more difficult to interpret biomarker data. These elements emphasize the need for advanced analytical tools capable of integrating several data dimensions while accounting for these confounders [32].

2.4. Potential of AI in Mitochondrial Biomarker Analysis

Given its capacity to integrate and interpret complex mitochondrial datasets, AI holds significant potential for addressing many of these challenges [33]. Through the identification of complex patterns and interactions among variables such as mtDNA-CN, ROS levels, and patient demographics, machine learning algorithms can predict oocyte quality and fertility results more precisely than traditional statistical methods [34].

Analysis of data from high-resolution mitochondrial imaging has demonstrated the effectiveness of deep learning methods, particularly convolutional neural networks (CNNs). These methods could be used to detect subtle structural or functional abnormalities in mitochondria that are not obvious to human observers [35].

Furthermore, a promising approach to thorough modeling of reproductive aging is AI-driven multi-omics integration [36]. Through the integration of proteomics, metabolomics, and mitochondrial genomes data, artificial intelligence frameworks can offer a comprehensive perspective on mitochondrial health and its correlation with reproductive capacity [37]. Personalized fertility treatment plans and non-invasive, precise prediction tools may be made possible by such methods [38,39].

3. OS as a Biomarker

3.1. Role of OS in Reproductive Aging

An imbalance between the generation of ROS and the antioxidant defense systems that counteract them results in OS [40]. Normal reproductive activities, including folliculogenesis, oocyte maturation, sperm capacitation, and embryo development, depend on physiological levels of ROS, whereas excessive ROS creation damages cells. This damage includes DNA fragmentation, protein oxidation, and lipid peroxidation, all of which are especially harmful to the reproductive system's highly specialized cells [41,42].

OS has been linked to age-related declines in ovarian reserve and oocyte quality in women [43]. Increased ROS buildup and decreased antioxidant capability in aging ovaries are linked to meiotic errors, aneuploidy, and granulosa cell death. OS is a major factor in men's sperm quality declining with age, leading to DNA breakage, decreased motility, and compromised fertilization ability [44].

OS in gametes can be directly assessed using a variety of techniques. While DNA fragmentation can be evaluated using TUNEL or Comet assays, ROS levels in sperm are often quantified using DCFDA labeling or chemiluminescence tests. Oxidative balance in oocytes is assessed by ROS imaging and antioxidant enzyme activity assays (e.g., SOD, catalase), and oxidative damage can also be deduced from DNA oxidation indicators or lipid peroxidation products. Similar biochemical tests are used to evaluate ROS levels and antioxidant capacity in granulosa and cumulus cells, which shed light on the follicular microenvironment and its capacity to promote oocyte development [45].

Gamete-Specific Impacts of OS

For functions including capacitation and hyperactivation, sperm require physiological amounts of ROS; nevertheless, too much ROS can harm sperm proteins, lipids, and DNA, decreasing motility and increasing morphological abnormalities. Male infertility, especially in older men, has been closely linked to elevated OS in seminal plasma.

Granulosa and cumulus cells' ability to function is hampered in ovarian follicles by OS in the follicular fluid, which changes the microenvironment surrounding the oocyte. In ART cycles, lower fertilization rates and lower-quality embryos are associated with elevated lipid peroxidation products in the follicle, such as malondialdehyde (MDA).

Oocytes are particularly vulnerable to oxidative injury due to their large cyto-plasmic volume and prolonged meiotic arrest. The consequences of aging on reproductive capacity can be exacerbated by excessive ROS, which can cause spindle integrity disruption, mitochondrial malfunction, and telomere shortening.

3.2. OS Biomarkers in Reproductive Aging

Several biomarkers have been proposed for the evaluation of OS within the reproductive system. ROS levels in follicular fluid, seminal plasma, or cumulus cells can be directly measured to ascertain the oxidative environment surrounding gametes [46,47]. Reduced implantation success, lower fertilization rates, and poorer embryo quality have been linked to increased ROS concentrations in ART [48,49].

Indirect indicators of oxidative damage are the markers of lipid peroxidation MDA and 4-hydroxynonenal (4-HNE). These have been reported to be present in increased quantities within infertile men's seminal plasma and women suffering from DOR's follicular fluid [50]. Oxidation of reproductive proteins required for gametic functionality is also suggested by markers of protein oxidation, such as advanced oxidation protein products (AOPPs) [51].

Measuring antioxidant capacity with specific enzymes such as catalase, glutathione peroxidase (GPx), and superoxide dismutase (SOD) or total antioxidant capacity (TAC) can yield more details on the oxidative equilibrium. These antioxidant defenses have been shown to decline with age and infertility in both sexes [52]. Table 2 summarizes the major biomarkers of OS associated with reproductive aging. Gametes meant for ART cannot be immediately subjected to OS evaluations since the majority of them still require destructive testing or invasive sampling. By combining label-free imaging, fast spectroscopic readouts, and non-invasive metabolic profiling, advances in AI-assisted analysis provide a mechanism to evaluate oxidative status in real time at the point of treatment while maintaining gamete integrity.

Table 2. Major biomarkers of OS relevant to reproductive aging, categorized by type (direct oxidative markers, lipid peroxidation, protein oxidation, and antioxidant status). Assessment methods, associations with gamete and embryo quality, and current challenges in clinical application are included.

Biomarker	Type	Assessment Method	Clinical Relevance	Limitations
ROS [53]	Direct oxidative marker	Fluorescence probes, EPR spectroscopy	Elevated ROS levels in gametes and reproductive fluids are linked to DNA damage, reduced fertilization rates, and poorer embryo quality in aging individuals	Highly unstable and short-lived; measurements can vary with handling time, oxygen exposure, and culture conditions

Table 2. *Cont.*

Biomarker	Type	Assessment Method	Clinical Relevance	Limitations
MDA [41]	Lipid peroxidation	TBARS assay, HPLC	Increased MDA in follicular fluid and seminal plasma correlates with membrane damage and reduced gamete viability in older patients	Not specific to reproductive tissues; TBARS can overestimate due to interference from other aldehydes
4-HNE [54]	Lipid peroxidation	Immunoassays, ELISA	Accumulates in oocytes during aging, contributing to spindle abnormalities and impaired embryo development	Limited clinical threshold data; cross-reactivity with similar aldehydes can affect accuracy
AOPPs [55]	Protein oxidation	Spectrophotometric assays	Elevated AOPPs in serum and follicular fluid are associated with subfertility and accelerated reproductive aging	Systemic OS can influence results; cannot differentiate between local and systemic protein oxidation sources
TAC [56]	Antioxidant status	FRAP, ABTS, ORAC assays	Reduced TAC in follicular fluid and seminal plasma correlates with diminished antioxidant defense and poor ART outcomes in older patients	Strongly influenced by recent diet, supplementation, and lifestyle factors; no universally accepted reference range for reproductive fluids

3.3. *Current Challenges in Biomarker Utilization*

Despite growing evidence that OS contributes to reproductive aging, the therapeutic use of OS biomarkers remains limited [57]. The variation in assay techniques used to assess ROS and antioxidant levels is a major issue that contributes to contradictory research outcomes. The assessment of OS is complicated by its dynamic character, which varies in response to clinical states, environmental exposures, and lifestyle factors [58].

Additionally, the intrusive collection of follicular fluid or cumulus cells for OS testing limits its usual use in reproductive clinics [59]. Men's semen collection is less intrusive, but interpretation is made more difficult by the variety of OS indicators in seminal plasma. A crucial first step in integrating biomarker assays into reproductive medicine is standardizing them and creating clinically meaningful reference ranges [60–62].

3.4. *Potential of AI in OS Biomarker Analysis*

By combining intricate datasets and identifying patterns that are difficult to identify using traditional techniques, artificial intelligence holds the potential to revolutionize the research of OS biomarkers [63]. To create prediction models of reproductive outcomes, ML algorithms can integrate clinical indicators, OS markers, antioxidant levels, and patient lifestyle factors [64].

Fluorescent ROS probes in gametes or embryos are examples of high-content OS imaging that deep learning techniques could examine to find minute oxidative signatures linked to aging [65]. AI frameworks can facilitate the integration of mitochondrial and telomere biomarkers with OS data, enabling a more comprehensive assessment of gamete quality and reproductive potential. Non-invasive, customized methods to track OS and improve the results of reproductive treatments may be made possible by these advancements [10].

4. Telomere Biology in Fertility

4.1. *Telomere Shortening and Reproductive Lifespan*

Telomeres, repetitive nucleotide sequences that cap the ends of chromosomes, function as a biological clock for cellular aging by progressively shortening with each cell division. The reduction in reproductive lifespan is closely related to this shortening [66]. Oocyte telomere attrition in females is linked to greater rates of infertility and miscarriage, as well as decreased ovarian reserve and oocyte quality. Male is adversely affected by spermatozoa with shortened telomeres, which have been linked to reduced sperm motility, increased DNA fragmentation, and lower fertilization rates [67].

Several well-established methods can be used to evaluate the integrity and length of the telomeres in gametes. While fluorescence in situ hybridization (FISH) can show telomere distribution, qPCR or terminal restriction fragment (TRF) analysis are typically used to quantify telomere length in sperm. Q-FISH is frequently used to assess oocyte telomeres because it enables the direct assessment of telomere length and the identification of dangerously short telomeres. The ability of granulosa and cumulus cells to support oocyte development and overall reproductive potential can be determined by measuring their telomere length using qPCR or FISH [68]. Current methods for measuring telomeres in gametes usually involve destructive sampling, which precludes the evaluated cells from being used in other clinical settings. Without sacrificing the viability of gametes for ART, quick, real-time telomere evaluation at the point of treatment may be possible by combining non-invasive optical or molecular profiling with AI-driven picture and data processing.

Gamete-Specific Telomere Dynamics

As paternal age increases, telomerase activity in spermatogonial stem cells tends to maintain or even increase telomere length in sperm. Nonetheless, telomeric DNA can still be harmed by severe OS, which can lead to fragmentation of sperm DNA and decreased embryo viability.

Follicle somatic cells in ovarian follicles, such as cumulus and granulosa cells, gradually shorten their telomeres as they age. Oocyte quality may be compromised if these supporting cells' telomeres are shortened, which could affect their capacity to protect and nourish the oocyte.

Due to the low telomerase activity after birth, oocytes show gradual telomere attrition throughout a woman's reproductive lifespan. Chromosome mis-segregation, meiotic spindle instability, and an elevated risk of miscarriage are all associated with oocytes with short telomeres. This attrition is further exacerbated by mitochondrial dysfunction and OS, creating a synergistic pathway that contributes to reproductive decline.

4.2. Male vs. Female Gametes: Telomere Dynamics

Male and female gametes have distinct telomere length dynamics as a result of differences in gametogenesis and telomerase activity. Since spermatogonial stem cells contain active telomerase, sperm telomeres often lengthen as paternal age increases [69]. However, oocytes lack considerable telomerase activity after birth, resulting in increasing telomere shortening with maternal age. This sexual dimorphism identifies distinct molecular mechanisms in gamete aging and emphasizes the significance of considering sex-specific telomere biology in reproductive research [70].

4.3. AI Approaches to Telomere Length Prediction

AI and ML techniques have emerged as very efficient methods for the analysis of telomere length from complex genomic and clinical data [71]. By integrating clinical traits and multi-omics data, AI models can precisely predict telomere length, enabling early detection of reproductive aging and risk stratification for infertility. These techniques may improve reproductive outcomes and allow for tailored fertility treatments by directing decisions regarding the timing and strategies of interventions [72].

5. AI in Reproductive Medicine

5.1. Current Applications of AI

AI has accelerated the transformation of reproductive medicine by enhancing clinical decision-making and diagnostic precision [73]. IVF selection is streamlined by embryo grading systems that assess embryo morphology and developmental potential using deep learning algorithms and sophisticated image analysis [74]. Furthermore, by examining patient clinical data and treatment parameters, prediction models have been created to forecast IVF success rates. AI-driven sperm quality evaluations in male fertility use pattern recognition and computer vision to detect sperm motility, morphology, and concentration more reliably and accurately than conventional techniques [75].

5.2. AI for Multi-Omics Integration

Reproductive biology is composed of complex interactions of the genome, proteasome, and metabolome. By integrating multi-omics datasets, AI techniques reveal new biomarkers and pathways involved in infertility and reproductive aging [76]. Extracting patterns and relationships between disparate sets of data that are routinely ignored by conventional analytical techniques, machine learning programs provide detailed insights into the health of gametes, embryo development, and processes of aging. Personalized reproductive health might be advanced by the integrated AI framework by customizing drugs based upon complex biological realities [77].

5.3. Case Studies and Existing AI Models in Reproductive Aging

Despite being a relatively recent focus, reproductive aging has prompted the development of several AI models. For example, by analyzing hormone patterns in combination with genetic markers, several studies have used machine learning to predict the decline of ovarian reserve [78]. Other models use imaging data to assess ovarian follicle quality and forecast when menopause will begin. These case studies, while still in their infancy, show how AI may advance our knowledge of and strategy for dealing with reproductive aging, opening the door for therapeutic applications that might prolong windows of fertility or maximize timing for fertility preservation [78]. Table 3 summarizes the key applications of AI in reproductive medicine.

Table 3. Key applications of AI in reproductive medicine.

Application Area	Description	Input Types	AI Techniques	Clinical Impact
Embryo Grading [74]	Automated assessment of embryo morphology and viability	Embryo images, time-lapse videos	Deep learning, CNNs	More consistent and objective embryo selection, leading to improved implantation and live birth rates in IVF
IVF Success Prediction [79]	Predicts likelihood of successful implantation and pregnancy	Patient clinical data, hormonal profiles	ML, predictive modeling	Enables individualized treatment protocols, potentially reducing cycle numbers and costs
Sperm Quality Analysis [80]	Evaluates sperm motility, morphology, and concentration	Sperm microscopy images, semen analysis	Computer vision, pattern recognition	Enhances diagnostic accuracy and reproducibility in male infertility assessment
Multi-Omics Integration [81]	Combines genomics, proteomics, metabolomics data for fertility insights	Genomic sequences, protein expression, metabolites	ML, data integration algorithms	Discovery of novel biomarkers and personalized therapies
Reproductive Aging Prediction [78]	DOR models and menopause onset	Hormonal profiles, genetic markers, imaging data	ML, regression models	Early detection of reproductive aging, fertility preservation decisions

5.4. AI for Integrating Complex Datasets in Reproductive Aging

The biological processes involved in reproductive aging are intricately linked and include OS, telomere attrition, and mitochondrial dysfunction. These processes are measured in a variety of gametes and supporting cells. Conventional studies cannot fully represent the biological complexity of the generated datasets since they are massive, multidimensional, and frequently non-linear [82]. AI provides the computing power to merge these diverse datasets—clinical, molecular, imaging, and functional—into logical models that can identify trends linked to less successful reproductive outcomes. To predict oocyte or sperm quality, aneuploidy risk, and embryo developmental potential, for example, machine learning can combine patient-specific reproductive features with data on mitochondrial activity, ROS levels, and telomere length. AI promotes tailored approaches to slow fertility decline and allows for a more comprehensive understanding of reproductive aging by combining intricate measures into useful insights (Figure 1) [72,83].

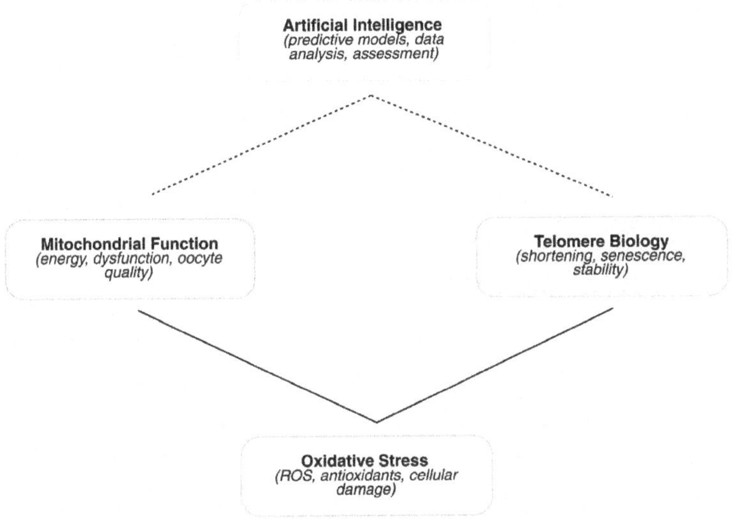

Figure 1. Schematic overview of the interplay between AI approaches and key mechanisms involved in reproductive aging. AI tools are applied to assess, predict, and monitor mitochondrial function, OS, and telomere biology. Solid arrows represent well-established mechanistic links, while dashed arrows indicate emerging or hypothesized connections. This schematic highlights how AI can integrate multifactorial biological data to provide insights into reproductive aging.

6. Challenges and Future Directions

6.1. Data Heterogeneity and Standardization

AI applications in reproductive aging are emerging, with existing models representing only the initial stages of development. ML has been used in several studies to predict DOR by examining hormone patterns in conjunction with genetic markers. Other models utilize imaging data to predict the onset of menopause and assess the health of ovarian follicles [77]. These early-stage case studies demonstrate how AI can improve our understanding and treatment of reproductive aging. This may lead to therapeutic applications that extend windows of viability or enhance timing for fertility maintenance [38].

6.2. Utilization of AI Models

Even though AI models, particularly deep learning networks, have a high predictive accuracy, their "black-box" nature makes clinical implementation difficult. Understanding how models make decisions, or explainability, is necessary to win over patients' and physicians' trust. Incorporating transparent reasoning techniques and developing interpretable AI frameworks will enable validation, regulatory approval, and ethical application in fertility care [84].

6.3. Explainability of AI Models

Reproductive medicine has used a number of different machine learning techniques, each with special benefits based on the kind and complexity of the data. CNNs are especially good at evaluating imaging data, including sperm morphology evaluations and time-lapse embryo movies. Their layered architecture makes it possible to identify tiny morphological variations that could be hard for human observers to notice by automatically extracting hierarchical image attributes. A CNN trained on more than 12,000 annotated embryo photos outperformed traditional morphological grading in one case study in terms of implantation prediction accuracy.

For tabular clinical data, such as patient information, hormone levels, and genetic markers, tree-based ensemble models like Random Forest are frequently utilized. Random Forest can handle diverse datasets with both continuous and categorical variables and minimize overfitting by merging several decision trees. For instance, a Random Forest model with significant cross-clinical generalizability was trained on a multi-center dataset of 2000 IVF cycles and was able to predict clinical pregnancy rates.

This strategy is expanded by gradient boosting algorithms like XGBoost, which construct trees one after the other with an emphasis on fixing the mistakes of the earlier ones. High prediction performance, effective management of missing data, and the capacity to identify intricate non-linear relationships are all hallmarks of XGBoost. With an area under the ROC curve (AUC) above 0.85 in validation cohorts, XGBoost models have been utilized in reproductive aging research to combine genetic, hormonal, and lifestyle data to estimate the likelihood of decreased ovarian reserve.

For these models to function at their best, access to well-annotated datasets is still essential. Training material can be obtained from publicly accessible sources, such as the Human Fertilization and Embryology Authority (HFEA) database for IVF results and curated imaging libraries for embryo development. To enable solid, repeatable AI research in reproductive medicine, collaborative data-sharing activities are necessary, as many high-quality datasets are still proprietary or limited.

6.4. Ethical and Legal Considerations

The application of AI in reproductive medicine raises important ethical and legal concerns [85]. Ensuring fair and responsible AI use requires addressing patient privacy, data security, informed consent, and biases in training data. Regulations specific to reproductive health applications are required to protect patient rights and advance equitable access to cutting-edge AI technologies [86].

6.5. Personalized Fertility Medicine Powered by AI

AI might transform future fertility treatment by supplying extremely personalized drugs [38]. Multi-dimensional information, like genetic and behavioral character traits, might be combined by AI to maximize therapy timing, personalize therapies based on each unique patient profile, and enhance results. Effective validation, ethical oversight, and continued innovation can unlock AI-led personalized fertility care [87].

6.6. Telomere Biology in Reproductive Aging: Measurement, Mechanisms, and Therapeutic Potential

Telomere length is increasingly recognized as an important biomarker of reproductive aging. It can be measured through different methods, each with their own advantages and disadvantages. Rapid, high-throughput analysis is possible using qPCR, although it only provides estimates of relative length. Although it allows for absolute length values, TRF analysis is less appropriate for small reproductive samples and necessitates substantial amounts of DNA. Individual gametes or embryos can be observed using Q-FISH, but more recent methods like telomere shortest length assay (TeSLA) and single telomere length analysis (STELA) improve the detection of critically short telomeres, which may be the most clinically relevant [88].

There is growing recognition that telomere dynamics differ by sex. Male sperm telomeres can be maintained or even extended over time by telomerase activity during spermatogenesis, while female oocytes incur progressive telomere attrition, which is made worse by mitochondrial malfunction and OS. With androgens affecting telomere stability through oxidative pathways and estrogen having been demonstrated to increase telomerase activity, hormonal regulation may also play a role [69].

Pharmacologic telomerase activators, antioxidant supplements, and lifestyle modifications to reduce OS are examples of potential telomere-targeted therapies that have shown some initial promise in preclinical animals. Though they are being investigated, more sophisticated strategies—like gene therapy to increase telomerase expression—need to be carefully evaluated for safety because of possible carcinogenic concerns. Using non-invasive biomarker screening to choose gametes or embryos with longer telomeres may improve the results of ART. Long-term safety and ethical issues must be weighed against these promising treatments, particularly when it comes to younger patient populations [89,90].

6.7. Limitations and Ethical Challenges of AI in Reproductive Medicine

Despite the promising advances in AI applications for reproductive medicine, there are important limitations that must be addressed before these technologies can be widely adopted in clinical practice. Given that AI models significantly depend on the caliber and representativeness of their training data, dataset bias is one of the main issues. Due to a lack of diversity in variables including age, ethnicity, and clinical conditions, many of the datasets currently in use may produce skewed forecasts that exacerbate healthcare inequities. For instance, when applied to underrepresented groups, models that were primarily trained on data from particular populations may perform poorly, which could lead to unequal outcomes for fertility care [91].

Model validation is another important concern. Thorough testing across several independent cohorts is necessary to determine the generalizability and dependability of AI models. However, single-center data and small sample sizes are common in reproductive medicine research, which restricts external validity. Comparing and evaluating various models is made more difficult by the lack of defined procedures for data gathering and result measurement [92].

Practical difficulties can arise when integrating AI models into clinical settings. Early-stage research occasionally ignores important steps like integration with current electronic health record systems, guaranteeing compatibility with clinical workflows, and offering sufficient user training. Furthermore, many AI algorithms are "black-box" in nature, which limits physicians' capacity to fully understand the predictions and confidently apply them to clinical decision-making [91].

Informed consent, algorithm openness, and patient privacy are ethical issues. The utilization of their data and the creation of AI-generated suggestions may not always be clear to patients. Additionally, AI may be used in ways that compromise patient autonomy or inadvertently reinforce preexisting biases [93].

Finally, securing governmental approval, protecting data, and defining who is responsible for AI blunders are some of the obstacles to real-world application. For example, it remains unclear who would be held accountable—the healthcare facility, the AI developer, or the clinician—if an AI model forecasts embryo viability inaccurately, resulting in a failed IVF cycle. Clinical professionals, data scientists, ethicists, and regulators must work together to address these intricate issues and guarantee that AI tools be used in reproductive care in a way that is safe, efficient, and morally sound [94].

7. Conclusions

This review underscores the essential link between mitochondrial dysfunction, OS, telomere biology, and fertility by illustrating the ways in which these interconnected processes determine gamete quality and reproductive duration for females and males. Key mechanisms of reproductive aging and poorer reproductive outcomes can be explained by telomere shortening acting as a cellular aging clock, OS causing molecular damage that compromises fertilization and embryo development, and mitochondrial impairment decreasing energy production and increasing ROS generation. By facilitating advanced analysis of sperm, precise IVF chance prognosis, better embryo grading, and incorporation of sophisticated multi-omics data, artificial intelligence has transformed reproductive medicine. Aging can now be better understood and managed due to these advances.

Data heterogeneity, model explainability requirements, and substantial ethical and regulatory challenges are just some of the challenges for the implementation of AI technology in this industry. AI technology solutions have to overcome these challenges for them to remain trustworthy, fair, and therapeutically valuable.

AI-centered methods of the future have unprecedented potential to provide customized diagnosis, customized fertility care, and precise reproductive age determination. It would take an interdisciplinary approach and innovation in technology to realize the full potential of AI and ultimately improve fertility and reproductive health outcomes across varied groups.

Author Contributions: Conceptualization, E.M. and E.D.; methodology, T.G. and S.S.; validation, I.T., C.P. and K.L.; investigation, A.P., A.Z. and A.G.; data curation, E.M.; writing—original draft preparation, E.M., T.G. and S.S.; writing—review and editing, A.P., A.Z., A.G., I.T., C.P., K.L. and E.D.; visualization, A.P.; supervision, A.P. and A.G.; project administration, E.D. All authors have read and agreed to the published version of the manuscript.

Funding: This research received no external funding.

Institutional Review Board Statement: Not applicable.

Informed Consent Statement: Not applicable.

Data Availability Statement: Data sharing is not applicable to this article as no new data were created or analyzed in this study.

Conflicts of Interest: The authors declare no conflicts of interest.

References

1. Moghadam, A.R.E.; Moghadam, M.T.; Hemadi, M.; Saki, G. Oocyte quality and aging. *JBRA Assist. Reprod.* **2022**, *26*, 105–122. [CrossRef]
2. Jimbo, M.; Kunisaki, J.; Ghaed, M.; Yu, V.; Flores, H.A.; Hotaling, J.M. Fertility in the aging male: A systematic review. *Fertil. Steril.* **2022**, *118*, 1022–1034. [CrossRef]
3. Le, M.T.; Nguyen, N.D.; Dang, H.N.T.; Nguyen, Q.H.V. Does diminished ovarian reserve impact oxidation-reduction potential in follicular fluid? *J. Int. Med. Res.* **2025**, *53*, 3000605251349926. [CrossRef] [PubMed]
4. Hochberg, A.; Esteves, S.C.; Yarali, H.; Vuong, L.N.; Dahan, M.H. Antimullerian hormone and antral follicle count thresholds for hyperresponse risk assessment in in vitro fertilization: A Hyperresponse Risk Assessment consensus study. *Fertil. Steril.* **2025**, *123*, 827–837. [CrossRef]

5. Moolhuijsen, L.M.E.; Visser, J.A. Anti-Mullerian Hormone and Ovarian Reserve: Update on Assessing Ovarian Function. *J. Clin. Endocrinol. Metab.* **2020**, *105*, 3361–3373. [CrossRef]
6. Wang, C.; Swerdloff, R.S. Limitations of semen analysis as a test of male fertility and anticipated needs from newer tests. *Fertil. Steril.* **2014**, *102*, 1502–1507. [CrossRef]
7. Cohen, J.; Silvestri, G.; Paredes, O.; Martin-Alcala, H.E.; Chavez-Badiola, A.; Alikani, M.; Palmer, G.A. Artificial intelligence in assisted reproductive technology: Separating the dream from reality. *Reprod. Biomed. Online* **2025**, *50*, 104855. [CrossRef] [PubMed]
8. Tao, X.; Zhu, Z.; Wang, L.; Li, C.; Sun, L.; Wang, W.; Gong, W. Biomarkers of Aging and Relevant Evaluation Techniques: A Comprehensive Review. *Aging Dis.* **2024**, *15*, 977–1005. [CrossRef]
9. Alowais, S.A.; Alghamdi, S.S.; Alsuhebany, N.; Alqahtani, T.; Alshaya, A.I.; Almohareb, S.N.; Aldairem, A.; Alrashed, M.; Bin Saleh, K.; Badreldin, H.A.; et al. Revolutionizing healthcare: The role of artificial intelligence in clinical practice. *BMC Med. Educ.* **2023**, *23*, 689. [CrossRef] [PubMed]
10. Hanassab, S.; Abbara, A.; Yeung, A.C.; Voliotis, M.; Tsaneva-Atanasova, K.; Kelsey, T.W.; Trew, G.H.; Nelson, S.M.; Heinis, T.; Dhillo, W.S. The prospect of artificial intelligence to personalize assisted reproductive technology. *NPJ Digit. Med.* **2024**, *7*, 55. [CrossRef]
11. Yildirim, R.M.; Seli, E. The role of mitochondrial dynamics in oocyte and early embryo development. *Semin. Cell Dev. Biol.* **2024**, *159–160*, 52–61. [CrossRef]
12. Almansa-Ordonez, A.; Bellido, R.; Vassena, R.; Barragan, M.; Zambelli, F. Oxidative Stress in Reproduction: A Mitochondrial Perspective. *Biology* **2020**, *9*, 269. [CrossRef]
13. Phan, O.T.H.; Trinh, T.T.C. Mitochondria in the reproduction system and mitotherapy in assisted reproductive technology: The importance of mitochondria selection. *Biomed. Res. Ther.* **2025**, *12*, 7054–7081. [CrossRef]
14. Ju, W.; Zhao, Y.; Yu, Y.; Zhao, S.; Xiang, S.; Lian, F. Mechanisms of mitochondrial dysfunction in ovarian aging and potential interventions. *Front. Endocrinol.* **2024**, *15*, 1361289. [CrossRef] [PubMed]
15. Zhang, W.; Wu, F. Effects of adverse fertility-related factors on mitochondrial DNA in the oocyte: A comprehensive review. *Reprod. Biol. Endocrinol.* **2023**, *21*, 27. [CrossRef] [PubMed]
16. Rickard, B.P.; Overchuk, M.; Chappell, V.A.; Kemal Ruhi, M.; Sinawang, P.D.; Nguyen Hoang, T.T.; Akin, D.; Demirci, U.; Franco, W.; Fenton, S.E.; et al. Methods to Evaluate Changes in Mitochondrial Structure and Function in Cancer. *Cancers* **2023**, *15*, 2564. [CrossRef]
17. Venturas, M.; Yang, X.; Sakkas, D.; Needleman, D. Noninvasive metabolic profiling of cumulus cells, oocytes, and embryos via fluorescence lifetime imaging microscopy: A mini-review. *Hum. Reprod.* **2023**, *38*, 799–810. [CrossRef]
18. Kupsco, A.; Bloomquist, T.R.; Hu, H.; Reddam, A.; Tang, D.; Goldsmith, J.; Rundle, A.G.; Baccarelli, A.A.; Herbstman, J.B. Mitochondrial DNA copy number dynamics and associations with the prenatal environment from birth through adolescence in a population of Dominican and African American children. *Mitochondrion* **2023**, *69*, 140–146. [CrossRef]
19. Zhang, D.; Keilty, D.; Zhang, Z.F.; Chian, R.C. Mitochondria in oocyte aging: Current understanding. *Facts Views Vis. Obgyn* **2017**, *9*, 29–38.
20. Lu, J.; Wu, L.; Wang, X.; Zhu, J.; Du, J.; Shen, B. Detection of Mitochondria Membrane Potential to Study CLIC4 Knockdown-induced HN4 Cell Apoptosis In Vitro. *J. Vis. Exp.* **2018**, *137*, e56317. [CrossRef]
21. Baig, J.; Pradeepkiran, J.A.; Reddy, P.H. Methods to Study Mitochondria: Techniques Used to Study the Effects of Age-Related Diseases Including Alzheimer's. *Curr. Protoc.* **2023**, *3*, e631. [CrossRef]
22. Afzal, S.; Abdul Manap, A.S.; Attiq, A.; Albokhadaim, I.; Kandeel, M.; Alhojaily, S.M. From imbalance to impairment: The central role of reactive oxygen species in oxidative stress-induced disorders and therapeutic exploration. *Front. Pharmacol.* **2023**, *14*, 1269581. [CrossRef]
23. Al-Saleh, I.; Coskun, S.; Al-Rouqi, R.; Al-Rajudi, T.; Eltabache, C.; Abduljabbar, M.; Al-Hassan, S. Oxidative stress and DNA damage status in couples undergoing in vitro fertilization treatment. *Reprod. Fertil.* **2021**, *2*, 117–139. [CrossRef] [PubMed]
24. Galeska, E.; Kowalczyk, A.; Wrzecinska, M.; Garcia, M.C.; Czerniawska-Piatkowska, E.; Gwozdziewicz, S.; Witkiewicz, W.; Dobrzanski, Z. The Importance of Mitochondrial Processes in the Maturation and Acquisition of Competences of Oocytes and Embryo Culture. *Int. J. Mol. Sci.* **2025**, *26*, 4098. [CrossRef] [PubMed]
25. Gualtieri, R.; Kalthur, G.; Barbato, V.; Di Nardo, M.; Adiga, S.K.; Talevi, R. Mitochondrial Dysfunction and Oxidative Stress Caused by Cryopreservation in Reproductive Cells. *Antioxidants* **2021**, *10*, 337. [CrossRef]
26. Yang, S.C.; Yu, E.J.; Park, J.K.; Kim, T.H.; Eum, J.H.; Paek, S.K.; Hwang, J.Y.; Lyu, S.W.; Kim, J.Y.; Lee, W.S.; et al. The Ratio of Mitochondrial DNA to Genomic DNA Copy Number in Cumulus Cell May Serve as a Biomarker of Embryo Quality in IVF Cycles. *Reprod. Sci.* **2021**, *28*, 2495–2502. [CrossRef]
27. Uribe, P.; Villegas, J.V.; Boguen, R.; Treulen, F.; Sanchez, R.; Mallmann, P.; Isachenko, V.; Rahimi, G.; Isachenko, E. Use of the fluorescent dye tetramethylrhodamine methyl ester perchlorate for mitochondrial membrane potential assessment in human spermatozoa. *Andrologia* **2017**, *49*, e12753. [CrossRef] [PubMed]

28. Lindsay, R.T.; Rhodes, C.J. Reactive Oxygen Species (ROS) in Metabolic Disease-Don't Shoot the Metabolic Messenger. *Int. J. Mol. Sci.* **2025**, *26*, 2622. [CrossRef]
29. Hu, L.L.; Liao, M.H.; Liu, Y.X.; Xing, C.H.; Nong, L.L.; Yang, F.L.; Sun, S.C. Loss of AMPK activity induces organelle dysfunction and oxidative stress during oocyte aging. *Biol. Direct* **2024**, *19*, 29. [CrossRef]
30. Koller, A.; Fazzini, F.; Lamina, C.; Rantner, B.; Kollerits, B.; Stadler, M.; Klein-Weigel, P.; Fraedrich, G.; Kronenberg, F. Mitochondrial DNA copy number is associated with all-cause mortality and cardiovascular events in patients with peripheral arterial disease. *J. Intern. Med.* **2020**, *287*, 569–579. [CrossRef]
31. Lemseffer, Y.; Terret, M.E.; Campillo, C.; Labrune, E. Methods for Assessing Oocyte Quality: A Review of Literature. *Biomedicines* **2022**, *10*, 2184. [CrossRef]
32. Singh, S.; Kriti, M.; Anamika, K.S.; Sarma, D.K.; Verma, V.; Nagpal, R.; Mohania, D.; Tiwari, R.; Kumar, M. Deciphering the complex interplay of risk factors in type 2 diabetes mellitus: A comprehensive review. *Metabol. Open* **2024**, *22*, 100287. [CrossRef]
33. Kitaoka, Y.; Uchihashi, T.; Kawata, S.; Nishiura, A.; Yamamoto, T.; Hiraoka, S.I.; Yokota, Y.; Isomura, E.T.; Kogo, M.; Tanaka, S.; et al. Role and Potential of Artificial Intelligence in Biomarker Discovery and Development of Treatment Strategies for Amyotrophic Lateral Sclerosis. *Int. J. Mol. Sci.* **2025**, *26*, 4346. [CrossRef]
34. Ferreira, T.; Rodriguez, S. Mitochondrial DNA: Inherent Complexities Relevant to Genetic Analyses. *Genes* **2024**, *15*, 617. [CrossRef]
35. Iqbal, M.S.; El-Ashram, S.; Hussain, S.; Khan, T.; Huang, S.; Mehmood, R.; Luo, B. Efficient cell classification of mitochondrial images by using deep learning. *J. Opt.* **2019**, *48*, 113–122. [CrossRef]
36. Theodorakis, N.; Feretzakis, G.; Tzelves, L.; Paxinou, E.; Hitas, C.; Vamvakou, G.; Verykios, V.S.; Nikolaou, M. Integrating Machine Learning with Multi-Omics Technologies in Geroscience: Towards Personalized Medicine. *J. Pers. Med.* **2024**, *14*, 931. [CrossRef]
37. Morabito, A.; De Simone, G.; Pastorelli, R.; Brunelli, L.; Ferrario, M. Algorithms and tools for data-driven omics integration to achieve multilayer biological insights: A narrative review. *J. Transl. Med.* **2025**, *23*, 425. [CrossRef] [PubMed]
38. Olawade, D.B.; Teke, J.; Adeleye, K.K.; Weerasinghe, K.; Maidoki, M.; Clement David-Olawade, A. Artificial intelligence in in-vitro fertilization (IVF): A new era of precision and personalization in fertility treatments. *J. Gynecol. Obstet. Hum. Reprod.* **2025**, *54*, 102903. [CrossRef] [PubMed]
39. Potiris, A.; Alyfanti, E.; Drakaki, E.; Mavrogianni, D.; Karampitsakos, T.; Machairoudias, P.; Topis, S.; Zikopoulos, A.; Skentou, C.; Panagopoulos, P.; et al. The Contribution of Proteomics in Understanding Endometrial Protein Expression in Women with Recurrent Implantation Failure. *J. Clin. Med.* **2024**, *13*, 2145. [CrossRef] [PubMed]
40. Liang, J.; Gao, Y.; Feng, Z.; Zhang, B.; Na, Z.; Li, D. Reactive oxygen species and ovarian diseases: Antioxidant strategies. *Redox Biol.* **2023**, *62*, 102659. [CrossRef]
41. Wang, Y.; Fu, X.; Li, H. Mechanisms of oxidative stress-induced sperm dysfunction. *Front. Endocrinol.* **2025**, *16*, 1520835. [CrossRef]
42. Gualtieri, R.; Kalthur, G.; Barbato, V.; Longobardi, S.; Di Rella, F.; Adiga, S.K.; Talevi, R. Sperm Oxidative Stress during In Vitro Manipulation and Its Effects on Sperm Function and Embryo Development. *Antioxidants* **2021**, *10*, 1025. [CrossRef]
43. Yan, F.; Zhao, Q.; Li, Y.; Zheng, Z.; Kong, X.; Shu, C.; Liu, Y.; Shi, Y. The role of oxidative stress in ovarian aging: A review. *J. Ovarian Res.* **2022**, *15*, 100. [CrossRef]
44. Potiris, A.; Moustakli, E.; Trismpioti, E.; Drakaki, E.; Mavrogianni, D.; Matsas, A.; Zikopoulos, A.; Sfakianakis, A.; Tsakiridis, I.; Dagklis, T.; et al. From Inflammation to Infertility: How Oxidative Stress and Infections Disrupt Male Reproductive Health. *Metabolites* **2025**, *15*, 267. [CrossRef] [PubMed]
45. Agarwal, A.; Qiu, E.; Sharma, R. Laboratory assessment of oxidative stress in semen. *Arab. J. Urol.* **2018**, *16*, 77–86. [CrossRef]
46. Castleton, P.E.; Deluao, J.C.; Sharkey, D.J.; McPherson, N.O. Measuring Reactive Oxygen Species in Semen for Male Preconception Care: A Scientist Perspective. *Antioxidants* **2022**, *11*, 264. [CrossRef] [PubMed]
47. Agarwal, A.; Aponte-Mellado, A.; Premkumar, B.J.; Shaman, A.; Gupta, S. The effects of oxidative stress on female reproduction: A review. *Reprod. Biol. Endocrinol.* **2012**, *10*, 49. [CrossRef]
48. Chen, Y.; Yang, J.; Zhang, L. The Impact of Follicular Fluid Oxidative Stress Levels on the Outcomes of Assisted Reproductive Therapy. *Antioxidants* **2023**, *12*, 2117. [CrossRef]
49. Moustakli, E.; Zikopoulos, A.; Skentou, C.; Katopodis, P.; Domali, E.; Potiris, A.; Stavros, S.; Zachariou, A. Impact of Reductive Stress on Human Infertility: Underlying Mechanisms and Perspectives. *Int. J. Mol. Sci.* **2024**, *25*, 11802. [CrossRef]
50. Nowicka-Bauer, K.; Nixon, B. Molecular Changes Induced by Oxidative Stress that Impair Human Sperm Motility. *Antioxidants* **2020**, *9*, 134. [CrossRef] [PubMed]
51. Liu, J.; Wen, S.; Lin, Y.; Yang, X.; Liu, Z.; Quan, S.; Song, Y. Advanced oxidation protein products change biological behaviors of rat endometrial epithelial cells by activating ERK/P38 signaling pathways. *Biol. Open* **2020**, *9*, bio048876. [CrossRef]
52. Gupta, S.; Finelli, R.; Agarwal, A.; Henkel, R. Total antioxidant capacity-Relevance, methods and clinical implications. *Andrologia* **2021**, *53*, e13624. [CrossRef] [PubMed]

53. Babić, N.; Peyrot, F. Molecular Probes for Evaluation of Oxidative Stress by In Vivo EPR Spectroscopy and Imaging: State-of-the-Art and Limitations. *Magnetochemistry* **2019**, *5*, 13. [CrossRef]
54. Mihalas, B.P.; De Iuliis, G.N.; Redgrove, K.A.; McLaughlin, E.A.; Nixon, B. The lipid peroxidation product 4-hydroxynonenal contributes to oxidative stress-mediated deterioration of the ageing oocyte. *Sci. Rep.* **2017**, *7*, 6247. [CrossRef] [PubMed]
55. Campara, K.; Rodrigues, P.; Viero, F.T.; da Silva, B.; Trevisan, G. A systematic review and meta-analysis of advanced oxidative protein products levels (AOPP) levels in endometriosis: Association with disease stage and clinical implications. *Eur. J. Pharmacol.* **2025**, *996*, 177434. [CrossRef]
56. Silvestrini, A.; Mancini, A. The Double-Edged Sword of Total Antioxidant Capacity: Clinical Significance and Personal Experience. *Antioxidants* **2024**, *13*, 933. [CrossRef] [PubMed]
57. Ibrahim, A.; Khoo, M.I.; Ismail, E.H.E.; Hussain, N.H.N.; Zin, A.A.M.; Noordin, L.; Abdullah, S.; Mahdy, Z.A.; Lah, N. Oxidative stress biomarkers in pregnancy: A systematic review. *Reprod. Biol. Endocrinol.* **2024**, *22*, 93. [CrossRef]
58. Giorgi, C.; Marchi, S.; Simoes, I.C.M.; Ren, Z.; Morciano, G.; Perrone, M.; Patalas-Krawczyk, P.; Borchard, S.; Jedrak, P.; Pierzynowska, K.; et al. Mitochondria and Reactive Oxygen Species in Aging and Age-Related Diseases. *Int. Rev. Cell Mol. Biol.* **2018**, *340*, 209–344. [CrossRef]
59. Da Broi, M.G.; Giorgi, V.S.I.; Wang, F.; Keefe, D.L.; Albertini, D.; Navarro, P.A. Influence of follicular fluid and cumulus cells on oocyte quality: Clinical implications. *J. Assist. Reprod. Genet.* **2018**, *35*, 735–751. [CrossRef] [PubMed]
60. Moustakli, E.; Zikopoulos, A.; Skentou, C.; Stavros, S.; Sofikitis, N.; Georgiou, I.; Zachariou, A. Integrative Assessment of Seminal Plasma Biomarkers: A Narrative Review Bridging the Gap between Infertility Research and Clinical Practice. *J. Clin. Med.* **2024**, *13*, 3147. [CrossRef]
61. Vashisht, A.; Gahlay, G.K. Understanding seminal plasma in male infertility: Emerging markers and their implications. *Andrology* **2024**, *12*, 1058–1077. [CrossRef]
62. Stavros, S.; Potiris, A.; Molopodi, E.; Mavrogianni, D.; Zikopoulos, A.; Louis, K.; Karampitsakos, T.; Nazou, E.; Sioutis, D.; Christodoulaki, C.; et al. Sperm DNA Fragmentation: Unraveling Its Imperative Impact on Male Infertility Based on Recent Evidence. *Int. J. Mol. Sci.* **2024**, *25*, 10167. [CrossRef]
63. Arya, S.S.; Dias, S.B.; Jelinek, H.F.; Hadjileontiadis, L.J.; Pappa, A.M. The convergence of traditional and digital biomarkers through AI-assisted biosensing: A new era in translational diagnostics? *Biosens. Bioelectron.* **2023**, *235*, 115387. [CrossRef]
64. Peng, J.; Geng, X.; Zhao, Y.; Hou, Z.; Tian, X.; Liu, X.; Xiao, Y.; Liu, Y. Machine learning algorithms in constructing prediction models for assisted reproductive technology (ART) related live birth outcomes. *Sci. Rep.* **2024**, *14*, 32083. [CrossRef] [PubMed]
65. Duanghathaipornsuk, S.; Farrell, E.J.; Alba-Rubio, A.C.; Zelenay, P.; Kim, D.S. Detection Technologies for Reactive Oxygen Species: Fluorescence and Electrochemical Methods and Their Applications. *Biosensors* **2021**, *11*, 30. [CrossRef]
66. Huang, X.; Huang, L.; Lu, J.; Cheng, L.; Wu, D.; Li, L.; Zhang, S.; Lai, X.; Xu, L. The relationship between telomere length and aging-related diseases. *Clin. Exp. Med.* **2025**, *25*, 72. [CrossRef] [PubMed]
67. Fragkiadaki, P.; Kouvidi, E.; Angelaki, A.; Nikolopoulou, D.; Vakonaki, E.; Tsatsakis, A. Evaluation of telomere length and telomerase activity on predicting in vitro fertilization treatment outcomes. *J. Assist. Reprod. Genet.* **2024**, *41*, 1463–1473. [CrossRef] [PubMed]
68. Montpetit, A.J.; Alhareeri, A.A.; Montpetit, M.; Starkweather, A.R.; Elmore, L.W.; Filler, K.; Mohanraj, L.; Burton, C.W.; Menzies, V.S.; Lyon, D.E.; et al. Telomere length: A review of methods for measurement. *Nurs. Res.* **2014**, *63*, 289–299. [CrossRef]
69. Fice, H.E.; Robaire, B. Telomere Dynamics Throughout Spermatogenesis. *Genes* **2019**, *10*, 525. [CrossRef]
70. Chico-Sordo, L.; Cordova-Oriz, I.; Polonio, A.M.; LS, S.M.; Medrano, M.; Garcia-Velasco, J.A.; Varela, E. Reproductive aging and telomeres: Are women and men equally affected? *Mech. Ageing Dev.* **2021**, *198*, 111541. [CrossRef]
71. Bakare, O.S. AI-Driven Multi-Omics Integration for Precision Medicine in Complex Disease Diagnosis and Treatment. *Int. J. Res. Publ. Rev.* **2025**, *6*, 5070–5084. [CrossRef]
72. Findikli, N.; Houba, C.; Pening, D.; Delbaere, A. The Role of Artificial Intelligence in Female Infertility Diagnosis: An Update. *J. Clin. Med.* **2025**, *14*, 3127. [CrossRef]
73. Wu, Y.C.; Chia-Yu Su, E.; Hou, J.H.; Lin, C.J.; Lin, K.B.; Chen, C.H. Artificial intelligence and assisted reproductive technology: A comprehensive systematic review. *Taiwan J. Obstet. Gynecol.* **2025**, *64*, 11–26. [CrossRef]
74. AlSaad, R.; Abusarhan, L.; Odeh, N.; Abd-Alrazaq, A.; Choucair, F.; Zegour, R.; Ahmed, A.; Aziz, S.; Sheikh, J. Deep learning applications for human embryo assessment using time-lapse imaging: Scoping review. *Front. Reprod. Health* **2025**, *7*, 1549642. [CrossRef] [PubMed]
75. Baldán, F.J.; García-Gil, D.; Fernandez-Basso, C. Revolutionizing Sperm Analysis with AI: A Review of Computer-Aided Sperm Analysis Systems. *Computation* **2025**, *13*, 132. [CrossRef]
76. Yetgin, A. Revolutionizing multi-omics analysis with artificial intelligence and data processing. *Quant. Biol.* **2025**, *13*, e70002. [CrossRef]
77. Wang, R.; Pan, W.; Jin, L.; Li, Y.; Geng, Y.; Gao, C.; Chen, G.; Wang, H.; Ma, D.; Liao, S. Artificial intelligence in reproductive medicine. *Reproduction* **2019**, *158*, R139–R154. [CrossRef]

78. Miao, H.; Liu, S.; Wang, Z.; Ke, Y.; Cheng, L.; Yu, W.; Yu, D.; Zhang, K.; Gao, Y.; Sun, Z. Artificial intelligence-derived retinal age gap as a marker for reproductive aging in women. *NPJ Digit. Med.* **2025**, *8*, 367. [CrossRef] [PubMed]
79. Wen, J.Y.; Liu, C.F.; Chung, M.T.; Tsai, Y.C. Artificial intelligence model to predict pregnancy and multiple pregnancy risk following in vitro fertilization-embryo transfer (IVF-ET). *Taiwan J. Obstet. Gynecol.* **2022**, *61*, 837–846. [CrossRef] [PubMed]
80. Ghayda, R.A.; Cannarella, R.; Calogero, A.E.; Shah, R.; Rambhatla, A.; Zohdy, W.; Kavoussi, P.; Avidor-Reiss, T.; Boitrelle, F.; Mostafa, T.; et al. Artificial Intelligence in Andrology: From Semen Analysis to Image Diagnostics. *World J. Mens. Health* **2024**, *42*, 39–61. [CrossRef]
81. Worheide, M.A.; Krumsiek, J.; Kastenmuller, G.; Arnold, M. Multi-omics integration in biomedical research—A metabolomics-centric review. *Anal. Chim. Acta* **2021**, *1141*, 144–162. [CrossRef] [PubMed]
82. Derevyanko, A.; Skowronska, A.; Skowronski, M.T.; Kordowitzki, P. The Interplay between Telomeres, Mitochondria, and Chronic Stress Exposure in the Aging Egg. *Cells* **2022**, *11*, 2612. [CrossRef]
83. Hew, Y.; Kutuk, D.; Duzcu, T.; Ergun, Y.; Basar, M. Artificial Intelligence in IVF Laboratories: Elevating Outcomes Through Precision and Efficiency. *Biology* **2024**, *13*, 988. [CrossRef]
84. Wadden, J.J. Defining the undefinable: The black box problem in healthcare artificial intelligence. *J. Med. Ethics* **2022**, *48*, 764–768. [CrossRef]
85. Rolfes, V.; Bittner, U.; Gerhards, H.; Krussel, J.S.; Fehm, T.; Ranisch, R.; Fangerau, H. Artificial Intelligence in Reproductive Medicine—An Ethical Perspective. *Geburtshilfe Frauenheilkd* **2023**, *83*, 106–115. [CrossRef]
86. Elendu, C.; Amaechi, D.C.; Elendu, T.C.; Jingwa, K.A.; Okoye, O.K.; John Okah, M.; Ladele, J.A.; Farah, A.H.; Alimi, H.A. Ethical implications of AI and robotics in healthcare: A review. *Medicine* **2023**, *102*, e36671. [CrossRef] [PubMed]
87. Sah, A.K.; Elshaikh, R.H.; Shalabi, M.G.; Abbas, A.M.; Prabhakar, P.K.; Babker, A.M.A.; Choudhary, R.K.; Gaur, V.; Choudhary, A.S.; Agarwal, S. Role of Artificial Intelligence and Personalized Medicine in Enhancing HIV Management and Treatment Outcomes. *Life* **2025**, *15*, 745. [CrossRef] [PubMed]
88. Fasching, C.L. Telomere length measurement as a clinical biomarker of aging and disease. *Crit. Rev. Clin. Lab. Sci.* **2018**, *55*, 443–465. [CrossRef]
89. Dragoumani, K.; Kletsas, D.; Chrousos, G.P.; Vlachakis, D.; Balatsos, N.A.A. Molecular and Environmental Modulators of Aging: Interplay Between Inflammation, Epigenetics, and RNA Stability. *Genes* **2025**, *16*, 796. [CrossRef]
90. Boccardi, V.; Marano, L. Aging, Cancer, and Inflammation: The Telomerase Connection. *Int. J. Mol. Sci.* **2024**, *25*, 8542. [CrossRef]
91. Ahmed, M.I.; Spooner, B.; Isherwood, J.; Lane, M.; Orrock, E.; Dennison, A. A Systematic Review of the Barriers to the Implementation of Artificial Intelligence in Healthcare. *Cureus* **2023**, *15*, e46454. [CrossRef] [PubMed]
92. Cabitza, F.; Campagner, A.; Soares, F.; Garcia de Guadiana-Romualdo, L.; Challa, F.; Sulejmani, A.; Seghezzi, M.; Carobene, A. The importance of being external. methodological insights for the external validation of machine learning models in medicine. *Comput. Methods Programs Biomed.* **2021**, *208*, 106288. [CrossRef] [PubMed]
93. Moulaei, K.; Akhlaghpour, S.; Fatehi, F. Patient consent for the secondary use of health data in artificial intelligence (AI) models: A scoping review. *Int. J. Med. Inform.* **2025**, *198*, 105872. [CrossRef] [PubMed]
94. Cestonaro, C.; Delicati, A.; Marcante, B.; Caenazzo, L.; Tozzo, P. Defining medical liability when artificial intelligence is applied on diagnostic algorithms: A systematic review. *Front. Med.* **2023**, *10*, 1305756. [CrossRef] [PubMed]

diagnostics

MDPI

Systematic Review

Advanced Deep Learning Approaches in Detection Technologies for Comprehensive Breast Cancer Assessment Based on WSIs: A Systematic Literature Review

Qiaoyi Xu [1,2,*], Afzan Adam [1], Azizi Abdullah [1] and Nurkhairul Bariyah [3]

[1] Center for Artificial Intelligence Technology, Faculty of Information Science and Technology, Universiti Kebangsaan Malaysia, Bangi 43600, Selangor, Malaysia; afzan@ukm.edu.my (A.A.); azizia@ukm.edu.my (A.A.)
[2] College of Intelligent Manufacturing, Zibo Vocational Institute, Zibo 255314, China
[3] Department of Pathology, Faculty of Medicine, Universiti Kebangsaan Malaysia, Jalan Yaacob Latif, Bandar Tun Razak, Cheras 56000, Wilayah Persekutuan Kuala Lumpur, Malaysia; p110546@siswa.ukm.edu.my
* Correspondence: p114345@siswa.ukm.edu.my

Abstract: Background: Breast cancer is one of the leading causes of death among women worldwide. Accurate early detection of lymphocytes and molecular biomarkers is essential for improving diagnostic precision and patient prognosis. Whole slide images (WSIs) are central to digital pathology workflows in breast cancer assessment. However, applying deep learning techniques to WSIs presents persistent challenges, including variability in image quality, limited availability of high-quality annotations, poor model interpretability, high computational demands, and suboptimal processing efficiency. **Methods:** This systematic review, guided by the Preferred Reporting Items for Systematic Reviews and Meta-Analyses (PRISMA), examines deep learning-based detection methods for breast cancer published between 2020 and 2024. The analysis includes 39 peer-reviewed studies and 20 widely used WSI datasets. **Results:** To enhance clinical relevance and guide model development, this study introduces a five-dimensional evaluation framework covering accuracy and performance, robustness and generalization, interpretability, computational efficiency, and annotation quality. The framework facilitates a balanced and clinically aligned assessment of both established methods and recent innovations. **Conclusions:** This review offers a comprehensive analysis and proposes a practical roadmap for addressing core challenges in WSI-based breast cancer detection. It fills a critical gap in the literature and provides actionable guidance for researchers, clinicians, and developers seeking to optimize and translate WSI-based technologies into clinical workflows for comprehensive breast cancer assessment.

Keywords: breast cancer; detection algorithm; whole slide images; deep learning; systematic literature review

1. Introduction

Breast cancer remains one of the most prevalent and deadly malignancies affecting women worldwide, posing a significant threat to both health outcomes and quality of life [1–3]. Despite remarkable advances in medical diagnostics and therapeutic strategies, the molecular heterogeneity and diverse clinical manifestations of breast cancer continue to complicate its detection and management [4]. Biomarker and lymphocyte detection are critical components in breast cancer assessment, offering essential guidance for diagnosis, classification, and prognosis [5].

Among these, the estrogen receptor (ER) serves as a key molecular marker for subtype classification and supports the development of personalized treatment regimens, directly influencing patient outcomes [6]. The proliferation index Ki-67 Antigen (Ki67) provides independent predictive value for treatment response, while the joint evaluation of ER and progesterone receptor (PR) further refines hormone therapy decisions [7]. Overexpression of human epidermal growth factor receptor 2 (HER2) correlates with increased tumor aggressiveness and recurrence risk, making HER2-positive cases suitable for targeted therapy. In addition, tumor-infiltrating lymphocytes (TILs) are considered reliable prognostic indicators, especially for triple-negative breast cancer (TNBC) patients, where TIL density correlates with both disease-free and overall survival [8]. Accurate identification of these biomarkers and immune features forms the foundation for effective clinical decision-making.

Recent advancements in whole-slide imaging (WSI) have enabled digital pathology to visualize entire tissue sections at ultra-high resolution, capturing both the spatial distribution of biomarkers and the microenvironmental context of lymphocytes [9,10]. These large-format digitized slides—typically prepared using Hematoxylin and Eosin (H&E) staining for structural visualization and Immunohistochemistry (IHC) for highlighting specific molecular targets—provide pathologists with richer information but also introduce significant technical challenges. The sheer volume of image data—often exceeding one billion pixels per slide—and the complex spatial patterns of diagnostic features render manual analysis time-consuming, subjective, and difficult to scale [11,12]. Traditional workflows depend heavily on expert interpretation, leading to potential variability and limited reproducibility in large-scale clinical studies.

To address these limitations, deep learning has emerged as a promising approach for automating WSI analysis. While segmentation tasks aim to label each pixel according to tissue type or structure [13], detection-based techniques are particularly well-suited for clinical applications. They generate interpretable, quantitative outputs such as cell counts, biomarker localization, and lymphocyte spatial distributions, which align more directly with diagnostic workflows [13,14]. This review focuses on detection-oriented methods in WSI analysis and their applications across four critical clinical tasks: diagnosis, classification, grading, and prognosis.

Nonetheless, the integration of deep learning into WSI-based breast cancer assessment remains nontrivial. The ultra-high resolution of WSIs demands substantial computational resources and presents design challenges for conventional model architectures [15,16]. Furthermore, WSIs exhibit a multi-scale nature—ranging from microscopic cell morphology to macroscopic tissue organization—necessitating models capable of learning across spatial hierarchies [17]. The analysis is further complicated by sparse diagnostic features, intersample heterogeneity, and staining variations. Compounding these issues is the scarcity of large, well-annotated datasets, which limits the scalability of supervised learning approaches [18]. Interpretability also remains a major concern, as the opaque decision-making processes of deep learning models reduce clinical trust [19]. Effective detection algorithms must therefore balance sensitivity to subtle morphological cues with robustness against noise and artifacts—especially when identifying key features such as biomarker expression and lymphocyte infiltration.

Despite a growing body of literature in this domain, existing reviews often remain narrowly focused. Many concentrate on segmentation techniques or algorithmic performance metrics, without sufficiently addressing the clinical integration of detection methods or their practical utility [20–22]. Additionally, critical issues such as dataset bias, computational burden, and feedback mechanisms from clinical deployment are frequently overlooked. This gap highlights the need for a more holistic and clinically grounded synthesis of detection-focused research in breast cancer WSIs.

To this end, this review aims to address three key research questions:

1. What types of datasets are used for comprehensive breast cancer assessment using WSIs?
2. What are the main challenges associated with comprehensive breast cancer assessment using WSIs?
3. How do WSIs impact the accuracy and reliability of advanced deep learning approaches for comprehensive breast cancer assessment?

Figure 1 summarizes the task types, datasets, AI models, and evaluation criteria that frame this review of deep learning-based breast cancer assessment using WSIs. This study systematically reviews the landscape of relevant approaches published between 2020 and 2024, following PRISMA guidelines [23]. It synthesizes recent methodological advancements, identifies unresolved challenges, and outlines future research directions. In particular, we emphasize the clinical significance of detection tasks, the scalability of AI-based diagnostic tools, and the potential for deep learning to transform biomarker discovery and personalized treatment planning in digital pathology.

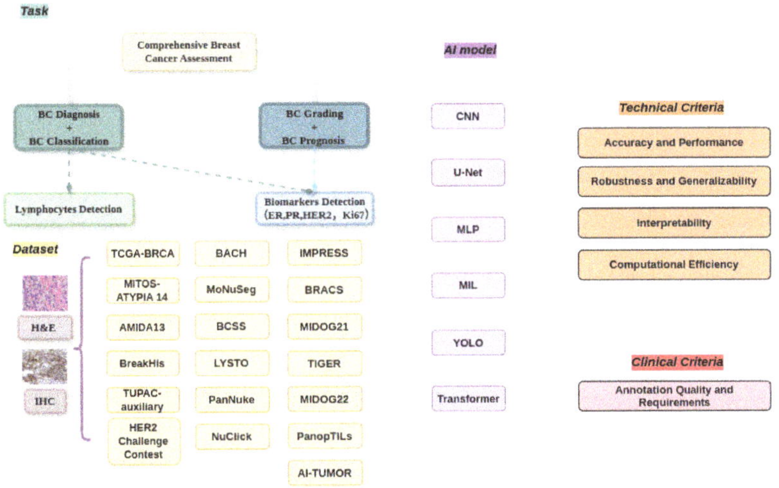

Figure 1. Overview of detection tasks, datasets, models, and evaluation criteria in WSI-based breast cancer assessment.

2. Methods

The study followed the PRISMA guideline [24] in this systematic literature review. PRISMA provides a consistent, repeatable process for locating, assessing, and selecting pertinent research. It also provides guidance on how to choose, recognize, and evaluate studies [25,26].

Figure 2 shows the PRISMA procedure used for this systematic literature review. The next subsection provides details on the review process.

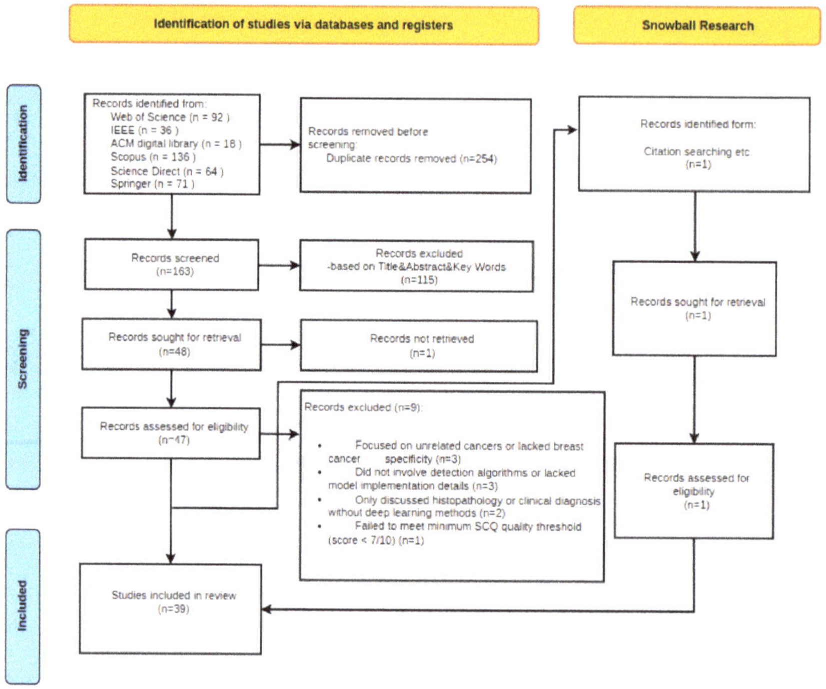

Figure 2. PRISMA flow diagram of the SLR.

2.1. Data Sources and Search Strategy

To identify relevant academic publications, 8 major bibliographic databases were used, including Scopus, IEEE Xplore Library, Web of Science, SpringerLink, ACM Digital Library, and ScienceDirect. Consequently, the systematic literature review focused on articles published between 2020 and 2024 to ensure the inclusion of the most recent and relevant research findings. The search strategy employed combinations of key terms like the following:

- "breast cancer detection" AND "deep learning"
- "breast cancer diagnosis" AND "deep learning"
- "convolutional neural networks" AND "breast cancer"
- "lymphocytes detection" OR "biomarkers detection" AND "breast cancer"
- "H&E stained images" AND "deep learning" AND "breast cancer"
- "immunohistochemistry" AND "deep learning" AND "breast cancer"
- "automated breast cancer diagnosis" OR "AI in breast cancer screening"

These search parameters were created to encompass the depth of knowledge regarding deep learning applications in the detection and analysis of breast cancer.

2.2. Selection Criteria

An exhaustive search strategy combining both automated and manual methods initially retrieved 417 academic publications. Throughout the entire screening process, the inclusion and exclusion criteria outlined in Table 1 were applied consistently. After eliminating 254 duplicate records, 163 unique publications were screened based on their titles, abstracts, and keywords. At this stage, 115 papers were excluded due to a lack of domain relevance or methodological inadequacy.

Table 1. Inclusion and exclusion criteria.

Inclusion Criteria	Exclusion Criteria
Articles related to advanced deep learning-based techniques for comprehensive breast cancer assessment, focusing on diagnosis, classification, grading, and prognosis	Duplicates
Emphasis on peer-reviewed journal articles and conference papers	Articles not addressing breast cancer detection, classification, grading, or prognosis strategies
Studies employing WSI techniques and related fields, particularly those focusing on breast cancer diagnosis and prognosis	Studies not related to WSI techniques and their application in breast cancer assessment
Articles that meet rigorous quality-assessment standards and have a clear focus on the two major tasks of breast cancer assessment	Articles not meeting quality-assessment standards
Articles addressing breast cancer-detection techniques through WSIs, focusing on key points like biomarkers and lymphocytes	Studies not utilizing WSIs or not focusing on the specified key points for breast cancer assessment

Following this, 48 full-text articles were retrieved for in-depth evaluation. One article was excluded due to inaccessibility, and the remaining 47 underwent full eligibility assessment. Nine additional studies were excluded for the following reasons: three did not focus specifically on breast cancer or its primary clinical tasks (e.g., detection, classification, prognosis); three lacked concrete details regarding deep learning algorithms or implementation strategies; two relied solely on conventional pathology without computational approaches; and one failed to meet the minimum quality threshold on the Standard Quality Checklist (SCQ).

This systematic and criteria-driven selection process resulted in 39 high-quality studies being included in the final review. The characteristics of these selected publications are summarized in Table 2, providing a foundation for subsequent quality assessment and synthesis.

Table 2. Summary of included studies with evaluation and data scale (LD = lymphocyte detection; BD = biomarker detection; - = not specified in the article).

Source	Year	Task	Model	Result	Dataset and Scale
1 [27]	2020	BD	AlexNet	F1 score = 0.73	Private Dataset 50 Ki67 WSIs 50 H&E WSIs
2 [28]	2020	LD	NucTraL + BCF	Accuracy = 0.9691	BreakHis Benign: 637 WSIs Malignant: 1390 WSIs
3 [29]	2020	LD	Deep-CNN + FSRM	Accuracy = 98.8%, F1 score = 0.967	BreakHis Benign: 2480 WSIs Malignant: 5429 WSIs

Table 2. *Cont.*

Source	Year	Task	Model	Result	Dataset and Scale
4 [30]	2020	LD	Faster R-CNN	F1 score: Scattered lymphocytes: 0.9615 Agglomerated lymphocytes: 0.8645 Artifact area: 0.8197	LYSTO 1228 WSIs
5 [31]	2021	BD	U-Net-piNET	F1 score: Ki67-: 0.868; Ki67+: 0.804	Private Dataset 1142 WSIs
6 [32]	2021	BD	U-Net	Pearson correlation coefficient of r = 0.95	Private Dataset 200 WSIs
7 [33]	2021	BD	DLS	AUC = 0.60	TCGA-BRCA 3274 WSIs
8 [34]	2021	LD	UBCNN	-	MoNuSeg 120 WSIs
9 [35]	2021	LD	Micro-Net + MLP	F1 score = 0.87	TCGA-BRCA 4281 nuclei images
10 [36]	2021	LD	UNMaSk	F1 score: H&E: 0.856 IHC: 0.9037	Private Dataset 178 WSIs
11 [37]	2021	LD	CNN	AUROC = 0.864	TCGA-BRCA 7075WSIs
12 [38]	2021	LD & BD	PathoNet	F1 score = 0.7928	SHIDC-BC-Ki-67 2357 WSIs
13 [39]	2021	LD	SegNet + U-Net	F1 score = 0.91	BCa 100 ROIs
14 [40]	2021	LD	WeakSTIL	-	TCGA-BRCA 286 WSIs
15 [41]	2021	LD	CNN	-	TCGA-BRCA 2358 WSIs
16 [42]	2022	LD	TDC-LC	F1 score = 0.892	LYSTO 19663 patches
17 [43]	2022	LD	DDTNet	F1 score = 0.907	TCGA-BRCA 865 WSIs
18 [44]	2023	BD	GAN+CNN+U-Net	-	Private Dataset 321 samples
19 [45]	2023	LD	CB-HVT Net	F1 score = 0.88	LYSTO & NuClick 21312 images
20 [46]	2023	LD	AC-Former	F1 score = 0.796	TCGA-BRCA 452 images
21 [47]	2023	LD	-	-	LYSTO 83 WSIs

Table 2. *Cont.*

Source	Year	Task	Model	Result	Dataset and Scale
22 [48]	2023	LD	CBAM-Residual U-Net	F1 score = 0.9	TNBC 81 WSIs
23 [49]	2023	LD	U-Net +Mask R-CNN	F1 score = 0.941	Private Dataset 63 WSIs
24 [50]	2023	LD	MobileNetV2 +U-Net	F1 score = 0.927	Private Dataset 30 WSIs
25 [51]	2023	LD	DC-Lym-AF	F1 score = 0.84	LYSTO & NuClick 871 images
26 [52]	2023	LD	FMDet	F1 score = 0.773	MIDOG21, MITOS-ATYPIA 14, AMIDA13, TUPAC-auxiliary 403 WSIs
27 [53]	2023	LD	DeepLabV3	F1 score = 71.23	OCELOT, TIGER 17041patches
28 [54]	2023	LD	BCF-Lym-Detector	F1 score: LYSTO: 0.93 NuClick: 0.84	LYSTO & NuClick 16326 images
29 [55]	2023	LD	CNN	F1 score: Immune cell: 0.82 Tumour cell: 0.92 Stromal cell: 0.81	Private Dataset 2549 images
30 [56]	2023	LD	PROACTING	AUC = 0.88	IMPRESS 1053 images
31 [57]	2024	BD	Based on CNN	AUC = 0.72	TCGA-BRCA 14435 images
32 [58]	2024	BD	ViT	F1 score = 0.9269	Her 2 challenge contest 172 WSIs
33 [59]	2024	LD	Cell-Tissue-ViT	F1 score = 0.7243	OCELOT 400 Patches
34 [60]	2024	LD	Tissue Context + Cell Refinement	F1-score = 0.7473	OCELOT 400 Patches
35 [61]	2024	LD	PathoNet	F1 score: SHIDC-B-Ki-67: 0.842 LSOC-Ki-67: 0.909	SHIDC-BC-Ki-67, LSOC-Ki-67 2447 WSIs
36 [62]	2024	LD	DeepMitosisNet	F1 score = 0.93	MITOS-ATYPIA 14 2127 images
37 [63]	2024	LD	CellViT	F1 score = 0.81	PanNuke 7959 images
38 [64]	2024	LD	YOLOv5	F1 score = 0.7438	TIGER 1879 ROIs
39 [65]	2024	LD	MuTILs	AUROC = 93.0	PanopTILs 1317 ROIs

2.3. Quality Assessment

Assessing the quality of evidence is crucial in a systematic literature review (SLR), as methodological biases may influence outcomes and lead to misinterpretation. To ensure the reliability and rigor of the included studies, this review adopted the Standard SCQ proposed by [66], which comprises ten evaluation items. Following the approach of [57], only studies that provided a "yes" response to at least seven SCQ items were included.

Among the 39 studies selected after quality filtering, the SCQ score distribution was as follows: 10 studies received a full score (10/10), 15 studies scored 9/10, 11 studies scored 8/10, and 3 studies met the minimum threshold with 7/10. Studies scoring below this threshold were excluded to maintain methodological rigor. This distribution reflects the overall quality consistency of the selected literature and ensures that only robust and dependable studies were included in the final synthesis. The SCQ evaluation and data extraction processes were closely integrated to enhance the validity and significance of the review outcomes. Table 3 outlines the SCQ criteria used in this study.

Table 3. Checklist for quality assessment.

Checklist for Quality Assessment	SCQ No
Is the report coherent and easy to read?	SCQ1
Is the research's purpose well-defined?	SCQ2
Is the procedure for gathering data clearly laid out?	SCQ3
Have the settings of diversity been thoroughly examined?	SCQ4
Can the study's conclusions be trusted?	SCQ5
Is there a connection between the information, analysis, and conclusion?	SCQ6
Is the process of experimentation and approach transparent?	SCQ7
Are the research methods sufficiently documented?	SCQ8
If they are credible, are they important?	SCQ9
Is it possible to duplicate the research findings?	SCQ10

2.4. Data Extraction and Synthesis

The study noted the pertinent information from each study, such as the publisher, authors, and year of publication, and gathered data for our SLR on the deep learning techniques used, reported accuracy, and assessment criteria. To answer the study's research questions, the authors particularly examined the results during the data synthesis phase. The authors used a variety of visualization approaches and tools, including tables and diagrams, to make this analysis easier.

3. Results and Meta-Analysis

The meta-analysis of the search results from our systematic literature review is shown in this section. It starts with a summary of the chosen articles before going into each of the study questions that were developed and stated in the introduction.

3.1. Overview of Selected Studies

Figure 3 provides a chronological overview of the articles selected for this SLR, detailing the number of publications related to advanced deep learning methods for breast cancer cell detection using digital pathology images from 2020 to 2024. The diagram indicates a growing trend in this research area over the past few years, particularly from 2023 to 2024, when the number of published articles significantly increased. Most of the articles considered for this study were published after 2023. Specifically, the highest number of articles published in a single year was 13 in 2023 and 9 in 2024, followed by 10 papers in 2021 and 4 papers in 2020. In contrast, only 2 papers were reviewed in 2022, which some literature attributes to the impact of the COVID-19 pandemic on research output.

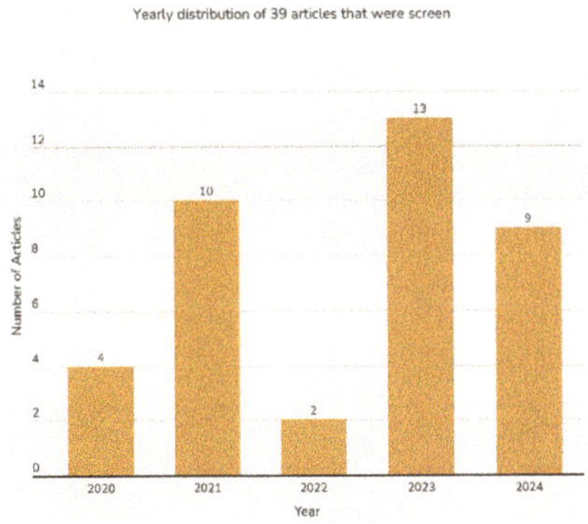

Figure 3. Diagram showing the number of articles published per year from 2020 to 2024.

3.2. Research Question 1: What Types of Datasets Are Employed for Comprehensive Breast Cancer Assessment Using WSIs?

This research evaluates 20 key WSIs datasets pivotal to advancing deep learning applications in breast cancer detection, diagnosis, classification, grading, and prognosis. These datasets, each contributing uniquely to comprehensive breast cancer assessment, reflect the rapid evolution and diversification of digital pathology resources.

The following attributes define the state of the breast cancer WSI datasets:

1. Scale and Origin:
    - The basic resources are large-scale public repositories such as TCGA-BRCA (3111 WSIs) [67].
    - Focused, high-resolution data are available from specialized datasets like PanNuke (200,000 nuclei across 19 tissue types) and BACH (400 patches, 30 WSIs) [68,69].
    - For particular study goals, derivative datasets (MoNuSeg, BCSS, TIGER) expand on primary sources [70].
2. Research Focus and Annotation Granularity:
    - Datasets cover a wide range of anatomical structures, such as nuclei in MoNuSeg and tumor-infiltrating lymphocytes in PanopTILs, to specific cellular structures.
    - Increasing model sophistication is reflected in the variation in annotation detail from whole-slide to pixel-level [71].
3. Multi-modal Integration:
    - Datasets that integrate clinical and genetic information with histopathological images, such as TCGA-BRCA, provide opportunities for more thorough and comprehensive analysis [72,73].
4. Ethical Considerations and Diversity:
    - More recent datasets, such as AI-TUMOR, highlight the diversity of patient demographics and the use of ethical data collection techniques [74].

Together, these datasets enable a wide range of deep learning uses, ranging from simple cell identification to intricate tumor categorization and prognostic modeling. In addition to driving innovation in deep learning architectures suited to the particular difficulties of breast cancer analysis, they act as benchmarks for model development and validation [75,76].

These datasets development follows the field's move toward more extensive, fully annotated resources on a wider scale. This pattern suggests a developing sector ready to use cutting-edge computational techniques to address the intricate, multidimensional character of breast cancer research, along with the integration of multimodal data and a growing emphasis on ethical issues.

Table 4 lists the various datasets and highlights their unique properties that were employed for WSI-based comprehensive breast cancer assessment. Each dataset plays a crucial role in advancing deep learning methodologies by providing diverse and detailed data for model training and validation.

Table 4. Key WSI datasets relevant to comprehensive breast cancer assessment.

Name	Year	Key Features	Contribution	Link
TCGA-BRCA [77]	-	3111 H&E-stained WSIs from 1086 female and 12 male breast cancer patients. Includes matched gene expression data and clinical information.	Widely used to create derivative datasets like MoNuSeg, BCSS, LYSTO, and TIGER.	https://portal.gdc.cancer.gov/projects/TCGA-BRCA (accessed on 18 July 2024)
MITOS-ATYPIA 14	2013	2400 high-power field (HPF) images from 11 breast cancer patients, scanned by two devices: 1200 at 1539 × 1376 pixels and 1200 at 1663 × 1485 pixels, all at 40× magnification.	Provides a comprehensive external test set for evaluating the robustness of mitosis-detection models across different imaging conditions.	https://mitos-atypia-14.grand-challenge.org/Description/ (accessed on 18 July 2024)
AMIDA13 [78]	2013	606 HPF images (311 training, 295 test) from 23 subjects, each 2000 × 2000 pixels (0.25 mm^2)	Established a benchmark for mitosis-detection algorithms, later integrated into larger datasets for broader impact.	-
BreakHis [79] (accessed on 18 July 2024)	2016	9109 breast tissue images from 82 patients at various magnifications (40×–400×). Includes 2480 benign and 5429 malignant samples, all 700 × 460 pixel RGB images. Samples collected via partial mastectomy.	Provides a diverse, well-annotated dataset for developing and evaluating breast cancer classification algorithms. Enables research on automated diagnosis across different magnifications and tumor types, potentially improving clinical diagnostic accuracy.	https://web.inf.ufpr.br/vri/databases/breast-cancer-histopathological-database-breakhis/ (accessed on 18 July 2024)
TUPAC-auxiliary [78]	2016	73 breast cancer WSIs from 3 pathology centers, scanned by 2 types of scanners at 40× magnification.	Integrates multi-center data, enhancing the scope of mitosis-detection research in breast cancer.	https://tupac.grand-challenge.org/ (accessed on 18 July 2024)
HER2 Challenge Contest [80]	2016	High-resolution breast cancer histology dataset. Comprises 100 gigapixel WSIs. Annotated with expert pathologist HER2 scores and percentage assessments.	Pioneering benchmark for automated HER2 quantification in digital pathology. Facilitates the development of AI tools to enhance diagnostic consistency and efficiency in breast cancer assessment.	https://warwick.ac.uk/fac/cross_fac/tia/data/her2contest/ (accessed on 18 July 2024)
BACH [81]	2018	Includes 400 H&E-stained patches (2048 × 1536 resolution) and 30 WSIs with pixel-level annotations	Useful for training models with pixel-level cancer type annotations	https://www.kaggle.com/datasets/truthisneverlinear/bach-breast-cancer-histology-images (accessed on 18 July 2024)
MoNuSeg [82]	2018	WSIs from 30 organs, creating 1000 × 1000 pixel sub-images with nuclear annotations.	Ensures variation in nuclear appearance, enhancing model training on diverse tissue samples.	https://monuseg.grand-challenge.org/Data/ (accessed on 18 July 2024)
BCSS [83]	2019	151 WSIs with representative regions of interest (ROI) selected, contributing to the TIGER dataset.	Helps in understanding tumor-infiltrating lymphocytes in HER2+ and triple-negative breast cancers.	https://bcsegmentation.grand-challenge.org/ (accessed on 18 July 2024)
LYSTO [47]	2019	LYSTO data set comprises 20,000 images from 43 patients with breast, colon, and prostate cancers. It's structured with a patient-level split: 19 for training, 9 for validation, and 6 for testing, ensuring diverse representation across cancer types and stages.	Enables development of cross-cancer lymphocyte-assessment algorithms. Patient-level data division supports robust AI model validation, advancing generalized lymphocyte-detection tools.	https://lysto.grand-challenge.org/ (accessed on 18 July 2024)

Table 4. *Cont.*

Name	Year	Key Features	Contribution	Link
PanNuke [84]	2020	Contains 200,000 nuclei categorized into five clinically significant classes, with high-resolution patches scanned at 20× or 40× magnification	Supports nuanced classification of different tissue types in breast cancer research	https://sites.google.com/view/panoptils (accessed on 18 July 2024)
NuClick [85]	2020	NuClick dataset comprises 871 images derived from 440 WSIs, strategically partitioned into 471 training, 99 validation, and 300 testing images. The dataset encompasses various cancer types, with careful consideration given to maintaining separation between patient samples across different sets.	Supports AI model development for cancer diagnostics with real-world applicability. Thoughtful data division prevents patient-level leakage, enhancing model reliability and clinical relevance.	https://github.com/navidstuv/NuClick (accessed on 18 July 2024)
IMPRESS [86]	2020	Large-scale linguistic dataset comprising over 25,000 sentence pairs. Utilizes a rich vocabulary of 3000+ lexical items with grammatical annotations. Generated using advanced natural language processing techniques, following established Natural language inference dataset formats.	Advances pragmatic inference research by providing a comprehensive benchmark for evaluating NLI models' understanding of presuppositions and implicatures. Facilitates the development of more nuanced language understanding systems capable of grasping subtle linguistic phenomena.	https://github.com/facebookresearch/Imppres?tab=readme-ov-file (accessed on 18 July 2024)
BRACS [87]	2021	4539 ROIs from 547 H&E WSIs, meticulously categorized into different lesion types.	Facilitates detailed subtyping in breast cancer research.	https://www.bracs.icar.cnr.it/ (accessed on 18 July 2024)
SHIDC-BC-Ki-67 [38]	2021	2357 tru-cut biopsy images of invasive ductal carcinoma, collected from 2017 to 2020. Comprises 1656 training and 701 test samples, all expertly annotated for Ki-67 markers.	Addresses the scarcity of comprehensive Ki-67 marked datasets in breast cancer research. Facilitates development of deep learning models for accurate Ki-67 assessment, potentially enhancing diagnostic precision and treatment planning for invasive ductal carcinoma.	https://shiraz-hidc.com/ki-67-dataset/ (accessed on 18 July 2024)
MIDOG21 [87]	2021	280 breast cancer WSIs at 8000 × 8000 pixels, scanned by 4 different devices.	Addresses scanner variability in mitosis detection, promoting robust algorithm development across diverse imaging equipment.	https://midog2021.grand-challenge.org/ (accessed on 18 July 2024)
TIGER [88]	2022	Includes H&E-stained WSIs of Her2 positive and Triple Negative breast cancer. TIGER comprises cases from clinical routine and a phase 3 clinical trial. Includes annotations for lymphocytes, plasma cells, invasive tumors, and stroma.	First challenge for fully automated assessment of TILs in breast cancer. Aims to validate AI-based TIL scores for clinical use.	https://tiger.grand-challenge.org/ (accessed on 18 July 2024)
MIDOG22 [89]	2022	50 canine mast cell tumor cases, scanned by a single device type.	Expands mitosis detection to veterinary pathology, offering cross-species validation for detection algorithms.	https://midog.deepmicroscopy.org/download-dataset/ (accessed on 18 July 2024)
PanopTILs [65]	2023	Includes annotations for 814,886 nuclei from 151 patients, with WSIs scanned at 20× magnification.	Enhances understanding of the role of TILs in breast cancer detection.	https://sites.google.com/view/panoptils (accessed on 18 July 2024)
AI-TUMOR [73]	2024	2500 WSIs with pixel-level annotations for tumor regions, normal tissue, and surrounding stroma.	Focuses on reducing biases in AI models, ensuring better generalizability.	https://github.com/nickryd/ATLAS/blob/main/README.md (accessed on 18 July 2024)

3.3. Research Question 2: What Are the Main Challenges Associated with Comprehensive Breast Cancer Assessment Using WSIs?

WSI has emerged as a pivotal component in the realm of digital pathology, particularly for the application of deep learning methodologies in the detection of breast cancer [90]. Nonetheless, numerous substantial obstacles hinder its optimal implementation. These obstacles encompass a spectrum of technical challenges associated with image processing and analytical procedures, as well as overarching issues pertaining to data integrity, and annotation practices. Table 5 summarizes the main issues raised in recent research papers, together with their descriptions, implications for breast cancer detection, and relevant research references.

Table 5. Main challenges in WSIs for comprehensive breast cancer assessment.

Challenge	Description	Impact on Breast Cancer Cell Detection	Source
Size and Complexity of WSIs	WSIs can be several gigabytes in size, containing millions of pixels that need to be processed.	Requires substantial computational resources, high-performance GPUs, and large memory capacities; storage and management of large datasets are logistically challenging.	[28–30]
Variability in Image Quality and Resolution	Inconsistencies in image quality and resolution across different scanners and datasets.	Leads to variations in training data quality, reducing model generalization and accuracy across different scanners.	[27,28,31,39,42,45,51,54,63,64]
Annotation Challenges	High-quality annotations are labor-intensive, time-consuming, and prone to variability.	Inconsistent annotations can introduce biases, affecting model robustness and generalizability.	[29,40,47,57,60,61]
Feature Extraction Difficulties	Complex and subtle patterns in breast cancer tissues are challenging to capture accurately.	Traditional methods often fall short, necessitating advanced deep learning techniques for accurate detection.	[29,30,32–38,40,41,43–60,62,63,65]

3.4. Research Question 3: How Do WSIs Affect the Accuracy and Reliability of Advanced Deep Learning Approaches for Comprehensive Breast Cancer Assessment?

WSI plays a critical role in enhancing the accuracy and reliability of deep learning techniques for comprehensive assessments of breast cancer [91]. Deep learning algorithms can examine complicated tissue structures and cellular configurations with more ease thanks to the high-resolution and finely detailed features of WSIs. This is crucial for distinguishing between cancerous and benign cells. However, as Table 6 summarizes, several critical variables related to WSIs significantly impact the accuracy and reliability of deep learning models when it comes to breast cancer diagnosis.

As Table 6 shows, these factors are interrelated and impact model performance. Reliability in various circumstances is contingent upon constant image quality and standardization, whereas high resolution improves detection accuracy but raises processing demands. Strong annotations and a wide range of training data are essential for the resilience and generalizability of the model. WSI resolution makes it easier to obtain the necessary detail for accurate analytical evaluations, but it also creates problems with data processing and standardization methods. It is crucial to guarantee that WSIs are of superior quality, coherent, and comprehensively annotated, while concurrently tackling the intricacies linked to data heterogeneity and standardization since it is essential to the creation of reliable models that may be successfully applied in clinical settings.

In summary, WSIs have a major influence on the precision and dependability of deep learning techniques used in the detection and assessment of breast cancer. Developing deep learning models that are therapeutically useful requires addressing these variables simultaneously. In order to further improve the accuracy and dependability of deep learning techniques in breast cancer evaluation utilizing WSIs, future research should concentrate on maximizing these factors.

Table 6. The impact of WSIs on the accuracy and reliability of deep learning methods for comprehensive breast cancer assessment.

Factor	Description	Impact on Accuracy and Reliability
Resolution of WSIs	High-resolution images provide detailed information, crucial for detecting subtle differences between normal and cancerous tissues, especially in early-stage cancers.	Enhances detection accuracy but increases computational requirements.
Quality and Consistency	Variations in staining, lighting, and scanner types can introduce noise and artifacts, affecting model predictions.	Inconsistent quality can lead to inaccuracies; standardization techniques are vital.
Availability of Annotated WSIs	High-quality annotations by expert pathologists are essential for training accurate models. Obtaining such annotations is resource-intensive.	Poor annotations reduce model accuracy; improving annotation quality is key.
Diversity and Generalizability of Training	Models trained on diverse WSIs, covering a range of tissue types and patient demographics, are more likely to generalize well across different clinical settings.	Enhances generalization and reliability, but lack of standardization can hinder performance.

4. Criteria for Comprehensive Breast Cancer-Assessment WSI Algorithms

A number of important factors must be considered when evaluating detection criteria for a thorough assessment of breast cancer based on WSI algorithms to guarantee efficacy, consistency, and clinical applicability. These criteria can be divided into two factors: technological and clinical. Each of these factors is vital in establishing the technology's overall value and suitability.

Technical Criteria:

1. Accuracy and Performance Metrics: According to [91], sensitivity, specificity, accuracy, recall, AUC, and F1 score are essential for accurately identifying cancer cells while reducing false positives.
2. Robustness and Generalizability: Algorithms must manage common problems like noise and artifacts while operating consistently over a range of datasets, scanners, and staining processes [92].
3. Interpretability and Explainability: Clinical trust depends on model openness and error analysis capabilities [93].
4. Computational Efficiency: Algorithms should be appropriate for a range of computational contexts, with respectable processing speeds and efficient resource consumption [94].

Clinical Criteria:

Annotation Quality and Requirements: Preference for algorithms that reduce reliance on resource-intensive annotations by performing well with minimum or semi-supervised learning [94].

Together, these criteria ensure that the algorithms chosen are not only sound from a methodological standpoint but also practical, significant, and useful in clinical settings. Through a methodical approach to these components, scientists and medical professionals can evaluate and choose algorithms that are suitable for the complex problems involved in WSIs-based breast cancer cell detection, improving diagnostic accuracy and patient outcomes. To drive progress in breast cancer-detection techniques, researchers must prioritize optimizing baseline models while also carrying out thorough assessments of those models. These models serve as essential baselines to assess the effectiveness of WSI-based detection techniques in clinical settings. Targeted optimization techniques can significantly enhance important characteristics like clinical relevance, accuracy, and robustness, addressing the many problems that come with assessing breast cancer. This systematic approach guarantees that the chosen algorithms enhance patient outcomes and boost diagnostic accuracy.

4.1. Baseline Models for Detection Technologies Applied in Comprehensive Breast Cancer Assessment Based on WSI Algorithms

To better visualize the methodological progression in WSI-based breast cancer detection over recent years, Figure 4 presents a Sankey diagram capturing the dynamic interplay between publication year, detection task, and model architecture from 2020 to 2024. Each stream represents a flow of research attention, where the thickness of the connection reflects the frequency of model usage for specific tasks. As shown in the figure, two major trends emerge: first, a shift in detection focus—from early emphasis on biomarkers to increasing attention on lymphocyte detection, and more recently, to frameworks addressing both targets simultaneously; and second, a transition in model design—from dominant use of Convolutional Neural Network (CNN) and U-Net toward more sophisticated or hybrid approaches involving Transformers and Generative Adversarial Network (GAN), reflecting growing demands for richer spatial modeling and generalization across WSI domains.

These evolving trends are closely reflected in the selection and adaptation of baseline model architectures for different detection tasks. Over the five-year span, CNN and U-Net remained dominant. CNNs were predominantly applied to biomarkers detection, where classification or sparse detection was needed to identify ER/PR/HER2-positive cells. In contrast, U-Net architectures were widely adopted for lymphocyte detection, due to their pixel-level precision and strong segmentation capabilities—critical for detecting densely distributed immune cells with indistinct boundaries. Notably, in tasks combining biomarkers and lymphocyte detection, U-Net-based frameworks were still preferred for their ability to support multi-task outputs, such as simultaneous localization and segmentation.

From 2022 onward, architectural diversification accelerated. Transformer-based models gained traction, especially in biomarker detection, by leveraging self-attention mechanisms to capture long-range contextual dependencies in high-resolution WSI data. Hybrid approaches, such as CNN+Transformer and GAN+CNN+U-Net, emerged around 2023, integrating the spatial locality of CNNs, the generative robustness of GANs, and the global modeling power of Transformers—enabling more adaptive and domain-generalizable detection systems. Meanwhile, lighter or exploratory models like Multilayer Perceptron (MLP), Multiple Instance Learning (MIL), and You Only Look Once (YOLO) appeared after 2021, though their use remained limited due to challenges in dense detection and precise localization on WSIs.

Evaluation metrics across these models varied with task and output granularity. Classification and sparse detection tasks typically employed AUC, accuracy, and F1-score, while segmentation-oriented models were assessed using Dice coefficient, IoU, and boundary-aware metrics. For multi-output detection models, task-specific metrics were reported independently, reflecting the complexity of comprehensive breast cancer assessment.

Overall, segmentation-centric models have remained the backbone of WSI-based detection. Their ability to handle high-resolution images through patch-based processing, preserve pixel-level detail, and support dense prediction tasks makes them especially suited for WSI applications, where targets are often overlapping, small, and structurally complex. The increasing use of hybrid and Transformer-based models reflects a broader trend toward unifying global and local representation learning for improved clinical utility.

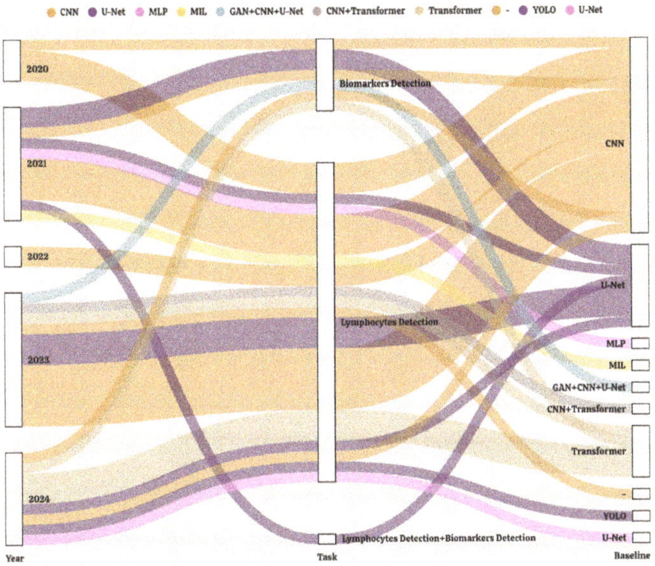

Figure 4. Evolution of baseline-detection models for breast cancer assessment in WSI from 2020 to 2024. (Flow width indicates the relative usage frequency of each model type, with thicker streams showing more widely adopted models. Different colors represent distinct model architectures tracked across the study period).

4.2. Optimizing and Improving Existing Baselines Based on Evaluation Criteria

A multidisciplinary approach is required to optimize current baseline models for breast cancer cell detection using WSI, considering technological and clinical factors. Several important categories can be used to group this optimization process:

4.2.1. Enhancing Model Performance

In the realm of deep learning-based detection techniques for computer-aided diagnosis (CAD) of breast cancer, strategies to enhance model performance have become increasingly diverse and sophisticated. Primarily, ensemble learning frameworks effectively improve detection accuracy and generalization by integrating various deep learning architectures such as U-Net, GANs, and CNNs [36,42–46,48–51,53–55,58,59,62,65]. Additionally, the application of multi-task learning paradigms, which allow models to jointly learn multiple related tasks such as lesion segmentation, classification, and malignancy grading within a unified architecture, has gained attention for its ability to leverage shared representations, reduce overfitting, and improve generalization across heterogeneous lesions. This approach not only provides more comprehensive pathological information but also enhances the model's robustness and diagnostic performance [43,53,56,59,61,63]. Furthermore, multimodal data fusion strategies integrate genomic data with WSIs [27,41], or combine multi-level data from cellular and tissue levels [37,57,60], significantly boosting diagnostic precision and interpretability by capturing complementary biological features. Training on cross-institutional, multi-center datasets enhances the model's domain adaptability, mitigating the adverse effects of data distribution shifts on performance [34].

Regarding model architectures, increasing network depth equips models with stronger feature extraction capabilities, enabling the capture of more complex pathomorphological features [30]. The introduction of diverse convolutional modules, such as residual convolutional blocks [38], parallel convolutional blocks [35], dilated convolutional blocks [51], and color deconvolution [50], further enhances the model's feature representation ability and multi-scale information capture. Recently, the integration of multiple attention mechanisms, including combinations of spatial attention, channel attention, and self-attention, has gained widespread application in medical image analysis, improving detection precision and efficiency by enhancing the model's focus on key regions and features.

Lastly, post-processing optimization techniques, including morphological opening operations, watershed algorithms [32,38], and advanced methods like HoVer-Net [63], further elevate the precision and consistency of detection outcomes, particularly in cell instance segmentation and separation of adhered structures. The synergistic effect of these methods is driving the gradual implementation and application of breast cancer CAD systems in clinical practice.

While recent advances have significantly improved detection accuracy, they often come at the expense of interpretability and computational efficiency. In deep learning-based CAD systems, increasing model complexity to boost performance tends to reduce transparency and raises deployment barriers. For example, models like CB-HVT Net, which integrate PVT, ResNet variants, and attention mechanisms, feature high parameter counts and computational demands that hinder real-time deployment [45,54]. These challenges highlight the need for balanced approaches that maintain strong accuracy while enhancing explainability and deployability.

4.2.2. Improving Robustness and Generalizability

In the realm of deep learning-based breast cancer-detection research, robustness enhancement strategies predominantly converge on two pivotal methodologies. Cross-disease data integration and validation, referring to the inclusion of datasets from multiple cancer types to expose the model to a broader range of pathological variations, substantially augments model robustness through the incorporation of multi-disease datasets and the execution of pan-cancer experiments [34,37,46,48,50,54]. This approach facilitates the model's acquisition of heterogeneous pathological features, thereby enhancing its discriminative capacity across diverse cancer types and elevating its adaptability within complex clinical milieus. Concurrently, the implementation of semi-supervised learning paradigms efficaciously addresses the constraints imposed by the paucity of annotated data [29]. By synergistically leveraging limited labeled datasets in conjunction with voluminous unlabeled data, this technique not only mitigates the reliance on extensive manual annotation processes but also markedly amplifies the model's generalization prowess in data-constrained environments.

However, while cross-disease integration can enhance the model's adaptability to diverse histopathological morphologies, it may also introduce label noise and inconsistencies in annotation standards. This, in turn, can lead to domain shift and reduce detection specificity for certain cancer types, such as breast cancer. For example, when independent models were constructed for five cancer types in TCGA and pan-cancer training was applied, the performance of pan-cancer models declined in certain tasks (e.g., PD-L1 prediction in STAD), suggesting that disease-specific signals may be diluted in a multi-cancer setting [37]. Moreover, many semi-supervised frameworks rely on heuristic thresholds or consistency regularization strategies, which often require task-specific tuning, thereby limiting their generalizability and scalability in real-world clinical applications.

4.2.3. Increasing Interpretability and Explainability

Interpretability techniques in deep learning have emerged as essential components for fostering trust, transparency, and clinical acceptability in breast cancer assessment. The Human-Interpretable Features (HIF) paradigm aims to bridge the semantic gap between model outputs and clinical understanding by aligning predictions with visually and diagnostically meaningful image features [37], whereas saliency-based visualization methods offer intuitive heatmaps that localize regions contributing most to the model's decision-making process, thereby enhancing interpretability for end-users [40]. While the integration of such methods has demonstrably improved the transparency and perceived reliability of AI-assisted diagnostic systems, several limitations persist. HIF-based strategies typically rely on predefined, handcrafted feature sets, which may insufficiently capture the complex and abstract representations encoded by deep neural networks, thus constraining their explanatory power and generalizability across datasets or imaging modalities. In parallel, saliency visualizations are often susceptible to input perturbations and architectural variations, producing unstable and sometimes misleading attributions. Moreover, the post hoc nature of most interpretability tools, coupled with a lack of standardized validation protocols, raises concerns regarding their clinical robustness and reproducibility. These limitations underscore an urgent need for the development of principled, rigorously evaluated interpretability frameworks that can yield consistent, meaningful, and clinically actionable explanations.

4.2.4. Optimizing Computational Efficiency

In research applying deep learning techniques to breast cancer assessment, various strategies have been employed to enhance model efficiency. The primary approach involves precise localization of ROI through methods such as Gaussian kernel annotation [32] and micro-block selection techniques [31,64], enabling models to focus on key pathological features. This not only improves accuracy but also reduces computational costs. Additionally, researchers have utilized pre-training strategies to optimize model architecture [29,31], accelerating model convergence, improving task initialization, and reducing parameter count and architectural complexity, thereby lowering computational demands while maintaining high performance. However, these efficiency-oriented strategies are not without limitations. ROI localization methods often rely on heuristic rules or expert-defined annotations, which may introduce bias and reduce scalability across datasets with varying staining characteristics or image resolutions. Moreover, such narrowly focused techniques risk omitting relevant contextual cues essential for accurate diagnosis. Similarly, the effectiveness of pre-training heavily depends on the relevance and quality of the source domain; mismatched pre-training can result in suboptimal initialization and diminished downstream performance. Furthermore, existing studies rarely provide systematic evaluations of the trade-offs between architectural simplification and diagnostic accuracy, leaving the optimal balance between efficiency and performance largely unexplored.

4.2.5. Addressing Data Quality and Annotation Challenges

In deep learning-based breast cancer-detection research, data quality and annotation challenges are primarily mitigated through two methodologies: weak supervision learning and segmentation map generation. Weak supervision enables models to extract features from limited or imprecise annotations, reducing dependence on fully annotated datasets [29,31,41]. Segmentation map generation techniques create synthetic annotations, providing finer-grained information on regions of interest, thus compensating for incomplete or noisy labels [39]. These approaches synergistically enhance model robustness and performance in the face of data quality and annotation challenges in breast cancer-detection tasks. However, both methods present notable limitations. Weakly supervised models are vulnerable to label noise and may overfit to coarse annotations, limiting their generalizability. Meanwhile, segmentation map generation often relies on heuristic or rule-based pseudo-labels that may introduce bias, particularly in complex tumor microenvironments. The lack of standardized validation procedures for these synthetic annotations also raises concerns regarding their clinical reliability and reproducibility.

Table 7 concisely summarizes the baseline models and their optimization strategies, aiding in the understanding of how these models can be improved to enhance the efficiency of comprehensive breast cancer assessment based on detection technologies.

Table 7. Baseline models for WSI detection technologies and the strategies for optimizing and improving these models based on specific criteria.

Criteria	Baseline Models	Optimization and Improvement Strategies
Accuracy and Performance Metrics	CNN, GAN, U-Net, Transformer, MIL, MLP	• Ensemble learning frameworks • Multi-task learning paradigms • Multimodal data fusion strategies • Cross-institutional training • Advanced convolutional modules • Multiple attention mechanisms
Robustness and Generalizability	CNN, U-Net, Transformer	• Cross-disease data integration and validation • Semi-supervised learning paradigms
Interpretability and Explainability	CNN, MIL	• HIF approach • Saliency visualization techniques
Computational Efficiency	CNN, U-Net, YOLO	• Precise localization of ROI • Pre-training strategies
Annotation Quality and Requirements	CNN, U-Net	• Weak supervision learning • Segmentation map generation techniques

5. Discussion and Potential Solutions for Improving WSIs for Breast Cancer Cell Detection

The application of advanced deep learning methodologies to WSIs for comprehensive breast cancer assessment represents a significant advancement in digital pathology. A systematic analysis of WSI datasets, associated challenges, and their impact on deep learning models has yielded five critical evaluation metrics: model performance, data integration and preprocessing, architectural optimization, robustness and generalizability, and interpretability and clinical application. This analytical framework provides a comprehensive evaluation of current technologies while illuminating future research trajectories.

The diversity of WSIs datasets, ranging from large-scale public repositories such as TCGA-BRCA to specialized high-resolution datasets like PanNuke and BACH, significantly influences model performance and data integration strategies. The multimodal nature of datasets such as TCGA-BRCA offers a robust foundation for developing comprehensive assessment models. However, dataset heterogeneity presents substantial challenges, particularly in terms of model generalizability. Innovative approaches have emerged to address these challenges. Notable among these is the integration of U-Net, GANs, and CNNs [43], which demonstrates exceptional performance in handling diverse data. Additionally, the multi-task learning paradigm described in [53] enhances model adaptability to varied WSIs data types through simultaneous segmentation, classification, and grading tasks.

The primary challenges in WSIs applications—including image size, quality variability, and annotation difficulties—directly impact data preprocessing strategies and model architecture design. These challenges have catalyzed innovative solutions. The panoramic segmentation method proposed by Liu et al. effectively addresses large-sized WSIs processing, markedly improving computational efficiency. In data integration and preprocessing, [27] showcases a multimodal fusion strategy combining genomic data with WSIs, enhancing diagnostic accuracy while partially mitigating data heterogeneity issues. Nevertheless, the efficient processing of large-scale WSIs data remains a significant challenge, necessitating further research into advanced preprocessing techniques.

The impact of WSIs on deep learning model accuracy and reliability reveals a dichotomy: high-resolution data enhances detection precision while simultaneously presenting computational and standardization challenges. This contradiction has driven innovations in model architectures. The introduction of residual convolutional blocks [38] significantly enhances feature extraction capabilities, while the attention mechanism described in [63] improves the model's capacity to identify key regions. These optimizations directly address the computational challenges posed by high-resolution WSIs while enhancing the model's ability to capture complex pathological features.

Regarding robustness and generalizability, cross-disease dataset integration [34] and semi-supervised learning methods [29] demonstrate significant advantages in managing diverse WSIs datasets and limited annotated data. These approaches enhance model adaptability across varied clinical settings and effectively address the challenge of WSIs data annotation difficulties.

Interpretability and clinical application remain significant hurdles for WSI-based deep learning models. HIF methods [37] and saliency visualization techniques [40] have advanced the interpretability of model outputs, crucial for fostering clinical trust and adoption. However, the seamless integration of these technologies into clinical workflows requires further investigation. The identified evaluation metrics not only provide a comprehensive assessment of existing models but also delineate key directions for future research. Significant opportunities persist in addressing WSIs dataset diversity, processing large-scale high-resolution data, and improving model robustness and interpretability.

6. Conclusions, Implication, and Recommendations for Future Research

This review has systematically examined deep learning-based detection methods for breast cancer using WSIs, highlighting substantial progress in model accuracy, robustness, and data efficiency. Nonetheless, significant challenges remain in computational scalability, interpretability, annotation quality, and clinical applicability. To address these issues, future research should be guided by both technical feasibility and clinical relevance. In the short term, efforts should focus on developing lightweight, interpretable architectures optimized for WSI-scale processing to support real-time, resource-aware deployment. Enhancing weakly supervised and semi-supervised learning frameworks through uncertainty modeling and confidence-guided label refinement represents a technically viable strategy for improving annotation robustness. Medium-term priorities include designing domain-adaptive and resolution-consistent models to address data heterogeneity across institutions and staining variations. In the long term, the establishment of clinically validated interpretability protocols and the construction of large-scale, standardized WSI datasets should be pursued to support reproducibility, benchmarking, and translational impact. Prioritizing these directions will facilitate a more effective alignment between algorithmic innovation and real-world clinical integration, advancing the role of AI in precision breast cancer diagnostics.

Author Contributions: Writing—original draft preparation and editing, Q.X.; Supervision, review, and editing, A.A. (Afzan Adam) and A.A. (Azizi Abdullah); Medical terminology and case validation, N.B. All authors have read and agreed to the published version of the manuscript.

Funding: This research was funded by the Ministry of Higher Education Malaysia through the Fundamental Research Grant Scheme (FRGS), grant code: FRGS/1/2024/ICT02/UKM/02/5.

Institutional Review Board Statement: Not applicable.

Informed Consent Statement: Not applicable.

Data Availability Statement: Not applicable.

Conflicts of Interest: The authors declare no conflicts of interest.

Abbreviations

The following abbreviations are used in this manuscript:

PRISM	Preferred Reporting Items for Systematic Reviews and Meta-Analyses
WSI	Whole Slide Image
WSIs	Whole Slide Images
ER	Estrogen Receptor
PR	rogesterone Receptor
HER2	Human Epidermal Growth Factor Receptor 2
Ki-67	Ki-67 Antigen
TIL	Tumor-Infiltrating Lymphocyte
H&E	Hematoxylin and Eosin
IHC	Immunohistochemistry
TNBC	Triple-Negative Breast Cancer
LD	Lymphocyte Detection
BD	Biomarker Detection
SCQ	Systematic Quality Criteria
SLR	Systematic Literature Review
HPF	High-Power Field
CNN	Convolutional Neural Network
GAN	Generative Adversarial Network
MLP	Multilayer Perceptron
MIL	Multiple Instance Learning
YOLO	You Only Look Once
CAD	Computer-Aided Diagnosis
ROI	Region of Interest
HIF	Human-Interpretable Features

References

1. Faroughi, F.; Fathnezhad-Kazemi, A.; Sarbakhsh, P. Factors Affecting Quality of Life in Women With Breast Cancer: A Path Analysis. *BMC Women's Health* **2023**, *23*, 578.
2. Khairi, S.S.M.; Bakar, M.A.A.; Alias, M.A.; Bakar, S.A.; Liong, C.Y.; Rosli, N.; Farid, M. Deep learning on histopathology images for breast cancer classification: A bibliometric analysis. *Healthcare* **2021**, *10*, 10. [CrossRef] [PubMed]
3. Saifullah, S.; Dreżewski, R. Enhancing breast cancer diagnosis: A CNN-based approach for medical image segmentation and classification. In *International Conference on Computational Science*; Springer: Berlin/Heidelberg, Germany, 2024; pp. 155–162.
4. Mahmoud, R.; Ordóñez-Morán, P.; Allegrucci, C. Challenges for triple negative breast cancer treatment: Defeating heterogeneity and cancer stemness. *Cancers* **2022**, *14*, 4280. [CrossRef]
5. El Bairi, K.; Haynes, H.R.; Blackley, E.; Fineberg, S.; Shear, J.; Turner, S.; De Freitas, J.R.; Sur, D.; Amendola, L.C.; Gharib, M.; et al. The tale of TILs in breast cancer: A report from the international immuno-oncology biomarker working group. *NPJ Breast Cancer* **2021**, *7*, 150. [PubMed]
6. Pauzi, S.H.M.; Saari, H.N.; Roslan, M.R.; Azman, S.N.S.S.K.; Tauan, I.S.; Rusli, F.A.M.; Aizuddin, A.N. A comparison study of HER2 protein overexpression and its gene status in breast cancer. *Malays. J. Pathol.* **2019**, *41*, 133–138.
7. Finkelman, B.S.; Zhang, H.; Hicks, D.G.; Turner, B.M. The evolution of Ki-67 and breast carcinoma: Past observations, present directions, and future considerations. *Cancers* **2023**, *15*, 808. [CrossRef]
8. Zahari, S.; Syafruddin, S.E.; Mohtar, M.A. Impact of the Cancer Cell Secretome in driving breast Cancer progression. *Cancers* **2023**, *15*, 2653. [CrossRef]
9. Gupta, R.; Le, H.; Van Arnam, J.; Belinsky, D.; Hasan, M.; Samaras, D.; Kurc, T.; Saltz, J.H. Characterizing immune responses in whole slide images of cancer with digital pathology and pathomics. *Curr. Pathobiol. Rep.* **2020**, *8*, 133–148.
10. Roostee, S.; Ehinger, D.; Jönsson, M.; Phung, B.; Jönsson, G.; Sjödahl, G.; Staaf, J.; Aine, M. Tumour immune characterisation of primary triple-negative breast cancer using automated image quantification of immunohistochemistry-stained immune cells. *Sci. Rep.* **2024**, *14*, 21417. [CrossRef]

11. Liu, Y.; Han, D.; Parwani, A.V.; Li, Z. Applications of artificial intelligence in breast pathology. *Arch. Pathol. Lab. Med.* **2023**, *147*, 1003–1013.
12. Shakhawat, H.; Hossain, S.; Kabir, A.; Mahmud, S.H.; Islam, M.M.; Tariq, F. Review of artifact detection methods for automated analysis and diagnosis in digital pathology. In *Artificial Intelligence for Disease Diagnosis and Prognosis in Smart Healthcare*; CRC Press: Boca Raton, FL, USA, 2023; pp. 177–202.
13. Li, X.; Li, C.; Rahaman, M.M.; Sun, H.; Li, X.; Wu, J.; Yao, Y.; Grzegorzek, M. A comprehensive review of computer-aided whole-slide image analysis: From datasets to feature extraction, segmentation, classification and detection approaches. *Artif. Intell. Rev.* **2022**, *55*, 4809–4878. [CrossRef]
14. Wu, Y.; Cheng, M.; Huang, S.; Pei, Z.; Zuo, Y.; Liu, J.; Yang, K.; Zhu, Q.; Zhang, J.; Hong, H.; et al. Recent advances of deep learning for computational histopathology: Principles and applications. *Cancers* **2022**, *14*, 1199. [CrossRef] [PubMed]
15. Carriero, A.; Groenhoff, L.; Vologina, E.; Basile, P.; Albera, M. Deep Learning in Breast Cancer Imaging: State of the Art and Recent Advancements in Early 2024. *Diagnostics* **2024**, *14*, 848. [CrossRef] [PubMed]
16. Duggento, A.; Conti, A.; Mauriello, A.; Guerrisi, M.; Toschi, N. Deep computational pathology in breast cancer. *Semin. Cancer Biol.* **2021**, *72*, 226–237. [CrossRef]
17. Luo, L.; Wang, X.; Lin, Y.; Ma, X.; Tan, A.; Chan, R.; Vardhanabhuti, V.; Chu, W.C.W.; Cheng, K.T.; Chen, H. Deep learning in breast cancer imaging: A decade of progress and future directions. *IEEE Rev. Biomed. Eng.* **2024**, *18*, 130–151. [CrossRef]
18. Al-Thelaya, K.; Gilal, N.U.; Alzubaidi, M.; Majeed, F.; Agus, M.; Schneider, J.; Househ, M. Applications of discriminative and deep learning feature extraction methods for whole slide image analysis: A survey. *J. Pathol. Inform.* **2023**, *14*, 100335. [CrossRef]
19. Hulsen, T. Explainable Artificial Intelligence (XAI): Concepts and Challenges in Healthcare. *AI* **2023**, *4*, 652–666. [CrossRef]
20. Mahmood, T.; Li, J.; Pei, Y.; Akhtar, F.; Imran, A.; Rehman, K.U. A brief survey on breast cancer diagnostic with deep learning schemes using multi-image modalities. *IEEE Access* **2020**, *8*, 165779–165809. [CrossRef]
21. Mridha, M.F.; Hamid, M.A.; Monowar, M.M.; Keya, A.J.; Ohi, A.Q.; Islam, M.R.; Kim, J.M. A comprehensive survey on deep-learning-based breast cancer diagnosis. *Cancers* **2021**, *13*, 6116. [CrossRef]
22. Wen, Z.; Wang, S.; Yang, D.M.; Xie, Y.; Chen, M.; Bishop, J.; Xiao, G. Deep learning in digital pathology for personalized treatment plans of cancer patients. *Semin. Diagn. Pathol.* **2023**, *40*, 109–119. [CrossRef]
23. Rabilloud, N.; Allaume, P.; Acosta, O.; De Crevoisier, R.; Bourgade, R.; Loussouarn, D.; Rioux-Leclercq, N.; Khene, Z.E.; Mathieu, R.; Bensalah, K.; et al. Deep learning methodologies applied to digital pathology in prostate cancer: A systematic review. *Diagnostics* **2023**, *13*, 2676. [CrossRef] [PubMed]
24. Page, M.J.; McKenzie, J.E.; Bossuyt, P.M.; Boutron, I.; Hoffmann, T.C.; Mulrow, C.D.; Shamseer, L.; Tetzlaff, J.M.; Akl, E.A.; Brennan, S.E.; et al. The PRISMA 2020 statement: An updated guideline for reporting systematic reviews. *BMJ* **2021**, *372*, n71. [CrossRef] [PubMed]
25. Knobloch, K.; Yoon, U.; Vogt, P.M. Preferred reporting items for systematic reviews and meta-analyses (PRISMA) statement and publication bias. *J. Cranio-Maxillofac. Surg.* **2011**, *39*, 91–92. [CrossRef] [PubMed]
26. Tricco, A.C.; Lillie, E.; Zarin, W.; O'Brien, K.K.; Colquhoun, H.; Levac, D.; Moher, D.; Peters, M.D.; Horsley, T.; Weeks, L.; et al. PRISMA extension for scoping reviews (PRISMA-ScR): Checklist and explanation. *Ann. Intern. Med.* **2018**, *169*, 467–473. [CrossRef]
27. Swiderska-Chadaj, Z.; Gallego, J.; Gonzalez-Lopez, L.; Bueno, G. Detection of Ki67 hot-spots of invasive breast cancer based on convolutional neural networks applied to mutual information of H&E and Ki67 whole slide images. *Appl. Sci.* **2020**, *10*, 7761. [CrossRef]
28. George, K.; Faziludeen, S.; Sankaran, P.; Joseph, P.K. Breast cancer detection from biopsy images using nucleus guided transfer learning and belief based fusion. *Comput. Biol. Med.* **2020**, *124*, 103954. [CrossRef]
29. Krithiga, R.; Geetha, P. Deep learning based breast cancer detection and classification using fuzzy merging techniques. *Mach. Vis. Appl.* **2020**, *31*, 63. [CrossRef]
30. Evangeline, I.K.; Precious, J.G.; Pazhanivel, N.; Kirubha, S.P.A. Automatic Detection and Counting of Lymphocytes from Immunohistochemistry Cancer Images Using Deep Learning. *J. Med Biol. Eng.* **2020**, *40*, 735–747. [CrossRef]
31. Geread, R.S.; Sivanandarajah, A.; Brouwer, E.R.; Wood, G.A.; Androutsos, D.; Faragalla, H.; Khademi, A. piNET: An automated proliferation index calculator framework for Ki67 breast cancer images. *Cancers* **2021**, *13*, 11. [CrossRef]
32. Krijgsman, D.; van Leeuwen, M.B.; van der Ven, J.; Almeida, V.; Vlutters, R.; Halter, D.; Kuppen, P.J.K.; van de Velde, C.J.H.; Wimberger-Friedl, R. Quantitative whole slide assessment of tumor-infiltrating CD8-positive lymphocytes in ER-positive breast cancer in relation to clinical outcome. *IEEE J. Biomed. Health Inform.* **2021**, *25*, 381–392. [CrossRef]
33. Gamble, P.; Jaroensri, R.; Wang, H.; Tan, F.; Moran, M.; Brown, T.; Flament-Auvigne, I.; Rakha, E.A.; Toss, M.; Dabbs, D.J.; et al. Determining breast cancer biomarker status and associated morphological features using deep learning. *Commun. Med.* **2021**, *1*, 14. [CrossRef] [PubMed]
34. Lu, X.; You, Z.; Sun, M.; Wu, J.; Zhang, Z. Breast cancer mitotic cell detection using cascade convolutional neural network with U-Net. *Math. Biosci. Eng.* **2021**, *18*, 673–695. [CrossRef] [PubMed]

35. Budginaite, E.; Morkunas, M.; Laurinavicius, A.; Treigys, P. Deep Learning Model for Cell Nuclei Segmentation and Lymphocyte Identification in Whole Slide Histology Images. *Informatica* **2021**, *32*, 23–40. [CrossRef]
36. Narayanan, P.L.; Raza, S.E.A.; Hall, A.H.; Marks, J.R.; King, L.; West, R.B.; Hernandez, L.; Guppy, N.; Dowsett, M.; Gusterson, B.; et al. Unmasking the immune microecology of ductal carcinoma in situ with deep learning. *NPJ Breast Cancer* **2021**, *7*, 19. [CrossRef]
37. Diao, J.A.; Wang, J.K.; Chui, W.F.; Mountain, V.; Gullapally, S.C.; Srinivasan, R.; Mitchell, R.N.; Glass, B.; Hoffman, S.; Rao, S.K.; et al. Human-interpretable image features derived from densely mapped cancer pathology slides predict diverse molecular phenotypes. *Nat. Commun.* **2021**, *12*, 1613. [CrossRef]
38. Negahbani, F.; Sabzi, R.; Jahromi, B.P.; Firouzabadi, D.; Movahedi, F.; Shirazi, M.K.; Majidi, S.; Dehghanian, A. PathoNet introduced as a deep neural network backend for evaluation of Ki-67 and tumor-infiltrating lymphocytes in breast cancer. *Sci. Rep.* **2021**, *11*, 8489. [CrossRef]
39. Diaz Guerrero, R.E.; Oliveira, J.L. Improvements in lymphocytes detection using deep learning with a preprocessing stage. In Proceedings of the 2021 IEEE 34th International Symposium on Computer-Based Medical Systems (CBMS), Aveiro, Portugal, 7–9 June 2021; pp. 178–182. [CrossRef]
40. Schirris, Y.; Engelaer, M.; Panteli, A.; Horlings, H.M.; Gavves, E.; Teuwen, J. WeakSTIL: Weak whole-slide image level stromal tumor infiltrating lymphocyte scores are all you need. *Proc. SPIE Med. Imaging: Digit. Comput. Pathol.* **2022**, *12039*, 120390B. [CrossRef]
41. Ektefaie, Y.; Yuan, W.; Dillon, D.A.; Lin, N.U.; Golden, J.A.; Kohane, I.S.; Yu, K.H. Integrative multiomics-histopathology analysis for breast cancer classification. *NPJ Breast Cancer* **2021**, *7*, 147. [CrossRef]
42. Zafar, M.M.; Rauf, Z.; Sohail, A.; Khan, A.R.; Obaidullah, M.; Khan, S.H.; Lee, Y.S.; Khan, A. Detection of tumour infiltrating lymphocytes in CD3 and CD8 stained histopathological images using a two-phase deep CNN. *Photodiagnosis Photodyn. Ther.* **2022**, *37*, 102676. [CrossRef]
43. Zhang, X.; Zhu, X.; Tang, K.; Zhao, Y.; Lu, Z.; Feng, Q. DDTNet: A dense dual-task network for tumor-infiltrating lymphocyte detection and segmentation in histopathological images of breast cancer. *Med. Image Anal.* **2022**, *78*, 102415. [CrossRef]
44. Chen, Y.; Li, H.; Janowczyk, A.; Toro, P.; Corredor, G.; Whitney, J.; Lu, C.; Koyuncu, C.F.; Mokhtari, M.; Buzzy, C.; et al. Computational pathology improves risk stratification of a multi-gene assay for early stage ER+ breast cancer. *NPJ Breast Cancer* **2023**, *9*, 40. [CrossRef] [PubMed]
45. Ali, M.L.; Rauf, Z.; Khan, A.; Sohail, A.; Ullah, R.; Gwak, J. CB-HVT Net: A Channel-Boosted Hybrid Vision Transformer Network for Lymphocyte Detection in Histopathological Images. *IEEE Access* **2023**, *11*, 115740–115750. [CrossRef]
46. Huang, J.; Li, H.; Wan, X.; Li, G. Affine-Consistent Transformer for Multi-Class Cell Nuclei Detection. In Proceedings of the 2023 International Conference on Computer Vision (ICCV 2023), Paris, France, 2–3 October 2023; pp. 21327–21336. [CrossRef]
47. Jiao, Y.; van der Laak, J.; Albarqouni, S.; Li, Z.; Tan, T.; Bhalerao, A.; Cheng, S.; Ma, J.; Pocock, J.; Pluim, J.P.W.; et al. LYSTO: The Lymphocyte Assessment Hackathon and Benchmark Dataset. *IEEE J. Biomed. Health Inform.* **2024**, *28*, 1161–1172. [CrossRef] [PubMed]
48. Shah, H.A.; Kang, J.M. An Optimized Multi-Organ Cancer Cells Segmentation for Histopathological Images Based on CBAM-Residual U-Net. *IEEE Access* **2023**, *11*, 111608–111621. [CrossRef]
49. Yosofvand, M.; Khan, S.Y.; Dhakal, R.; Nejat, A.; Moustaid-Moussa, N.; Rahman, R.L.; Moussa, H. Automated Detection and Scoring of Tumor-Infiltrating Lymphocytes in Breast Cancer Histopathology Slides. *Cancers* **2023**, *15*, 3635. [CrossRef]
50. Huang, P.W.; Ouyang, H.; Hsu, B.Y.; Chang, Y.R.; Lin, Y.C.; Chen, Y.A.; Hsieh, Y.H.; Fu, C.C.; Li, C.F.; Lin, C.H.; et al. Deep-learning based breast cancer detection for cross-staining histopathology images. *Heliyon* **2023**, *9*, e13171. [CrossRef]
51. Rauf, Z.; Sohail, A.; Khan, S.H.; Khan, A.; Gwak, J.; Maqbool, M. Attention-guided multi-scale deep object detection framework for lymphocyte analysis in IHC histological images. *Microscopy* **2023**, *72*, 27–42. [CrossRef]
52. Wang, X.; Zhang, J.; Yang, S.; Xiang, J.; Luo, F.; Wang, M.; Zhang, J.; Yang, W.; Huang, J.; Han, X. A generalizable and robust deep learning algorithm for mitosis detection in multicenter breast histopathological images. *Med. Image Anal.* **2023**, *84*, 102703. [CrossRef]
53. Ryu, J.; Puche, A.V.; Shin, J.; Park, S.; Brattoli, B.; Lee, J.; Jung, W.; Cho, S.I.; Paeng, K.; Ock, C.Y.; et al. OCELOT: Overlapped Cell on Tissue Dataset for Histopathology. In Proceedings of the IEEE/CVF Conference on Computer Vision and Pattern Recognition, Paris, France, 2–3 October 2023; pp. 23902–23912. [CrossRef]
54. Rauf, Z.; Khan, A.R.; Sohail, A.; Alquhayz, H.; Gwak, J.; Khan, A. Lymphocyte detection for cancer analysis using a novel fusion block based channel boosted CNN. *Sci. Rep.* **2023**, *13*, 14047. [CrossRef]
55. Makhlouf, S.; Wahab, N.; Toss, M.; Ibrahim, A.; Lashen, A.G.; Atallah, N.M.; Ghannam, S.; Jahanifar, M.; Lu, W.; Graham, S.; et al. Evaluation of Tumour Infiltrating Lymphocytes in Luminal Breast Cancer Using Artificial Intelligence. *Br. J. Cancer* **2023**, *129*, 1747–1758. [CrossRef]

56. Aswolinskiy, W.; Munari, E.; Horlings, H.M.; Mulder, L.; Bogina, G.; Sanders, J.; Liu, Y.H.; van den Belt-dusebout, A.W.; Tessier, L.; Balkenhol, M.; et al. PROACTING: Predicting Pathological Complete Response to Neoadjuvant Chemotherapy in Breast Cancer from Routine Diagnostic Histopathology Biopsies with Deep Learning. *Breast Cancer Res.* **2023**, *25*, 142. [CrossRef] [PubMed]
57. Genc-Nayebi, N.; Abran, A. A systematic literature review: Opinion mining studies from mobile app store user reviews. *J. Syst. Softw.* **2017**, *125*, 207–219. [CrossRef]
58. Kabir, S.; Vranic, S.; Al Saady, R.M.; Khan, M.S.; Sarmun, R.; Alqahtani, A.; Abbas, T.O.; Chowdhury, M.E.H. The utility of a deep learning-based approach in Her-2/neu assessment in breast cancer. *Expert Syst. Appl.* **2024**, *238*, 122051. [CrossRef]
59. Li, Z.; Li, W.; Mai, H.; Zhang, T.; Xiong, Z. Enhancing Cell Detection in Histopathology Images: A ViT-Based U-Net Approach. In *Graphs in Biomedical Image Analysis, and Overlapped Cell on Tissue Dataset for Histopathology, 5th MICCAI Workshop, Proceedings of the 5th International Workshop on Graphs in Biomedical Image Analysis (GRAIL) / Workshop on Overlapped Cell on Tissue—Cell Detection from Cell-Tissue Interaction Challenge (OCELOT), MICCAI 2023, Vancouver, BC, Canada, 23 September–4 October 2023*; Ahmadi, S.A., Pereira, S., Eds.; Lecture Notes in Computer Science; Springer: Berlin/Heidelberg, Germany, 2024; Volume 14373, pp. 150–160. [CrossRef]
60. Millward, J.; He, Z.; Nibali, A. Dense Prediction of Cell Centroids Using Tissue Context and Cell Refinement. In *Graphs in Biomedical Image Analysis, and Overlapped Cell on Tissue Dataset for Histopathology, 5th MICCAI Workshop, Proceedings of the 5th International Workshop on Graphs in Biomedical Image Analysis (GRAIL) and the Workshop on Overlapped Cell on Tissue (OCELOT), MICCAI 2023, Vancouver, BC, Canada, 23 September–4 October 2023*; Ahmadi, S.A., Pereira, S., Eds.; Lecture Notes in Computer Science; Springer: Berlin/Heidelberg, Germany, 2024; Volume 14373, pp. 138–149. [CrossRef]
61. Karol, M.; Tabakov, M.; Markowska-Kaczmar, U.; Fulawka, L. Deep Learning for Cancer Cell Detection: Do We Need Dedicated Models? *Artif. Intell. Rev.* **2024**, *57*, 53. [CrossRef]
62. Lakshmanan, B.; Anand, S.; Raja, P.S.V.; Selvakumar, B. Improved DeepMitosisNet Framework for Detection of Mitosis in Histopathology Images. *Multimed. Tools Appl.* **2023**, *83*, 43303–43324. [CrossRef]
63. Hoerst, F.; Rempe, M.; Heine, L.; Seibold, C.; Keyl, J.; Baldini, G.; Ugurel, S.; Siveke, J.; Gruenwald, B.; Egger, J.; et al. CellViT: Vision Transformers for Precise Cell Segmentation and Classification. *Med. Image Anal.* **2024**, *94*, 103143. [CrossRef]
64. Marzouki, A.; Guo, Z.; Zeng, Q.; Kurtz, C.; Loménie, N. Optimizing Lymphocyte Detection in Breast Cancer Whole Slide Imaging through Data-Centric Strategies. *arXiv* **2024**, arXiv:2405.13710.
65. Liu, S.; Amgad, M.; More, D.; Rathore, M.A.; Salgado, R.; Cooper, L.A.D. A panoptic segmentation dataset and deep-learning approach for explainable scoring of tumor-infiltrating lymphocytes. *NPJ Breast Cancer* **2024**, *10*, 52.
66. Keele, S. *Guidelines for Performing Systematic Literature Reviews in Software Engineering*; Technical Report, Version 2.3, EBSE-2007-01; Software Engineering Group, School of Computer Science and Mathematics; Keele University: Keele, UK; Department of Computer Science, University of Durham: Durham, UK, 2007.
67. Tafavvoghi, M.; Bongo, L.A.; Shvetsov, N.; Busund, L.T.R.; Møllersen, K. Publicly available datasets of breast histopathology H&E whole-slide images: A scoping review. *J. Pathol. Inform.* **2024**, *15*, 100363.
68. Abdel-Nabi, H.; Ali, M.; Awajan, A.; Daoud, M.; Alazrai, R.; Suganthan, P.N.; Ali, T. A Comprehensive Review of the Deep Learning-Based Tumor Analysis Approaches in Histopathological Images: Segmentation, Classification and Multi-Learning Tasks. *Clust. Comput.* **2023**, *26*, 3145–3185. [CrossRef]
69. Basu, A.; Senapati, P.; Deb, M.; Rai, R.; Dhal, K.G. A survey on recent trends in deep learning for nucleus segmentation from histopathology images. *Evol. Syst.* **2024**, *15*, 203–248.
70. Wang, L.; Pan, L.; Wang, H.; Liu, M.; Feng, Z.; Rong, P.; Chen, Z.; Peng, S. DHUnet: Dual-branch hierarchical global–local fusion network for whole slide image segmentation. *Biomed. Signal Process. Control* **2023**, *85*, 104976.
71. Liu, S.; Amgad, M.; Rathore, M.A.; Salgado, R.; Cooper, L.A.D. A panoptic segmentation approach for tumor-infiltrating lymphocyte assessment: Development of the MuTILs model and PanopTILs dataset. *MedRxiv* **2022**. [CrossRef]
72. Mondello, A.; Dal Bo, M.; Toffoli, G.; Polano, M. Machine learning in onco-pharmacogenomics: A path to precision medicine with many challenges. *Front. Pharmacol.* **2024**, *14*, 1260276.
73. Rydzewski, N.R.; Shi, Y.; Li, C.; Chrostek, M.R.; Bakhtiar, H.; Helzer, K.T.; Bootsma, M.L.; Berg, T.J.; Harari, P.M.; Floberg, J.M.; et al. A platform-independent AI tumor lineage and site (ATLAS) classifier. *Commun. Biol.* **2024**, *7*, 314.
74. Liu, Y.; He, X.; Yang, Y. Tumor immune microenvironment-based clusters in predicting prognosis and guiding immunotherapy in breast cancer. *J. Biosci.* **2024**, *49*, 19.
75. Ahmed, F.; Abdel-Salam, R.; Hamnett, L.; Adewunmi, M.; Ayano, T. Improved Breast Cancer Diagnosis through Transfer Learning on Hematoxylin and Eosin Stained Histology Images. *arXiv* **2023**, arXiv:2309.08745.
76. Nasir, E.S.; Parvaiz, A.; Fraz, M.M. Nuclei and glands instance segmentation in histology images: A narrative review. *Artif. Intell. Rev.* **2023**, *56*, 7909–7964.
77. National Cancer Institute. TCGA-BRCA Project. Available online: https://portal.gdc.cancer.gov/projects/TCGA-BRCA (accessed on 18 July 2024).

78. Veta, M.; Van Diest, P.J.; Willems, S.M.; Wang, H.; Madabhushi, A.; Cruz-Roa, A.; Gonzalez, F.; Larsen, A.B.L.; Vestergaard, J.S.; Dahl, A.B.; et al. Assessment of algorithms for mitosis detection in breast cancer histopathology images. *Med. Image Anal.* **2015**, *20*, 237–248.
79. Spanhol, F.A.; Oliveira, L.S.; Petitjean, C.; Heutte, L. A dataset for breast cancer histopathological image classification. *IEEE Trans. Biomed. Eng.* **2015**, *63*, 1455–1462. [CrossRef]
80. Qaiser, T.; Mukherjee, A.; Reddy Pb, C.; Munugoti, S.D.; Tallam, V.; Pitkäaho, T.; Lehtimäki, T.; Naughton, T.; Berseth, M.; Pedraza, A.; et al. Her 2 challenge contest: A detailed assessment of automated HER 2 scoring algorithms in whole slide images of breast cancer tissues. *Histopathology* **2018**, *72*, 227–238. [CrossRef] [PubMed]
81. Aresta, G.; Araújo, T.; Kwok, S.; Chennamsetty, S.S.; Safwan, M.; Alex, V.; Marami, B.; Prastawa, M.; Chan, M.; Donovan, M.; et al. Bach: Grand challenge on breast cancer histology images. *Med. Image Anal.* **2019**, *56*, 122–139. [CrossRef] [PubMed]
82. Kumar, N.; Verma, R.; Anand, D.; Zhou, Y.; Onder, O.F.; Tsougenis, E.; Chen, H.; Heng, P.A.; Li, J.; Hu, Z.; et al. A Multi-Organ Nucleus Segmentation Challenge. *IEEE Trans. Med. Imaging* **2020**, *39*, 1380–1391. [CrossRef] [PubMed]
83. Ortega-Ruiz, M.A.; Roman-Rangel, E.; Reyes-Aldasoro, C.C. Multiclass Semantic Segmentation of Immunostained Breast Cancer Tissue with a Deep-Learning Approach. *medRxiv* **2022**. [CrossRef]
84. Gamper, J.; Koohbanani, N.A.; Benes, K.; Graham, S.; Jahanifar, M.; Khurram, S.A.; Azam, A.; Hewitt, K.; Rajpoot, N. Pannuke dataset extension, insights and baselines. *arXiv* **2020**, arXiv:2003.10778.
85. Koohbanani, N.A.; Jahanifar, M.; Tajadin, N.Z.; Rajpoot, N. NuClick: A deep learning framework for interactive segmentation of microscopic images. *Med. Image Anal.* **2020**, *65*, 101771. [CrossRef]
86. Jeretic, P.; Warstadt, A.; Bhooshan, S.; Williams, A. Are natural language inference models IMPPRESsive? Learning IMPlicature and PRESupposition. *arXiv* **2020**, arXiv:2004.03066.
87. Brancati, N.; Anniciello, A.M.; Pati, P.; Riccio, D.; Scognamiglio, G.; Jaume, G.; De Pietro, G.; Di Bonito, M.; Foncubierta, A.; Botti, G.; et al. BRACS: A Dataset for BReAst Carcinoma Subtyping in H&E Histology Images. *arXiv* **2021**, arXiv:2111.04740.
88. Grand Challenge. Tiger Challenge. 2022. Available online: https://tiger.grand-challenge.org/ (accessed on 18 July 2024).
89. Aubreville, M.; Stathonikos, N.; Donovan, T.A.; Klopfleisch, R.; Ammeling, J.; Ganz, J.; Wilm, F.; Veta, M.; Jabari, S.; Eckstein, M.; et al. Domain generalization across tumor types, laboratories, and species—Insights from the 2022 edition of the Mitosis Domain Generalization Challenge. *Med. Image Anal.* **2024**, *94*, 103155. [CrossRef]
90. Madoori, P.K.; Sannidhi, S.; Anandam, G. Artificial Intelligence and Computational Pathology: A comprehensive review of advancements and applications. *Perspectives* **2023**, *11*, 30. [CrossRef]
91. Kumar, N.; Gupta, R.; Gupta, S. Whole slide imaging (WSI) in pathology: Current perspectives and future directions. *J. Digit. Imaging* **2020**, *33*, 1034–1040. [CrossRef] [PubMed]
92. Wagner, S.J.; Matek, C.; Boushehri, S.S.; Boxberg, M.; Lamm, L.; Sadafi, A.; Winter, D.J.E.; Marr, C.; Peng, T. Built to last? Reproducibility and reusability of deep learning algorithms in computational pathology. *Mod. Pathol.* **2024**, *37*, 100350. [CrossRef] [PubMed]
93. Nasarian, E.; Alizadehsani, R.; Acharya, U.R.; Tsui, K.L. Designing interpretable ML system to enhance trust in healthcare: A systematic review to proposed responsible clinician-AI-collaboration framework. *Inf. Fusion* **2024**, *108*, 102412. [CrossRef]
94. Hossain, M.S.; Shahriar, G.M.; Syeed, M.M.M.; Uddin, M.F.; Hasan, M.; Hossain, M.S.; Bari, R. Tissue artifact segmentation and severity assessment for automatic analysis using WSI. *IEEE Access* **2023**, *11*, 21977–21991. [CrossRef]

MDPI AG
Grosspeteranlage 5
4052 Basel
Switzerland
Tel.: +41 61 683 77 34

Diagnostics Editorial Office
E-mail: diagnostics@mdpi.com
www.mdpi.com/journal/diagnostics

www.ingramcontent.com/pod-product-compliance
Lightning Source LLC
LaVergne TN
LVHW070502061126
851858LV00011B/277